Pediatric Nursing

made
Incredibly
Easy!

Second Edition

Clinical Editor
Mikki Meadows-Oliver

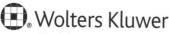

. Wolters Kluwer

Health

Philadelphia • Baltimore • New York • London
Buenos Aires • Hong Kong • Sydney • Tokyo

Staff

Acquisitions Editor
Shannon W. Magee

Product Development Editor
Maria McAvey

Production Project Manager
Marian Bellus

Editorial Assistant
Zachary Shapiro

Design Coordinator
Joan Wendt

Creative Services Director
Doug Smock

Senior Marketing Manager
Mark Wiragh

Manufacturing Coordinator
Kathleen Brown

Prepress Vendor
Absolute Service, Inc.

2nd Edition

Copyright © 2015 Wolters Kluwer Health.

Care has been taken to confirm the accuracy of the information presented and to describe generally accepted practices. However, the authors, editors, and publisher are not responsible for errors or omissions or for any consequences from application of the information in this book and make no warranty, expressed or implied, with respect to the currency, completeness, or accuracy of the contents of the publication. Application of this information in a particular situation remains the professional responsibility of the practitioner; the clinical treatments described and recommended may not be considered absolute and universal recommendations.

The authors, editors, and publisher have exerted every effort to ensure that drug selection and dosage set forth in this text are in accordance with the current recommendations and practice at the time of publication. However, in view of ongoing research, changes in government regulations, and the constant flow of information relating to drug therapy and drug reactions, the reader is urged to check the package insert for each drug for any change in indications and dosage and for added warnings and precautions. This is particularly important when the recommended agent is a new or infrequently employed drug.

Some drugs and medical devices presented in this publication have Food and Drug Administration (FDA) clearance for limited use in restricted research settings. It is the responsibility of the health care provider to ascertain the FDA status of each drug or device planned for use in his or her clinical practice.

LWW.COM

Library of Congress Cataloging-in-Publication Data

Pediatric nursing made incredibly easy! — 2nd edition.
   p. ; cm.
  Includes bibliographical references and index.
  ISBN 978-1-4511-9254-4
  I. Lippincott Williams & Wilkins, issuing body.
  [DNLM: 1. Nursing Care—methods—Handbooks.
2. Adolescent. 3. Child. 4. Infant. 5. Pediatric
Nursing—methods—Handbooks. WY 49]
  RJ245
  618.92'00231—dc23

2014009310

RRS1405

Contents

Contributors and consultants

Peggy Baikie, DNP, RN, PNP-BC, NNP-BC
Program Manager/Nurse Practitioner,
  Denver Health
Adjunct Faculty, Metropolitan State
  University of Denver
Denver, CO

Nancy Banasiak, MSN, PNP-BC, APRN
Pediatric Nurse Practitioner, Yale-New
  Haven Hospital
Associate Professor, Yale University
  School of Nursing
New Haven, CT

Vera C. Brancato, EdD, MSN, RN
Professor of Nursing
Alvernia University
Reading, PA

**Rosalynn Bravo-Cavoli, APRN, MS, CPNP,
  AE-C**
Pediatric Nurse Practitioner, Pulmonary
  Clinic
Connecticut Children's Medical Center
Hartford, CT
Clinical Instructor, Yale University
  School of Nursing
New Haven, CT

Doreen S. DeAngelis, RN, MSN
Nursing Instructor
Penn State Fayette, The Eberly Campus
Lemont Furnace, PA

Cheryl L. DeGraw, RN, MSN, CRNP
Nursing Instructor
Central Carolina Technical College
Sumter, SC

Shelia Savell, PhD, RN
Nursing Department Chair
Hallmark College
San Antonio, TX

Martha M. Z. Shemin, MS, RN
Nursing Instructor
Facilitator for Parent-Child Health
  Nursing Course
Holy Name Medical Center School of
  Nursing
Teaneck, NJ

Ralph Vogel, RN, PhD, CPNP
Clinical Assistant Professor (retired)
University of Arkansas for Medical
  Sciences
College of Nursing
Little Rock, AR

Julee Waldrop, DNP, FNP, PNP, PMHS, CNE
Associate Professor
University of Central Florida
Orlando, FL

Karen Wilkinson, MN, ARNP
Pediatric Nurse Practitioner
Wilkinson Consulting
Seattle, WA

Foreword

The first edition of *Pediatric Nursing Made Incredibly Easy!* was published in 2005. Since the initial publication, there have been many advances in pediatric health care and within the nursing profession. Much of that knowledge has been captured here in this revised and updated second edition of *Pediatric Nursing Made Incredibly Easy!* Revising this edition required a team of dedicated nurse experts from different regions of the country who worked to ensure that this book contained relevant information that is useful in everyday practice.

In order to provide safe, quality care to the pediatric patient, nurses need to have an understanding of some common pediatric conditions. The primary goal of the second edition of *Pediatric Nursing Made Incredibly Easy!* is to provide the nurse interested in pediatrics with increased knowledge about pediatric health care conditions as they relate to nursing practice. This edition of *Pediatric Nursing Made Incredibly Easy!* provides an introduction to topics essential to pediatrics for nurses with limited pediatric experience and serves as a refresher for nurses already caring for children in a variety of settings. This book is also a valuable resource for students on their pediatric clinical rotations. Students will appreciate the easy-to-read format and the "Advice from the experts." Even the most experienced nurses will find a means to enhance their knowledge.

All 15 chapters have revised, and I am sure that the revisions have significantly enhanced the scope and value of the book. The second edition of *Pediatric Nursing Made Incredibly Easy!* begins with a chapter introducing the reader to pediatric nursing. This chapter defines the role of the pediatric nurse, the philosophy of family-centered care, and standards of care for pediatric nursing. The next chapter reviews factors that influence growth and development, how to assess and manage pain in the pediatric patient, and the needs of the hospitalized and special needs child. The next three chapters review developmental aspects of pediatric care related to infants, early childhood, middle childhood, and adolescence. Chapters 6 to 15 review commonly encountered pediatric conditions relevant to various body systems—for example, cardiovascular, respiratory, and gastrointestinal. Each chapter provides you with an abundance of practical, useful information.

An easy-to-read format and witty artwork are presented to aid and engage the reader. Illustrations are presented to help you visualize the pathophysiology of the condition. "Memory joggers" provide useful tips to help you remember important information. In addition, the second edition of *Pediatric Nursing Made Incredibly Easy!* has several icons to draw your attention to important issues.

Advice from the experts—presents information from skilled practitioners

It's all relative—provides topics for education for patients and their families

Growing pains—offers age and stage description, expectations, and dangers

Cultured pearls—notes unique aspects of care by cultural groups.

After reading each chapter, you can test how much you've learned with the "Quick quiz" at the end of each chapter. You will then realize how valuable a resource this book is and how much this material applies to your pediatric practice!

Mikki Meadows-Oliver, PhD, RN, PNP-BC
Associate Professor
Yale University School of Nursing
President, National Association of Pediatric
  Nurse Practitioners

1

Introduction to pediatric nursing

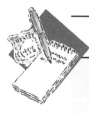

Just the facts

In this chapter, you'll learn:

♦ the role of the pediatric nurse

♦ the philosophy of family-centered care

♦ standards of care for pediatric nursing

♦ types of family structures

♦ sociocultural influences that affect pediatric health.

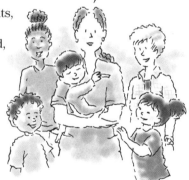

Pediatric nursing includes babies and teens and everyone in between!

Role of the pediatric nurse

Pediatric nursing involves providing care for infants, children, and adolescents on a continuum from health to illness to recuperation and, when needed, rehabilitation.

However, providing care to the pediatric population doesn't stop with the pediatric patient; pediatric nursing should incorporate parents and other family members into the child's care. This philosophy is known as *family-centered care.*

Family-centered care

Family-centered care acknowledges the parents as the constant in the child's life and as experts in the care of their child, whether in the hospital or at home. In family-centered care, the family's input is the major driving force behind the development of the child's care plan.

In addition, the needs of the child and his family are taken into account in family-centered care. Interventions are geared toward respecting, supporting, and encouraging the family's ability to participate in the care of their child throughout illness and recovery.

Power to the people

Empowering and enabling are two important concepts in family-centered care. *Empowering* is allowing parents to maintain, or helping them to develop, a sense of control over their child's care. *Enabling* refers to the practices that help family members to acquire the new skills necessary to meet the needs of their child.

These two concepts foster the teamwork between the family and health care professionals that serves to benefit the child, both physically and emotionally. (See *Benefits of family-centered care.*)

Standards of care

Pediatric nursing care is governed by standards. The American Nurses Association (ANA), the National Association of Pediatric Nurse Practitioners (NAPNAP), and the Society of Pediatric Nurses (SPN) have developed a document which outlines the scope and standards of pediatric nursing practice to ensure that each pediatric patient receives safe and effective care. (See *Standards of pediatric nursing care and professional performance.*)

Room for improvement

In 2010, there were 74.1 million children younger than 18 years old living in the United States. Children younger than 16 years of age compose 24% of the total population. Although children's health has improved dramatically over the last century, there's still work to be done.

Childhood morbidity and mortality rates, key indicators of the health of a population, provide the nurse with essential information about how and where to direct care for individual patients and the community at large.

Childhood morbidity

Morbidity is defined as the number of people in a population who are faced with a specific health problem at a particular point in time. Because these statistics aren't compiled on an annual basis, it's difficult to compare them from year to year. It is important to remember that it is during the middle childhood and early adolescent times that the children are usually healthy, but they develop habits that will influence their health later in life.

Morbidity rates for many illnesses that previously caused severe problems for children, such as poliomyelitis and measles, have been dramatically reduced through immunizations. Other conditions studied in relation to morbidity include obesity, injuries, acute illness, HIV infection, and sexually transmitted infections (STIs).

Benefits of family-centered care

Family-centered care benefits the child and family as well as the health care professional.

Benefits to families
• Less stress and heightened feelings of confidence and competence in caring for their children
• Less dependence on professional caregivers
• Empowerment to develop new skills and expertise in the care of their children

Benefits to health care professionals
• Greater job satisfaction
• Empowerment to develop new skills and expertise in pediatric nursing

Acute isn't cute

The most common causes of acute illness in childhood include:
- respiratory illness (50%)
- injuries (15%)
- infections and parasitic disease (11%).

Standards of pediatric nursing care and professional performance

By adhering to these guidelines, jointly developed by the ANA, NAPNAP, and the SPN, the pediatric nurse can serve as an advocate for patients and their families. These guidelines should be upheld to ensure that professional care is provided to all patients.

Scope of practice

The scope of practice section of the document discusses the different areas of pediatric nursing practice and the different settings where pediatric nurses practice. Also discussed in this section are education and certification of pediatric nurses.

The Differentiated Areas of Pediatric Nursing Practice include:
- The Pediatric Nurse: Generalist
- The Advanced Practice Pediatric Nurse
- Pediatric Clinical Nurse Specialist (PCNS)
- Pediatric Nurse Practitioner (PNP)
- Neonatal Nurse Practitioner (NNP)

The Settings for Pediatric Nursing Practice include:
- Inpatient and Acute Care Settings
- Perioperative and Surgical Settings
- Hospice and Palliative Care Settings
- Ambulatory Care Settings
- Community Health and School Settings
- Transport Settings
- Camp Settings

Standards of care

Comprehensive pediatric nursing care focuses on helping children and their families and communities achieve their optimum health potentials. This goal is best achieved within the framework of family-centered care and the pediatric nursing process, including primary, secondary, and tertiary care coordinated across health care and community settings. The jointly published document includes 16 standards that govern the practice of the pediatric nurse.
- Standard 1. Assessment
- Standard 2. Diagnosis
- Standard 3. Outcomes Identification
- Standard 4. Planning
- Standard 5. Implementation
- Standard 5a. Coordination of Care and Case Management
- Standard 5b. Health Teaching and Health Promotion, Restoration, and Maintenance
- Standard 5c. Consultation
- Standard 5d. Prescriptive Authority and Treatment
- Standard 5e. Referral
- Standard 6. Evaluation
- Standard 7. Quality of Practice
- Standard 8. Professional Practice Evaluation
- Standard 9. Education
- Standard 10. Collegiality
- Standard 11. Collaboration
- Standard 12. Ethics
- Standard 13. Research, Evidence-Based Practice, and Clinical Scholarship
- Standard 14. Resource Utilization
- Standard 15. Leadership
- Standard 16. Advocacy

American Nurses Association, National Association of Pediatric Nurse Practitioners, & Society of Pediatric Nurses. (2008). *Pediatric nursing: Scope of practice*. Washington, DC; American Nurses Association.

Risky business

Factors that place children at risk for increased morbidity include:
- chronic illness
- homelessness
- low birth weight
- poverty
- adoption from a foreign country
- time spent in day-care centers.

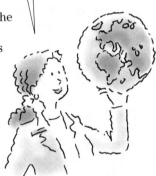

Most nations with a lower infant mortality rate have national health programs in place.

Childhood mortality

Mortality refers to the number of deaths from a specific cause in a given year. Accidents are the leading cause of death in all age-groups of children (older than age 1) in the United States.

Infant mortality rates are the number of infant deaths during the first year of life per 1,000 live births. Infant mortality rates have decreased dramatically in the United States, but the nation still lags behind other developed countries that have even lower infant mortality rates.

Many of the nations with lower infant mortality rates also have national health programs in place. Researchers aim to improve these vital statistics for all populations in the United States.

National health initiatives

The current focus on health promotion and disease prevention has prompted national initiatives, such as *Healthy People 2020*, aimed at improving children's health.

Solid start

For the past three decades, the U.S. Department of Health and Human Services (DHHS) has issued a national health agenda called *Healthy People*, aimed at improving the health of people living in the United States. The *Healthy People* goals were developed to provide evidence-based, 10-year national objectives for improving health. The first set of national targets for health was released in 1979 and was entitled, *Healthy People: The Surgeon General's Report on Health Promotion and Disease Prevention*. The target date for the attainment of these goals was 1990. Since then, the goals have been updated every 10 years.

Building on success

Healthy People 2020 (http://www.healthypeople.gov/2020/default .aspx) was released in December 2010, with the stated mission to identify nationwide health improvement priorities by increasing public awareness of determinants of health, disease, and disability; providing measureable goals and objectives to determine progress in attaining the health improvement priorities; engaging multiple sectors to improve practices based on evidence and knowledge; and identifying critical research, evaluation, and data collection. Thirteen new topics or priority areas were added for *Healthy People 2020* that were not included in *Healthy People 2010*. Of the 13 areas, several are particularly relevant to children and adolescents: adolescent health; early and middle childhood; lesbian, gay, bisexual, and transgender (LGBT) health; and sleep health.

In kids' corner

The *National Vaccine Program* is a health initiative that's especially significant to children's health. National Vaccine Plan serves as a guide to ensure all Americans have access to vaccines so that disease can be prevented.

Healthy People 2020 objectives

Healthy People 2020 aims to have a society where people live longer and healthier lives. There are over 417 objectives related to the pediatric population. Here are some of the *Healthy People 2020* objectives related to the pediatric population:
• Increase the number of individuals going to a single health care provider for care.
• Increase the number of adolescents getting yearly physical, dental, and vision examinations.
• Increase number of adolescents involved in extracurricular activities at school.
• Increase the number of adolescents who have a positive adult role model to talk to.
• Increase number of children with disabilities who receive adequate care.
• Increase the number of schools that have adequate health education for children in schools.
• Increase education related to unintentional injury, use of tobacco products, unplanned pregnancy, STIs, alcohol use or other drugs, inadequate nutrition, and lack of physical activity.
• Increase use of vehicle restraint usage in all age-groups.
• Increase the number of moms breast-feeding and support for them while breast-feeding.
• Increase amount of time children spend in daily physical education and recess at school.

• Increase number of children who limit screen time activities to 2 hours or less per day.
• Increase number of high school students who get sufficient sleep.
• Increase number of students who are free of substance abuse.
• Maintain and increase vaccination coverage for all ages of children.
• Reduce number of adolescents affected by violent crime.
• Reduce number of children and adolescents with high blood pressure.
• Reduce number of otitis media cases.
• Reduce number of new cases of HIV/AIDS cases.
• Reduce number of cases of immunization-preventable diseases.
• Reduce incidence of bullying and violence among all age-groups.
• Reduce rate of fetal and infant deaths.
• Reduce number of children who have dental caries.
• Reduce number of hospital visits or emergency department (ED) visits for children who have asthma.
• Reduce number of adolescents who are binge drinkers.

Look, Mom! I'm meeting two *Healthy People 2020* objectives at once! I'm getting my 30 minutes of physical activity, and I'm alcohol and drug-free.

A closer look at the family

Family is defined as the structure, or the relationship between individuals, that provides the financial and emotional support needed for social functioning. Individuals don't have to have blood relationships in order to be a family. Today, many different family structures exist in our society: the nuclear family, binuclear family, and the blended family. Each type of family may provide a unique set of challenges to the nurses who care for their children. When conducting a pediatric history, remember to ask about who lives in the home.

Nuclear family

A *nuclear family* (also known as a *traditional family*) consists of spouses and their child or children (biological or adopted). The nuclear family serves as a support system for its members, who share roles and responsibilities as well as financial obligations. One disadvantage of some nuclear families is the absence of additional support that may be needed in times of crisis.

A *binuclear family* is becoming more common as more parents remarry and share custody and care of the children. A binuclear family consists of each parent and their new spouses, sharing custody and raising of the child. Each couple has their own household in which the child spends his or her time. The child may have to learn two sets of rules—which can sometimes be quite confusing.

Blended family

A *blended family* consists of parents with a child or children from a previous relationship who marry and live together.

Add two or more children, mix well . . .

A blended family provides emotional support and allows for shared roles within the household. It also provides the opportunity for the family members to learn how to work together and discover new ways of accomplishing tasks.

. . . but don't spread too thin

Financial responsibilities can be shared but can also produce strain if support must be provided to the previous spouse or children of either adult, or both.

Cohabitation family

A *cohabitation family* is one in which two adults and a child or children live together as a nuclear family while the adults remain unmarried. This type of family provides emotional and financial support to its members. However, the risk exists that one individual may feel threatened by the partner's real or perceived lack of commitment.

Extended family

An *extended family* (also called a *multigenerational family*) includes at least one parent; a child or children; and any combination of grandparents, aunts, uncles, or cousins. In this type of family, the group provides the support.

A potential disadvantage of an extended family is the conflict that may arise about roles; confusion may occur about which adult is viewed as the child's mother or father, or who should make decisions regarding the child's care.

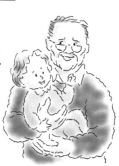

Single-parent family

A *single-parent family* is composed of one parent living at home with a child or children. Because of such factors as the rise in divorce rates, the single-parent family is becoming more common.

Being a single parent can be rewarding—and exhausting!

Bonded . . .

In a single-parent family, the parent and child are each other's source of support. This can create close bonds but can also lead to strain for the single parent in terms of the parental role he or she plays. If a child becomes ill, child care difficulties may arise. There may also be financial constraints related to limited income.

. . . and ready for a nap

The single parent can become exhausted from being responsible for all of the tasks involved in raising children. Single parenting can also lead to low self-esteem, as the parent tries—and sometimes fails—to provide everything for the child that some two-parent families are able to provide.

Communal family

In a *communal family*, adults and their children choose to live with a group of people (not relatives) who become the extended family. The relationship is usually one of religious beliefs or social values. The parent usually gives up the parental role, and the leader of the group makes decisions for the child. Disadvantages of this family structure include the tendency to provide medical care within the group rather than seeking outside for professional help for health-related matters.

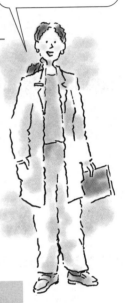

Foster care is based on the idea that the foster home will be a temporary one for the child.

Foster family

A *foster family* is designed to care for a child whose biological or adoptive parents can't do so. Foster parents may or may not be related to the child in foster care. If the foster parents are related to the child, the placement is generally referred to as kinship care. Ideally, foster care is provided on a temporary basis until the biological or adoptive parent can resume his or her role. Unfortunately, the foster child may be shuffled from foster family to foster family, lacking the stability that comes from being with the same family (biological, adoptive, or foster) for an extended period. It can also be difficult to determine who's responsible for making decisions about the foster child's health care.

Sociocultural influences on pediatric health

Sociocultural influences on pediatric health include:
- ethnicity
- socioeconomic factors
- religion
- school
- peers
- the family's health-related beliefs and practices.

Ethnicity

Ethnicity refers to belonging to or believing in a group with the same customs, languages, and characteristics. The United States is known for its ethnic diversity. The pediatric nurse must be aware that different ethnic groups tend to view health care differently.

Father knows best

In some ethnic groups, the adult male is the decision maker. When a child is brought in for treatment, no decisions can be made until he arrives.

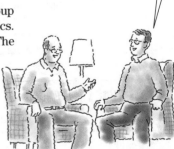

My family doesn't make decisions without me. In my ethnic group, what the man says, goes.

Grin and bear it

Other ethnic groups believe that pain shouldn't be shown. Children from these ethnic groups may be up and walking or conversing, or may appear stoic, despite being in pain. This can make it difficult for the nurse to assess, or even detect, pain.

Hold the pickles, hold the meat

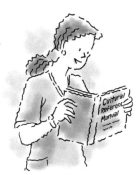

Diet is another area in which ethnic influence can be strong. For instance, caffeine and meat products may be removed from the diet.

The pediatric nurse should do a thorough assessment of the family's beliefs in order to provide the most complete care and avoid offending the family. Remember, not every member of the culture will participate in all aspects of the culture. This is why it is important to do a cultural assessment. (See *Putting cultural care into practice*.)

Socioeconomic factors

Socioeconomic influences on pediatric health result from income levels that don't meet the needs of the child and family. *Poverty* is the lack of money or resources necessary for survival. Approximately 22% of children in the United States, or 16.4 million children, live in families with incomes below the federal poverty level. People who live in areas with low socioeconomic levels have fewer accessible health care facilities available to them.

Planes, trains, and automobiles

The availability of transportation to a health care facility can have a tremendous impact on whether parents or caregivers will seek care for themselves and their children.

Cultured pearls

Putting cultural care into practice

Awareness and knowledge are the first steps toward incorporating cultural care into your daily nursing practice. To facilitate cultural care on your practice setting, develop a cultural reference manual that includes:
• brief descriptions of pertinent cultures
• views on health, illness, diet, and other matters
• lists of interpreters (including American Sign Language interpreters), ethnic community services, and other sources for quick reference.

Calling in sick

Another area of concern arises when both parents work, as is common in today's economy. One or both parents may not be able to afford to take time off from work to bring their child to the health care provider's office or hospital, or may risk their job by doing so. If they can't take time off, and health care isn't available after working hours, the child may not receive the care he or she needs.

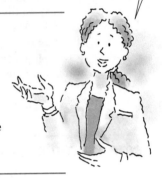

When both parents work because of socioeconomic reasons, they may not be able to take time off for their child's illness.

Religion

Religious beliefs can affect when, where, and even if an individual will seek health care. Because religious beliefs guide health care practices for many people, the pediatric nurse must be aware of what beliefs the individual holds and should help ensure that these needs are met in a way that provides the child with the needed care.

School

School typically reinforces the concepts of right and wrong, or moral values. School commonly helps children learn rules and regulations and introduces them to the concept of an authority figure other than their parents.

A child who has a negative experience with school may fear the hospital setting, thinking it will be the same as school. The child whose school experiences are positive will be likely to apply these experiences to the health care environment. It is important for the pediatric nurse to remember that some children are homeschooled.

A bad experience at school can lead to more than detention. It can make kids fear hospitals, too.

Peer influences

Peer relationships are the relationships a child has with other individuals in the same age-group. A child's ability to be part of a peer group is influenced by his having the same beliefs or attitudes as the others in his group. With the use of social media and cellular phones, friends are only a screen away. Nurses must remember that with the use of social media, there is a potential for cyberbullying.

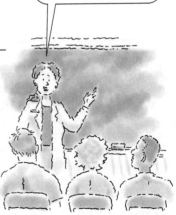

A child may try to change his beliefs or behaviors to feel a part of the group or norm. He may partake in behaviors that risk his health to conform to the group. For example, a child's experimentation with smoking, drinking alcohol, or using drugs can be heavily influenced by the behaviors of his peers.

Health-related beliefs and practices

Health-related beliefs and practices of the family have a strong influence on how often they will seek health care for their child. If family members hesitate to seek health care for themselves, they commonly won't seek care for their child until he becomes seriously ill.

Once bitten

Sometimes, a family's health-related beliefs and practices are based on previous experiences with health care. Negative experiences can make family members reluctant to seek care for themselves and for their child.

These experiences may include:
• real or perceived poor quality of care
• real or perceived insensitivity of health care professionals
• physical or emotional pain or trauma
• death of a family member in a health care facility.

The pediatric nurse can help to make a family's health-related beliefs more positive by:
• asking family members about their past health care experiences and acknowledging their concerns
• stressing the ways the current situation differs from past situations
• encouraging family members to participate actively in their child's health care and praising them for the care they're already providing.

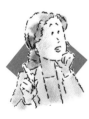

Quick quiz

1. The phrase *infant mortality rates* refers to the:
   A. number of children faced with any given health problem.
   B. number of infant deaths in any given year.
   C. nutritional health of a population of infants.
   D. socioeconomic status of a population of infants.

Answer: B. Infant mortality rates refer to the number of infant deaths per 1,000 live births in any given year.

2. A child is admitted for surgery. On your admission assessment, the mother tells you that her family is composed of herself, the patient (her daughter), her new husband, and her stepson. What type of family is this?

    A. Nuclear family
    B. Cohabitation family
    C. Blended family
    D. Foster family

Answer: C. A family composed of a mother with children from a previous relationship who marries a father with children from a previous relationship is called a *blended family.*

3. A 5-year-old is in the hospital after having an appendectomy. A full liquid diet is ordered for the child. A carbonated soda, chicken broth, milk, and ice cream are on his food tray. The mother states that the child isn't permitted to have these foods because she doesn't allow him to have foods containing sugar. Which action is the nurse's best response?

    A. Explain to the mother that these are the only foods allowed after surgery.
    B. Respect the mother's wishes and remove the food.
    C. Discuss the nutritional value of these foods after surgery.
    D. Review with the mother what foods are allowed and include her in the menu selection.

Answer: D. By allowing the mother to participate in making decisions about the child's care, the nurse is fostering family-centered care.

4. Relationships that a child has with others in his age-group are known as:

    A. peer relationships.
    B. family relationships.
    C. sibling relationships.
    D. caregiver relationships.

Answer: A. Peers are those in a person's own age-group. Peers can heavily influence the behavior of a child as he attempts to conform to the norms of the group.

Scoring

✩✩✩ If you answered all four items correctly, congratulations! Your introduction to pediatric nursing is empowering.

✩✩ If you answered three items correctly, good work! Tell your peers you have a well-centered grasp of pediatric nursing.

✩ If you answered fewer than three items correctly, don't get morbid! You have 14 more chapters to create a positive pediatric nursing experience.

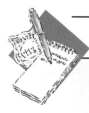

2

Concepts in pediatric nursing care

Just the facts

In this chapter, you'll learn:

♦ factors influencing growth and development

♦ methods of preparing and administering medications to children

♦ how to assess and manage pain in the child

♦ needs of the hospitalized and special needs child.

Principles of growth and development

Growth and development occur throughout the life span. *Growth* implies an increase in size, such as height and weight. *Development* refers to the acquisition of skills and abilities that takes place throughout life. (See *Patterns of development*, page 14.)

Growth and development are essential parts of the pediatric nursing assessment. Problems that may initially seem insignificant might actually have severe consequences in later life if not dealt with early.

> Whether you're 5 or 50, growth and development continue to occur.

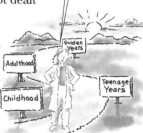

Stages of development

There are five stages of development during childhood:

Infancy is the period from birth until age 1.

The *toddler stage* is the period from ages 1 to 3.

The *preschool stage* lasts from ages 3 to 6.

School-age refers to children ages 6 to 12.

Adolescence is the period from ages 13 to 19. Some experts now consider the period of adolescence from ages 10 to 25 due to recent research on brain development.

Patterns of development

This chart shows the patterns of development and their progression and gives examples of each.

Pattern	Path of progression	Examples
Cephalocaudal	From head to toe	Head control precedes the ability to walk.
Proximodistal	From the trunk to the tips of the extremities	The neonate can move his arms and legs but can't pick up objects with his fingers.
General to specific	From simple tasks to more complex tasks (mastering simple tasks before advancing to those that are more complex)	The child progresses from crawling to walking to skipping.

Factors that influence growth and development

From birth on, children normally accomplish a series of developmental tasks during the stages of growth. As a child matures, he develops a readiness to master new, age-appropriate tasks.

Task master

A child's ability to master these tasks is affected by environmental, social, cultural, and relational factors. Without the appropriate stimuli or environment, these tasks might not be accomplished, and development may be arrested or may occur in a maladaptive manner.

Family

The family in which a child is raised greatly influences his development. For example, a child who has been abused or neglected may experience delays in learning trust as well as disorders of attachment and problems with feeding and sleeping. Repeated episodes of maltreatment or emotional deprivation have been shown to also have a physical impact, decreasing a child's rate of growth.

Health status

A child's physiologic state can significantly affect his development. Children with chronic health conditions may experience developmental lags in acquiring skills relating to cognition, communication, adaptation, and social and motor functioning. The extent to which a health condition affects a child's development depends on the severity of the illness.

Socioeconomic status

A family's socioeconomic status can have a significant impact on a child's growth and development.

Ain't got no culture

Parents who must work long hours to provide basic necessities may have little time or money to help their child achieve his highest level of functioning through enriching experiences. Travel as well as cultural and educational outings—to the library, museum, or zoo—may not be possible.

> I'm singing the blues. My parents can't afford lessons. Who knows how far my talent would have taken me!

I could have been a contender

A lack of time and funds can also limit a child's ability to pursue such special interests as art, music, and sports.

Cultural background

A family's cultural beliefs and circumstances also affect a child's growth and development. Culture influences the way children are socialized, learn values, and experience the world. The child's developing beliefs, customs, mode of communication and dress, and actions are influenced by and vary according to culture.

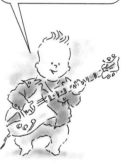

Normal to me, taboo to you

Practices vary from culture to culture; what's acceptable in one culture may be taboo in another. It's extremely important for nurses to become knowledgeable about and respectful of cultural beliefs that differ from their own. This knowledge enables nurses to develop strategies for effective interventions. (See *Cultural influences on developmental assessment*, page 16.)

> Ya know, I think I need to take it easy and get some more sleep so I can reach my highest potential.

Basic necessities

A child must have such basic necessities as sleep, rest, and proper nutrition to reach his highest potential.

Children need more sleep than adults, and nurses should keep in mind that sleep deprivation can impact performance on growth and development assessments. Chronic sleep deprivation yields negative physiologic consequences.

Amount of sleep needed for healthy growth and development

(Recognize each child is different and may require more or less depending on circumstances such as illness, body metabolism, etc.)

Age	Number of hours needed	Sleep patterns
Newborns 1 to 4 weeks	15 to 16 hours/day	No recognizable sleep patterns established yet
Infants 1 to 12 months	14 to 15 hours/day	Most babies sleep 4 to 6 hours at a time, eventually taking two to three naps per day.
Toddlers 1 to 3 years	12 to 14 hours/day	8 to 10 hours at night and one long nap per day
Preschoolers 3 to 6 years	10 to 12 hours/day	Most sleep at night. By 5 years old, most children no longer take naps.
School age 6 to 12 years	10 to 11 hours/day	School-age children may still need a nap occasionally.
Teens 13 to 19 years	8 to 10 hours/day	Most teens need additional sleep during growth times.

Cultured pearls

Cultural influences on developmental assessment

Tools for measuring development might not take into account cultural influences. For example, Southeast Asian children may be considered delayed in the area of personal-social development on the Denver II test because of a lack of familiarity with games such as pat-a-cake, a game well-known to other cultures.

No single tool can take into account all the factors that contribute to the patient's development. Variables that will impact assessment of a child's development must be considered when performing developmental screenings.

Brain food

Nutritional deprivation can seriously interfere with brain development. Nutritional guidelines, such as the MyPlate guidelines from the U.S. Food and Drug Administration (FDA), should be taught to children and their parents to help them achieve optimum nutrition needed for normal growth and development. (See *www .ChooseMyPlate.gov*.)

Teach your children well

Beginning in infancy and continuing throughout the early years of childhood, the nurse, parents, and other significant people in the child's life can teach habits of healthy eating and living. These healthy habits may prevent serious health problems as the child grows.

> Teach parents and children good nutritional habits. Bon appetit!

Other influences

Other influences on growth and development include genetics and heredity as well as the inborn personality or temperament of the child.

MyPlate food guide for young children

These sample daily food plans from www.ChooseMyPlate.gov were designed specifically for children ages 2 to 5 and 6 to 11 by the U.S. Department of Agriculture.

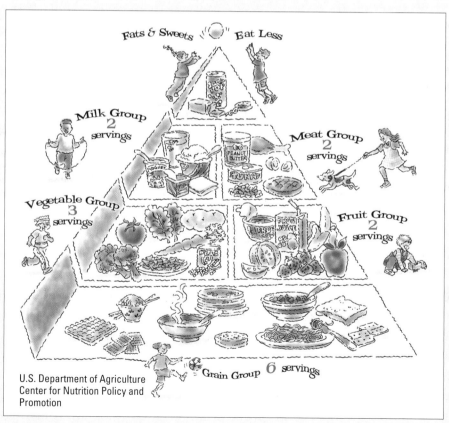

Fats & Sweets — Eat Less

Milk Group
2
servings

Meat Group
2
servings

Vegetable Group
3
servings

Fruit Group
2
servings

Grain Group 6 servings

U.S. Department of Agriculture
Center for Nutrition Policy and
Promotion

Theories of development

According to most theories of personality and cognitive development, certain tasks must be mastered before a child can advance to other, more advanced tasks. This process is similar to the patterns of biological development (cephalocaudal, proximodistal, general to specific). (See *Theories of development*.)

Psychosocial development

A developmental framework for the entire life span was first proposed by Erik Erikson in 1959. Erikson's *psychosocial theory* has been further refined but essentially remains the same today.

Erikson believed that the psychosocial development of an individual is a function of *ego* (the conscious part of the personality—and the part that most immediately controls thought

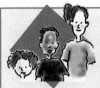

Growing pains

Theories of development

The child development theories discussed in this chart shouldn't be compared directly because they measure different aspects of development. Erik Erikson's psychosocial-based theory is the most commonly accepted model for child development, although it can't be empirically tested.

Age-group	Psychosocial theory	Cognitive theory	Psychosexual theory	Moral development theory
Infancy (birth to age 1)	Trust versus mistrust	Sensorimotor (birth to age 2)	Oral	Not applicable
Toddlerhood (ages 1 to 3)	Autonomy versus shame and doubt	Sensorimotor to preoperational	Anal	Preconventional
Preschool age (ages 3 to 6)	Initiative versus guilt	Preoperational (ages 2 to 7)	Phallic	Preconventional
School age (ages 6 to 12)	Industry versus inferiority	Concrete operational (ages 7 to 11)	Latency	Conventional
Adolescence (ages 13 to 19)	Identity versus role confusion	Formal operational thought (ages 11 to 20)	Genitalia	Postconventional

and behavior) as well as social and biologic processes. At given times in the life cycle, the interaction between these processes cause psychosocial crises by placing a demand on the individual. In order for the person to grow, he must resolve these crises and master the task at hand.

He trusts me, he trusts me not

These tasks occur in eight different stages, five of which pertain to childhood. Each stage is characterized by a specific positive identity issue, such as trust in the infancy stage, and a contrasting negative attribute that may emerge from that issue, such as mistrust in the infancy stage. The prominence of either positive or negative attributes determines mastery of the crisis.

Weighing the pros . . .

If the positive attribute emerges, the individual has a better chance of experiencing unimpaired development.

. . . and the cons

If the negative attribute predominates, the individual may have problems with later attitudes and personal strength. Some negative attributes are, however, necessary to completely master the task at hand. As the person deals with each task, he assumes both increased vulnerability and increased potential, which garners new strength and pushes him on to the next level.

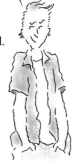

Hey, it isn't my fault if my attitude stinks. Blame it on my predominant negative attribute. (Can I get grounded for that?)

Hopeful today, caring tomorrow

Optimal development depends on the proper resolution of each task in the appropriate sequence. For example, the trust developed in infancy leads to a sense of hope, which forms a foundation for the emerging trait of fidelity in adolescence, and an ability to care in adulthood.

Stages of psychosocial theory

The five childhood stages of psychosocial theory are:

trust versus mistrust (birth to age 1). The child develops trust as the primary caregiver meets his needs.

autonomy versus shame and doubt (ages 1 to 3). The child learns to control his body functions and becomes increasingly independent, preferring to do things himself.

initiative versus guilt (ages 3 to 6). The child learns about the world through play and develops a conscience.

industry versus inferiority (ages 6 to 12). The child enjoys working on projects and with others and tends to follow rules;

competition with others is keen, and forming social relationships takes on greater importance.

🖐 *identity versus role confusion (ages 12 to 19).*
Changes in the child's body are taking place rapidly, and
the child is preoccupied with how he looks and how others
view him; while trying to meet the expectations of his
peers, he's also trying to establish his own identity.

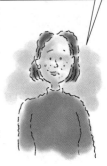

Who am I? What's
my role? Will my skin
ever clear up? I made
it through Erikson's
other four stages,
but I could have done
without number five!

Cognitive development

According to Jean Piaget, cognitive or intellectual acts occur
when an individual is adapting to and organizing the perceived environment around him. Piaget thought a child moves
through four stages of cognitive development. As he moves
through each stage, he builds on structures gained from the
previous stages, moving from relatively simple to very complex
operations.

Some people never grow up!

Piaget noted that all individuals have the capability to achieve the
most advanced levels of functioning, although not all will reach
the final stages of development.

No problem too big

It's through experience with the environment that development
is pushed ahead. The child incorporates new ideas, skills, and
knowledge into familiar patterns of thought and action.

When faced with a problem that's new or too complex to fit
into his existing pattern of thought, the child *accommodates*
(draws on past experiences that are closest to his current problem
to solve it).

Sensorimotor stage

The sensorimotor stage spans birth to age 2. During this stage, the
child progresses from reflex activity, through simple repetitive behaviors, to imitative behaviors. Concepts to be mastered include:
• *object permanence*—the understanding that objects and events
continue to exist, even when they can't be seen, heard, or touched
directly
• *causality*—the relationship between cause and effect
• *spatial relationships*—the recognition of different shapes and
the relationships between them (for example, placing a round
object in a round hole).

Preoperational stage

The preoperational stage starts at age 2 and ends around age 7. This stage is marked by *egocentricity* (the child can't comprehend a point of view different from his own). It's a time of magical thinking and increased ability to use symbols and language. Concepts to be mastered include:
• *representational language and symbols*—re-presenting a reality into internal knowledge through language acquisition, using symbolic play such as riding a broom like horse
• *transductive reasoning*—generalization to the extent that items that share characteristics are labeled the same.

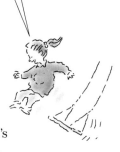

Look at me! I'm flying! (If this is just magical thinking, I'm in big trouble.)

Concrete operational stage

During the concrete operational stage (ages 7 to 11), the child's thought processes become more logical and coherent. He can use inductive reasoning (using facts gathered from one or more specific experiences to draw a general conclusion about a situation) to solve problems but still can't think abstractly. The child is less self-centered during this stage. Concepts to be mastered include sorting, ordering, and classifying facts to use in problem-solving.

Formal operational thought stage

The formal operational thought stage, which runs from ages 11 to 20, is characterized by adaptability and flexibility. The adolescent can think abstractly, form logical conclusions from his observations, and establish and test hypotheses. Concepts to be mastered include abstract ideas and concepts, possibilities, inductive reasoning, and complex deductive reasoning.

Psychosexual development

Development of human sexuality is influenced by physical, emotional, and cultural aspects in the society in which we live. This sexuality is part of the total person, which develops over time. It's expressed through many avenues, including a person's attitudes, feelings, beliefs, and self-image.

Sexual feelings

Sigmund Freud theorized that sexual feelings are present in some form from the newborn period through adulthood. He felt human nature has two sides: rational intellect and irrational desires. Freud's theory of psychosexual development is fairly controversial, yet it is still used. He focused more on the abnormal mind and function rather than on the normal functioning of children and tied the development of personality to sexual development.

Id, ego, and superego

According to the psychosexual theory, personality is composed of three entities:

👆   The *id*, the largest portion of the mind, is the center of our primitive instincts and requires immediate gratification. (The neonate is the epitome of the id.)

✌️   The *ego* develops in infancy and is the conscious, rational part of the personality; it's less inward seeking than the id, and recognizes the larger picture. (The ego acts as a censor to the id; if there's conflict between the id and the ego, neuroses may develop.)

🖐️   The *superego* represents the person's conscience and ideals; therefore, it's in continuous battle with the id.

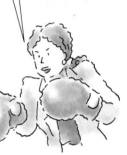

Between the id, ego, and superego, there's always a battle going on. Are you up for the challenge?

Five stages of development

Freud proposed five stages of development; these stages center around the early years of the person's life and the parent-child relationship. At each stage, sexual energy, what Freud called *instinctual libido*, is focused on a different area of the body.

Each stage also centers on a conflict that must be resolved before the child can progress to the next stage. If the conflict isn't resolved, the child becomes fixated in that stage and development is arrested.

So many stages, so little time. Thanks to Dr. Freud, I have my work cut out for me.

I can't get no . . . satisfaction

Satisfaction must be achieved before a person can move on to the next stage. If he isn't fully satisfied, it's possible he may never fully complete the stage.

How the individual responds to others depends on which stage he's in. This was a hallmark theory in the field of psychology, although it's relatively limited in its scope.

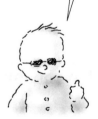

Oral stage

In the oral stage (birth to age 1), the child seeks pleasure through sucking, biting, and other oral activities. Oral stimulation reduces tension and provides sensual satisfaction.

Anal stage

The anal and urethral areas are of great interest in the anal stage (ages 1 to 3). The child goes through toilet training and learns to control his excreta.

Phallic stage

During the phallic stage (ages 3 to 6), the child is interested in his genitalia and various sensations and discovers the difference between boys and girls. The child may love the opposite-sex parent and consider the parent of the same sex a rival. This is known as the *Oedipal* (boys) or *Electra* (girls) *complex*.

Latency period

In the latency period (ages 6 to 12), the child expands on traits developed in earlier stages and concentrates on playing and learning. The child doesn't focus on a particular area of the body during this stage.

The Oedipal or Electra complex resolves, and the child forms close relationships with other children of the same age and gender. Energy is directed toward physical and intellectual quests.

Genitalia stage

The production of sex hormones becomes intense during the genitalia stage (ages 12 and older), and the reproductive system reaches maturation. During this stage, the adolescent develops the capacity for object love and maturity.

Moral development

Lawrence Kohlberg's ideas of moral reasoning (the basis for ethical behavior) are based on the work of Piaget and the American philosopher John Dewey.

Born free . . . of morals, that is!

Kohlberg's theory is based on the premise that, at birth, all beings are devoid of morals, ethics, and honesty. Then, through different stages, the family, and then the larger society, instills values, morality, and a sense of right and wrong. As the child's intelligence and ability to interact with others mature, his patterns of moral behavior mature as well.

Kohlberg, along with Piaget, believed that most moral development occurs through social interaction; he felt that development could be promoted through formal education.

Can we talk?

According to Kohlberg, it's important to present a person with moral dilemmas for discussion, which helps him see the reasonableness of the next higher stage and progress toward it. Kohlberg based this discussion approach on the insight that a person develops as a result of cognitive conflicts in his current stage.

Three levels of moral development

Kohlberg proposed three levels of moral development through which the person must pass. As the child comprehends and understands a stage, he can then progress to the next stage.

Preconventional level of morality

At the preconventional level (ages 2 to 7), the child attempts to follow rules set by those in authority. He tries to adjust his behavior according to good and bad and to right and wrong.

Conventional level of morality

At the conventional level (ages 7 to 12), the child seeks conformity and loyalty. He attempts to justify, support, and maintain the social order, and he follows fixed rules.

Postconventional autonomous level of morality

At the postconventional level (ages 12 and older), the adolescent strives to construct a personal and functional value system independent of authority figures and his peers.

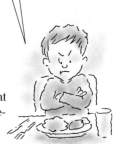

I'm trying to follow my parents' rules, but this preconventional stuff isn't easy.

Caring for the hospitalized child

Everyone has stress—even kids. We all have to find a way to deal with it.

Hospitalization is a major stressor for any individual, but especially for a child. The child is in an unfamiliar surrounding, with unfamiliar people. His routine is disrupted, and he isn't able to do things he normally does.

Added to these stressors are the fear, pain, and discomfort associated with the child's illness or injury and, in many cases, the diagnostic and therapeutic interventions used to treat the child. What's more, even a minor illness may be perceived by the family as life-threatening. This perception can trigger fears that may overwhelm the family's coping skills and lead to crisis.

Developmentally appropriate interventions should be geared toward helping the child and his family cope with this very stressful time.

No place like home

Separation of the child from his parents, siblings, and usual support systems further adds to the emotional stress and discomfort a child feels when hospitalized. Parents (and siblings) should be encouraged and allowed to spend as much time as possible with the hospitalized child. When policy permits, arrangements should be made for a parent to spend the night in the child's room or close by.

Minimizing the trauma of hospitalization

Preparing a child for hospitalization and any interventions will help the child cope more effectively and make it easier for him to trust the health care professionals responsible for his care.

Always be prepared

When possible, it's ideal to prepare the child for admission to the hospital. The timing of the preparation and the amount of teaching given depend on the child's age, developmental stage, personality, and the length of the procedure or treatment.

Young children may need only a few hours of preparation, whereas the older child may benefit from several days of preparation. The use of developmentally appropriate activities will also help the child cope with the stress of hospitalization. (See *The importance of play*.)

Specialist on the job

Many hospitals have a *child life specialist* on staff, who can arrange a preadmission visit for the child and his parents. During these visits, the child and his parents tour the pediatric unit, helping to familiarize the child with the sights, sounds, and smells of the hospital. The child life specialist, an expert in child development, then explains, step-by-step, what the child can expect—especially relating to any planned procedures—and can also stay with the child during those procedures.

Keep it in the family

To reduce the fear that accompanies hospitalization, the nurse can help the child and family cope by:
- explaining procedures
- answering questions openly and honestly
- minimizing separation from the parents
- structuring the environment to allow the child to retain as much control as possible.

Patient- and family-centered care is an approach to health care that recognizes that the child patient and the family are integral members of the health care team. It allows the family to remain as involved as possible and helps give the child and his family a sense of control in a difficult and unfamiliar situation. It may also help

---

The importance of play

One of the most important aspects of a child's life is play. Play can become even more important to a child who's hospitalized. It can serve several functions:
- Play is an excellent stress reducer and tension reliever. It allows the child freedom of expression to act out his fears, concerns, and anxieties.
- Play provides a source of diversional activity, alleviating separation anxiety.

- Play provides the child with a sense of safety and security because, while he's engaging in play, he knows that no painful procedures will occur.
- Developmentally appropriate play fosters the child's normal growth and development, especially for children who are repeatedly hospitalized for chronic conditions.
- Play puts the child in the driver's seat, allowing him to make choices and giving him a sense of control.

alleviate separation anxiety and reassure the child that all care is intended to help him get better. The child needs reassurance that the illness isn't his fault and that fear is a normal response. All children should be encouraged to express their feelings.

Caring for the special needs child

All children go through times in their lives when parents, family, and others need to adapt to certain outside influences. How the child copes with these influences, either positive or negative, is determined by his strengths, personality, developmental stage, and support systems.

Chronic illness and disability

When a child has a chronic illness or is disabled, family members experience additional stress that has lasting implications for the child, his parents, and his siblings.

Flexibility required

Chronic or terminal illnesses, disabilities, or acute conditions that impact daily living require the family and the child to adapt their normal process of living and being; they also require health care professionals to adapt their usual way of providing care.

On the rise

Almost 20% of the pediatric population has a condition that would qualify them as having a special health care need. This percentage is increasing because of improved technology, health care, and treatments that increase survival rates.

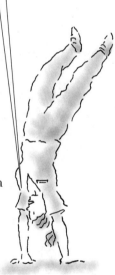

Always stay flexible when providing care to children with special needs.

Barriers to optimal care level

Children with special needs commonly require continuous and complex care. Oversight of care is usually provided by specialists who may or may not take into account alterations in development or the child's response to the illness. Occasionally, this may mean that the child doesn't receive preventive health services. Other barriers to optimal health care in the special needs child include financial, health care system, and knowledge barriers. For these reasons, it's especially important for the nurse to help ensure that the child is up-to-date on immunizations, well-child checkups, and routine health care.

Impact on the family

The diagnosis of a chronic condition may cause extreme distress in the family. Parents grieve over the loss of their "healthy" child and may perceive him as vulnerable. This view may hinder the child in meeting the tasks required for him to grow and develop as normally as possible. Helping the family understand the condition and its impact on normal growth and development will help the child achieve his highest level of functioning. The complexity of care that a special needs child may have also increases the burden of care on the family or may further isolate a family from outside support systems. This added stress may increase the risk for child abuse and other forms of victimization to the child.

Hey, what about me?

Having a sibling with a chronic condition may elicit feelings of stress, helplessness, guilt, or depression. Siblings should be included in the family assessment of coping and should be provided with appropriate support. Older siblings commonly participate in providing care to a special needs child at home as much as the parents do. They must be included when providing care and teaching to the child.

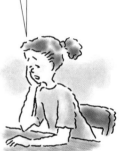

When you have a sick brother or sister, it's easy to get lost in the shuffle.

Nursing strategies

Care and nursing interventions should be adapted to the child's level of development.

Consult the experts

Parents and families are the people that know the most about their child. When planning interventions, the nurse should take into consideration the family's expertise in providing care for their child; the parents should be consulted for advice about the child's routine, care preferences, and special needs.

Be all that you can be

The child should receive special needs care, as appropriate, and interventions aimed at promoting the child's ability to reach his maximum potential.

A little help, please

It's important to remember that a child with a disability or chronic illness faces many challenges. Encouraging the use of such resources as support groups will help the child and family interact with others who are experiencing, or who have managed, the same issues.

Understanding that the child's condition realigns the hopes and expectations of the family and the assigned roles within that family, the nurse can help provide interventions to help the child and family cope. To this end, the nurse can show respect and caring by:
• supporting family coping strategies
• providing education in a forthright, honest manner
• brokering access to health services
• promoting preventive health measures.

Caring for the terminally ill child

The dying child elicits many different emotions in the child, family, and nurse. A perception exists in our society that children aren't supposed to die. For the nurse, this can be a painful and awkward situation.

Dealing with a terminal illness

An understanding of how the child and his family have managed health and illness in the past may provide the nurse with clues about how the family will cope with having a dying child.

Impact on the family

The death of a child is viewed by most people as the worst possible thing that can happen to a parent. Family members of a terminally ill child must deal with a range of emotions while still trying to deal with everyday needs, such as those related to jobs, the household, and the needs of their other children.

> It's difficult to imagine how parents must feel when their child is terminally ill.

To stay or to go—that is the question

These stressors can bring families closer together, but they can also tear families apart. It isn't unusual for parents to have marital stress after the death of a child, at a time when they need each other's support more than ever. Recent statistics show less than one-third of marriages end in divorce after the death of a child.

It's a roller coaster ride

Parents may experience a range of emotions, from fear and anger (sometimes directed at health care providers) to guilt and disabling grief even before their child dies. Siblings may feel unloved or forgotten, as their parents focus their attention on the dying child. They may then feel guilty about having those feelings.

Nursing strategies

The child who's dying has the same emotional and developmental needs as any other child of the same age—as well as other needs related to his poor prognosis. The nurse should develop care plans based on family input to meet these needs at the child's developmental level—realizing that the ill child may have some regression in his or her developmental level. Adaptations in care must be made and must be based on the child's physiologic and psychological status.

Growing pains

Concepts of death in childhood

A child's concept of death depends on his developmental stage.

Developmental stage	Concept of death	Nursing considerations
Infancy	• None	• Help parents understand that the infant or very young child may react to the emotions of others and may show changes in behavior, sleeping, or feeding patterns. • Be aware that the older infant will experience separation anxiety and may express fear through crying. • Help the family cope with death so they can be available to the infant or young child.
Early childhood	• Knows the words "dead" and "death" but the concept of forever may not have value • Reactions are influenced by the attitudes of parents	• Help the family members (including siblings) cope with their feelings. • Reassure the child and siblings that the illness is not their fault nor is it a punishment. • Allow the child to express his own feelings in an open and honest manner. • Help parents deal with potential aggressive or regressive behaviors if the child is unable to verbalize his feelings.
Middle childhood	• Understands universality and irreversibility of death • May have a fear of parents dying	• Use play to facilitate the child's understanding of death. • Ask questions to help facilitate a discussion with the child. Address any distortions or erroneous views of death. • Allow siblings to express their feelings.
Late childhood	• Begins to incorporate family and cultural beliefs about death • Explores views of an afterlife • Faces the reality of own mortality	• Provide opportunities for the child to verbalize his fears. • Help the child discuss his concerns with his family.
Adolescence	• Adult perception of death, but still focused on the "here and now"	• Use opportunities to open discussion about death. • Allow expression of feelings of guilt, confusion, and anxiety. Encourage the youth to not repress emotions. • Support and maintain self-esteem.

Tell me no lies

Communication should be honest. Understanding the developmental level of the child in relation to his concept of death will help foster appropriate communication techniques. (See *Concepts of death in childhood*.)

A positive and helpful approach should be maintained, and the family should be included in all aspects of care. All procedures and therapies should be explained before carrying them out.

Maximum control

Pain control is an essential component in the management of a terminally ill child. The nurse should serve as the child's advocate to ensure that the child receives the most effective pain management possible.

Helping families cope

The nurse can help the family cope during this very difficult time by:
• encouraging all family members to express their feelings, even though they might be difficult to hear
• allowing families to spend as much time as possible with the dying child (including overnight stays)
• allowing and encouraging parents to continue to take an active role in their child's care.

Strong like a bull? Not always!

The nurse can also help the family cope by:
• reminding parents that they don't always have to be strong and that asking for help is a sign of strength, not weakness
• helping parents to talk with their child about dying in a developmentally appropriate manner if he's ready to do so
• providing parents and siblings with information about support groups and professionals who can help them with their grief
• contacting other health care professionals (social workers, child life specialists, play therapists, art and music or pet therapists) and volunteers who may be able to help the child, his siblings, and his parents with coping and with concrete daily needs (such as transportation, sibling care, and special arrangements)
• reassuring parents that you understand how difficult this must be but avoiding such phrases as "I know how you feel"
• remaining as accessible and available as possible and facilitating contact and communication with other individuals on the child's health care team.

Nurses have the unique opportunity to impact the child in every stage of life. Using the principles of caring for the whole person will help the child and his family deal with the most difficult stage, that of the dying child.

An art, music, or play therapist can help a child cope.

Pain in the pediatric patient

> Hey, give me a break! I have no idea that I'll feel all better in 10 minutes. I live in the here and now, baby! Whaah!

Pain is a subjective experience; for infants and children, it's possibly the most bewildering and frightening occurrence in their young lives. Until age 3 or so, children can't grasp abstract concepts, such as time, cause and effect, and quantification. Consequently, it's impossible for them to understand why pain occurs or that relief is just around the corner. They know only that something hurts right now.

My kingdom for a word

What makes the experience particularly distressing is that infants and young children lack the language skills needed to tell someone that they're in pain, where it hurts, and how much, or to ask for help.

In this respect, infants and children are uniquely dependent on the ability of their parents and health care providers to recognize the physiologic and behavioral signs of pain and to react by relieving their pain. Similarly, children could reasonably expect these same caregivers to anticipate and prevent or minimize painful experiences whenever possible.

Assessing pain

A growing number of health professionals who work with children talk about pain as a fifth vital sign, one that should be assessed early and often to ensure prompt, effective relief.

Assessing pain in infants and young children requires the cooperation of the parents and the use of age-specific assessment tools. If the child can communicate verbally, he can also aid the process.

Health history and physical examination

Normal clinical assessment involves a health history that includes a description of any pain and palliative measures and a comprehensive physical examination. When assessing infants and children, you must rely on parents for the health history and background on experience with pain.

Wanna play 20 questions?

To help you better understand the child's pain, ask the parents these questions:
• What kinds of pain has your child had in the past?
• How does your child usually respond to pain?
• How do you know your child is in pain?
• What do you do when he's hurting?

- What does your child do when he's hurting?
- What works best to relieve your child's pain?
- Is there anything special you'd like me to know about your child and pain?

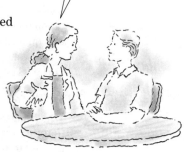

Anything you can tell me will help me understand your child's pain.

No wonder they call 'em vital

The child's vital signs can be pain indicators. Elevated pulse, blood pressure, or respirations can be signs of pain and stress. However, findings here must be viewed in conjunction with other assessment data because nonpainful stimuli can elicit changes in vital signs as well. For example, just touching an infant can speed or calm the child's pulse rate.

Assessment tools

A number of proven assessment tools have been designed for a young patient. Many of these tools seek to quantify the child's pain, one of the harder things to accomplish during assessment and observation. Using an assessment tool will help, but quantifying pain in the infant or preverbal child will still be difficult.

Where's that toolbox?

Pain assessment tools are described as being *unidimensional* (measuring or assessing one indicator) or *multidimensional* (measuring or assessing multiple indicators). Composite measures of pain include physiologic, behavioral, sensory, and cognitive indicators. These tools tend to be especially useful when assessing children under age 3 or older children with cognitive deficits.

Painful measures

Because of the complexity of assessing pain in infants, there's no single pain measurement tool that works well for all patients. However, four multidimensional tools for measuring pain in infants have proved to be quite effective. These four tools are the:

 CRIES Neonatal Postoperative Pain Measurement Scale

 Neonatal Infant Pain Scale

 Premature Infant Pain Profile (See *Measuring pain in infants.*)

 COMFORT Scale.

The CRIES inventory is one of the easier tools to use. Five separate factors are scored on a scale of 0 to 2. Infants with a score of 0 would be pain-free. A total score of 10 would indicate extreme pain.

All of the assessment tools for infants and young children were developed to help assess acute pain. Currently, no tools exist to help measure chronic pain in infants and young children. The

Memory jogger

To help you stay focused when assessing pain in the young patient, remember the mnemonic QUEST:

Q—Question the child's parents (and the child, too, if he's old enough to respond).

U—Use appropriate pain assessment tools.

E—Evaluate the child's behavior.

S—Secure the parents' active participation in treatment.

T—Take the cause of the pain into consideration.

Measuring pain in infants

Assessing pain in infants and young children can be challenging for health care providers. This chart describes four assessment tools that can help you meet this challenge.

Assessment tool	Factors measured
CRIES Neonatal Postoperative Pain Measurement Scale	• Crying (C) • Oxygen saturation (R—requires oxygen to maintain saturation above 95%) • Heart rate and blood pressure (I—increased) • Expression (E) • Sleeplessness (S)
Neonatal Infant Pain Scale	• Facial expression • Crying • Breathing patterns • State of arousal • Movement of arms and legs
Premature Infant Pain Profile	• Gestational age • Heart rate • Oxygen saturation • Behavioral state • Brow bulge • Eye squeeze • Nasolabial furrow
COMFORT Scale	• Alertness • Calmness • Respiratory distress • Crying • Physical movement • Muscle tone • Facial tension • Blood pressure (mean arterial pressure [MAP]) baseline • Heart rate baseline

variability of pain response and the pathology of chronic pain in infants and young children make measurement very difficult.

Speaking of pain

For the child capable of speaking, typically age 3, the task is somewhat easier. Several simple and effective pain-measuring scales can help the child identify a level of pain. These include a:
• faces pain-measuring scale
• visual analog scale
• chip pain-measuring tool. (See *Measuring pain in young children*, page 34.)

Measuring pain in young children

For children who are old enough to speak and understand sufficiently, three useful tools can help them communicate information for measuring their pain. Here's how to use each one:

Faces scale (examples: Faces Pain Scale, Wong-Baker FACES® Pain Rating Scale, etc.)

The child age 3 and older can use any of the faces scales to rate his pain. When using this tool, make sure he can see and point to each face and then describe the amount of pain each face is experiencing. If he's able, the child can read the text under the picture; otherwise, you or his parent can read it to him.

Avoid saying anything that might prompt the child to choose a certain face. Then, ask the child to choose the face that shows how he's feeling right now. Record his response in your assessment notes.

 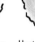

| Happy because he doesn't hurt at all | Hurts just a little bit | Hurts a little more | Hurts even more | Hurts a whole lot | Hurts the most |

Visual analog scale

A visual analog pain scale is simply a straight line with the phrase "no pain" at one end and the phrase "the most pain possible" at the other. Children who understand the concept of a continuum can mark the spot on the line that corresponds to the level of pain they feel.

No pain   The most pain possible

Chip tool

The chip tool uses four identical chips to signify levels of pain and can be used for the child who understands the basic concept of adding one thing to another to get more. If available, you can use poker chips. If not, simply cut four uniform circles from a sheet of paper. Here's how to present the chips:

• First say, "I want to talk with you about the hurt you might be having right now."

• Next, align the chips horizontally on the bedside table, a clipboard, or other firm surface where the child can easily see and reach them.

• Point to the chip at the child's far left and say, "This chip is just a little bit of hurt."

• Point to the second chip and say, "This next chip is a little more hurt."

• Point to the third chip and say, "This next chip is a lot of hurt."

• Point to the last chip and say, "This last chip is the most hurt you can have."

• Ask the child, "How many pieces of hurt do you have right now?" (You won't need to offer the option of "no hurt at all" because the child will tell you if he doesn't hurt.)

• Record the number of chips. If the child's answer isn't clear, talk to him about his answer; then record your findings.

Behavioral responses to pain

Behavior is the language infants and children rely on to convey information about their pain. Areas of behavior that change because of pain include body positioning, facial expression, patterns of eating and sleeping, attention level, and vocalization.

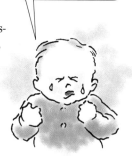

Can you tell I'm in pain? Until I can say it, this is the best way I can let you know.

Look at that face!

In an infant, facial expression is the most common and consistent behavioral response to all stimuli, painful or pleasurable, and may be the single best indicator of pain for the provider and the parent. Studies indicate that facial expression is a more reliable pain indicator than crying, heart rate, or body position and movement.

Facial expressions that tend to indicate that the infant is in pain include:
- mouth stretched open
- eyes tightly shut
- brows and forehead knitted (as they are in a grimace)
- cheeks raised high enough to form a wrinkle on the nose.

Older signs

In young children, facial expression is joined by other behaviors to convey pain. In these patients, look for such signs as:
- narrowing of the eyes
- grimace or fearful appearance
- frequent and longer lasting bouts of crying, with a tone that's higher and louder than normal
- less receptiveness to comforting by parents or other caregivers
- holding or protecting the painful area.

It takes a little detective work to solve a crying mystery. Thank goodness the parents can offer some clues!

Hush-a-bye, why do you cry?

Enlist the parents' help in interpreting the child's crying. Pain may be the cause, but hunger, anger, fear, or a wet diaper can also elicit crying. Typically, parents can distinguish among the different cries of their child and help narrow down the possible causes.

Crying associated with pain is distinguished by frequency, duration, pitch, and intensity. Cries of pain are usually short, sharp, higher in pitch, tense, harsh, nonmelodious, and loud.

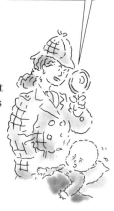

Silent cry

On the other hand, some infants don't cry in response to pain, even pain associated with an invasive procedure. Also, some treatments make crying impossible. Intubated infants, for example, can't produce an audible cry because the endotracheal tube passes through their vocal cords. However, these infants still exhibit the facial expressions that accompany crying—mouth opened wide and eyes tightly closed, insinuating crying.

Looks can be deceiving

It's a mistake to rely too heavily on observed behavior alone when assessing pain in young patients. Some children will suffer pain rather than report it or allow others to see that they're in pain. Others are adept at distracting themselves and may appear pain-free. Some children may have been conditioned to not show pain because of negative consequences if they do. Some children will sleep soundly, not because they have no pain, but because they're physically and emotionally exhausted.

Translation needed

A child who has mastered the rudiments of language can provide some useful information. However, keep in mind that his language skills are very basic and that he may not understand words you use; you may call it pain, but he may think of it as a hurt or boo-boo. Find the words that work best by talking with his parents and with the child himself.

> I have a boo-boo on my doo-dah and it's foo-foo! Do you need a translation? Ask my Mommy.

Check the mirror

Remember that children who are just learning to talk have a great deal more skill in reading the facial expressions and body language of their parents and caregivers. After all, they've been reading this language since birth.

Be sure your expression and body posture are conveying a message consistent with your words. If you or his parents appear concerned, he may feel there's something to fear, and this may color his description of the pain he's feeling.

Managing pain

Infants and young children may experience acute pain, cancer pain, or chronic pain associated with an underlying disorder. Pain management is most effective when it prevents, limits, or avoids noxious stimuli and involves administering analgesics.

Regardless of the underlying cause, pain management for these young patients seeks to:
• identify and relieve existing pain
• anticipate and prevent or minimize pain related to hospitalization, procedures, and treatments
• optimize pharmacologic and nonpharmacologic interventions to reduce stress, increase comfort, and enhance healing.

Pharmacologic intervention

Pharmacologic therapy is the mainstay of pain management for an infant or a child. Selection of the medications, dosages, and administration routes depends on the specific needs of the patient.

Opioid analgesics

Opioid analgesics are highly effective pain relievers and constitute the core of most pharmacologic interventions to manage acute pain (especially postoperative pain) in infants and children.

Choose your weapon . . .

Tramadol (Ultram), morphine (MS Contin), and fentanyl (Duragesic) are among the opioids used most commonly in these patients. While they're thought to be equivalent, morphine may provide better sedation and a lower risk of chest wall rigidity than fentanyl. Tramadol has less respiratory depression than morphine but is not quite as strong.

OK, guys, this is it. Get ready to wipe out some pain.

. . . and pick a route

Opioid analgesics are available in oral, sublingual, rectal, nasal, subcutaneous, transdermal, intravenous (I.V.), and intraspinal forms, which makes it relatively easy to find an acceptable route.

Although we've learned much about the pharmacodynamics and pharmacokinetics of opioids in young children, many practitioners still resist prescribing them.

Hip hooray for PCA!

Patient-controlled analgesia (PCA) can be useful in managing pain in the young patient, provided the parents are involved and they (and, if appropriate, the child) are trained in the theory and proper use of this equipment. PCA allows the patient to maintain a therapeutic level of the prescribed opioid analgesic at all times. It has proven effective in children ages 5 and older.

Parent-controlled analgesia is an effective way to allow the use of I.V. PCA for children younger than age 5 and for those with a developmental delay.

Nonopioid analgesics

Nonopioid analgesics, which include acetaminophen and nonsteroidal anti-inflammatory drugs (NSAIDs), are prescribed to manage mild to moderate pain. In instances of severe pain, nonopioid analgesics can be used in conjunction with opioid analgesics to reduce the required dosage of the opioid drug.

Infants and children metabolize nonopioid analgesics in a similar manner and rate as adults; consequently, the selection criteria, effects, and possible adverse effects are comparable to adults.

Acetaminophen anyone?

Acetaminophen is the drug of choice for treating mild pain. It has the added benefit of helping reduce fever and is very safe, even for neonates. Acetaminophen has few adverse effects or contraindications. However, long-term use can increase the risk of liver damage, and overdosing can be lethal. It's also possible to reach a point at which additional doses no longer provide an analgesic effect. On the plus side, acetaminophen is available in suppository, liquid, and chewable tablet form, making it easy to administer and appropriate for most situations. Caution the parents to not use combination medications (such as cough and cold remedies that may also contain acetaminophen) to prevent the risk of overdose.

Who said NSAIDs?

NSAIDs relieve mild to moderate pain, reduce fever and also act as anti-inflammatory agents. Commonly prescribed NSAIDs, such as ibuprofen (Advil or Motrin), naproxen (Naprosyn), tolmetin (Tolectin), indomethacin (Indocin), and ketorolac (Toradol), are approved for use in children. Possible adverse effects of NSAIDs include inhibition of platelet aggregation and GI irritation.

Combining or alternating therapy

Although alternating ibuprofen and acetaminophen is a very common practice, it is not recommended. Current studies looking at fever management have not found any significant advantage for alternating medications versus using a single medication. Studies of alternating the two for pain management in children are limited. The American Academy of Pediatrics does not recommend combining or alternating medications due to the risk of confusion causing an inappropriate or over dose to be given.

Adjuvant therapy

Adjuvant therapy is defined as a pharmacologic agent that is added to another medication to increase its effect. Although there are very few studies of the effectiveness of adjuvant therapy in infants and children, doctors prescribe a range of medications as adjuvant therapy, usually when treating cancer pain in infants and children. Positive results from such therapy have made adjuvant therapy more acceptable as a constructive facet of pain management in other chronic conditions as well, such as neuropathies, headache, myofascial pain, and recurrent abdominal pain.

Types of drugs used for adjuvant therapy, and their therapeutic effects, include:

• antianxiety medications, such as lorazepam (Ativan), diazepam (Valium), and midazolam (Versed), which are used to enhance the effect of opioids

• anticonvulsants, such as phenytoin (Dilantin), carbamazepine (Tegretol), and gabapentin (Neurontin), which are used to treat neuropathies caused by certain diseases or trauma

• corticosteroids, which help alleviate severe inflammation and bone pain

• neuroleptic drugs, which are antipsychotic, tranquilizing, sedative, and analgesic, to help relieve pain associated with cancer, certain neuralgias, phantom limb, and muscular discomfort

- tricyclic antidepressants, such as amitriptyline (Elavil), which are sometimes used to manage headache and chronic pain
- topical or local anesthetics, which are given before procedures, such as I.V. insertion, to reduce procedural pain.

Many of the previously mentioned medications can have serious side effects or even a paradoxical response. Make sure you help the parents understand the importance of using the medication properly and to report any adverse effects right away.

Nonpharmacologic interventions

For the infant, child, or youth, nonpharmacologic interventions pick up where drug therapies stop—by reducing stress and anxiety and increasing comfort and security. Typically, these measures are just as critical to the patient's well-being as pain relief.

Nonpharmacologic interventions cause no adverse effects, require no special equipment, and can be used at any time. These interventions have another benefit: They can give the parents an opportunity to shine in the care of their child.

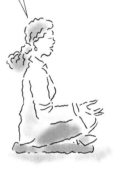

There's nothing like a little relaxation to relieve stress in patients—and in nurses too!

Cognitive-behavioral therapies

Cognitive-behavioral interventions for the infant include positioning, containment or swaddling, distraction, touching, and gentle massage.

Wrap 'em up

Placing an infant in a midline or supine position has a calming effect, as does wrapping him snugly in a soft blanket. Providing distraction—for example, with a bedside mobile or a safe, colorful toy or stuffed animal—helps the infant focus on something enjoyable rather than his pain.

You're getting sleepy—very sleepy

For a toddler, distraction, hypnosis, guided imagery, gentle massage, snuggling with Mom and Dad, and curling up in bed listening to a story are all methods of moving the child's focus away from his pain toward more serene, safe, and comforting thoughts.

Physical therapy

Thermotherapy is the most common form of physical therapy used with infants. Applying warm and cold to painful areas can make them feel better. Heat promotes circulation, and cold helps reduce swelling and provides a limited amount of numbing.

Complementary therapies

Complementary therapies, such as music or aromatherapy, are gaining acceptance because of the influence music and aromas can have on emotions and state of mind.

Charms to soothe

For the infant or child, soothing music has a calming effect and can help him drift off to sleep at nap time. More lively music can stimulate memories or encourage singing, which distract the child for a time. Smells that remind him of Mom, Dad, or Grandma's house can be comforting as well.

Sucking on sucrose

For the infant, nonnutritive sucking using a pacifier, a pacifier dipped in sucrose, or a small bottle of water containing sucrose is effective in reducing pain associated with procedures. Nonnutritive sucking with or without sucrose can be used to calm the infant before the procedure as well as afterward.

A little music goes a long way toward soothing or distracting a child in pain. (And he probably won't even notice if you're off-key!)

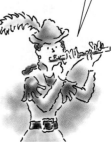

Preparing pediatric medications

Medications are used throughout the life span to treat health problems (including pain), combat disease, and promote health. Many health care professionals have expressed concerns about medication use in infants and children. These concerns are gradually beginning to fade, primarily because our understanding of medications' pharmacokinetics and pharmacodynamics in infants and young children has significantly improved in recent years.

Pharmacokinetics and pharmacodynamics

The *pharmacokinetic* (how a drug acts and how it moves through the body) and *pharmacodynamic* (study of drug mechanisms that produce biochemical or physiologic changes in the body) properties of medications include:
- absorption—how the drug is absorbed or moved into the bloodstream
- distribution—how the drug is distributed or transferred to another site
- protein-binding capacity—a measure of the drug's efficiency
- metabolism—the process of converting the drug into a useful form
- elimination—the removal of the drug from the body.

Children aren't little adults. Their bodies absorb, distribute, and metabolize medications differently.

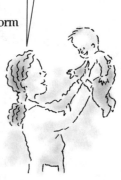

Medication metabolism in young children

It's important to understand how the unique physiology of young children affects pharmacokinetics and pharmacodynamics. Infants and young children are still developing physiologically, which affects the way their bodies absorb, distribute, and metabolize drugs. The metabolism of an infant or young child differs significantly from that of an older patient.

Acid, protein, and water . . . oh my!

A better understanding of how medications are used and metabolized in children will lead to safer medication administration in the pediatric population:
• Because gastric acidity doesn't stabilize until approximately age 3, the absorption and concentration of drugs that require an acid environment to be fully assimilated may be affected.
• Protein-binding, which aids in the distribution of drugs in the body, is lower in infants and children than in older patients.
• Compared to adults, infants have proportionately more water weight and extracellular water, less fat, and less muscle tissue. In infants, hepatic (liver) metabolism is slower and renal clearance is delayed. These factors can increase the potential for drug toxicity.

Dosage calculations

To calculate and verify the safety of pediatric drug dosages, use either the *dosage per kilogram of body weight* method or the *body surface area (BSA)* method. Other methods, such as those based on age, are less accurate and typically aren't used.

Whichever method you use, remember that, as a nurse, you're professionally and legally responsible for checking the safety of a prescribed dose before administration. (See *Trio of timesaving tips.*)

Dosage per kilogram of body weight

Many pharmaceutical companies provide information about safe drug dosages for pediatric patients in milligrams per kilogram of body weight. This measurement is the most accurate and common way to calculate pediatric dosages.

Pediatric dosages are usually expressed as *mg/kg/day* or *mg/kg/dose*. Based on this information, you can determine the pediatric dose by multiplying the child's weight in kilograms by the required number of milligrams of drug per kilogram.

Shifting weight

Most pediatric patients' weights are measured in kilograms. If you must convert from pounds to kilograms before calculating the dosage per kilogram of body weight, remember that 1 kg equals 2.2 lb.

Real world problems

The following example shows how to use proportions to convert pounds to kilograms, how to calculate a *mg/kg/dose* for one-time or as-needed (p.r.n.) medications, and how to

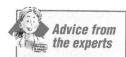

Advice from the experts

Trio of timesaving tips

When calculating safe pediatric dosages, save time and prevent errors by following these three suggestions:

🖐 Carry a calculator for use when solving equations.

✌ Consult a formulary or drug handbook to verify a drug dose. (When in doubt, call the pharmacist.)

🖖 Keep your patient's weight in kilograms at his bedside so you won't have to estimate it or weigh him in a rush.

calculate *mg/kg/day* for doses given around the clock to maintain a continuous drug effect.

Penicillin problem

The doctor orders penicillin V potassium oral suspension 56 mg/kg/day in four divided doses for a patient who weighs 55 lb. The suspension that's available is penicillin V potassium 125 mg/5 ml. What volume should you administer for each dose?

Here's how to solve this problem using ratios and fractions:
• First, convert the child's weight from pounds to kilograms by setting up this proportion:

$$X : 55 \text{ lb} :: 1 \text{ kg} : 2.2 \text{ lb}$$

• Multiply the extremes and the means:

$$X \times 2.2 \text{ lb} = 1 \text{ kg} \times 55 \text{ lb}$$

• Solve for X by dividing each side of the equation by 2.2 lb and canceling units that appear in both the numerator and the denominator.

$$\frac{X \times \cancel{2.2 \text{ lb}}}{\cancel{2.2 \text{ lb}}} = \frac{1 \text{ kg} \times 55 \cancel{\text{ lb}}}{2.2 \cancel{\text{ lb}}}$$

$$X = \frac{55 \text{ kg}}{2.2}$$

$$X = 25 \text{ kg}$$

The child weighs 25 kg.

• Next, determine the total daily dosage by setting up a proportion with the patient's weight and the unknown dosage on one side and the ordered dosage on the other side:

$$\frac{25 \text{ kg}}{X} = \frac{1 \text{ kg}}{56 \text{ mg}}$$

• Cross-multiply the fractions:

$$X \times 1 \text{ kg} = 56 \text{ mg} \times 25 \text{ kg}$$

• Solve for X by dividing each side of the equation by 1 kg and canceling units that appear in both the numerator and the denominator:

$$\frac{X \times \cancel{1 \text{ kg}}}{\cancel{1 \text{ kg}}} = \frac{56 \text{ mg} \times 25 \cancel{\text{ kg}}}{1 \cancel{\text{ kg}}}$$

$$X = \frac{56 \text{ mg} \times 25}{1}$$

$$X = 1,400 \text{ mg}$$

- The child's daily dosage is 1,400 mg. Now, divide the daily dosage by four doses to determine the dose to administer every 6 hours:

$$X = \frac{1,400 \text{ mg}}{4 \text{ doses}}$$

$$X = 350 \text{ mg/dose}$$

The child should receive 350 mg every 6 hours.

- Lastly, calculate the volume to give for each dose by setting up a proportion with the unknown volume and the amount in one dose on one side and the available dose on the other side:

$$\frac{X}{350 \text{ mg}} = \frac{5 \text{ ml}}{125 \text{ mg}}$$

- Cross-multiply the fractions:

$$X \times 125 \text{ mg} = 5 \text{ ml} \times 350 \text{ mg}$$

- Solve for X by dividing each side of the equation by 125 mg and canceling units that appear in both the numerator and denominator:

$$\frac{X \times \cancel{125 \text{ mg}}}{\cancel{125 \text{ mg}}} = \frac{5 \text{ ml} \times 350 \cancel{\text{ mg}}}{125 \cancel{\text{ mg}}}$$

$$X = \frac{5 \text{ ml} \times 350}{125}$$

$$X = \frac{1,750 \text{ ml}}{125}$$

$$X = 14 \text{ ml}$$

You should administer 14 ml of the drug at each dose.

> I guess my math teacher was right. You really do have to solve for X in the real world.

Dosage by BSA

The BSA method is used to calculate safe pediatric dosages for a limited number of drugs. (It's also used to calculate safe dosages for adult patients receiving extremely potent drugs that need to be administered with absolute precision, such as antineoplastic or chemotherapeutic agents.)

Advice from the experts

What's in a nomogram?

BSA is critical when calculating dosages for pediatric patients or for drugs that are extremely potent and need to be given in precise amounts. The nomogram shown here lets you plot the patient's height and weight to determine the BSA. Here's how it works:

• Locate the patient's height in the left column of the nomogram and his weight in the right column.

• Use a ruler to draw a straight line connecting the two points. (The point where the line intersects the surface area column indicates the patient's BSA in square meters.)

• For an average-sized child, use the simplified nomogram in the box. Just find the child's weight in pounds on the left side of the scale and then read the corresponding BSA on the right side.

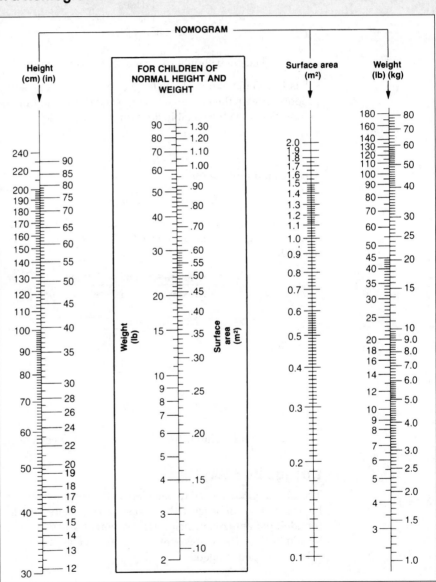

The plot thickens

Calculating dosages by BSA is done in two steps:
- Plot the patient's height and weight on a chart (called a *nomogram*) to determine the BSA in square meters (m^2). (See *What's in a nomogram?*)
- Multiply the BSA by the prescribed pediatric dose in $mg/m^2/day$. Here's the formula:

$$\text{child's dose in mg} = \text{child's BSA in } m^2 \times \frac{\text{pediatric dose in mg}}{m^2/day}$$

The BSA method is also used to calculate a child's dose based on the average adult BSA—1.73 m^2—and an average adult dose. The formula looks like this:

$$\text{child's dose (mg)} = \frac{\text{child's BSA in } m^2}{\text{average adult BSA (1.73 } m^2)} \times \text{average adult dose}$$

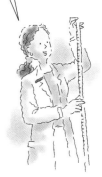

I have the height. Now I need the weight and the BSA. Will this be on the final exam?

Administering pediatric medications

The methods used to prepare drugs and administer them to pediatric patients differ from the methods used for adults, depending on which route is used. There are specific administration guidelines and precautions for each route as well. (See *Giving medications to children*, page 46.)

Oral route

Infants and young children who can't swallow tablets or capsules are given oral drugs in liquid form. When a liquid preparation isn't available, you may, generally, crush a tablet and mix it with a small amount of liquid. However, it's important that you don't:
- mix crushed tablets in essential fluids, such as infant formula, because this could lead to feeding refusal
- crush enteric-coated drugs or timed-release capsules or tablets because crushing destroys the coating that causes drugs to release at the right time or prevent stomach irritation.

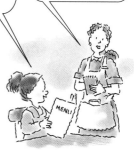

Ah, yes. I think the apple juice will go quite nicely with my acetaminophen today.

Allowing choices gives the child a sense of control.

A spoonful of sugar

These suggestions will help to make administering pills and liquids easier for the child and the nurse:
- Allow the child as much choice as possible (for instance, which pill to take first or which beverage to drink).

• If the liquid drug is prepared as a suspension or as an insoluble drug in a liquid base, mix it thoroughly before you measure and administer it to ensure that none of the drug remains settled out of the solution.

• If the child can drink from a cup, measure and give liquid medications in a cup that's calibrated in metric and household units.

• If the child is very young or can't drink from a cup, use a medication dropper, syringe, or hollow-handle spoon.

• For the infant, slowly instill liquid medication by dropper along the side of his tongue, or offer it through a nipple. Hold the infant with his head elevated to prevent aspiration.

Nasal route

Administering a nasal medication to a child may not be as difficult as it sounds. Parents can also be instructed in giving nose drops and giving medication with a nasal inhaler.

Drop in the bucket?

To administer nose drops:

• Warm the medication to room temperature and warn the child that he may taste the medication.

• Wash your hands.

• Draw up the proper amount of medication into the dropper.

• Have the child gently blow his nose if he's able, or clean away secretions with a washcloth.

• Tilt the child's head back. (In small children, this can be accomplished by having the child lie on his back with a small pillow placed between the shoulders and tilting his head back over the top of the pillow.)

• Push up gently on the child's nose.

• Instruct the child to breathe through his mouth while the medication is being placed in the nose. (For infants, be sure to instill the drops in one naris at a time because infants are obligate nose breathers.)

• Without touching the dropper to the nose, aim the dropper toward the back of the nostril and place the correct number of drops in each side of the nose.

• Keep the head tilted back for at least 1 minute (count to 60) and then allow the child to spit out any medication that has run down the back of his throat.

The nose knows

To give medication with a nasal inhaler:

• Wash your hands.

• Place the tip of the inhaler inside the child's nostril.

• Have the child inhale; then administer the medication.

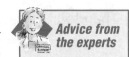

Advice from the experts

Giving medications to children

When giving oral and parenteral medications to children, safety is essential. Keep these points in mind:

• Check the child's mouth to make sure he has swallowed the oral medication.

• Carefully mix oral drugs that come in suspension form.

• Give intramuscular (I.M.) injections in the vastus lateralis muscle of infants who haven't started walking.

• Don't inject more than 1 ml into I.M. or subcutaneous sites.

• Rotate injection sites.

- Have the child hold his breath for a few seconds and then exhale through his mouth.
- Don't allow the child to blow his nose for at least 3 minutes.

Up your nose with a . . . sprayer

To administer a nasal spray:
- Wash your hands.
- Plug one nostril and place the tip of the sprayer a short distance into the opposite nostril.
- Have the child hold his breath; then administer the medication.
- Tell the child to hold his breath for a few more seconds and then exhale through his mouth.
- Make sure the child keeps his head tilted back for at least 1 minute, and don't allow him to blow his nose.

Optic route

The administration of eye drops or eye ointment can be difficult for the child because of his natural instinct to blink. Tell the child and parents that eye ointment may cause blurred vision for a short time.

The eyes have it

To administer eye drops or ointments:
- Warm the medication to room temperature.
- Wash your hands.
- Clean the eye of all secretions and residual medication.
- Tilt the child's head back and have the child look at the ceiling.
- Using your thumb and index finger, gently pull back the lower lid to expose the conjunctival sac.
- Without touching the dropper or bottle to the eye, administer the drops into the conjunctival sac, not directly into the eye. When administering an eye ointment, apply the ointment from the inner canthus to the outer canthus of the eye.
- Have the child close his eyes for a few minutes; then wipe away excess ointment.
- If a second type of eye drop or an eye ointment is required, wait 5 minutes before administering the second medication.

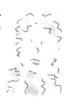

> Always prepare the child and the parent for blurred vision before instilling eye ointment. Knowing what to expect makes interventions less frightening.

Otic route

Because younger children are more prone to developing ear infections than older children or adolescents, eardrops may be used frequently in young children. Medications that are cold may cause dizziness and nausea when placed into the ear; therefore, always warm the medication to body temperature by placing it between your hands for several minutes.

In one ear . . .

To administer eardrops:
• Wash your hands.
• Place the child on his side, with the affected ear facing up.
• Clean away secretions or residual medication.
• Straighten the ear canal. (In children younger than age 3, hold the ear and gently pull down and back. In children older than 3, gently pull the pinna up and back.)
• Instill the correct number of drops into the ear without touching the dropper to the ear. (Try to let the drops run down the side of the canal rather than dropping into the center of the canal.)
• Have the child lie on his side for at least 1 minute.

Take special care of how you hold a baby's ear when administering eardrops.

Rectal route

Rectal suppositories may be needed for a child who has been vomiting or who can't receive his medications orally. The rectal suppository should be firm. If it isn't, run it under cold water before unwrapping it.

How it's supposed to go

To administer a suppository:
• Wash your hands.
• Remove the suppository from its wrapper.
• Assist the child into the Sims' position (on his left side with his right knee flexed and close to his chest).
• Dip the suppository into water or a water-soluble lubricant such as K-Y jelly.
• Wearing gloves, gently separate the buttocks to expose the anus.
• Gently insert the smooth, rounded end of the suppository into the anal orifice.
• Push the suppository into the rectum (approximately 1″ [2.5 cm]) until there's no resistance. (Use your smallest finger in a child younger than age 3.)
• Remove your finger, ensuring the suppository remains in place.
• Hold the child's buttocks together for 5 minutes to prevent expulsion of the medication.
• Keep the child in the Sims' position for approximately 20 minutes.

NG, OG, or gastrostomy route

Administration of nasogastric (NG), orogastric (OG), and gastrostomy medications or feedings follows the same principles. Tube placement is checked by inserting 5 cc of air into the tube while simultaneously listening for a "whoosh" sound over the stomach. This sound ensures that the tube hasn't slipped out of place before administering the medication or feeding. Alternatively, you may check for stomach contents, using pH paper. The medication or formula should be warmed to room temperature to decrease the likelihood of discomfort.

Past the lips, past the gums . . .

To administer NG, OG, or gastrostomy medications or feedings:
• Wash your hands.
• Aspirate and measure stomach contents to determine the amount of residual stomach contents and then return the contents to the stomach to prevent an electrolyte imbalance.
• Pinch or clamp the tubing closed to prevent air from entering the stomach.
• Remove the plunger from the barrel of the syringe and attach the barrel to the gastric tube.
• Fill the tube with the medication or formula.
• Allow the medication or formula to infuse slowly, holding the tube no more than approximately 6″ (15.2 cm) above the stomach.
• Flush with water (use a minimal amount, no more than 30 cc) to clean the tubing and prevent obstruction.
• Clamp the end of the tubing when finished.

Inhalation route

Aerosol medications are commonly used in treating respiratory illnesses such as asthma or bronchiolitis. Advantages of using this route include delivering the medication directly to the site of action, a faster onset of action, and less systemic side effects. The most commonly used methods of giving aerosolized medications are via a metered-dose inhaler or through a nebulizer.

Using an inhaler

Most children are not able to coordinate the steps required to use a metered-dose inhaler properly and therefore need to use a spacer with the inhaler. Teach the parents and the child the steps for ensuring all the medication is delivered to the airways. Many inhalers have a counter attached so it is easy to know how many doses are available. To use an inhaler with a spacer:
• Take off the protective caps of both the inhaler and the spacer.
• Shake the inhaler to ensure the medication is mixed.
• Place the inhaler into the open end of the spacer, opposite the spacer mouthpiece or mask.
• Have the child completely exhale by blowing out all his breath.
• Put the spacer mouthpiece in the child's mouth and have him seal his lips around it (or place the mask around the mouth and nose).

- Push the inhaler canister once to release the medication into the spacer.
- Have the child breathe in slowly through his mouth, inhaling the medication that is trapped in the spacer. Some spacers will make a sound if the child breathes in too fast.
- If the child is able, tell the child to hold his breath for 10 seconds.
- Take the spacer out of the child's mouth (or the mask away from the face) and have him breathe out slowly.
- Wait at least 1 full minute before taking any additional puffs that may be ordered.
- If using a steroid inhaler, teach the child to rinse his mouth after finishing the dose.
- Replace the caps. Rinse the spacer and inhaler canister routinely to prevent a buildup of medication.

If using a mask spacer for an infant or young child, have the parent place the inhaler in the soft ring opposite the mask and then place the mask securely over the child's nose and mouth to form a good seal. Keep the mask firmly in place while the child takes six breaths. Wait 1 minute between each puff ordered.

Using a nebulizer

Nebulizers work by turning the medication into an aerosol mist that is easily breathed in. In many cases, nebulizers are not needed if an inhaler is used properly. To use a nebulizer, teach the parent or older child how to use the machine properly.

- Hook up the hose to the air compressor.
- Fill the medication cup with the proper dose of medication.
- Attach both the hose and the mouthpiece to the medication cup.
- Place the mouthpiece in the child's mouth.
- Have the child breathe in through his mouth until all the medication is gone. This can take approximately 10 to 15 minutes.

A mask may be used for smaller children. Nose clips may also be used if it is hard for the child to remember to only breathe through his mouth. Also teach the parents and child to rinse out the medication cup and mouthpiece and let them air dry after each use.

I.M. and S.C. routes

I.M. and subcutaneous (S.C.) routes are commonly used when medications are better absorbed outside of the gastric system. Children commonly fear needles and need reassurance when receiving parenteral medications. Help the child cope by explaining how he can help, applying ice on the injection site, or teaching distraction techniques.

Allowing the parents to hold and comfort the child may make the job easier for you and less traumatic for the child. If time

Needle and syringe selection

This chart will help you select the most appropriate needle and syringe size to use when administering medications by the I.M. or S.C. route to children. Children usually require the smallest gauge possible.

Route	Needle size	Syringe size
S.C.	• 25G to 29G • ⅜″ to ⅝″	1 ml to 3 ml
I.M.	• 23G to 25G • ⅝″ to 1″	1 ml to 5 ml

permits, consider using a topical skin anesthetic (such as EMLA cream) to numb the skin. (See *Needle and syringe selection*.)

S.C. P's and Q's

To administer an S.C. injection:
• Wash your hands.
• Select the site for administration; the typical areas used are the abdomen, the lateral and posterior aspects of the upper arm or thigh, the scapular area of the back, and the upper ventrodorsal gluteal areas. (For frequent S.C. administration, plan rotation sites before the injections are given.)
• Clean the area with alcohol.
• Grasp subcutaneous tissue between the thumb and forefinger.
• Insert the needle at a 45-degree angle. (If using a prepackaged syringe with a short needle, a 90-degree angle may be used.)
• Aspirate for blood; if none is seen, slowly inject the medication, limiting the volume to 0.5 ml.
• Withdraw the needle and massage the area to increase absorption.

I.M.-formation

To administer an I.M. injection:
• Wash your hands.
• Select the muscle for injection. (Don't inject into the gluteus muscle until the child learns to walk, at which point the muscle will be fully developed.) (See *I.M. injection sites in children*, page 52.)
• Spread the skin taut between your thumb and forefinger. (In smaller children, grasp the muscle to increase muscle mass and prevent striking the bone.)
• Insert the needle at a 90-degree angle, using a quick, darting action to reduce puncture pain.
• Inject the medication slowly.
• Withdraw the needle quickly and massage the area.

I.M. injection sites in children

When selecting the best site for a child's I.M. injection, consider the child's age, weight, and muscle development; the amount of subcutaneous fat over the injection site; the type of drug you're administering; and the drug's absorption rate.

Vastus lateralis and rectus femoris

For a child younger than age 3, you'll typically use the vastus lateralis or rectus femoris muscle for an I.M. injection. Constituting the largest muscle mass in this age-group, the vastus lateralis and rectus femoris have fewer major blood vessels and nerves.

Ventrogluteal and dorsogluteal

For a child who can walk and is older than age 3, use the ventrogluteal and dorsogluteal muscles. Like the vastus lateralis, the ventrogluteal site is relatively free of major blood vessels and nerves. Before you select either site, make sure that the child has been walking for at least 1 year to ensure sufficient muscle development.

Deltoid

For a child older than 18 months who needs rapid medication results, consider using the deltoid muscle. Because blood flows faster in the deltoid muscle than in other muscles, drug absorption should be faster.

Be careful if you use this site because the deltoid doesn't develop fully until adolescence. In a younger child, it's small and close to the radial nerve, which could be injured during needle insertion.

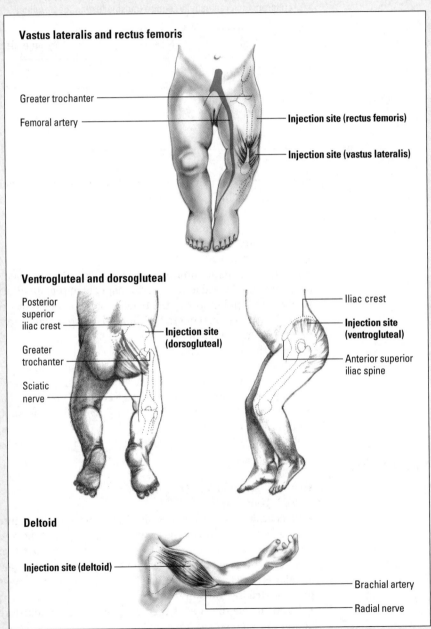

Vastus lateralis and rectus femoris

Greater trochanter
Femoral artery
Injection site (rectus femoris)
Injection site (vastus lateralis)

Ventrogluteal and dorsogluteal

Posterior superior iliac crest
Greater trochanter
Sciatic nerve
Injection site (dorsogluteal)
Iliac crest
Injection site (ventrogluteal)
Anterior superior iliac spine

Deltoid

Injection site (deltoid)
Brachial artery
Radial nerve

Performing intraosseous administration

In an emergency, intraosseous drug administration may be used for a critically ill child younger than age 6. Insert a bone marrow needle (or spinal needle with stylette, trephine, or standard 16G to 18G hypodermic needle) into the anteromedial surface of the proximal tibia ⅜" to 1¼" (1 to 3 cm) below the tibial tuberosity. To avoid the epiphyseal plate, direct the needle at a perpendicular or slightly inferior angle.

After penetrating the bony cortex and inserting the needle into the marrow cavity, you'll feel no resistance, you'll be able to aspirate bone marrow, the needle will remain upright without support, and the infusion will flow freely without subcutaneous infiltration. If bone or marrow obstructs the needle, replace the needle by passing a second one through the cannula.

When the needle is properly inserted, stabilize and secure it with gauze dressing and tape. Discontinue when a secure I.V. line is established.

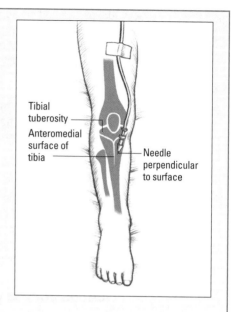

Tibial tuberosity

Anteromedial surface of tibia

Needle perpendicular to surface

Intraosseous route

At times, venous access in a child may be a challenge. For the critically ill child in cardiac arrest or shock, the administration of fluids and medications may be lifesaving. For the child in whom venous access can't be quickly established, intraosseous infusion may be necessary. (This occurs most commonly in children younger than age 5.) Fluids and medications that are infused into the medullary space of the long bones quickly enter the venous circulation. (See *Performing intraosseous administration.*)

The most common site for intraosseous infusion is the medial surface of the proximal tibia. Other sites include the distal tibia and the distal femur.

When the needle has been placed into the bone, fluid resuscitation should be instituted by injecting fluid under pressure via a syringe. Standard I.V. pumps and tubing may be used to deliver the fluids. Gravity may help infuse the fluid if the patient is hemodynamically stable. It's important to remember that extravasation is common around the site, especially with prolonged placement and pressure infusion.

I.V. therapy

I.V. therapy commonly is used to give both fluids and medications to an ill child. Extreme caution and care must be taken in giving the prescribed amounts of fluids and medications. The rate of flow should be checked frequently, and a pump system is recommended. Because extravasation of fluid or phlebitis may develop quickly, the site must be checked frequently.

Access granted

The venous system may be accessed either peripherally or centrally. After the access device is in place, the site must be kept secure and protected to provide the necessary fluids and medications.

On a short leash

The nurse must consider the sensitivity of the child's skin and limit the use of tape. The nurse should also consider the child's developmental needs, such as the desire to explore, and take steps to ensure his safety while giving him as much freedom as possible after the I.V. is in place.

Venous access devices

Commonly used peripheral I.V. sites include the hands and arms; however, in some children, these might not be the most readily accessible peripheral sites.

By foot or by scalp . . . we shall prevail

The feet (greater saphenous vein) or even a scalp vein in the neonate may be used. Always use the smallest needle size possible. For children, this is typically a 24G or 25G needle.

Have no fear—no tourniquet here

Smaller children may be fearful of a tourniquet. In this instance, venous distention may be obtained simply by grasping and applying pressure to the area proximal to the vein.

Long-term I.V. therapy

Long-term I.V. therapy is best accomplished with a vascular access device. Such devices include infusion ports, catheters, and cannulas. The type that's most appropriate in a particular situation depends on the type and length of treatment as well as the diagnosis. Children with cancer who require chemotherapy, blood transfusions, fluids, and nutrition are usually given an implantable device such as a port. This type of device allows for frequent access to the venous system with venipuncture and multiple I.V. lines.

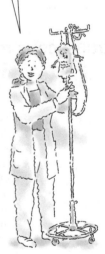

A mobile child is a happy child. Most kids can become experts at getting around with an I.V. pole. It just takes a little teaching and some supervision.

Check, check, and check again

Such devices as central venous catheters also provide access for drawing blood. These catheters may remain in place for months. The nurse must check the site frequently for signs and symptoms of infection, patency, proper functioning, and placement.

Infusion pumps

Infusion pumps are commonly used in pediatric patients. The pump doesn't depend on gravity for flow; instead, it maintains a preselected volume delivery by adding pressure to the system when necessary. If the pressure required to deliver the fluid exceeds a maximum pressure limit, an alarm sounds.

Infiltrate and irritate

Unfortunately, the use of pumps carries the danger of infiltration or vein irritation caused by the medication or solution administered under pressure. When the pump has delivered the exact volume prescribed, an alarm sounds. Many facility policies dictate the time lapse allowed for checking the pump, the I.V. site, and the volume of solution infused.

Calculating pediatric fluid needs

Children's fluid needs are proportionally greater than those of adults, so children are more vulnerable to changes in fluid and electrolyte balance. Because their extracellular fluid has a higher percentage of water, children's fluid exchange rates are two to three times greater than those of adults, leaving them more susceptible to dehydration.

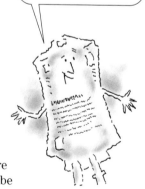

Go ahead—calculate me. It's just a matter of choosing among weight, metabolism, and BSA.

Calculation trio

Determining and meeting the fluid needs of children are important nursing responsibilities. You can calculate the number of milliliters of fluid a child needs based on:
• weight in kilograms
• metabolism (calories required)
• BSA in square meters.
   Although results may vary slightly, all three methods are appropriate. Keep in mind that fluid replacement can also be affected by clinical conditions that cause fluid retention or loss. Children with these conditions should receive fluids based on their individual needs.

Fluid needs based on weight

You may use three different formulas to calculate a child's fluid needs based on his weight.

Fluid formula for tiny tots . . .

A child who weighs less than 10 kg requires 100 ml of fluid per kilogram of body weight per day. To determine this child's fluid needs, first convert his weight from pounds to kilograms. Then multiply the results by 100 ml/kg/day.

Here's the formula:

weight in kg × 100 ml/kg/day = fluid needs in ml/day

. . . middleweights . . .

A child weighing 10 to 20 kg requires 1,000 ml of fluid per day for the first 10 kg plus 50 ml for every kilogram over 10. To determine this child's fluid needs, follow these steps:
• Convert his weight from pounds to kilograms.
• Subtract 10 kg from the child's total weight and then multiply the result by 50 ml/kg/day to find the child's additional fluid needs. Here's the formula:

(total kg − 10 kg) × 50 ml/kg/day = additional fluid need in ml/day

• Add the additional daily fluid need to the 1,000 ml/day required for the first 10 kg. The total is the child's daily fluid requirement:

1,000 ml/day + additional fluid need = fluid needs in ml/day

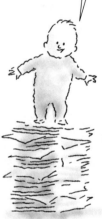

You won't need a mountain of papers to figure out my fluid needs.

. . . and bigger kids too

A child weighing more than 20 kg requires 1,500 ml of fluid for the first 20 kg plus 20 ml for each additional kilogram. To determine this child's fluid needs, follow these steps:
• Convert the child's weight from pounds to kilograms.
• Subtract 20 kg from the child's total weight and then multiply the result by 20 ml/kg to find the child's additional fluid needs. Here's the formula:

(total kg − 20 kg) × 20 ml/kg/day = additional fluid need in ml/day

• Because the child needs 1,500 ml of fluid per day for the first 20 kg, add the additional fluid need to 1,500 ml. The total is the child's daily fluid requirement:

1,500 ml/day + additional fluid need = fluid needs in ml/day

Real-world problem

This problem will give you some real-world experience with calculating fluid needs based on weight.

Maintenance mystery

How much fluid should you give a 44-lb patient over 24 hours to meet his maintenance needs?
• First, convert 44 lb to kilograms by setting up a proportion with fractions. (Remember that 1 kg equals 2.2 lb.)

$$\frac{44 \text{ lb}}{X} = \frac{2.2 \text{ lb}}{1 \text{ kg}}$$

• Cross-multiply the fractions and then solve for X by dividing both sides of the equation by 2.2 lb and canceling units that appear in both the numerator and denominator.

$$X \times 2.2 \text{ lb} = 44 \text{ lb} \times 1 \text{ kg}$$

$$\frac{X \times \cancel{2.2 \text{ lb}}}{\cancel{2.2 \text{ lb}}} = \frac{44 \cancel{\text{ lb}} \times 1 \text{ kg}}{2.2 \cancel{\text{ lb}}}$$

$$X = \frac{44 \text{ kg}}{2.2}$$

$$X = 20 \text{ kg}$$

• The child weighs 20 kg. Now, subtract 10 kg from the child's weight and multiply the result by 50 ml/kg/day to find the child's additional fluid need:

$$X = (20 \text{ kg} - 10 \text{ kg}) \times 50 \text{ ml/kg/day}$$

$$X = 10 \cancel{\text{ kg}} \times 50 \text{ ml/}\cancel{\text{kg}}\text{/day}$$

$$X = 500 \text{ ml/day additional fluid need}$$

• Next, add the additional fluid need to the 1,000 ml/day required for the first 10 kg (because the child weighs between 10 and 20 kg).

$$X = 1,000 \text{ ml/day} + 500 \text{ ml/day}$$

$$X = 1,500 \text{ ml/day}$$

The child should receive 1,500 ml of fluid in 24 hours to meet his fluid maintenance needs.

Fluid needs based on calories

You can calculate fluid needs based on calories because water is needed for metabolism. A child should receive 120 ml of fluid for every 100 kilocalories (kcal; also called *calories*) of metabolism.

> What a nice change. I'm counting calories, and it has nothing at all to do with my thighs!

Calorie-conscious calculation

To calculate fluid requirements based on calorie requirements, follow these steps:
• Find the child's calorie requirements. You can take this from a table of recommended dietary allowances for children, or you can have a dietitian calculate it.
• Divide the calorie requirements by 100 kcal because fluid requirements are determined for every 100 calories.
• Multiply the results by 120 ml (the amount of fluid required for every 100 kcal). Here's the formula:

$$\text{fluid requirements in ml/day} = \frac{\text{calorie requirements}}{100 \text{ kcal}} \times 120 \text{ ml}$$

Real-world problem

This problem will help sharpen your skills for calculating fluid needs based on calories. Use the preceding information to solve it.

Daily dilemma

Your pediatric patient uses 900 calories/day. What are his daily fluid requirements?
• Set up the formula inserting the appropriate numbers and substituting X for the unknown amount of fluid:

$$X = \frac{900 \text{ kcal}}{100 \text{ kcal}} \times 120 \text{ ml}$$

$$X = 9 \times 120 \text{ ml}$$

$$X = 1,080 \text{ ml}$$

The patient needs 1,080 ml of fluid per day.

Fluid needs based on BSA

Another method for determining pediatric maintenance fluid requirements is based on the child's BSA.

To calculate the daily fluid needs of a child who isn't dehydrated, multiply the BSA by 1,500, as shown in this formula:

$$\text{fluid maintenance needs in ml/day} = \text{BSA in m}^2 \times 1,500 \text{ ml/day/m}^2$$

Real-world problem

This problem gives you a taste of the process used to calculate fluid needs based on BSA. Use the preceding formula to solve it.

Your patient is 36″ tall and weighs 40 lb. If his BSA is 0.72 m², how much fluid does he need each day?

• Set up the equation, inserting the appropriate numbers and substituting X for the unknown amount of fluid. Then solve for X:

$$X = 0.72 \ \cancel{m^2} \times 1,500 \ \text{ml/day/}\cancel{m^2}$$

$$X = 1,080 \ \text{ml/day}$$

The child needs 1,080 ml of fluid per day.

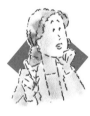

Quick quiz

1. A 2-year-old can be expected to sleep:
    A.   12 to 14 hours a day with most of it during the night and one long nap during the day.
    B.   14 to 15 hours a day, usually 4 to 6 hours at a time and two to three naps during the day.
    C.   10 to 12 hours a day with no naps.
    D.   8 to 10 hours a day with one nap during the day.

Answer: A. A toddler can be expected to sleep 8 to 10 hours a night with a long nap during the day to equal 12 to 14 hours. Infants sleep more total hours throughout the day but in shorter time frames. By the time a child reaches kindergarten, he sleeps a long time at night and typically does not need a nap. Teens require 8 to 10 hours of sleep daily but may need a nap during periods of growth.

2. According to Erikson's theory of psychosocial development, a 7-year-old who enjoys working with others and helping his parents on weekend projects is in what stage?
    A.   Autonomy versus shame and doubt
    B.   Initiative versus guilt
    C.   Industry versus inferiority
    D.   Identity versus role confusion

Answer: C. Industry versus inferiority occurs from approximately ages 6 to 12. During this time, the child enjoys being helpful and relationships become more important. Autonomy versus shame and doubt occur through toddlerhood. Initiative versus guilt happens in 3- to 6-year-olds, and identity versus role confusion occurs during adolescence.

3.   The nurse is caring for a 6-year-old who is terminally ill. She recognizes at this age, the child:

    A.   has no concept of death whatsoever.

    B.   knows the words "dead" and "death" but the concept of forever has no value.

    C.   understands the universality and irreversibility of death.

    D.   has an adult perception of death but is focused on the here and now.

Answer: B. A 6-year-old is in early childhood and cannot grasp the concept of forever but does know words relating to death. As he matures, the more concrete the concept of death becomes. It isn't until adolescence that the child has an adult perception of death yet he remains focused on the present.

Scoring

⭐⭐⭐   If you answered all three items correctly, bravo! You've mastered the complex tasks in this chapter.

⭐⭐   If you answered two items correctly, good for you! You're on your way to a higher stage of functioning in pediatric nursing.

⭐   If you answered fewer than two items correctly, there's no need for a bruised ego! A second look at the chapter will be less painful.

③

Infancy

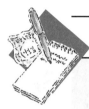

Just the facts

In this chapter, you'll learn:

♦ progression of system, physical, and psychological development in infancy

♦ nutrition and sleep guidelines for infancy

♦ injury prevention strategies

♦ common infant health issues.

A closer look at the infant

Infancy, the period from birth to age 1 year, is a time of many changes. During the first year of life, the infant progresses from a neonate, totally dependent on the world around him, to a baby who can interact with and process change within his surroundings. Tremendous physiologic, cognitive, and emotional development also occurs.

> Before you know it, you'll be able to interact with others and notice the changes around you.

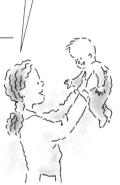

System development

From birth to age 1 year, remarkable changes occur in the infant's neurologic, cardiovascular, respiratory, and immune systems.

Neurologic system

The central nervous system (CNS) is the fastest growing system during the infancy stage, as brain cells continue to develop in both size and number. The effects of a poor environment, including nutritional deprivation, can't be reversed when experienced during this early stage.

Hold your head up!

Myelinization refers to the development of a myelin sheath around nerve fibers. Myelin enables quick, efficient transmission of nerve impulses. Myelinization of the neurons occurs in a cephalocaudal (head-to-toe) direction, although it takes up to 2 years for the entire process to be completed. An infant progresses from being unable to hold up his head to being able to hold himself in an upright position, sit, and keep his head erect.

> I think my neurons are starting to myelinate. Today, I hold my head up. Tomorrow, the world!

Extreme CNS makeover

As myelinization reaches the extremities, the infant can put weight on his legs and use them to stand up. As the brain and CNS develop, more sophisticated cognitive and behavioral skills follow.

Converge, stare, and search

Vision development is also tremendous. At birth, the newborn prefers facial features, but by 8 weeks, the baby is alert to moving objects and is attracted to bright colors and lighted objects, such as toys with flashing lights and an otoscope light. Convergence and following with the eyes are jerky and inexact. By ages 4 to 6 months, the baby has bifocal vision and can stare and search. By age 1 year, distance vision and depth perception have markedly improved.

Cardiovascular and respiratory systems

The cardiovascular and respiratory systems undergo dramatic changes at birth. Because of placental oxygenation, the fetus shunts a majority of blood away from the lungs while in utero.

> As soon as I get out of here, my heart and lungs will start to function just like my mom's!

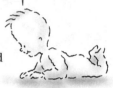

Cardiopulmonary drama

At birth, a cascade of physiologic changes occur, and deoxygenated blood begins to circulate to the lungs, where it receives oxygen and is then pumped out to the rest of the body through the left ventricle of the heart. Within moments, the cardiovascular and respiratory systems are functioning at essentially the same way as those of an adult.

Immune system

The immune system develops over the first year of life. The neonate depends on maternal antibodies received in utero or via breast milk for immunologic protection. By ages 6 to 8 weeks, an antigen-antibody response is maturing and can be triggered, for example, by immunizations, and by age 9 months, the infant is developing his own immunity.

Physical development

The physical growth and development that take place during infancy are astounding. Although patterns of growth and development will occur in a predictable order, it's important to remember that the rate at which they occur may vary among children of the same age. Also remember that the most reliable way to interpret growth measurements is to follow their trend over time using growth charts. Pediatric growth charts have been used in the United States since 1977. Growth charts consist of a series of percentile curves that depict the distribution of selected body measurements in infants and children. Many infants have their length, weight, and head circumferences measured and plotted on standardized growth charts. Centers for Disease Control and Prevention (CDC) recommends that nurses and other pediatric health care providers use the World Health Organization's (WHO) growth standards to monitor growth for infants and children ages 0 to 2 years in the United States and use the CDC growth charts for children age 2 years and older in the United States.

Height, weight, and head circumference

Intrauterine growth is assessed by measuring height, weight, and head circumference. These parameters are also the basis of growth evaluation for the rest of the infant and toddler period.

Height

Until the child is age 24 months, height, or length, is measured in the supine position, from the top of the head to the bottom of the heel. When measuring the infant, it's important to keep his body as straight as possible to achieve an accurate measurement. An infant's length is best measured using a stadiometer.

Trunk first, legs to follow

At the end of the first year, the infant's birth length has increased by 50%, with growth of approximately 1″ (2.5 cm) per month for the first 6 months, followed by about ½″ (1.3 cm) per month for the second 6 months. Most of this growth occurs in the trunk rather than in the legs.

Weight

Weight ideally is measured on an infant scale with a bucket-type area in which the infant can lie down or sit. Weight is the primary indicator of nutritional status; changes in weight can also be used to assess hydration status. The average infant will double his birth weight by age 5 months, and triple it by age 1 year.

Head circumference

Head circumference, or occipital frontal circumference, is measured by placing a measuring tape around the largest diameter of

Advice from the experts

Measuring height and head circumference

These illustrations show the correct (supine) positioning for measuring length and the proper location for measuring head circumference.

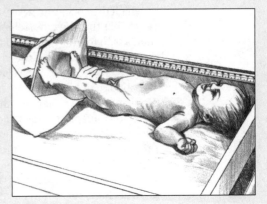

Measuring height

Because of an infant's tendency to be flexed and curled up, these tips will help make assessing an infant's height (length) both easy and accurate:
• Using one hand, hold the infant's head in the midline position.
• Hold the knees together with your other hand and gently press them down toward the table until they're fully extended.
• Using an infant stadiometer, measure the length from the top of the infant's head to his heels.

Measuring head circumference

To obtain an accurate head circumference measurement:
• Use a paper measuring tape to avoid stretching (as can happen with a cloth tape).
• Use landmarks—typically, place the tape just above the infant's eyebrows, and around the occipital prominence at the back of the head to measure the largest diameter of the head.
• Take into consideration the shape of the infant's head and make adjustments as needed to measure the largest diameter.

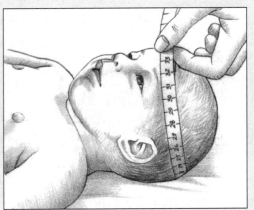

the head, from the frontal bone of the forehead to the occipital prominence at the back of the head.

Don't get a big head

A head circumference that's smaller, or lags behind the height and weight of an infant, may indicate inadequate brain growth. A head circumference that increases rapidly may indicate an increase in ventricular fluid and intracranial pressure (hydrocephalus). (See *Measuring height and head circumference*.)

Locating the fontanels

The locations of the anterior and posterior fontanels are depicted in this illustration of the top of a neonatal skull.

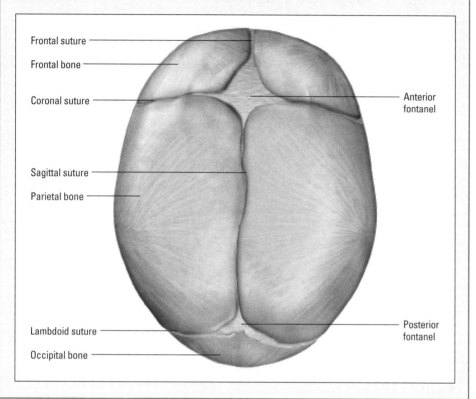

Frontal suture

Frontal bone

Coronal suture

Anterior fontanel

Sagittal suture

Parietal bone

Lambdoid suture

Posterior fontanel

Occipital bone

Fontanel changes

Fontanels are the two openings between the bones in the neonate's skull. (See *Locating the fontanels*.)

The *anterior fontanel* is formed at the intersection of the sagittal, frontal, and coronal suture lines. The average size of the anterior fontanel is 2 cm by 2 cm at birth. It remains open for up to 18 months and gradually closes as the head grows.

The *posterior fontanel* is formed at the intersection of the sagittal and lambdoid suture lines. The average size of the posterior fontanel is 1 cm by 1 cm at birth. It's usually closed by age 2 months.

Growing pains

Sequence of tooth eruption

A child's primary teeth typically erupt in a predictable order, as described here:

Age	Tooth eruption
6 to 10 months	Central lower incisors
8 to 10 months	Central upper incisors
9 to 13 months	Lateral upper incisors
10 to 16 months	Lateral lower incisors

Palpation and pulsation

In infancy, the fontanels are assessed by palpation. The fontanel should feel soft and flat. You may be able to see pulsations at the anterior fontanel; this is a normal finding. A bulging or tense fontanel may indicate increased intracranial pressure. A sunken fontanel indicates dehydration. The nurse may auscultate the fontanel to assess for bruits.

Teeth

Most neonates don't have teeth. Occasionally, a "natal tooth" will be present at birth and should be evaluated by a pediatric dentist because they may become loose and pose a risk of aspiration. Neonatal teeth are teeth that erupt within the first 28 days of life.

A little drool, a big eruption

The average age at first tooth eruption is 8 months. Most infants start drooling and mouthing hard objects months beforehand. (See *Sequence of tooth eruption.*)

Gross motor development

Gross motor skills refer to the child's development of skills that require the use of large muscle groups. (See *Developmental milestones.*) They include:
• posture
• head control

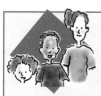

Growing pains

Developmental milestones

This chart shows the major gross and fine motor skills the infant should master as he progresses through the first year of life.

Age	Gross motor skills	Fine motor skills
1 month	• Can hold head parallel momentarily but still has marked head lag • Back is rounded in sitting position, with no head control	• Strong grasp reflex • Hands remain mostly closed in a fist
2 months	• In prone position, can lift head 45 degrees off table • In sitting position, back is still rounded but with more head control	• Diminishing grasp reflex • Hands open more often
3 months	• Displays only slight head lag when pulled to a seated position • In prone position, can use forearms to lift head and shoulders 45 to 90 degrees off table • Can bear slight amount of weight on legs in standing position	• Grasp reflex now absent • Hands remain open • Can hold a rattle and clutch own hand
4 months	• No head lag • Holds head erect in sitting position, back less rounded • In prone position, can lift head and chest 90 degrees off table • Can roll from back to side	• Regards own hand • Can grasp objects with both hands • May try to reach for an object without success • Can move objects toward mouth
5 months	• No head lag • Holds head erect and steady when sitting • Back is straight • Can put feet to mouth when supine • Can roll from stomach to back	• Can voluntarily grasp objects • Can move objects directly to mouth
6 months	• Can lift chest and upper abdomen off table, bearing weight on hands • Can roll from back to stomach • Can bear almost all of weight on feet when held in standing position • Sits with support	• Can hold bottle • Can voluntarily grasp and release objects
7 months	• Can sit, leaning forward on hands for support • When in standing position, can bear full weight on legs and bounce	• Transfers objects from hand to hand • Rakes at objects • Can bang objects on table
8 months	• Can sit alone without assistance • Can move from sitting to kneeling position	• Has beginning pincer grasp • Reaches for objects out of reach
9 months	• Creeps on hands and knees with belly off floor • Pulls to standing position • Can stand, holding on to furniture	• Refining pincer grasp • Use of dominant hand may become evident

(continued)

Developmental milestones *(continued)*

Age	Gross motor skills	Fine motor skills
10 months	• Can move from prone to sitting position • Stands with support; may lift a foot as if to take a step	• Refining pincer grasp
11 months	• Can cruise (take side steps while holding on to furniture) or walk with both hands held	• Can move objects into containers • Deliberately drops object to have it picked up • Neat pincer grasp
12 months	• Cruises well, may walk with one hand held • May try to stand alone	• May attempt to build a two-block tower • Can crudely turn pages of a book • Uses cup alone

- sitting
- creeping/crawling
- standing
- walking.

The infant will attain gross motor control in a cephalocaudal manner, progressing from the head to the toes. He can lift the head, then sit, stand, and, eventually, walk.

Fine motor development

Fine motor skills refer to the infant's ability to use his hands and fingers to grasp an object. As the infant grows, he begins to refine his fine motor skills to grab small objects and feed himself.

Normal infant reflexes

Much of a neonate's behavior is controlled by reflexes. At ages 4 to 8 weeks old, many of these reflexes reach their peak—especially the sucking reflex, which affords nutrition (and, therefore, survival) and psychological pleasure.

At age 3 months, the most primitive reflexes begin to disappear, except for the protective and postural reflexes (blink, parachute, cough, swallow, and gag), which remain for life. (See *Infant reflexes*.)

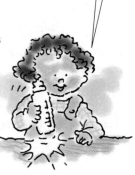

I'm 7 months old. Banging things on tables is my job.

Infant reflexes

This chart lists normal infant reflexes, how they're elicited, and the age at which they disappear.

Reflex	How to elicit	Age at disappearance
Trunk incurvature	When a finger is run laterally down the neonate's spine, the trunk flexes and the pelvis swings toward the stimulated side.	2 months
Tonic neck (fencing position)	When the neonate's head is turned while he's lying supine, the extremities on the same side extend outward while those on the opposite side flex.	2 to 3 months
Grasping	When a finger is placed in each of the neonate's hands, the neonate's fingers grasp tightly enough to be pulled to a sitting position.	3 to 4 months
Rooting	When the cheek is stroked, the neonate turns his head in the direction of the stroke.	3 to 4 months
Moro (startle reflex)	When lifted above the crib and suddenly lowered (or in response to a loud noise), the arms and legs symmetrically extend and then abduct while the fingers spread to form a "C."	4 to 6 months
Sucking	Sucking motion begins when a nipple or gloved finger is placed in the neonate's mouth.	6 months
Babinski's	When the sole on the side of the small toe is stroked, the neonate's toes fan upward.	2 years
Stepping	When held upright with the feet touching a flat surface, the neonate exhibits dancing or stepping movements.	Variable

Psychological development

Psychological development involves language development and socialization as well as play and cognitive development.

Language development and socialization

Language development and socialization begin as soon as the neonate is born. Initially, the neonate communicates primarily through crying and socializes through some of the reflexive behaviors such as the grasp reflex. However, he'll make tremendous strides in these areas during his first year of life.

Cry me a river

The infant cries to express needs. During the first 3 months, crying usually signals a physiologic need such as hunger. As the

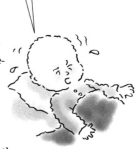

I cry, therefore I am . . . expressing my needs; trying to get attention; or feeling frustrated, afraid, or just plain cranky.

infant grows, he may cry for attention, from fear, or from frustration during the trials of mastering new skills. Parents usually become adept at translating their child's cry.

Infants who cry frequently and are difficult to console may be at increased risk for abuse. To help parents prepare for and effectively deal with crying infants, the pediatric nurse should:
• reinforce that there are times when infants cry for no reason at all
• assess how parents cope with fussy periods and offer support as needed
• teach parents comforting techniques, such as holding, swaddling, and massaging.

Smile and say "eh"

An infant's vocalization develops from cries. By age 2 months, the infant can produce single-vowel sounds, such as "ah" and "eh," and he begins to develop a social smile. The social smile is the infant's first social response; it initiates social relationships, signals the beginning of thought processes, and further strengthens the bond between parent and child. By ages 3 to 4 months, the infant can coo and gurgle and laugh in response to his environment.

Stranger danger

By age 6 months, the infant begins to experiment with sounds and attempts to imitate others. He can discern one face from another and exhibits stranger anxiety—he's wary of strangers and clings to or clutches his parents. Separation anxiety may also develop at this period and peaks around 9 months.

I'd like to buy a vowel

By ages 7 to 9 months, the infant can verbalize all vowels and most consonants but speaks no intelligible words. He'll focus intently on the mouth of someone speaking to him. He can also understand simple commands such as the word "no." He may imitate the expressions of others and may be able to play pat-a-cake. He can recognize and respond to his own name.

Infant of few words

By ages 10 to 12 months, the infant can say about 5 words but can understand up to 100 words. He can wave good-bye and enjoys rhythm games. If the child experiences delays in vocalization, he should be evaluated for hearing loss. (See *Language and social development*.)

Growing pains

Language and social development

This chart highlights the language and social development of an infant from birth to age 1 year.

Age	Behaviors
0 to 2 months	• Listens to voices; quiets to soft music, singing, or talking • Distinguishes mother's voice after 1 week, father or other primary caregiver by 2 weeks • Prefers human voices to other sounds • Produces vowel sounds "ah," "eh," and "oh" • Begins to smile socially
3 to 4 months	• Coos and gurgles • Babbles in response to someone talking to him • Babbles for own pleasure with giggles, shrieks, and laughs • Says "da," "ba," "ma," "pa," and "ga" • Vocalizes more to a real person than to a picture • Responds to caregiver with social smile by 3 months
5 to 6 months	• Notices how his speech influences actions of others • Makes "raspberries" and smacks lips • Begins learning to take turns in conversation • Talks to toys and self in mirror • Recognizes names and familiar sounds
7 to 9 months	• Tries to imitate more sounds; makes several sounds in one breath • Begins learning the meaning of "no" by tone of voice and actions • Experiences early literacy; enjoys listening to simple books being read • Enjoys pat-a-cake • Recognizes and responds to his name and names of familiar objects
10 to 12 months	• May have a few word approximations, such as "bye-bye" and "hi" • Follows one-step instructions such as "go to daddy" • Recognizes words as symbols for objects • Says "ma-ma-ma" and "da-da-da"

> Da, ba, ma, pa, ga. That's all I've got. I'm 4 months old.

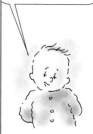

Play

Play is an integral part of the socialization process. From birth to age 3 months, infants enjoy having their body parts touched and moved and looking at objects with contrasting colors. They develop the ability to grasp objects and move them, so rattles are great toys at this time.

Growing pains

Cognitive development and play

This chart shows the infant's development of two cognitive skills, object permanence and causality. It includes play, an integral part of infant development.

Age	Object permanence	Causality	Play
0 to 4 months	• Objects out of sight are out of mind • Continues to look at hand after object is dropped out of it	• Creates bodily sensations by actions (for example, thumbsucking)	• Grasps and moves objects such as a rattle • Looks at contrasting colors
4 to 8 months	• Can locate a partially hidden object • Visually tracks objects when dropped	• Uses causal behaviors to recreate accidentally discovered interesting effects (for example, kicking the bed after the chance discovery that this will set in motion a mobile above the bed)	• Reaches and grasps an object and then will mouth, shake, bang, and drop the object (usually in this order)
9 to 12 months	• Object permanence develops • Can find an object when hidden but can't retrieve an object that's moved in plain view from one hiding place to another • Knows parent still exists when out of view but can't imagine where they might be (separation anxiety may arise)	• Understanding of cause and effect leads to intentional behavior aimed at getting specific results	• Manipulates objects to inspect with eyes and hands • Has ability to process information simultaneously instead of sequentially • Ability to play peek-a-boo demonstrates object permanence

Mimicking Mommy

From ages 4 to 9 months, infants explore the world by using their senses: looking and touching. They tend to put everything within reach in their mouths. They enjoy being read to and will display more reciprocal play, such as talking back to and mimicking adult vocalizations.

Social butterfly

By ages 9 to 12 months, increased mobility allows infants to seek out new stimuli, including people, for interaction. They enjoy social games, such as peek-a-boo, tickling, and swinging.

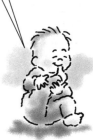

This isn't bad. Maybe a little salt will help when I'm older.

Cognitive development

Cognitive development refers to the intellectual abilities of a child—his thinking, reasoning, and ability to problem-solve and understand. Cognitively, the infant develops the ability to perform very sophisticated mental operations. Even the neonate can process and react to stimuli in the environment around him.

Over time, he develops social skills and a sense of *object permanence* (the realization that objects continue to exist even when they can't be seen) and *causality* (understanding that a particular action, or cause, leads to an effect). (See *Cognitive development and play.*)

Trust begins to develop during this stage. Temperament emerges as the infant displays the inborn characteristics that influence activity level, response to new people and situations, and adaptability to change.

I can't see my mom, but I know she still exists. Where did she go? Hey, I'm only 9 months old—that stuff comes later.

On stage with Piaget

According to Jean Piaget's stages of early cognitive development, infants are in the sensorimotor stage, which lasts from birth to age 2 years. In this stage, infants are discovering relationships between their bodies and the environment. They rely on their senses to learn about the world around them, and they learn that the external world isn't an extension of themselves.

Maintaining health

Keeping an infant healthy involves:
- providing proper nutrition
- ensuring adequate sleep and rest
- providing a safe environment.

Nutrition guidelines

Breast milk or iron-fortified infant formula is recommended for the first 12 months of life. Human milk consumed through breast-feeding is considered optimal for neonates. Even so, not all mothers can or choose to breast-feed. Medical conditions, cultural background, anxiety, use of certain medications, drug abuse, and other factors can prevent a woman from breast-feeding. In these cases, bottle-feeding with iron-fortified infant formula is an acceptable alternative.

Breast-feeding

Breast-feeding is widely supported in the medical community. The American Academy of Pediatrics (AAP) and the American Dietetic Association recommend breast-feeding exclusively for the first 6 months and then in combination with infant foods until at least age 1 year. (See *Advantages of breast-feeding*.)

I demand my 10 to 15!

How long a breast-fed infant nurses at each feeding is very individual. In general, a neonate should nurse on demand, approximately 8 to 10 times per day for at least 10 to 15 minutes at each breast. The duration of feeding may increase and the frequency may decrease as the infant gets older and after solid foods are introduced.

Parents should be assured that they can feel confident their infant is receiving enough breast milk if he's growing appropriately. Keep in mind that intake is adequate if:
• weight loss after birth is normal (less than 10% of birth weight)
• the infant regains the weight lost after birth by age 2 weeks
• the infant has six to eight wet diapers or more per day
• there's a minimum weight gain of 15 g (0.5 oz) per day in the first 2 months of life.

Advantages of breast-feeding

It's a well-known fact that breast-feeding is best for an infant. Here are some of the reasons.

Passive immunity
Human milk provides passive immunity from mother to infant. *Colostrum* is the first fluid secreted from the breast (within the first few days after delivery) and provides immune factor and protein to the neonate. Many components of breast milk protect against infection—it contains antibodies (especially immunoglobulin A) and white blood cells that protect the infant from some forms of infection. Breast-fed babies also experience fewer allergies and food intolerances as well as a lower risk for obesity in childhood.

Digestibility
Breast milk provides essential nutrients in an easily digestible form. It contains *lipase*, which breaks down dietary fat, making it easily available to the infant's system.

Brain development
The lipids in breast milk are high in linoleic acid and cholesterol, which are needed for brain development.

Low protein content
Cow's milk contains proportionally higher concentrations of electrolytes and protein than are needed by human infants. It must be cleared by the immature kidneys and thus isn't recommended until a baby is at least 12 months old.

Convenient and cost-free
The woman who breast-feeds saves the money and time that would be needed to buy and prepare formula.

It's all relative

Tips for preparing formula

Provide parents with these tips for properly preparing infant formula:
• Wash your hands before preparing formula.
• If your water source is safe, mix formula with room temperature tap water.
  If your water source is not safe or you are unsure, use fluoridated bottled water or boil water for no longer than 1 minute then let it cool for 30 minutes to room temperature.
• Wash utensils in warm, soapy water and rinse them well to ensure they're safe to use.
• Avoid using microwave ovens to warm formula; they fail to sanitize utensils and cause uneven heating, which increases the risk of burns.
• Discard a prepared bottle of formula after it's been offered to the infant or has sat at room temperature for longer than 1 hour.
• Cover and store opened cans of liquid formula in the refrigerator; discard after 48 hours.

Recommended vitamin supplements

Breast-fed infants should receive oral supplementation of vitamin D, 400 units per day. At 4 months of age, exclusively breast-fed infants should also be supplemented with 1 mg/kg per day of oral iron until iron-containing complementary foods are introduced.

Formula feeding

Formula feedings can provide adequate nutrition when the mother shouldn't or can't breast-feed her infant. Some mothers may feel guilty about being unable to breast-feed or about making the decision not to breast-feed. The pediatric nurse should support, and never judge, the mother who can't or who chooses not to breast-feed and should reassure her about the nutritional value of infant formulas.

Infant formulas are constituted to provide the proper variety and amount of carbohydrates, protein, fats, and micronutrients needed for healthy growth and development. The U.S. Food and Drug Administration regulates the composition, labeling, and inspection of infant formula to ensure infant safety. (See *Tips for preparing formula*.)

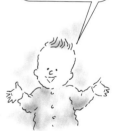

Oops! I think that was diaper number seven. I'm definitely getting enough breast milk.

No moo cows, please

Women are strongly urged to use commercially prepared formulas rather than regular cow's milk because cow's milk:
• doesn't meet all of an infant's nutritional needs
• can be difficult to digest
• can strain the infant's renal system.

Unlocking the secret formula

Most formulas are based on cow's milk proteins, although preparations based on soy proteins and casein hydroxylate are available for infants who can't tolerate cow's milk–based preparations. There are also special formulas for infants with such diseases as phenylketonuria and other metabolic disorders.

Formula comes in powder form, concentrated liquid, and ready-to-feed forms. Ready-to-feed formulas are convenient and prevent problems based on incorrect dilution and preparation but are more expensive.

Special care should be used so that formula isn't improperly mixed or stored, which can be hazardous to the infant.

Weaning

The American Academy of Pediatrics and the American Dental Association recommend that infants be weaned from the bottle to the cup by age 1 year. In preparation for weaning, and to promote the developmental step toward independent feeding, the cup should be introduced by age 9 months in all infants. This is usually done gradually, by omitting one bottle at a time and replacing it with a cup over a period of several days to weeks.

Slow and steady to bottle-ready

How long a mother continues to breast-feed is an individual choice; if a mother chooses or needs to switch from breast to bottle, it is accomplished similarly to the weaning from bottle to cup. One breast-feeding session per day is replaced with a bottle-feeding until, over a period of days to weeks, the transition occurs.

This gradual weaning approach helps prevent engorgement in the mother and decreases her risk of mastitis. An infant can also be weaned from breast-feeding to a cup, eliminating the need for bottles.

When an infant reaches 4 to 6 months of age, you can start feeding him solid foods. The trick is getting it in his mouth!

Introducing solid foods

The age at which solid foods are introduced into an infant's diet depends on such factors as the nutritional need for iron, the infant's physiologic capability to digest starch, and his physical ability to chew and swallow.

Rice is nice

By age 4 to 6 months, an infant should be mature enough to begin eating iron-fortified cereal mixed with formula or breast milk. Rice cereal is the best to begin with because it's least likely to cause allergies. (See *Solid foods and infant age*.)

Solid foods and infant age

This table gives an overview of solid foods that are appropriate for the developing infant.

Age	Type of food	Rationale
4 to 6 months	Rice cereal mixed with breast milk or formula is a traditional choice; however, strained vegetables (offered first) and fruits are just as good.	Rice cereal is easy to digest and less likely than wheat to cause an allergic reaction. Vegetables are offered first because they may be more readily accepted than if introduced after sweet fruits.
7 to 8 months	Strained meats, cheese, yogurt, rice, noodles, pudding	Provide an important source of iron and add variety to the diet
8 to 9 months	Finger foods (bananas, soft crackers)	Promote self-feeding
10 months	Mashed egg yolk (no whites until age 1); bite-size cooked food (no foods that may cause choking)	Use of bite-size pieces to decrease risk of choking (Avoiding foods that may cause choking is the safest option, even though the infant chews well.)
12 months	Foods from the adult table (chopped or mashed according to the infant's ability to chew foods)	Provide a nutritious and varied diet that should meet the infant's nutritional needs

Fingers before forks

By about age 8 or 9 months, the infant should be able to sit up and grasp objects, so introducing finger foods at this time can help promote self-feeding. (See *Teaching points for feeding and nutrition.*)

Sleep and rest guidelines

The AAP recommends that all infants be positioned on their backs for every sleep (including naps) until they can roll over and determine their own sleeping position. Since its inception, this simple maneuver has significantly decreased the incidence of sudden infant death syndrome (SIDS). In addition to providing safe sleep guidelines for the prevention of SIDS, the AAP recommendations focus on safe sleeping environments to prevent sudden unexpected infant deaths (SUIDs)

It's all relative

Teaching points for feeding and nutrition

Stress these feeding and nutrition points to the parents of an infant:
• Watch for behaviors that indicate feeding preferences. If the infant rejects a food initially, offer it again later and many more times as tastes change!
• Keep the infant in an upright feeding position.
• Don't try to make the infant eat more to finish the serving or portion.
• Initially, offer iron-fortified rice cereal.
• Introduce new foods one at a time, waiting 5 to 7 days between them so that if a food allergy develops, it will be apparent which food triggered the allergic reaction.
• Avoid grapes and grape halves and cut up hot dogs until the infant has adequate chewing and swallowing skills.
• Limit 100% pure fruit juice to no more than 4 oz per day.
• Avoid other sweetened beverages.
• If the infant has a history of food allergies, delay offering eggs, wheat-based products, peanut and tree nuts–based products, and citrus fruits.
• Avoid honey and other unpasteurized products because they may put infants at risk for infantile botulism.

caused by entrapment, suffocation, and asphyxiation. Soft materials, even if covered by a sheet, should not be placed in the crib under a sleeping infant. Objects such as quilts, bumper pads, comforters, and blankets should be kept out of infant's sleeping environment. Clothing designed to keep infant warm without covering the head (such as a sleep sac) can be used. There is no evidence that wedges, positioners, special mattresses, and special sleep surfaces reduce the risk of SIDS or that they are safe.

Because of an increased risk of entrapment or suffocation, infants should not be placed to sleep on beds. Room sharing without bed sharing is recommended to decrease the risk of SIDS. Bed rails should not be used due to a risk of strangulation. The sleep area should be kept free from dangling cords, window-covering cords, or electrical wires. Sitting devices such as car seats, strollers, and swings are not recommended for routine sleep. If a baby is being carried in a sling, it is essential that the head and face be visible and that the infant's nose and mouth are clear of obstructions.

To sleep, per chance to . . . wake up and eat!

Certain expectations for sleeping through the night can be made for each age-group in infancy:
• From birth to age 4 months, an infant will wake to feed at night from 0 to 3 times. Because breast milk is digested faster than formula, breast-fed infants commonly will wake up to feed more frequently than bottle-fed infants.
• At ages 4 to 6 months, infants are beginning to be physiologically capable of sleeping (without feeding) for 6 to 8 hours at night. Infants may awaken during this sleep period but should be able to calm themselves and return to sleep. (See *Sleep requirements in infancy*.)

Napping

From birth to age 3 months, infants may take many naps per day. However, an infant shouldn't be allowed to sleep longer than 4 hours at a time during the day because this will lead to more nighttime awakenings to feed.

From ages 4 to 9 months, the infant will have transitioned to two naps per day (one in the morning and one in the afternoon). Total naptime should add up to about 2 to 3 hours. By ages 9 to 12 months, most infants will have transitioned to only one nap, for a total of 1 to 2 hours of napping time.

Dental hygiene

Gentle care can be given to the infant's gums and new teeth. Wiping the teeth and gums with a soft washcloth and water alone provides adequate cleaning when the infant has only a few teeth.

Growing pains

Sleep requirements in infancy

This chart shows the amount of sleep per 24 hours (including nighttime and naps) needed by infants from ages 1 week to 12 months.

Age	Hours of sleep per day
1 week	16½
1 month	15½
3 months	15
6 months	14½
9 months	14
12 months	13¾

Hold the paste

Once teeth have erupted, they can be cleaned with a small, soft-bristled toothbrush and water. Toothpaste shouldn't be used because the infant would swallow it. Ingesting fluoridated toothpaste can cause nausea and fluorosis, a gray discoloration of the permanent teeth.

A dental home should be established by 12 months of age, but dental care begins with the first tooth eruption. Fluoride supplements may be needed in areas where the water supply contains inadequate fluoride (less than 0.3 ppm) or none at all. The American Academy of Pediatric Dentistry recommends that fluoride supplements be given to infants who need them beginning at age 6 months.

Preventing dental caries during infancy

In addition to being a condition associated with dietary factors, early childhood caries can be transmitted from mother to baby by the bacteria *Streptococcus mutans*. To keep an infant's smile healthy, teach the parents how to avoid dental caries with these tips:

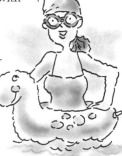

While pooling in here is fun, pooling around the teeth is no laughing matter.

• Don't put an infant to bed with a bottle at night or at naptime because pooling of carbohydrate-rich fluids (including breast milk and formula) or other sweetened liquid around the infant's teeth can cause decay. If an infant must be put to bed with a bottle, fill the bottle with water only.
• Don't allow the infant to carry a bottle filled with milk, formula, juice, or other sweetened liquid to use as a pacifier throughout the day. Again, frequent exposure to carbohydrate-rich liquids to the teeth can occur, leading to decay. Bottles that contain liquids other than water should be offered only at mealtimes.
• Transition the infant to a cup beginning around 9 months and completed by the time of his first birthday. Cup-drinking doesn't permit pooling of liquids around the teeth.
• Don't offer the infant a pacifier dipped in sugar or honey.
• Provide regular care of the infant's teeth and gums.
• Encourage mothers to chew gum or mints with xylitol listed as the first ingredient (3 to 5 times daily) because xylitol has been shown to inhibit the growth of *S. mutans*.

Injury prevention

Injury prevention during infancy centers around automobile safety, preventing aspiration and falls, and childproofing the infant's environment.

Child passenger safety

The use of child restraints in automobiles has reduced the risk of injury by 71% to 82% compared to just using a seat belt for the same-age child. Infants and toddlers should always ride in a rear-facing car safety seat until age 2 years or until the child achieves the highest weight or height allowed by the manufacturer of the car seat.

Aspiration

Because infants become adept at placing objects in their mouths for exploration, they're at risk for aspiration. To prevent aspiration:
• Feed infants in a slightly upright position.
• Burp infants in an upright or prone position.
• Cut solid foods into very small pieces when the infant starts eating solids.
• Avoid foods and other things that can be choking hazards. (See *Choking hazards*.)

Choking hazards

These foods can easily cause choking and should be avoided during infancy:
• hot dogs
• nuts
• popcorn
• hard candy
• ice cubes
• grapes
• uncooked vegetable chunks
• lumps of peanut butter.

Falls

Even a neonate is at risk for falling. As the child becomes mobile, the risk of falls increases. To prevent falls, encourage parents to:
• never leave an infant unattended, especially on a changing table, bed, sofa, or counter
• place gates at the top and bottom of staircases
• put up window guards or other window safety devices on windows above the first floor level
• avoid placing infants in walkers because they can tumble over an uneven surface or the leg of a chair or table or fall down stairs.

Childproofing

After an infant is mobile, it's too late to childproof. Here are some tips for childproofing, based on the infant's age.
At birth:
• Turn down the thermostat on the water heater to 120° F (48.9° C) or lower. (See *Dangers of high temperature water*.)

Here's a great strategy for childproofing. Get down on your hands and knees, crawl around a bit, and see how much trouble you could get into!

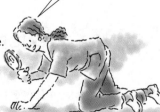

Dangers of high temperature water

Teach your patients' parents to cool it—the water heater thermostat, that is!

When the hot water temperature is set at 150° F (65.6° C), it takes only 2 seconds of exposure for an adult to suffer a full-thickness burn. Because infants have thin skin, it takes even less time for them to suffer a full-thickness burn.

By turning the water temperature down to a maximum of 120° F (48.9° C), parents can drastically reduce the risk of injury; at 120° F, it takes 10 minutes for a burn to occur.

- To prevent an accidental scalding burn, never drink hot liquids while holding the infant.
- To prevent drowning, never leave the infant alone in the bath.
- Install smoke detectors.
- Install a carbon monoxide monitor outside the infant's room.
- Use flame-retardant pajamas.
- Remove firearms from the home. (If this isn't an option, use trigger locks or lock the firearm and ammunition in separate areas.)

  By age 4 months:
- Cover all electrical outlets.
- Tape down all electrical cords (or place them behind furniture).
- Install childproof locks on all cabinets.
- Place all medicines and cleaning agents in high cabinets with locks to prevent accidental ingestions.
- Remove all breakable items from tabletops and shelves within the infant's reach.
- Keep small toys and other small items off the floor.

Accidental ingestions

Although not a common cause of death in infancy (16 deaths in 2011), accidental ingestions are easily preventable by placing all toxic substances such as cleaning supplies and medications in upper or locked cabinets. In addition, the American Association of Poison Control Centers has a national poison emergency hotline that can be called toll-free 24 hours a day: 1-800-222-1222. Every household should have this number in an easy to find location or already entered into the phone so that it can be accessed quickly.

Health problems

Health concerns during infancy include:
- colic
- failure to thrive
- regurgitation
- SIDS.

Colic

Time spent crying per day increased from birth and peaks for all infant around 6 weeks of age and then starts to decline. Some infants cry more than others. *Colic* is defined as a daily period of crying for 3 hours or longer, during which the infant is virtually inconsolable. These episodes usually occur in the late afternoon or evening. About 10% to 20% of infants suffer from colic.

What causes it

No one knows for sure what causes this behavior.

How it happens

Although long thought to be related to the gastrointestinal (GI) tract, current theories about the origins of colic lean toward CNS maturation. The process of CNS maturation can cause difficulties with the infant's ability to self-regulate (especially relating to overstimulation and an inability to self-calm).

What to look for

In an otherwise healthy infant, he may have colic if he:
• cries and is inconsolable
• fails to calm in response to normally calming maneuvers (holding, rocking)
• isn't hungry (refuses the breast or bottle)
• doesn't need changing (has a dry diaper)
• has no fever or other medical reason for crying.

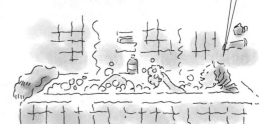

A warm bath can be very soothing. It works for an infant with colic, too!

Complications

Colic produces no complications unless a caregiver gets so frustrated that she harms the infant. Fussy infants who are difficult to care for are at increased risk for abuse.

How it's treated

Colic is a clinical diagnosis, meaning no tests exist to help diagnose colic. There's no medical cure for colic, except time. Most infants "outgrow" it or sufficiently mature so that symptoms disappear or markedly improve by age 3 months.

What to do

Because of the potential for abuse when caregivers become frustrated with an inconsolable infant, the pediatric nurse should make every effort to help parents deal effectively with an infant with colic.

Decreasing rapidly changing stimulation seems to be the most effective intervention for an infant with colic. Any strategy might work, but the key is to keep the stimulation consistent for at least 5 minutes so the infant can adjust to it. Rapidly trying different "fixes" only increases stimulation and makes matters worse. (See *Tips for reducing colic.*)

When all else fails and parents are at their wits' end, suggest that they place the infant on his back in the bassinet or crib, shut the door, leave the room, and do something to calm down (for example, meditation, listening to music). The parents should be encouraged to call a family member, friend, or the infant's health care provider if help is needed to cope with the crying. The parent should not return to the infant's room until he or she is calm enough to care for the infant.

Failure to thrive

Failure to thrive (FTT) is a state of undernutrition diagnosed when an infant isn't growing at the expected rate. FTT is characterized by failure to maintain weight for length above the 5th percentile on age-appropriate growth charts. It can also be detected from a deviation in an already established growth curve.

What causes it

The cause of FTT is often multifactorial including medical, psychosocial, and environmental factors.

How it happens

If caloric intake is less than that required for nutritional needs, growth and development suffer. Inadequate calorie intake is often caused by problems with feeding. Family issues such as a parent with mental health problems, lack of knowledge or poverty, as well as neglect or abuse can also be associated with FTT.

FTT caused by inadequate calorie absorption may be due to malabsorptive pathology or metabolic disorders. Excessive use of calories can occur with chronic illness such as congenital heart disease or chronic pulmonary disease of prematurity.

It's all relative

Tips for reducing colic

Providing parents with these tips may help them relieve their infant's colic behavior.

Provide rhythmic movement
• Front-carrying sling
• Infant swing
• Car ride in approved safety seat
• Walking with the infant on your shoulder

Try alternative positioning
• Swaddling
• Prone position over parent's knees

Reduce environmental stimuli
• Quiet, soothing music
• No sudden, loud noises
• No smoking

Provide tactile stimuli
• Pacifier
• Warm bath
• Massage

What to look for

An absence of weight gain or a loss of weight is the first growth parameter to be affected; a drop in height percentile is the next sign, followed by a drop in head circumference. A drop in percentile over time or between visits warrants further investigation.

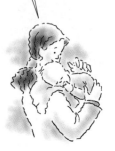

You're a little too little, little one.

What tests tell you

No definitive tests for FTT exist. However, after taking a history and performing a comprehensive exam, you should be able to determine whether medical causes are a possibility. All possible medical or pathologic causes should be ruled out.

Complications

Complications of FTT can include developmental delay, growth retardation, impaired bonding, and altered family relationships.

How it's treated

All factors impacting the infant's nutrition should be addressed. If a pathologic cause is determined, treatment focuses on the underlying disease process. If indicated, treatment is also directed toward changing the surroundings. A change in the infant's environment might be as drastic as removing him from the home or as simple as educating a caregiver on breast-feeding or proper mixing of formula or reading the infant's cues more accurately.

What to do

When providing care to an infant hospitalized with FTT, the nurse should:
• weigh the child on admission to determine baseline weight and continue to weigh daily during treatment
• properly feed and interact with the child to promote nutrition and growth and development
• provide the infant with visual and auditory stimulation to promote normal sensory development
• teach the parents effective parenting skills to increase their knowledge of routine child care practices, such as comfort measures, age-appropriate developmental tasks, and play activities
• praise the parents for positive interactions with the infant and avoid judgmental statements and actions.

Regurgitation

Regurgitation, also referred to as *spitting up* or a *wet burp*, is considered normal infant behavior. Most infants will spit up at least occasionally.

What causes it

Regurgitation in infants is most commonly caused by swallowing air or by overfeeding. However, it can also be caused by gastro-esophageal reflux disease or pyloric stenosis.

How it happens

A wet burp involves either dribbling of undigested liquids from the mouth and esophagus, or the expulsion of those liquids with the force of a burp.

What to look for

Spitting up in infancy may be characterized by:
• white, curdled liquid plopping or running out of the corners of the mouth or, occasionally, coming from the nose
• a "burp" of air that sometimes precedes the regurgitation.
  The infant with regurgitation may:
• be fussy during feedings
• grimace, cry, and pull away from the bottle or breast
• occasionally refuse to eat.

What tests tell you

Testing can rule out gastroesophageal reflux disease and pyloric stenosis, two common causes of regurgitation in infants.

Probing the problem

The definitive test for gastroesophageal reflux is called a *pH probe*. Because the pH of the stomach is so acidic (pH of 1 to 3), a probe placed in the esophagus will demonstrate the presence of stomach acid if reflux if present.

Slow stomach

If projectile vomiting is reported, pyloric stenosis may be suspected. An ultrasound of the area may demonstrate delayed or slowed stomach emptying, a thickened sphincter, or complete closure of the sphincter. Surgical treatment is necessary.

Complications

Complications of regurgitation are rare but it may include aspiration pneumonia and failure to gain weight.

How it's treated

If an infant is growing well, is generally happy, and isn't bothered by spitting up, regurgitation can be left to improve with time.

Memory jogger

When caring for an infant with re-gurgitation, remember to BERP him:

B—Burp the infant frequently.

E—Evaluate feeding.

R—Reassure caregivers that the condition will improve with time.

P—Prevent aspiration.

If the infant isn't growing well, is refusing to feed, is unhappy, or has been diagnosed with gastroesophageal reflux or pyloric stenosis, drug therapy or even surgery may be necessary.

What to do

When providing care to an infant with regurgitation:
• Evaluate feeding methods (amount of burping, air in nipple with formula feeding).
• Burp the infant frequently; feed smaller amounts more frequently and don't overfeed.
• Place or hold infant in an upright position after feeding to help food stay down.
• Reassure caregivers that spitting up may improve with time.

Sudden infant death syndrome and sleep-related infant deaths

SIDS is the sudden death of a previously healthy infant when the cause of death isn't confirmed by a postmortem examination. It's the most common cause of death between ages 1 month and 1 year. However, the incidence of SIDS has declined dramatically by more than 50% since 1990, which is mostly attributed to the 1992 initiative to put babies on their backs, called the "Back to Sleep Campaign" now relabeled the "Safe Sleep Campaign." The safe sleep campaign focuses on a safe sleeping environment that reduces the risk of all sleep-related deaths including SIDS.

What causes it

Although the exact cause of SIDS is unknown, currently a triple-risk model includes development, vulnerabilities, and environmental stressors. Several factors, including exposure to tobacco smoke and long QT syndrome, have been shown to be associated with an increased risk of SIDS. (See *Risk factors for SIDS.*)

How it happens

Current theories focus on neurologic immaturity related to the infant's inability to sense and regulate oxygenation status, ultimately leading to respiratory arrest. The syndrome can't be prevented or explained; the infant usually dies during sleep without noise or struggle.

What to look for

Autopsy findings may show pulmonary edema, intrathoracic petechiae, and other minor changes suggesting chronic hypoxia.

Risk factors for SIDS

• Prematurity
• Low birth weight
• Twin or triplet
• Race/ethnicity (Native Americans and African-Americans are at highest risk—possibly related to infant sleep position preferences)
• Male gender
• In utero exposure to nicotine or alcohol
• Age between 1 and 4 months
• Passive smoke exposure
• History of respiratory compromise

What tests tell you

There are no tests to diagnose SIDS. A thorough postmortem investigation must rule out all other causes of death.

Complications

Sudden death is the sole medical complication of SIDS. However, SIDS affects the family members of the infant who dies of SIDS. Parents may need counseling or some other form of help to cope with their loss.

How it's treated

There is, of course, no way to treat a condition that, by its definition, is sudden death without warning. There are, however, measures that can be taken to decrease the risk of SIDS and other sleep-related infant deaths including:
• putting the infant on his back to sleep for every sleep; side sleeping is not advised
• using a firm sleep surface
• room sharing without bed sharing
• removing pillows, quilts, stuffed toys, or any other soft surfaces from the infant's crib or sleeping environment
• keeping the infant warm while sleeping, but not overheated
• not smoking, drinking alcohol, and using illicit drugs
• breast-feeding
• considering offering a pacifier at nap and bedtime
• immunizing per recommendations.

What to do

When dealing with a family whose infant has just died of suspected SIDS in the emergency room:
• Be aware that assessment, planning, and implementation related to the parents' needs should begin as soon as they arrive in the emergency department.
• Provide the family with a room (for privacy) and a staff member who can stay with them and provide support.
• Stay calm and let the parents express their feelings. (In their need to blame someone or something for the tragedy, they may express anger at emergency department personnel, each other, or anyone involved with the infant's care.)
• Prepare the family for how the infant will look and feel.
• Let the parents touch, hold, and rock the infant, if desired. Allow them to say good-bye.
• Contact spiritual advisors, significant others, or other support systems
• Provide literature on sudden unexplained infant death and support groups.

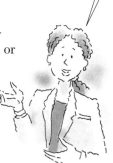

It's important to let the family of an infant who has died of SIDS express their feelings.

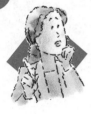

Quick quiz

1.   A social milestone that infants should acquire by ages 2 to 3 months is:

    A.   grasping at objects.
    B.   smiling.
    C.   stranger anxiety.
    D.   vocalizing "mama."

Answer: B. Smiling is a social communication milestone that should be reached by ages 2 to 3 months.

2.   Which finger food is appropriate for an 8-month-old infant?

    A.   Cheerios
    B.   Grapes
    C.   Mixed nuts
    D.   Raw carrot slice

Answer: A. Infants are developmentally ready to eat solids by age 6 months, when they can maintain their posture in an upright position to decrease the risk of choking.

3.   The best assessment of whether an infant is receiving enough formula or breast milk is if he:

    A.   burps well.
    B.   doesn't cry after feeding.
    C.   has six or more wet diapers per day.
    D.   sleeps all night.

Answer: C. Infants receiving adequate formula or breast milk for hydration and growth will void and wet six to eight diapers daily.

4.   Which of these interventions decreases the risk of SIDS?

    A.   Feeding the infant in an upright position
    B.   Not giving a bottle in bed at night
    C.   Putting an infant on his back to sleep
    D.   Raising the head of the crib

Answer: C. Putting the infant on his back to sleep has decreased the prevalence of SIDS and will decrease the individual infant's risk as well.

Scoring

   ☆☆☆ If you answered all four items correctly, terrific! You've developed a strong sense of infant development.

      ☆☆ If you answered three items correctly, good job! Treat yourself to a play break and then read on.

        ☆ If you answered fewer than three items correctly, don't cry over spilled milk! Take a nap and review the chapter again.

4

Early childhood

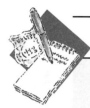

Just the facts

In this chapter, you'll learn:

♦ physical, psychological, and cognitive development of toddlers and preschoolers

♦ developmental theories in the toddler and preschool years

♦ common concerns of parents of toddlers and preschoolers

♦ injury prevention for toddlers and preschoolers

♦ health problems of toddlers and preschoolers.

Toddlerhood

Toddlerhood, from ages 1 to 3 years, is the stage in which children start displaying independence and pride in their accomplishments. They intensely explore their environment, trying to figure out how things work. It's also the time when they begin to display negativism and have temper tantrums.

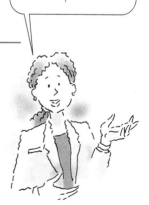

The "terrible two's" don't have to be terrible. "No" may be a toddler's favorite word, but he'll also take pride in every little accomplishment.

Physical development

During the toddler stage, physical growth is characterized by:

• growth rate that slows during the second year of life
• possible limited food intake, which may concern parents, so they need to be reassured this is normal
• steady growth on a growth curve that's more steplike than linear, demonstrating growth "spurts."

Height, weight, and head circumference

From ages 1 to 2:
- Toddlers grow approximately 3½″ to 5″ (9 to 12.5 cm) per year (with growth mostly in the legs, rather than in the trunk, like infants).
- Toddlers gain about 8 oz (227 g) per month.
- Head circumference increases about 1″ (2.5 cm) per year.
- Anterior fontanel usually closes (between 12 and 18 months).

Two's take off

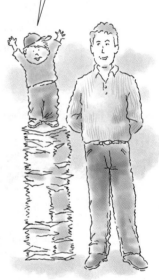

I'm only 2 but I'm halfway there. A few more growth spurts ought to do it!

By age 2:
- Birth weight has usually quadrupled; average weight is 27 lb (12.3 kg).
- Head circumference is usually equal to chest circumference.
- The child is about half of adult height, with an average height of 34″ (86.4 cm).

Three's relax

From ages 2 to 3, toddlers:
- grow 2″ to 2½″ (5 to 6.5 cm)
- gain about 3 to 5 lb (1.5 to 2.5 kg)
- show slowed increases in head circumference (less than ½″ [1.3 cm] per year).

Teeth

By approximately 33 months, all deciduous teeth have erupted and the child has about 20 teeth. The child should already be brushing with a small, soft-bristled toothbrush (with parental supervision) and may use a scant amount of fluoride toothpaste or, if needed, fluoride supplements.

Gross motor development

Gross motor activity develops rapidly in toddlers. One-year-olds can:
- walk alone using a wide stance
- begin to run but fall easily.
    By age 2, the toddler can:
- run without falling most of the time
- throw a ball overhand without losing his balance
- jump with both feet
- walk up and down stairs
- use push and pull toys.

Fine motor development

Fine motor development begins slowly; however, by age 2, the toddler has generally mastered some fairly complex fine motor skills.

A 1-year-old can:
• grasp a very small object.

A 2-year-old can:
• build a tower of four blocks
• scribble on paper
• drop a small pellet into a small, narrow container
• use a spoon well and drink well from a covered cup
• undress himself.

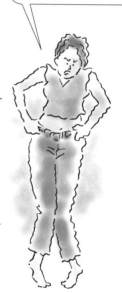

A toddler can undress himself, so what's my problem? I guess 2-year-olds are **too** smart **to** wear jeans that are **two** sizes **too** small.

Psychological development

A child develops a more elaborate vocabulary, a sense of autonomy, and socially acceptable play skills during the toddler stage.

Language development and socialization

As the toddler learns to understand and, ultimately, communicate with the spoken word, he develops the social skills that will allow him to interact more effectively with others.

Language

During toddlerhood, the ability to understand speech is much more developed than the ability to speak.

Now we're talking

By age 1:
• The child uses one-word sentences or *holophrases* (real words that are meant to represent entire phrases or ideas).
• The toddler has learned about four words.
• Twenty-five percent of the 1-year-old's vocalization is understandable.

Talk about progress!

By age 2:
• The number of words learned has increased from about four (at age 1) to approximately 300.
• The child uses multiword (two- to three-word) sentences.
• Sixty-five percent of speech is understandable.
• Frequent, repetitive naming of objects helps toddlers to learn appropriate words for objects.

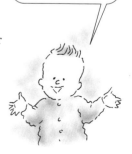

Foo, da-da, po-po, moop. Hey, I'm only 1. If you got 25% of that, I'm right on target.

Socialization

During toddlerhood, children develop social skills that determine the way they interact with others. As the toddler develops psychologically, he can:
- differentiate himself from others
- tolerate being separated from a parent
- withstand delayed gratification
- control his bodily functions
- acquire socially acceptable behaviors
- communicate verbally
- become less egocentric.

Erikson's developmental theory

As discussed in chapter 2, Erikson believed that each developmental stage is characterized by a particular psychosocial crisis (positive versus negative) that must be resolved before the child can master the task at hand.

Putting the "no" in autonomous

According to Erikson's developmental theory, *autonomy versus doubt and shame* is the developmental task of toddlerhood. In this context, Erickson maintains that:
- Toddlers are in the final stages of developing a sense of trust (the task from infancy) and are ready to start asserting some control, independence, and autonomy.
- Negativism is displayed in the toddler's quest for autonomy.
- *Ritualism*, a need to maintain sameness and reliability, gives the toddler a sense of comfort.
- The child's significant other is the "paternal" person in his (or her) life.
- Development of the ego creates a conflict for the child, specifically, how to deal with the impulses of the *id* (which requires immediate gratification), while learning socially acceptable ways to interact with the environment.
- Development of the *superego*, or conscience, begins with the incorporation of the morals of society. (See *Toddler development*.)

Play

Play is the work of children. It's through play that the child learns about his own capabilities and develops the skills needed to interact with others and his environment.

Growing pains

Toddler development

At the toddler stage, children begin to master:
- individuation (differentiation of self from others)
- separation from parents
- control of body functions
- communication with words
- acquisition of socially acceptable behaviors
- lesser egocentricity when interacting with others.

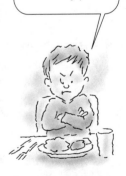

No! No! No! (I'm on a quest for my autonomy— whatever that means. How am I doing?)

New rules, new game

During the toddler stage:
• Play changes considerably as the toddler's motor skills develop; he uses his physical skills to push and pull objects; to climb up, down, in, and out; and to run or ride on toys.
• A short attention span requires frequent changes in toys and play media.
• Toddlers increase their cognitive abilities by manipulating objects and learning about their qualities, which makes tactile play (with water, sand, finger paints, clay) important. (See *Toddler toys*.)
• Many play activities involve imitating behaviors the child sees at home, which helps them learn new actions and skills.
• Play becomes more social but not necessarily interactive.

Parallel play

During the toddler stage, children commonly play with others without actually interacting. In this type of *parallel play*, children play side by side, commonly with similar objects. Interaction is limited to the occasional comment or trading of toys. This form of play helps the toddler develop the social skills needed to move into more interactive play.

Cognitive development

According to Piaget's developmental theory, a child moves from the sensorimotor stage of infancy and early toddlerhood (birth to age 2) to the longer, preoperational stage (ages 2 to 7). Piaget made several observations about this transitional time in the young child's life.
• *Tertiary circular reactions* refers to the 13- to 18-month-old child's use of *active experimentation* (trial and error); he uses newly acquired skills and knowledge to reach previously unattainable goals and discover new objects and areas.

Familiar at home, foreign at the store

• The toddler may be aware of the relationship between two events (cause and effect) but may not be able to transfer that knowledge to a new situation. (For example, a toddler might need to reinvestigate the function of a familiar object or the identity of a familiar person over and over again when he encounters that object or person in a new, out-of-context setting.)

That's using my head

• From about ages 18 to 24 months, the toddler will look for new ways to accomplish tasks through mental calculations.

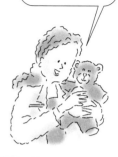

A toddler's favorite toy can change at the drop of a hat.

Toddler toys

Safe toys that promote a toddler's exploration include:
• play dough and modeling clay
• building blocks
• plastic, pretend housekeeping toys, such as pots, pans, and play food
• stackable rings and blocks of varying sizes
• toy telephone
• wooden puzzles with big pieces
• textured or cloth books
• plastic musical instruments and noise-makers
• toys that roll, such as cars and trains
• tricycle or riding car
• fat crayons and coloring books
• stuffed animals with painted faces (button eyes can pose a choking hazard).

• Object permanence advances as toddlers are more aware of the existence of objects that are out of sight, such as behind closed doors, in drawers, and under tables.
• Toddlers begin to use language and are able to think about objects or people when they aren't present.

Sincerest form of flattery

• Imitation displays deeper meaning and understanding of the toddler's role in the family as the child observes and helps with household activities and identifies with the same-sex parent.
• Toddlers begin to use *preoperational thought*, with increasing use of words as symbols.
• Problem solving, creative thinking, and some understanding of cause and effect begin during the toddler years.

> I'm hungry and I want my mom. If I make lots of noise, my mom will wake up and the French toast is mine! How's that for problem solving?

Keys to health

Guidelines for nutrition, sleep and rest, and dental hygiene should be followed to maintain a toddler's good health.

Nutrition

Nutrition guidelines for toddlers include:
• a decrease in protein requirements from infancy (to 1.2 g/kg/day)
• caloric requirement of approximately 100 kcal/kg/day
• considerable need for vitamins and minerals, such as iron, calcium, and phosphorus.

Developing healthy eating habits

The eating habits learned during the toddler years can set the stage for many years to come. Positive experiences with food and family meals are likely to set a foundation for a healthy, pleasurable "relationship" with food. On the other hand, negative experiences—power struggles, unpleasantness, food given or withheld to control behavior—may predispose the toddler to future food-related problems, such as overeating, extremely picky eating, and even an increased risk for eating disorders.

You eat what you are

A toddler's developing eating habits are influenced by a range of factors, including:
• physiologic anorexia, which occurs at approximately age 18 months (when growth slows), and results in decreased appetite and a picky, fussy eater with strong taste preferences

• need to imitate family members (toddlers may refuse to eat a particular food that parents or siblings choose not to eat)
• being easily overwhelmed by large portions
• inability to sit through a long meal without becoming fidgety or disruptive at times
• food used as a reward or sign of approval (which may encourage overeating for nonnutritive reasons)
• food that's forced or mealtimes that are consistently unpleasant (which may keep the child from developing the sense of pleasure usually associated with eating).

Food preparation

Most toddlers eat the same food that's prepared for the rest of the family. Here are a few "toddler truisms" to help make mealtime enjoyable:
• Serving size should be approximately 1 T of solid food per year of age (or one-fourth to one-third the adult portion size) so as not to overwhelm the child with larger portions.
• Frequent, nutritious snacks are more likely to promote proper nutrition than are three large meals per day.
• Most toddlers prefer to feed themselves; they're skillful at handling finger foods but are still messy with soft foods as they're learning to use a spoon.

Sleep and rest

Parents are usually pleased to hear that most toddlers sleep through the night without awakening. A consistent routine, such as a set bedtime, a light snack, reading, and a security object, helps toddlers prepare for sleep.

Good night, sleepyhead

Sleep requirements change slightly as a toddler grows and approaches the preschool stage.
• From ages 1 to 2, a toddler needs 10 to 15 hours of sleep every 24 hours.
• The 2- to 3-year-old needs 10 to 12 hours of sleep per night.
• During toddlerhood, naps gradually decrease to one per day; at age 3, toddlers usually don't need a nap.

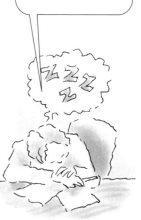

It's just about the time when toddlers stop needing to take naps (around age 3) that their parents could really use them!

Dental hygiene

When teeth begin to break through the gumline, a child should begin brushing his teeth with a small, soft-bristled toothbrush (with parental assistance). Fluoride toothpaste should be avoided until the child is 2 years old. When used earlier, before the child can spit out toothpaste, ingested fluoride leads to fluorosis, which can discolor teeth.

Fluoride

Fluoride is a mineral that reduces the incidence of tooth decay. It's found naturally in water, certain foods, and drinks made with fluoridated water.

Unless the water supply has adequate fluoride (more than 0.6 ppm), children age 2 and older may need to receive a daily fluoride supplement. Before recommending fluoride supplements, consider other potential fluoridated water sources such as the child care center or a relative's house that the child frequents. When administering supplements or teaching the caregiver to do so, keep in mind that:
• The supplement should be taken on an empty stomach and the child shouldn't eat or drink for 30 minutes afterward.
• The supplement should remain in the child's mouth for 30 seconds before swallowing (if possible).
• Use of fluoride products can lead to accidental poisoning; fluoride-containing toothpastes, supplements, and rinses must be stored out of the reach of young children.

Low-cariogenic diet

A low-cariogenic diet is important for developing strong, healthy teeth because caries need fermentable sugars, especially sucrose, to develop. The following information will help parents identify and minimize high-cariogenic foods in their child's diet:
• Sticky or hard foods are more cariogenic than others because they remain in the mouth longer.
• Refined table sugar, honey, molasses, corn syrup, and dried fruits such as raisins are highly cariogenic.
• It's more important to limit the frequency of sugar consumption than the total amount consumed.

Timing is everything

• Sweets that are consumed immediately after a meal are less damaging than sweets that are eaten as snacks.
• "Early childhood caries" (ECC) may occur when a child is routinely given a bottle of milk or juice at naptime or bedtime or uses the bottle as a pacifier while awake (a bottle of water may be used if needed). Breast-feeding has also been associated with ECC when the child frequently falls asleep at the breast.

Coping with concerns

A toddler is prone to developing troubling behaviors relating to toilet training, temper tantrums, and discipline. Negativism and periods of separation anxiety may manifest through physical behaviors such as temper tantrums.

Toilet training

For toilet training to be successful, the child must display three signs of toilet training readiness:

First, the child must have control of the rectal and urethral sphincters.

Second, the child must have a cognitive understanding of what it means to hold his stool and urine until he can go to a certain place at a certain time.

Third, the child must have a desire to delay his immediate reward for a more socially accepted action.

It's in his head, too

Physical readiness for toilet training occurs at ages 18 to 24 months when myelinization of pyramidal tracts and conditioned reflex sphincter control are intact. Despite physical readiness, however, many children aren't cognitively ready to begin toilet training until they're between ages 36 and 42 months.

Ready, set, go potty!

When physically and cognitively ready, the child can start toilet training. The process can take 2 weeks to 2 months to complete successfully. It's important to remember that there's considerable variability from one child to another. Other signs of readiness for toilet training include:
• periods of dryness for 2 hours or more, indicating bladder control
• child's ability to walk well and remove clothing
• cognitive ability to understand the task
• facial expression or words suggesting that the child knows when he's about to defecate.

Step by step

Steps to toilet training include:
• teaching words for voiding and defecating
• teaching the purpose of the toilet or potty chair
• changing the toddler's diapers frequently to give him the experience of feeling dry and clean
• helping the toddler make the connection between dry pants and the toilet or potty chair
• placing the child on the potty chair or toilet for a few moments at regular intervals and rewarding successes
• helping the toddler understand the physiologic signals by pointing out behaviors they display when they need to void or defecate
• rewarding successes but not punishing failures.

Temper tantrums

As they assert their independence, toddlers demonstrate "temper tantrums" or violent objections to rules or demands. These tantrums include such behaviors as lying on the floor and kicking his feet, screaming, and holding his breath.

Hush little baby, don't throw a fit

Tantrums can occur at any time of the day but commonly occur before bedtime. The active toddler may have trouble slowing down and, when placed in bed, resists staying there.

Assessment of temper tantrums in a toddler should include the following questions:
- How often do tantrums occur?
- What circumstances provoke tantrums?
- How does the child behave during tantrums?
- How does the child behave between tantrums?
- Are expectations of the parent consistent with the child's developmental age?
- Have there been any recent changes in the home?
- Does the child have other behavior problems?

Dealing with tantrums

Dealing with a child's temper tantrums can be a challenge for parents who may be frustrated, embarrassed, and exhausted by their child's behavior. If tantrums occur in public places, parents may feel as if they're being judged by others and viewed as inept at parenting and unable to control their child's behavior.

Annoying but normal

The nurse should reassure parents that temper tantrums are a normal occurrence in toddlers and that the child will outgrow them as he learns to express himself in more productive ways. This type of reassurance should be accompanied by some concrete suggestions for dealing effectively with temper tantrums:
- Provide a safe and childproof environment.
- Hold the child to keep him safe if his behavior is out of control.
- Give the toddler frequent opportunities to make developmentally appropriate choices.
- Give the child advance warning of request to help prevent tantrums.
- Remain calm and be supportive of a child having a tantrum.
- Ignore tantrums when the toddler is seeking attention or trying to get something he wants.

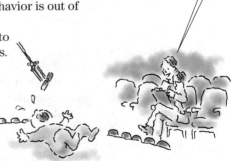

Sometimes, ignoring a temper tantrum is the best—and only—thing to do. I suggest a good pair of earplugs.

• Help the toddler find acceptable ways to vent his anger and frustration.

Stop the insanity! A toddler's negativism can push a parent's patience to the limits.

When to get help

Parents should be advised to seek help from a health care provider when problematic tantrums:
• persist beyond age 5
• occur more than five times per day
• occur with a persistent negative mood
• cause property destruction
• cause harm to the child or others.

Negativism

Negativism refers to persistent negative responses to requests and is typical of toddlers as they strive for autonomy. "No" and "Me do" become the responses to almost everything, and the toddler's emotions are very strongly expressed with rapid mood swings.

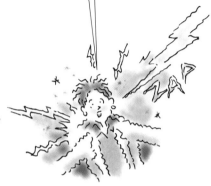

No, non, nein!

Negativism commonly becomes exasperating for parents, who may find it easier to give in to the behavior than to deal with it constructively. Unfortunately, this reinforces the child's negative ways of interacting with others.

Apple or grape?

Negativism can usually be reduced by giving the child appropriate choices. It's hard to say "no" when the question is, "Would you like apple juice or grape juice?"

Discipline

Toddlers must be under direct supervision of a caregiver at all times. A childproof environment must be provided as they can move quickly and skillfully and are always exploring their surroundings.

Frustration-free zone

Most discipline for toddlers involves taking measures to make the environment safe and age-appropriate, which reduces the frequency of frustration-producing situations that require a "no" from parents.

Tackle the triggers

Behavior management for toddlers includes attending to their needs to reduce fatigue and hunger triggers, as most inappropriate behavior occurs when the toddler is tired or hungry.

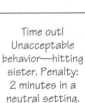

Tell me, Tommy, how do you feel about the potty chair?

Discipline guidelines include:
• setting up routines and creating and adhering to a consistent schedule
• providing an environment that limits opportunities for negative behavior and giving positive feedback for good behavior
• using behavior modification, or positive reinforcement, for good behavior and brief time-outs (with reasonable limits) for inappropriate behavior
• recognizing individuality in the toddler's temperament
• allowing toddlers to start attempting to solve some of their own problems
• understanding and recognizing feelings of frustration, boredom, and anger
• having the patience to allow toddlers to express themselves and to provide distraction when they're bored
• avoiding physical punishment, threats, and criticism (remembering that toddlers' behaviors are generally the result of normal development, such as exploring and experimenting with their environment).

Time-outs

When using time-outs in response to a toddler's inappropriate behavior, keep these guidelines in mind:
• Make sure the child knows the rules ahead of time.
• Give the child a simple explanation of why the behavior requiring a time-out is unacceptable.
• Place the child in a neutral or uninteresting environment.
• Limit the time-out to 1 minute per year of age (anything longer becomes frustrating and loses its intended effect).
• Reset the timer for one additional time-out if the child acts unacceptably.
• If the child is having trouble resolving his behavior problem on his own, try discussing the offense calmly and constructively and, if appropriate, helping the child determine ways to "fix" the result of the bad behavior (such as clean up a mess or apologize to a hurt friend).
• After a successful time-out, praise the child for his improved behavior.

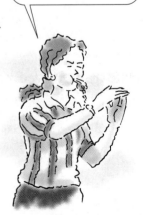

Time out! Unacceptable behavior—hitting sister. Penalty: 2 minutes in a neutral setting.

Separation anxiety

Stranger fear and separation anxiety are expected and normal reactions from an infant with a healthy parent-child attachment. As the child matures to toddler age, he may still protest being left with someone other than a parent, close friend, or relative.

Parents should be reassured that separation anxiety is a normal, expected behavior that is actually necessary for developmental growth, and that children usually progress beyond these fears with time and support.

Anxiety antidote

The following information and advice will help parents deal with their toddler's separation anxiety:
• Toddlers should be allowed to explore at their own rate with close adult supervision. They're normally ready to venture away from their parents for short periods and are curious about strangers.
• A toddler should be allowed to "warm up" to a new person. To do so, the parent should hold or stand near the child at a "safe" distance from the stranger, allowing the child to observe the new person from the safety of his parent's presence. (If the parent welcomes the new person, the toddler will likely do the same.)

Separation from parents can be a major stressor for toddlers, and this stress can be even more severe when a child is ill or hospitalized. To toddlers, nurses (and other health care professionals) are not only strangers but also strangers in a strange environment.

Slow, low, small, and clear

These measures can reassure a toddler who's hospitalized or undergoing a medical procedure:
• Start by talking to the parent in a soft voice while maintaining a safe distance from the child; avoid sudden movements or reaching for the child.
• Approach the child at his eye level; you may be more likely to be accepted in a stance that makes you appear smaller and less threatening.
• Minimize separation between the child and parent to the extent possible. (A parent's presence during a painful or frightening procedure, such as an injection, blood drawing, or intravenous [I.V.] insertion, will reassure the child that nothing truly bad will happen to him.)
• If separation can't be helped (such as in the operating room or during a radiologic examination), tell the child where his parent is waiting for him, and reassure the child that his parent knows exactly where he is.

- If a child is hospitalized and his parents must leave the hospital, reassure the child that his parents will return, and tell him when they'll return in terms he can understand (for example, "Your parents will be back after *Sesame Street*" or "Your parents will be back at lunchtime").

Preschool

During the preschool stage (ages 3 to 5), children are gaining new initiative and independence and have well-developed language skills.

Physical development

Physical development is slow and steady during the preschool stage, with most growth occurring in the long bones of the arms and legs.

Height and weight

- Preschoolers grow about 2½″ to 3″ (6.5 to 7.5 cm) per year; their average height is 37″ (94 cm).
- Weight gain is 3 to 5 lb (1.5 to 2.5 kg) per year; the average preschooler weighs 32 lb (14.5 kg).

Teeth

By the preschool years, the development of the child's primary (or *deciduous*) teeth is complete. Prepare the child and parents for the loss of these "baby" teeth and replacement with secondary (or *permanent*) teeth, which usually begins to occur at age 6 years.

Gross motor development

A 3-year-old can:
- stand on one foot for a few seconds
- climb stairs with alternating feet
- jump in place
- perform a broad jump
- dance, but with somewhat poor balance
- kick a ball
- ride a tricycle.

Fabulous 4 and 5

A 4-year-old can:
- hop, jump, and skip on one foot
- throw a ball overhand
- ride a tricycle or bicycle with training wheels.

A 5-year-old can:
• skip, using alternate feet
• jump rope
• balance on each foot for 4 to 5 seconds.

Fine motor development

A 3-year-old can:
• build a tower of 9 to 10 blocks and a 3-block bridge
• copy a circle and a cross
• draw a circle with facial features (but usually not a stick figure)
• use a fork well.
    A 4- or 5-year-old can:
• build a tower of 10 blocks
• copy a square and trace a cross and a diamond
• draw a person or stick figure with three or more parts
• use scissors to cut out a picture following an outline
• lace shoes (may be unable to tie a bow).

Psychological development

During the preschool years, the child functions more socially as he is able to learn and follow rules and perhaps has entered a daycare or nursery school setting, which enhances social development.

Many of the thought processes a preschooler will go through are essential to prepare him for kindergarten and the school years ahead.

Psychosocial development

According to Erikson's psychosocial theory, children between ages 3 and 5 have mastered a sense of autonomy and are now facing the task of *initiative versus guilt*. During this time:
• The child's significant other is the family.
• A conscience begins to develop, and dealing with the concept of right and wrong becomes a major task for preschoolers.
• A sense of guilt arises when the child feels that his imagination and activities are unacceptable or that they clash with his parents' expectations.
• The preschooler uses simple reasoning and can tolerate longer periods of delayed gratification.

Language development and socialization

By the time a child reaches preschool age:
• His vocabulary increases to about 900 words by age 3 and 2,100 words by age 5.

- He or she may talk incessantly and ask many "why" questions.
- He usually talks in three- or four-word sentences by age 3; by age 5, he speaks in longer sentences that contain all parts of speech.

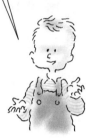

Why is the sky blue? Why do I have a baby brother? Why do I keep asking why?

Come one; come all

Socialization continues to develop as the preschooler's world expands beyond himself and his family. Significant others now include grandparents, siblings, and preschool teachers (although parents remain central). Regular interaction with same-age children is necessary for the preschooler to further develop social skills.

Play

Play changes as children move into preschool years, and the parallel play of toddlerhood is essentially replaced by more interactive, cooperative play.

Ch-, ch-, ch-, ch-, changes!

Other changes in play include:
- more *associative play*, in which there's interaction between the children as they play together
- better understanding of the concept of sharing
- enjoyment of large motor activities, such as swinging, riding tricycles or bicycles, and throwing balls
- more dramatic play, in which the child lives out the dramas of human life (in the context of the preschool years) and may have imaginary playmates. (See *Preschool play.*)

Cognitive development

Preschoolers exhibit preoperational thought by using symbols or words to represent objects and people and by thinking about objects and people as well.

Preschool play

Suggested play activities for preschoolers include:
- running and jumping in an open space
- creative play with dress-up clothes, pretend kitchens, and dolls
- art activities with paints, paper, crayons, blunt scissors, and markers
- trips to the museum, park, fire station, zoo, library, and shopping mall
- swimming and other individual sports and activities to encourage gross motor development
- puzzles and toys to aid fine motor development and stimulate imagination.

Piaget's cognitive theory divides the preoperational phase into two stages during the preschool years: *the preconceptual phase* and the *intuitive thought phase.*

It's all about me!

The preconceptual phase, from ages 2 to 4, begins in the toddler stage and extends into the preschool stage. During this phase, the child is able to:
• form beginning concepts that aren't as complete or logical as an adult's are
• make simple classifications
• rationalize specific concepts but not the idea as a whole
• exhibit *egocentric thinking* (evaluating each situation based on his feelings or experiences, rather than the feelings of others).

Call it children's intuition

The *intuitive thought phase* begins at age 4 and extends into school age (age 7). During this phase, the child:
• can classify, quantify, and relate objects (but can't yet understand the principles behind these operations)
• uses intuitive thought processes (but isn't able to fully see the viewpoints of others)
• uses many words appropriately (but without true understanding of their meaning).

Moral and spiritual development

Kohlberg's *preconventional phase* of moral development spans the preschool and school age stages, extending from ages 4 to 10. During this phase:
• Conscience emerges and emphasis is on external control.
• The preschooler's moral standards are those of others, and he understands that these standards must be followed to avoid punishment for inappropriate behavior or gain rewards for good or desired behavior.
• The preschooler behaves according to what freedom is given or what restriction is placed on his actions.
• Children ages 4 to 7 are more focused on meeting their own personal needs than on the desires of others.

Spirituality

Children learn about faith and religion from significant people in their lives, such as their parents or religious teachers.

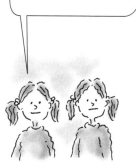

Today I learned a moral standard. It's wrong to put your sister's head in the toilet because your mom won't let you watch TV for a whole week if you do.

Friends at the top

Although preschoolers can imagine the physical characteristics of a supreme being, they commonly treat Him as an imaginary friend. They can understand the basic plot of simple religious stories but typically don't grasp the underlying meanings. Religious principles are best learned from concrete images in picture books and small statues such as those seen at a place of worship.

During this stage, children may view an illness or hospitalization as a punishment for some real or perceived bad behavior.

Keys to health

Guidelines for nutrition, sleep, and dental hygiene should be followed in order to maintain a preschooler's good health.

Nutrition

The daily caloric requirement for preschoolers is 85 to 90 kcal/kg/day or about 1,700 to 1,800 calories per day. Daily fluid intake should average 100 ml/kg, depending on the preschooler's activity level.

Make pleasant conversation

By age 5, the focus on the "social" aspects of eating can begin. Parents should encourage table conversation, good table manners, and a willingness to try a variety of foods. Preschoolers are old enough to help with meal preparation and cleanup and usually enjoy doing so.

No food fights

Parents should be discouraged from using food as a bribe, reward, or threat, which can set the stage for unhealthy attitudes about food and eating.

Food preferences

Many 3- to 4-year-olds have strong taste preferences. The child may want to eat only one thing, or a narrow range of foods, over and over. Emphasis should be placed on the quality of the food eaten rather than the quantity to prevent emotional struggles over food.

To promote healthy eating habits, parents should encourage the child to eat fruits and vegetables (raw are usually preferred over cooked).

Sleep and rest

By the time a child reaches the preschool stage, sleep patterns have been established (during toddlerhood). Normal sleep patterns for preschoolers consist of 10 to 12 hours at night and, if not already stopped at age 3, one daytime nap or rest period.

Monsters under the bed

Despite these well-established patterns, sleep-related problems may reappear during preschool years, including:
• Dreams and nightmares become more real as magical thinking increases and a vivid imagination develops.
• Problems falling asleep may occur due to overstimulation, separation anxiety, fear of the dark or monsters, or use of medications such as stimulants.
• Nighttime waking may occur due to nightmares and night terrors as well as the child's inability to soothe and comfort himself.
• Sleepwalking may occur if the child hasn't had enough sleep or is experiencing unusual stress.

Dental hygiene

Preschoolers have developed the fine motor skills needed to use a toothbrush properly and should be encouraged to brush two to three times daily. Parents should still supervise the child's brushing (assisting, as necessary) and perform flossing. As in toddlerhood, cariogenic foods should be avoided.

The preschool years are an excellent time to encourage good dental hygiene habits. Parents should administer fluoride supplements if the water supply isn't fluoridated. In addition, they should schedule a first dental visit so the child can become comfortable with the routine of preventive dental care. The child should then visit the dentist at 6- to 12-month intervals.

Coping with concerns

Parents may be concerned about their preschoolers in the areas of discipline and fears. They may also have concerns about their child's readiness to start formal schooling.

Discipline

Parents commonly have questions about how best to discipline young children. Here are some pointers about appropriate methods of discipline:
• Authority figures should administer discipline firmly, consistently, and fairly.

- The child should be given simple explanations about why a certain behavior isn't appropriate.
- Time-outs (generally 1 minute per year of age) can be used to help the child relieve intensity, regain control, and think about his inappropriate behavior.
- Discipline shouldn't be confused with punishment. Discipline refers to the process of managing behaviors—good and bad—to achieve desired outcomes. Punishment is a single action taken in response to a specific behavior.

Fears

Children experience more fears during the preschool years than at any other time. Common fears include:

- the dark
- ghosts
- being left alone
- animals (particularly large dogs)
- body mutilation, blood oozing out of cuts (children consider bandages very important to keep body contents inside)
- pain and objects or persons associated with painful experiences.

Preschoolers are commonly afraid of large animals.

Who you gonna call? Ghostbusters!

No amount of logical persuasion will help allay these fears, which leaves many parents perplexed about how to help. Parents can help their child overcome his fears by:

- actively involving him in finding practical solutions to dealing with his fears, such as using a night-light and keeping the closet door open or closed (to keep monsters under control)
- desensitizing the child to the object of his fear by exposing him to the object in a safe situation (for example, allowing him to watch a large dog interact with children who aren't fearful but never forcing him to approach or touch one unless he's ready)
- giving it time (by age 5 or 6, most children will have overcome these types of fears).

Preschool and kindergarten readiness

Factors to consider when assessing for preschool readiness include:

- visual, perceptual, cognitive, social, and behavioral abilities (such as gross and fine motor skills, visual processing, spatial-body awareness, auditory language, memory, general knowledge,

It's all relative

Selecting an appropriate preschool

Criteria to consider when selecting a preschool include accreditation, daily activity schedule, teacher qualifications, overall environment, and parent recommendations.

Accreditation
• Is the preschool up-to-date with its state license?
• Does the National Association for the Education of Young Children accredit the preschool?
• Does the preschool clearly define its goals and philosophy of teaching?

Daily activity schedule
• Does your child prefer to play outdoors or indoors?
• Are plenty of rest periods or quiet activities scheduled throughout the day?
• Are the children stimulated by a variety of activities or are they easily distracted by visitors because of boredom?
• Are the children encouraged to express themselves individually?
• Are nutritionally balanced snacks and meals provided?

Teacher qualifications
• Are the teachers trained in early childhood development?
• Is there a high staff turnover rate?
• Do the teachers appear friendly and approachable?
• Are the teachers actively engaged with the children or are they passively supervising?

Environment
• Does an adult always supervise the children?
• Will your child work well with the noise level in the preschool?
• Is the preschool clean, and are good sanitary habits practiced there?
• Are emergency plans in place and updated regularly in the event of a fire, medical emergency, or other crisis?

Parent recommendations
• What are the opinions of other parents whose children attend the preschool?
• Have other parents expressed concerns or reported problems with the preschool?

cognitive development, temperament, attention-activity, and social readiness)
• physical, sensory, mental, or emotional handicaps. (See *Selecting an appropriate preschool.*)

Kindergarten
In general, a child is ready for kindergarten when he:
• can dress himself (except for tying shoes)
• can copy a square
• can count six objects when asked "How many?"
• knows the letters of the alphabet and can count to 20
• can answer simple questions such as "What's a table made of?"
• can manage his emotions and behavior when away from home

• can control his own behavior by using words to solve problems (instead of fists or feet) and learns that better results come from talking than hitting
• has sufficient language and listening skills, such as speaking in full sentences, using correct language with ease, and defining objects by their use
• can verbally communicate his needs, wants, and thoughts
• can follow simple directions
• can work independently
• can approach new activities with enthusiasm
• can take turns and share.

Injury prevention

Injuries are the number one cause of death in toddler and preschool age-groups. For this reason, much emphasis should be placed on injury prevention and safety awareness.

Aspiration

Aspiration can easily occur in toddlers because they're still exploring their environments with their mouths. Toddlers may ingest small objects, while the small size of their oral cavities increases the risk of aspiration while eating. Preventive measures include:
• learning the Heimlich maneuver (making sure the maneuver is age-appropriate)
• avoiding large, round chunks of meat such as hot dogs (slicing them into short, lengthwise pieces is a safer option)
• avoiding fruit with pits, fish with bones, hard candy, chewing gum, nuts, popcorn, whole grapes, and marshmallows
• keeping easily aspirated objects out of a toddler's environment
• being especially cautious about what toys the child plays with (choosing sturdy toys without small, removable parts). (See *Aspiration risks*.)

Burns

Burns can easily occur in toddlers and preschoolers because they're tall enough to reach the stovetop and can walk to a fireplace or a woodstove to touch.

Hot stuff

Preventive measures include:
• setting the hot water heater thermostat at a temperature less than 120° F (49° C)

It's all relative

Aspiration risks

Toddlers explore their environment by putting things in their mouths. Foods and other items that can place a toddler at risk for aspiration include:
• small foods, such as popcorn, peanuts, whole grapes, cherry tomatoes, chunks of hot dogs, raw carrots, hard candy, bubble gum, long noodles, dried beans, and marshmallows
• small toys, such as broken latex balloons, button eyes, beaded necklaces, and small wheels
• common household items, such as broken zippers, pills, bottle caps, and nails and screws.

- checking bath water temperature before a child enters the tub
- keeping pot handles turned inward and using the back burners on stovetop
- keeping electric appliances toward the backs of counters
- placing burning candles, incense, hot foods, and cigarettes out of reach
- avoiding the use of tablecloths so the curious toddler doesn't pull it to see what's on the table (possibly spilling hot foods or liquids on himself)

> If it's too hot for you, it's too hot for the child. Always check the temperature before putting the child in the tub.

Hot potato

- teaching the child what "hot" means and stressing the danger of open flames
- storing matches and cigarette lighters in locked cabinets, out of reach
- burning fires in fireplaces or wood stoves with close supervision and using a fire screen when doing so
- securing safety plugs in all unused electrical outlets and keeping electrical cords tucked out of reach
- teaching preschoolers who can understand the hazards of fire to "stop, drop, and roll" if his clothes are on fire

The great escape

- practicing escapes from home and school with preschoolers
- visiting a fire station to reinforce learning
- teaching preschoolers how to call 911 (for emergency use only)

Drowning

Toddlers and preschoolers are quite susceptible to drowning because they can walk onto docks or pool decks and stand or climb on seats in a boat. Drowning can also occur in mere inches of water, resulting from falls into buckets, bathtubs, hot tubs, toilets, and even fish tanks.

Water, water, everywhere

Preventive measures include:
- close adult supervision of any child near water, including bathtubs and toilets
- teaching children never to go into water without an adult and never to horseplay near the water's edge
- using child-resistant pool covers and fences with self-closing gates around backyard pools

Memory jogger

Remember tips on preventing drowning when you think of the word WATER.

Wear life jackets
Adult supervision
Teach water safety
Empty buckets
Reinforce safety with pool covers

• emptying buckets when not in use and storing them upside down
• using U.S. Coast Guard–approved child life jackets near water and on boats.

> *If parents make a fashion statement by wearing their life jackets, their child will follow suit.*

Falls

Falls can easily occur as gross motor skills improve and the toddler and preschooler are able to move chairs to climb onto counters, climb ladders, and open windows.

Movin' on up

Preventive measures include:
• providing close supervision at all times during play
• keeping crib rails up and the mattress at the lowest position
• placing gates across the tops and bottoms of stairways
• installing window locks on all windows to keep them from opening more than 3.5″ (7.6 cm) without adult supervision
• keeping doors locked or using childproof doorknob covers at entries to stairs, high porches or decks, and laundry chutes
• removing unsecured scatter rugs
• using a nonskid bath mat or decals in bathtub or shower
• avoiding the use of walkers, especially near stairs
• always restraining children in shopping carts and never leaving them unattended
• providing safe climbing toys and choosing play areas with soft ground cover and safe equipment
• teaching the difference between acceptable and unacceptable places for climbing.

Motor vehicle and bicycle injuries

Motor vehicle and bicycle injuries can easily occur in toddlers and preschoolers because they may be able to unbuckle seat belts, resist riding in a car seat, or refuse to wear a bicycle helmet.

Look both ways

Preventive measures include:
• educating parents about the proper fit and use of bicycle helmets and requiring the child to wear a helmet every time he rides a bicycle

It's all relative

Car safety seat guidelines

Proper installation and use of a car safety seat are critical. In addition to the weight and age guidelines outlined in the chart below, these guidelines for booster seat use will help ensure a child's safety while riding in a vehicle:

• Always make sure belt-positioning booster seats are used with both lap and shoulder belts.

• Make sure the lap belt fits low and right across the lap/upper thigh area and the shoulder belt fits snug, crossing the chest and shoulder to avoid abdominal injuries.

• All children younger than age 12 should ride in the back seat.

Weight and age	Seat type	Seat position
Up to 2 years or 20 lb	Infant-only or rear-facing convertible	Rear-facing
Up to 2 years and over 20 lb	Rear-facing convertible	Rear-facing
Over 2 years and 20 to 40 lb	Rear-facing convertible (until meeting seat manufacturer's limit for maximum weight and height), then forward-facing	Forward-facing with harness, placed in back seat
4 to 8 years and over 40 lb	Belt-positioning booster seat	Forward-facing

• teaching the preschooler never to go into a road without an adult
• not allowing a child to play on a curb or behind a parked car
• checking the area behind vehicles before backing out of the driveway (small children may not be visible in rearview mirrors because of blind spots, especially in larger vehicles)
• providing a safe, preferably enclosed, area for outdoor play (and keeping fences, gates, and doors locked)
• educating parents on the use of child safety seats for all motor vehicle trips and ensuring proper use by having the seats inspected (many local fire departments offer free inspections). (See *Car safety seat guidelines.*)

Poisoning

As a toddler's gross motor skills improve, he's able to climb onto chairs and reach cabinets where medicines, cosmetics, cleaning products, and other poisonous substances are stored.

Please don't eat the daisies

Preventive measures include:
• keeping medicines and other toxic materials locked away in high cupboards, boxes, or drawers
• using child-resistant containers and cupboard safety latches
• not storing a large supply of toxic agents
• teaching that medication is not a candy or treat (even though it might taste good)
• teaching the child that plants outside aren't edible and keeping houseplants (also explained as inedible) out of reach
• promptly discarding empty poison containers and never reusing them to store a food item or other poison
• always keeping original labels on containers of toxic substances
• having the poison control center number (1-800-222-1222) prominently displayed on every telephone, including cell phones.

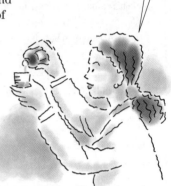

It's a dilemma. Medicines need to taste good so children will take them, but children need to learn that medicines aren't treats, no matter how good they taste.

Suffocation

Suffocation can easily occur in toddlers and preschoolers exposed to objects that can occlude the airway. A child may place such an object over his head or get tangled in an object such as a cord or string. Suffocation can also occur if a child becomes enclosed in a small space with a limited oxygen supply.

Preventive measures are extremely important and include:
• storing plastic bags, latex balloons, strings, and ribbons out of the child's reach
• never allowing the child to play with latex balloons, which can burst into small pieces that can be easily aspirated (supervised play with Mylar balloons is acceptable)
• keeping strings and cords (such as those on hooded clothing or window coverings) out of the child's reach
• discarding old appliances, such as refrigerators and ovens, or removing the doors from old appliances that must be stored (to prevent a child from becoming trapped)
• choosing safe toy boxes or chests without heavy, hinged lids.

Health problems

Toddlers and preschoolers may suffer from a range of health problems, including lead poisoning. Unfortunately, they may also be subjected to neglect and abuse.

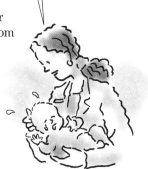

A delay in bonding, for whatever reason, may create a risk for abuse.

Child abuse and neglect

Child abuse and neglect can occur as acts of commission or omission by a caregiver. These acts can prevent children from actualizing their potential for growth and development.

What causes it

Risk factors that may predispose a child to abuse or neglect may involve the parent or the child.

Vicious cycle

Risk factors involving the parent include:
- history of being abused as a child
- substance abuse
- low self-esteem
- difficulty controlling aggressive impulses
- being a domestic violence victim or abuser
- youth or inexperience
- having limited support
- having unrealistic expectations of the child
- being overly demanding or overprotective.

It was an accident

Risk factors involving the child include:
- being unresponsive or overactive
- having frequent accidents, illnesses, or slow recovery from illness
- being excessively negative
- being born prematurely.
   Other risk factors include a history of abuse of the child's siblings and stressful environmental factors, such as divorce, poverty, unemployment, and inadequate housing.

How it happens

Child abuse is a widespread problem and is part of a larger problem of violence. Many children die each day as a result of maltreatment:
- Approximately 35% of all child abuse cases involve parental substance abuse.

• One of every four parents who grew up in a violent home goes on to seriously injure a child.
• As domestic violence rates increase, the number of children who suffer from abuse will likely increase as well (children of battered women are at higher risk for abuse than other children).
• Many child abusers were abused as children and may not know healthier ways to discipline a child or to show love.

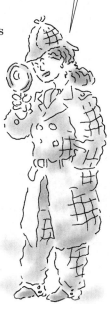

Every finding is a clue when you suspect abuse.

It's the law

If abuse is suspected, health care providers, including doctors, nurses, and dentists, are legally required to report their suspicions to Child Protective Services.

What to look for

Physical indicators of abuse and neglect include:
• unexplained fractures (children younger than walking age rarely have fractures because their bones are still pliable)
• bruises with specific patterns, over soft tissue areas, back, or genitals, in various stages of healing (because bruising caused by accidents most commonly occurs over bony prominences in children)
• bald spots (however, most infants normally have a bald spot over the occipital prominence of the skull since the inception of the "Back to Sleep" campaign to prevent sudden infant death syndrome [SIDS])
• welts from belt buckles or other distinctive instruments
• cigarette burns as well as "glove-," "sock-," or doughnut-shaped burns from dipping extremities in hot water or holding a child's bottom in hot water
• human bite marks larger than 1″ (2.5 cm) (because they would not likely come from another child at that size)
• retinal hemorrhages indicating shaken baby syndrome (different from scleral hemorrhages)
• inappropriate dress, poor hygiene, or untreated medical needs
• failure to thrive.

Acting it out

Behavioral indicators include:
• withdrawn, passive, apathetic, or depressed moods
• habit-related disorders such as excessive sucking or rocking.

When things don't add up

Other findings include:
• conflicting reports from caregiver and child about how injuries occurred

- inappropriate delay in seeking treatment for injuries
- inconsistency between the history of the injury and the child's developmental level
- inappropriate response of the child to the injuries.

What tests tell you

There's no definitive test to detect child abuse or negligence. However, many laboratory tests and X-rays may be indicated, such as:
- hemoglobin and lead levels, because children who have been abused may not have had routine health care and are at higher risk for anemia and lead poisoning
- complete blood count to rule out any blood disorders
- laboratory studies to rule out sexually transmitted diseases whenever sexual abuse is suspected
- radiographic studies to diagnose suspicious injury or trauma
- skeletal X-ray survey to examine the entire body for evidence of fractures occurring at various times with various levels of healing. (X-rays may indicate previous nonaccidental trauma that is ongoing and predates the incident that brought the child to the health care provider's attention.)

Calling in the cavalry

Child Protective Services should be contacted to document the suspected injuries. When visible lesions are present, color photographs should be taken and the image should include:
- ruler for accurate measurement
- name of child
- name of person taking photo
- written description of lesion.

Complications

Complications of child abuse and neglect come in various forms depending on severity. Children can suffer a wide range of physical complications and lasting emotional effects.

How it's treated

Child abuse is treated by first identifying it as a problem. After the injury is treated, the child's safety must be ensured if there's any suspicion of abuse or violence.

What to do

The nurse should always be assessing children and care providers for potential domestic violence. In individual instances:
- Complete a thorough assessment of all body systems while comforting and reassuring the child to the extent possible.

• Carefully assess the child's emotional status.
• Document history and assessment objectively and with clear descriptions.
• Report suspected cases to Child Protective Services following the protocols of your facility (all health care providers are mandated reporters).
• Notify the parent that you're required by law to report your concerns and assessments.

The "A" team

• Collaborate with the multidisciplinary health care team about immediate and long-term interventions to prevent further abuse.
• Work with the caregiver on changing the situation that led to the abuse and refer him or her to an agency or program that specializes in working with similar families.
• Teach the parents relevant child development principles, give them anticipatory guidance, and serve as their role model.
• Provide the child with positive attention and age-appropriate play activities.
• Reassure the child that nothing that happened was his fault and that you're there to help, not hurt him.

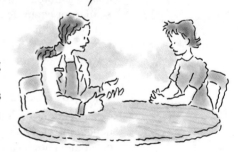

I need to take a thorough history of your child to assess for lead poisoning.

Lead poisoning

Lead poisoning, or *plumbism*, is a toxic condition that's caused by ingestion or inhalation of lead or lead-containing compounds. Children at risk for lead poisoning are those between the ages of 6 months and 6 years; the incidence peaks from ages 2 to 3.

What causes it

Lead poisoning can result from:
• chronic ingestion of lead-based paint, dust, or caulking chips in older homes
• ingestion of particles that fall from work clothes of parents who have at-risk jobs, such as those in construction, lead smelting, or ceramic and stained glass making
• inhalation of fumes from leaded gasoline or batteries
• use of unglazed pottery or ceramics
• drinking water from older, lead-containing plumbing
• certain folk remedies
• deficient parental interaction and supervision, such as insufficient feeding and poor hygiene practices.

How it happens

Children can ingest lead from numerous sources within the environment. Poisoning can occur from repeated exposure over a period of time, with toxic effects generally seen when more than 0.5 mg of lead is absorbed daily. Occasionally, a child may ingest large amounts of lead at one time by swallowing something that contains lead or being given a large dose of lead such as that found in a traditional Mexican folk remedy (azarcon [lead tetroxide]). Venous blood lead levels are used to gauge the severity of the lead poisoning.

What to look for

Risk screening for lead poisoning should begin at age 6 months, with a verbal risk assessment performed at every well-child visit until age 6. Children should receive a capillary fingerstick to screen for elevated blood lead levels at ages 1 and 2 years (and beyond if at risk for lead poisoning).

A little snooping

Ask questions about the child's exposure to well water, the proximity of the residence to major highways, the parents' occupations and hobbies, and whether and how often folk remedies are used.

Casting judgment

During the assessment, care should be taken not to judge or blame parents who may already be feeling guilty or even fearful that their children might be removed from their home.

Clinical assessment

In addition to the verbal assessment for risk of environmental exposure, the child should be assessed for symptoms of lead ingestion, including:
• failure to gain weight
• developmental lags
• behavioral changes, such as *pica* (ingestion of nonedible substances), lethargy, and decreased interest in surroundings
• vague symptoms that come and go, including weakness; irritability; weight loss; vomiting; personality changes; constipation; headache; and colicky, abdominal pain.

What tests tell you

A child with a blood lead level greater than 5 mcg/dl requires intervention such as parental education and an environmental assessment for the source of the lead exposure.

Complications

Complications include learning disabilities, such as language and speech impairments; behavioral problems, such as aggression and restlessness; and, at high levels, seizures, coma, and even death.

How it's treated

Treatment goals include separating the child from the lead source and reducing the blood lead levels.

Chelation 'til completion

For children with venous blood levels of 45 mcg/dl or higher, pharmacologic treatment is necessary. Pharmacologic treatment consists of chelation therapy to remove lead from the circulating blood.

Chelation therapy involves the administration of chelating agents such as succimer (Chemet) or dimercaprol (BAL in Oil). These agents bind with the lead and excrete it from the body. (As it's removed from the blood, lead is released from the organs to establish a new equilibrium with the blood lead level.)

Chelation therapy should be used for children with levels of 45 mcg of lead per deciliter of blood or above.

What to do

- Administer chelating medication as ordered.
- Teach parents how to eliminate sources of lead from the child's environment and to discourage children from eating dirt or paint chips.
- Encourage good nutrition because this will reduce the chances of lead absorption.
- Instruct parents on medication administration and age-appropriate growth and developmental needs (assist with referrals for developmental programs as appropriate).

In addition, provide parents with these prevention tips:
- Allow tap water to run for 2 minutes before using it for drinking, cooking, or mixing formula.
- Don't store food in an open can nor use cookware or ceramic dishes that may contain lead.
- Teach the child to carefully wash his hands with hot, soapy water before eating.

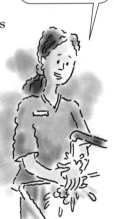

I always wash my hands before chow time!

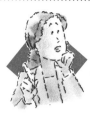

Quick quiz

1. What Erikson psychosocial stage do toddlers try to master?
   A. Trust versus mistrust
   B. Autonomy versus doubt and shame
   C. Initiative versus guilt
   D. Industry versus inferiority

Answer: B. According to Erikson's developmental theory, *autonomy versus doubt and shame* is the developmental task of toddlerhood.

2. At mealtime, a toddler:
   A. generally tries a variety of different foods willingly.
   B. should only eat commercially prepared, pureed baby food.
   C. can sit in his high chair for long periods of time.
   D. should be served approximately 1 T of food per year of life.

Answer: D. Serving size should be approximately 1 T of solid food per year of age (or one-fourth to one-third the adult portion size) so the child isn't overwhelmed with larger portions.

3. What's the average weight and height for a preschooler?
   A. 8 lb and 21″
   B. 18 lb and 26″
   C. 32 lb and 37″
   D. 54 lb and 45″

Answer: C. The average weight and height of a preschooler is 32 lb and 37″.

4. When a toddler is playing, he'll most likely:
   A. play with similar objects near, rather than with, another child.
   B. become more interactive with children around him.
   C. willingly share his toys with other children.
   D. play with one toy for a while because of his long attention span.

Answer: A. During the toddler stage, children typically play with others without actually interacting. In this type of *parallel play,* children play side-by-side, usually with similar objects.

5.   To help prevent aspiration of foods, toddlers and preschoolers should avoid which types of food?

A.   Small pieces of cooked, lean meat
B.   Round chunks of meat such as hot dogs
C.   Cooked vegetables, such as lima beans and corn
D.   Frozen desserts such as ice cream

Answer: B. To help prevent aspiration, avoiding large, round chunks of meat such as hot dogs is advisable. (Slicing them into short, lengthwise pieces is a safer option.)

Scoring

☆☆☆   If you answered all five items correctly, hooray! You've mastered the tasks of early childhood.

☆☆   If you answered three or four items correctly, yippee! Buy yourself a new toy and read on.

☆   If you answered fewer than three items correctly, don't have a tantrum! Take a nap and give it another try.

5

Middle childhood and adolescence

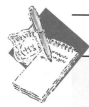

Just the facts

In this chapter, you'll learn:

♦ physical, psychosocial, cognitive, and moral development of school-age children and adolescents

♦ keys to health maintenance in middle childhood and adolescence

♦ common concerns of school-age children and adolescents and their parents

♦ injury prevention for school-age children and adolescents

♦ common health problems during middle childhood and adolescence.

School can be joyful and yet physically and psychologically challenging.

School age

School age, or *middle childhood*, refers to the stage of a child's life from ages 6 to 12. The school-age years can be a spectacular journey filled with joys and successes as the child continues to grow and mature.

They can also be marked by challenges, as the child struggles to make sense of physical and psychological changes, his emerging identity, and the way he sees himself and is viewed by others (especially his peers).

Physical development

Physical growth at this time in a child's life is relatively slow and smooth.

Height and weight

Growth slows considerably during middle childhood. During this stage, height increases an average of 2″ (5 cm) per year, and weight increases an average of 6 lb (2.5 kg) per year. However, during this time, the typical school-age child slims down and becomes more agile and graceful.

Ladies first

Girls tend to develop slightly faster than boys; although boys are, on average, taller and heavier than girls until the adolescent growth spurt.

> Physical growth is slower during school age, but grace and agility make a stellar appearance.

Fine motor skills

By age 7, the brain has nearly completed its growth (at approximately 90%) and basic neuromuscular mechanisms are in place.

No more excuses

Development of small-muscle and eye-hand coordination increases, leading to the skilled handling of tools, such as pencils and papers for drawing and writing. The child can then spend the remainder of this period refining physical and motor skills and coordination.

Pubertal changes

The pubertal growth spurt begins in girls at about age 10 and in boys at about age 12.

Jumpin' in feet first

Different areas of the body reach their peak growth at different times. Changes are easily recognized in the feet, which are the first part of the body to experience a growth spurt. Increased foot size is followed by a rapid increase in leg length and then trunk growth.

> My friends may call me Big foot today, but they'll call me a star when my legs hit their peak growth and it's nothing but net!

Leggy and hippy

During this time, leg growth increases more dramatically than trunk growth in boys. In addition, although girls have a greater growth spurt in hip width, boys exceed girls in other areas of bone growth.

No turning back

In addition to bones, gonadal hormone levels increase and cause the sexual organs to mature.

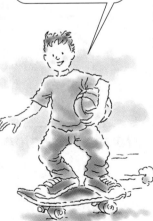

Preparation for menses

In girls, the first menstruation, called *menarche*, usually starts around age 12 but can occur as early as age 9 and still be considered normal. The menstrual cycle may be irregular at first.

Secondary sexual characteristics may start to develop—including breasts, hips, and pubic hair—and girls may experience a sudden increase in height. Nurses may find that this provides an excellent opportunity to educate school-age girls about breast self-examination and sexual responsibility.

Teeth

Loss of primary teeth and eruption of the first secondary teeth occur during the school-age years. Because of their size, secondary teeth may, for a while, appear disproportionately large in relation to the child's other, smaller facial features.

Psychological development

Attending school marks an acceleration in the separation of the child from his parents. It introduces the child to a new set of authority figures (teachers, school administrators) and strengthens the concept of peer relationships.

Psychosocial development

The school-age child enters Erikson's stage of industry versus inferiority. In this stage, the child wants to work and produce, accomplishing and achieving tasks. However, if too much is expected of him, or if he feels unable to measure up to set standards, the negative attributes of inadequacy and inferiority may prevail.

Language development and socialization

The school-age child has an efficient vocabulary and begins to correct previous mistakes in usage. He begins to understand the double meanings of words and becomes proficient at giving others directions without using physical signals.

Pick a clique

In the first and second grades, peers are increasingly significant to the child. His need to find his place within a group becomes important.

Same-sex cliques are established during this period, and competition becomes more common, as does bragging over accomplishments. The child may be overly concerned with peer rules;

however, parental guidance continues to play an important role in the child's life.

Handle with care: Sensitive to ridicule

The child's world expands as interests and activities outside the home take on an expanded role in his life. He's more independent, inside and outside the home. He understands the reasons for rules and becomes more sensitive to criticism and ridicule.

Play

The child's personality has become structured, and he's ready to be a partner in play with his friends. The child in this age-group typically has two to three best friends, who may change frequently. Most of his energies are devoted to school and his friends.

Cognitive development

School and learning are viewed by the school-age child as an exciting experience. The major developmental tasks at this time are achievement in school and acceptance by peers. Expectations in the classroom have intensified, and require concentration, attendance, and complex auditory and visual processing.

The school-age child is in Piaget's concrete-operational period, a time in which the child uses thought processes to experience and understand events and actions. Children at this age are less egocentric and can see things from another's point of view.

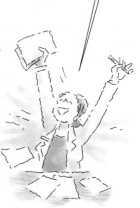

A school-age child's enthusiasm for learning is contagious!

Try to remember

Reorganization of the *frontal brain*, which is used for selective attention, occurs between ages 5 and 7. The ability to reason and memorize improves, and the child tends to use mnemonic strategies to remember new information. In addition, the following occurs:

• Magical thinking diminishes around this time, and the child has a much better understanding of cause and effect.

• The child begins to accept rules but may not necessarily understand them.

• Memory skills are continually improving, along with an increased attention span. The child is ready for basic reading, writing, and arithmetic.

• Abstract thinking begins to develop during the middle elementary school years.

• Parents remain very important during this time. Adult reassurance of the child's competence and basic self-worth is essential.

Moral and spiritual development

In general, the first level of moral thinking is put into practice at the elementary school level, and the school-age child is in Kohlberg's conventional level. The child behaves according to socially acceptable norms because an authority figure tells him to do so. This obedience is compelled by the threat of punishment (external factors).

"Because I said so"

At ages 11 to 12, as the child begins to approach adolescence, school and parental authority is questioned and, occasionally, even challenged or opposed. The importance of the peer group intensifies, and rough, bold, or even brazen behavior becomes increasingly common. The peer group becomes the source of behavior standards and models.

Mom's still the bomb

Parental guidance, love, and support are absolutely essential for the development of values during this time. The child at this age needs the opportunity to make decisions within defined boundaries. Ideally, those boundaries are set by responsible adults in the child's life.

Earth-bound

Spiritual lessons should be taught in concrete terms during this stage. Children have a hard time understanding supernatural religious symbols. Repeated religious rituals, such as praying and attending church services, may comfort them.

Keys to health

During the school-age years, the child's understanding of cause and effect, coupled with his need for parental (and peer) approval, provides an excellent opportunity to continue teaching about the need to make healthy lifestyle choices. Parents should continue to teach their children about the importance of:
• proper nutrition
• sleep and rest
• exercise
• dental hygiene.

Nutrition

Children should be encouraged to eat a variety of healthy foods, such as lean meats, fruits, vegetables, and grains, to ensure proper nutritional intake.

Memory jogger

When it comes to teaching children about being healthy, tell parents to remember these things to care for their PEDS:

Proper nutrition

Exercise

Dental hygiene

Sleep.

Developing healthy eating habits

Encouraging healthy eating habits now (during school age and, ideally, before) will lay a stable foundation for adolescence, when caloric needs increase. Childhood obesity is increasing, and measures should be taken to avoid high-fat, high-sugar, low-protein foods. (See *Encouraging proper nutrition.*)

Sleep and rest

Requirements for sleep and rest are unique and relate to the child's activity level and physical health. School-age children generally don't require an afternoon nap, and compliance at bedtime becomes easier. Children should develop healthy sleep habits by not having a television in their bedrooms.

Things that go bump in the night

Sleepwalking and sleeptalking may begin during this stage, and parents should take measures to ensure the child's physical safety during these episodes. Nightmares are usually related to a real event in the child's life and can usually be eradicated by resolving any underlying fears the child might have.

Exercise and activity

Exercise and other forms of physical activity should be encouraged to help the child begin healthy habits for a lifetime. Doing so may also prevent childhood obesity.

Children who are interested in sports should be encouraged to join sport teams or participate in sporting events. Sport teams and events are usually same-sex events at this age level, making them less intimidating. Those who aren't interested in team sports and whose family are unable to meet the time or financial demands should be encouraged to participate in regular family play, walks, or bike rides. Children should learn the importance of daily activity, and parents should limit sedentary activities such as playing video games.

Clicking the remote doesn't count

Parents should encourage physical exercise after school instead of more sedentary activities such as watching television or playing video games.

Dental hygiene

During the school-age years:
• Teeth should be brushed at least twice a day and, if possible, after meals.
• Drinking water should contain fluoride or fluoride supplements should be given.

It's all relative

Encouraging proper nutrition

To ensure that children continue to develop and maintain healthy eating habits, encourage parents to:

• stock the pantry and refrigerator with healthy choices for after-school snacks (raw vegetables, low-fat yogurts, fresh fruits)
• avoid taking children to fast-food establishments where high-fat foods are abundant
• teach children how to read nutrition labels while shopping at the grocery store
• involve children in planning and preparing meals for the family
• offer candy and other sweets as an infrequent privilege rather than a reward for good behavior
• change their own eating habits to model good dietary habits for their children.

- Flossing should be taught, and parents should monitor for method and compliance until the child is 8 years old.
- Regular dental cleanings should be scheduled every 6 months.

Coping with concerns

During school age, the child's life revolves around home and family, school, and peers. School-age children (and their parents) are commonly faced with concerns about school and after-school supervision.

School phobias

School phobias may also be called *school refusal* or *school avoidance*. A child's refusal to go to school may be a sign of a separation anxiety, which occurs in families that are particularly close and caring or in a child who relies heavily on the support of his family. It may also occur after a particular trauma, such as the death of a pet, illness within the family, or a move to a new school.

In these cases, the child may be more fearful of leaving home than he is of going to school. He may, for example, be afraid that something bad will happen to a parent, sibling, or pet if he isn't there to protect them.

Scary school

Refusal to go to school may also be related to fear of the school itself and what the child experiences there. Parents should talk to their child and try to determine the underlying cause of his fear. Possible reasons for school phobias include:
- being the target of a bully
- anxiety about academic achievement
- having problems adapting to the school structure.

Stealing

Stealing is attractive to the younger school-age child who simply wants items for himself. The child has a limited sense of what belongs to someone else and will commonly lie to cover up the offense.

Low on dough

A sense of responsibility for one's actions begins to take shape at the end of middle childhood. Stealing at the end of middle childhood is commonly a sign that something is lacking in that child's life. Possible causes include a lack of:
- financial means
- attention from a parent or caregiver
- sense of property rights.

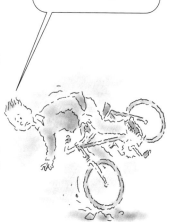

I know Mom will get upset because I'm not wearing a helmet, but at least I'm not stealing!

What's yours is mine

Parents should recognize the child's property rights and offer some privacy in this regard, when possible. A child who knows that his own property is respected is more likely to understand the importance of respecting the property of others.

Adolescence

Adolescence is defined as the developmental stage between ages 13 and 19.

Physical development

Adolescence is a time of change. As physical changes occur, adolescents struggle with the conflict between asserting their independence and still relying on their parents.

Terrible teens

Many adults view the changes that occur during adolescence with great fear and trepidation. Although not always the case, it may be a turbulent time for the adolescent and his parents.

Height and weight

During this time, a teenager's weight almost doubles and his height increases by 15% to 20%. Girls may grow 3″ to 6″ (7.5 to 15 cm) per year until age 16. Boys may grow 3″ to 6″ per year until age 18. Major organs double in size; the exception is the lymphoid tissue, which decreases in mass.

Boys attain greater strength and muscle mass, but motor coordination lags behind growth in stature and musculature. Motor coordination catches up as strength improves.

> Sure, I have the strength and the muscles—so how much longer do I have to wait for this coordination stuff?

Development of secondary sex characteristics

The pituitary gland is stimulated at puberty to produce androgen steroids responsible for secondary sex characteristics. (See *Beginning sexual maturity in girls* and *Beginning sexual maturity in boys,* page 133.)

It's a girl thing

Female secondary sexual development during puberty involves increases in the size of the ovaries, uterus, vagina, labia, and

(Text continues on page 134.)

Growing pains

Beginning sexual maturity in girls

Breast development and pubic hair growth are the first signs of sexual maturity in girls. These illustrations show the development of the female breast and pubic hair in puberty.

Breast development

Stage 1
Only the *papilla* (nipple) elevates (not shown).

Stage 2
Breast buds appear; the areola is slightly widened and appears as a small mound.

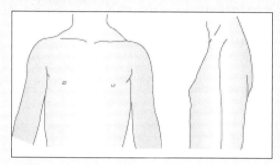

Stage 3
The entire breast enlarges; the nipple doesn't protrude.

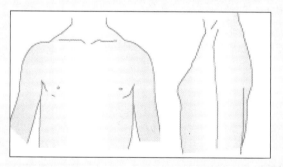

Stage 4
The breast enlarges; the nipple and the papilla protrude and appear as a secondary mound.

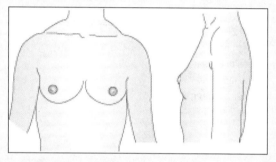

Stage 5
The adult breast has developed; the nipple protrudes and the areola no longer appears separate from the breast.

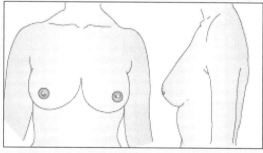

(continued)

Beginning sexual maturity in girls *(continued)*

Pubic hair development

Stage 1
No pubic hair is present.

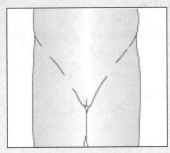

Stage 2
Straight hair begins to appear on the labia and extends between stages 2 and 3.

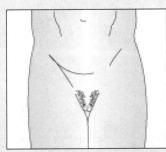

Stage 3
Pubic hair increases in quantity; it appears darker, curled, and more dense and begins to form the typical (but smaller in quantity) female triangle.

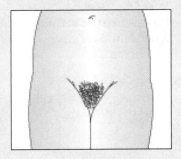

Stage 4
Pubic hair is more dense and curled; it's more adult in distribution but less abundant than in an adult.

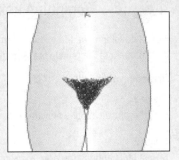

Stage 5
Pubic hair is abundant, appears in an adult female pattern, and may extend onto the medial part of the thighs.

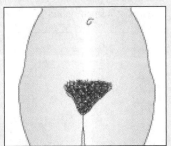

Growing pains

Beginning sexual maturity in boys

Genital development and pubic hair growth are the first signs of sexual maturity in boys. The illustrations below show the development of the male genitalia and pubic hair in puberty.

Stage 1
No pubic hair is present.

Stage 2
Downy hair develops laterally and later becomes dark; the scrotum becomes more textured, and the penis and testes may become larger.

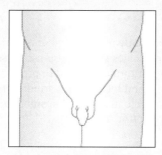

Stage 3
Pubic hair extends across the pubis; the scrotum and testes are larger; the penis enlarges in length.

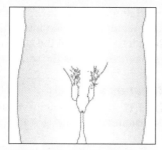

Stage 4
Pubic hair becomes more abundant and curls, and the genitalia resemble those of adults; the glans penis has become larger and broader, and the scrotum becomes darker.

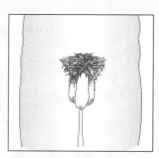

Stage 5
Pubic hair resembles an adult's in quality and pattern, and the hair extends to the inner borders of the thighs; the testes and scrotum are adult in size.

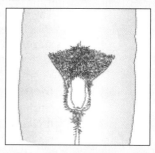

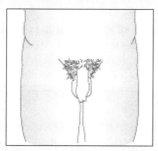

breasts. The first visible sign of sexual maturity is the appearance of breast buds. Body hair appears in the pubic area and under the arms, and menarche occurs. The ovaries, present at birth, remain inactive until puberty.

Boys will be boys . . . until they're men

Male secondary sexual development consists of genital growth and the appearance of pubic and body hair.

Androgens and estrogens

The trigger that starts puberty is unknown. What's clear is that, for some reason, the hypothalamus produces gonadotropin-releasing hormone, which triggers the anterior pituitary gland to produce follicle-stimulating hormone (FSH) and luteinizing hormone (LH). FSH and LH initiate the ovulation cycle in girls and promote testicular maturation and sperm production in boys.

Tanner staging

The development of secondary sex characteristics occurs in an anticipated sequence for girls and boys, and is divided into distinct stages, called *Tanner stages*. Although the timing of the stages is different for each individual, the sequence remains the same.

Menstruation and spermatogenesis

During early adolescence (ages 11 to 14), most girls achieve menarche. Most boys achieve active spermatogenesis at ages 12 to 15.

Teeth

The secondary (permanent) teeth are all present during the early adolescent years. The four third molars (also called *wisdom teeth*) may need to be extracted if impaction occurs.

Psychological development

Psychological development during adolescence revolves around socialization. As the teen ventures into the world outside his own family and is exposed to other viewpoints, peers become increasingly important and independence is tested.

Psychosocial development

Adolescence is the period of identity development, according to Erikson, as the child enters the stage of identity versus role confusion. Changes in the adolescent's body are taking place rapidly, and he's preoccupied with how he looks and with how others view him. While trying to meet the expectations of his peers, he's also trying to establish his own identity.

Early adolescence

During early adolescence, the teen begins to show more interest in the opposite sex, although the peer group usually consists of same-sex friends.

That's what friends are for

Friends become much more important, and interest in family and family activities decreases.

Rebel with a question

Conformity to peer group standards is of utmost importance at this time. This may lead to rebellion and questioning of parental (and other adult) authority.

Middle adolescence

The teen becomes more self-assured during middle adolescence, and independent decision-making skills are tested.

The young and the tasteless

Activities outside the home take on even greater importance, and the teenager commonly defines himself by whatever the peer group has defined. He wears what other teens in his group wear, he speaks using the common language the peer group has decided on, and his taste in music and other preferences go along with the crowd.

When girls no longer have cooties

It's at this time that relationships with the opposite sex are established.

Late adolescence

During the late teen years, adolescent rebellion has diminished. The young adult has a fairly strong sense of who he is but may not yet have committed to a particular occupation or role in life.

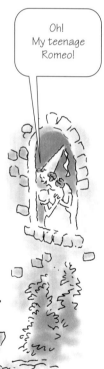

Oh! My teenage Romeo!

Cognitive development

During adolescence, the teen moves from the concrete thinking of childhood into Piaget's stage of *formal operational thought*. The teen can now reason logically about abstract concepts and derive conclusions from hypothetical premises.

I can see clearly now . . .

He can imagine events in the future instead of focusing on the present (as in childhood). Because the future becomes a possibility, the teen may be more receptive to education that focuses on health promotion and can concentrate on future benefits as a result of current behaviors.

One step forward, two steps back

Although abstract thinking becomes more refined, the teen may revert back into concrete thinking during times of stress.

Moral and spiritual development

Kohlberg's conventional level of moral development continues into early adolescence. At this level, the child does what's right because it's the socially acceptable action. At this level, the child continues to advance in moral reasoning as his cognition develops.

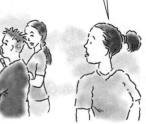

You guys go ahead—I have to do my homework. (Did I say that? It must be that postconventional level of moral development stuff.)

In with the in-crowd

The teen becomes increasingly dependent on his peer group for approval and associates good behavior with "fitting in" with the crowd. Morality may be dependent on the situation and relationship. Commonly, peer pressure will override the teen's own moral reasoning.

At long last—my own person

As adolescence ends, the teen enters Kohlberg's *postconventional*, or *principled, level of moral development*. He starts to question and discard status quo, and chooses values for himself, not necessarily what's dictated by his peers. Although he may appreciate the peer group's opinions, he's now capable of forming a moral decision independent of the group.

Hey, Dad. Can I have the car keys and $20 for gas so I can be an adult and go vote?

What's the meaning of life?

The teen formulates questions about the larger world as he considers religion, philosophy, and the values held by parents, friends, and others. Adolescents are suspicious about parental religious views, and curiosity about other religious beliefs is normal. They sort through and adopt those religious beliefs that are consistent with their moral character.

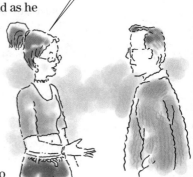

Look, Mom, I'm legal!

Their worldview becomes solidified during this time. The teen may be considered a young adult and societal laws reinforce this. By age 18, he's allowed to vote, and by age 21, he's considered a full adult with all of the rights and responsibilities that go along with that status. Even so, the adolescent remains somewhat dependent on his parents for finances and for help in meeting the adult responsibilities given to him.

Keys to health

Health issues during adolescence include nutrition, sleep and rest, exercise, and dental hygiene.

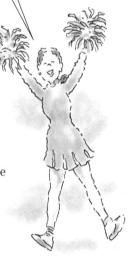

Iron, protein, keep me strong!
I hope these cramps don't last too long!

Nutrition

Because physical changes are so drastic during adolescence, nutritional needs are greater than at any other time in a person's life.

Run a little, eat a lot

Activity plays a large role in a teen's caloric requirements for maintaining weight. An active teenager playing sports for several hours per day may need in excess of 3,000 kcal per day, whereas an inactive adolescent girl may have to take in fewer than 2,000 kcal to prevent weight gain. In addition, iron and protein needs increase as girls begin the menstruation cycle and boys begin to develop lean muscle mass.

Got milk?

Because bone growth is so critical during adolescence, teens need to ensure the proper intake of calcium and vitamin D. Starting in the preteen years through adolescence, daily calcium intakes should be between 1,200 and 1,500 mg/day. To achieve adequate levels, they need to consume at least three servings of calcium-fortified foods per day. Thus, it is important for providers to ask teens if they regularly consume dairy foods or other calcium-containing foods such as broccoli, spinach, tofu, or legumes.

Teens continue to select their own meals and form food preferences, making it even more important for parents to offer nutritionally balanced snacks and meals that will become lifelong choices for teens.

Sleep and rest

Sleep requirements increase slightly from the school-age years because of physical growth spurts and high activity levels in adolescents.

Use 'em or lose 'em

Sleep needs vary from person to person, but teens require at least 8 hours of sleep each night, and those 8 hours can't be made up or stored. Therefore, "catch-up" sleep on the weekends isn't effective in replenishing a teen's sleep store.

Exercise

Physical fitness and exercise are important for several health-related reasons. With adolescent obesity on the rise in the United States, regular aerobic exercise can help maintain a healthy weight and prevent excessive gain. It also promotes a healthy cardiovascular system by reducing and preventing high blood pressure and hyperlipidemia.

Running from depression

Physical fitness may also help prevent periods of depression and help foster relationships between peers that have common sports activities.

Dental hygiene

Good dental hygiene should consist of brushing at least twice daily, flossing once daily, and professional cleanings twice per year. Teens should avoid snacks with high sucrose levels and sticky candies that could cause dental caries.

> Physical fitness helps prevent depression, high blood pressure, and parental nagging!

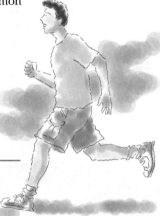

Coping with concerns

Adolescents and their parents are typically faced with a range of concerns that may be intensified by the teen's need for peer approval and his desire to assert his independence.

Acne

During adolescence, acne is caused by blockage of follicles as a result of excessive sebum or bacteria. Acne has been associated with hormones due to the prevalence of flare-ups during a girl's premenstrual period.

Acne is found primarily on the face but can also appear on the chest and back. It's usually seen by the naked eye and treated with topical agents or antibiotics for inflammatory lesions.

> Adolescent acne should be taken seriously. Sometimes, it makes me feel socially isolated and depressed.

No laughing matter

Acne can be devastating during this time of life when appearance is of the utmost concern. Even mild to moderate acne can have lasting negative effects on self-esteem and a teen's ability and willingness to develop friendships and other relationships. In severe cases, embarrassment and isolation can lead to depression.

For these reasons, acne should be considered a serious problem that warrants intervention rather than a "phase" that a teen should simply "wait to grow out of."

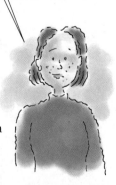

Body piercings and tattoos

Teens use body piercings and tattoos to make a "statement" about their sense of style and to express their individuality. For health reasons, such as risk of hepatitis C, piercings and tattoos should be performed by an experienced, licensed person. It's important not to pass judgment on the teen who chooses to get a tattoo or piercing. Rather, consider his choice an opportunity to provide education on the subject which, in turn, helps the teen make an informed decision.

Cigarette smoking

Cigarette smoking among teens is reaching epidemic proportions; 1 out of 4 high school seniors have smoked cigarettes in the past month; 1 out of 10 adolescent males use smokeless tobacco. According to the American Lung Association, nearly 5,000 teenagers will start smoking on any given day, with close to 2,000 of those teens becoming routine smokers.

Dangling the bait

Peer influence and family practices have a tremendous influence on teen smoking. Teens may start smoking to "look cool" or "fit in" with their peer groups, despite their knowledge of the deadly health consequences. Tobacco companies have been involved in court battles in an attempt to defend their advertising practices. Those opposing the large manufacturers claim that marketing programs unfairly target teens as potential smokers.

A slippery slope

Tobacco use can be associated with increasingly risky behaviors, such as alcohol use, drug use, and experimenting with sexual conduct. The American Lung Association has instituted a voluntary program in the public school systems that uses peer counseling to educate teens on the dangers and health consequences of smoking.

Injury prevention

When a child reaches school age, he's no longer under his parents' constant supervision. Because of this unfamiliar freedom, school-age children and adolescents can sustain a range of serious, sometimes life-threatening, injuries.

Firearms

Firearm safety is a major concern due to the teen's belief that "it won't happen to me." Their curiosity about how a gun operates could have deadly consequences. Parents should educate teens on the safe use of a firearm but always practice safe gun storage.

A loaded gun should never be stored in the home, and the ammunition and unloaded gun should be securely stored in separate areas. Parents should consider using trigger locks on their firearms.

Motor vehicle accidents

Motor vehicle accidents are one of the leading causes of death among teens. During the late teen years, the adolescent is, by law, "ready" to get a driver's license. However, with greater privilege comes increased responsibility. Nurses can prevent motor vehicle accidents through education. Teens may be reluctant to listen to their parents but may engage in a conversation with another trusted authority figure.

Will parallel parking be on the final exam?

State law requires teens to pass written and practical driving tests before being issued a temporary driver's license. Most states and some public high schools offer driver education classes as part of their curriculum. Some states have graduated drivers' licenses for new teen drivers. New drivers typically must pass through three stages in order to receive their full driver's license: obtaining a learner's permit, progression to a probationary license, and the proceeding to a full driver's license. Graduated drivers' licenses often limit nighttime, expressway, and unsupervised driving during early stages. The restrictions lift with time, concluding with the teen receiving a full driver's license.

Texting while driving

Distracted driving leads to accidents. Unfortunately, about 44% of teens 16 years old or older report texting while driving, and of these teens, they had a higher incidence of infrequent seat belt use, riding with a driver who has been drinking, and drinking and driving themselves than those teens who did not text while driving.

Buckled up for safety

A teen should be shown that wearing a seat belt, no matter what seat he's in, can drastically reduce the risk of life-threatening injuries in the event of an accident. He should also be encouraged to use a helmet when operating such motor vehicles as a motorcycle and a moped.

> Driving plus drugs or alcohol equals disaster. Sometimes, those words mean more when they come from a nurse.

A deadly mix

Perhaps the greatest emphasis should be placed on educating the adolescent about the risks of mixing driving with alcohol or drug use. Not only is the combination illegal, but it also impairs the driver's judgment and could have deadly consequences.

Risk-taking behaviors

Teenagers are still maturing, both cognitively and emotionally. A lack of maturity may lead them to take unwise chances in an attempt to be accepted by their peers.

Risky business

Teens have an "it can't happen to me" attitude and feel they're invincible. They may take risks to seek attention from others because of failures in school, rejection by peers, neglect at home, or a combination of these factors. A teen tends to be less of a risk taker if he has established autonomy and respects his parents and other authority figures.

Sports injuries

Although there's the potential for injury in any sport, most injuries occur during recreational sporting events rather than during organized competitions. Serious injuries are generally more common during recreational and individual sports.

In any case, although injuries are usually random events, the risk of injury can be decreased by improving playing conditions, demanding compliance with rules and protective equipment, and providing diligent coaching and supervision.

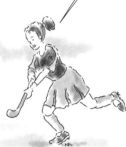

There's safety in numbers. Sports injuries are less common in team sports.

Injury protection

The nurse can help prevent sports injuries through education about safety equipment and potential risk. Teens need to be encouraged to use helmets when skateboarding or riding bicycles and snowmobiles. They should be encouraged to wear other protective equipment, such as pads and mouthguards, when playing contact sports.

Slow down, you move too fast

Because a teen's body is physically maturing, he needs to realize his own limitations to avoid straining or overextending himself until his body is more able to perform a physically challenging task. After experiencing an injury, a teen must be encouraged to follow rehabilitation instructions to prevent further injury or reinjury.

Health problems

Several serious health problems can affect school-age children and adolescents. Some of these problems may be life-threatening.

Alcohol and drug abuse

Alcoholism is a chronic disorder most commonly described as the uncontrolled intake of alcoholic beverages. *Psychoactive drug abuse and dependence* is the use of illegal drugs or misuse of legal drugs, including narcotics, stimulants, depressants, antianxiety agents, and hallucinogens. Alcoholism and drug abuse impair physical and mental health, social and familial relationships, and the ability to uphold responsibilities related to school and jobs.

It's old school

Today, children aren't waiting until college, or even high school, to take a first drink of alcohol or "experiment" with drugs. Alcohol and drugs are readily available to school-age children, making substance abuse a problem of enormous proportions.

What causes it

Numerous biological, psychological, and sociocultural factors may cause alcoholism and drug abuse. Family background may play a significant role, as the child of one alcoholic parent is seven to eight times more likely to become an alcoholic than a peer without such a parent.

> A positive adult role model is the best antidote for negative peer influences.

Psychologically speaking

Psychological factors that may cause alcohol or drug abuse may include:
• inadequate coping skills, leading to the urge to reduce anxiety and tension through the use of substances
• a desire to avoid responsibility
• an inability to deal effectively with loneliness or boredom
• a need to bolster self-esteem.

Socioculturally speaking

Sociocultural factors that may cause alcohol or drug abuse include:
• the availability of alcohol and drugs
• group or peer pressure
• societal attitudes that condone alcohol or drug use.

What to look for

Substance abuse is defined as a maladaptive pattern of substance use (drug or alcohol) leading to clinically significant impairment or distress. This impairment or distress manifests as one or more of the following (occurring within a 12-month period):
• recurrent substance use resulting in a failure to fulfill major role obligations at work, school, or home

- recurrent substance use in situations in which using the substance is physically hazardous
- recurrent substance-related legal problems
- continued substance use despite persistent or recurrent social or interpersonal problems caused by or exacerbated by the effects of the substance.

Ups and downs

Chronic substance abusers may present with a variety of minor complaints, such as mood swings and depression, malaise, and an increased incidence of infection.

Something smells fishy

The effects on personal appearance include poor personal hygiene, unexplained injuries (such as cigarette burns), and nutritional deficiencies.

I've got a secret

The teen or child may be secretive about his disorder and may engage in suspicious behaviors, such as lying and stealing money, to support his habit. The school may report multiple, unexplained absences; poor classroom performance; and behavior pattern changes. When confronted about his behavior, he may deny the problem or become angry and violent toward others.

Acute intoxication

With acute alcohol or drug intoxication, look for one or any number of the following:
- decreased inhibitions
- euphoria followed by depression or hostility
- impaired judgment
- incoordination
- respiratory depression
- slurred speech
- unconsciousness
- vomiting.

What tests tell you

Urine, blood, and saliva tests can confirm drug use and blood alcohol level, determine the amount and type of substance taken, and reveal complications.

Complications

Most body tissues can be adversely affected by the heavy intake of alcohol, and death can occur from abrupt alcohol withdrawal. (See *Complications of alcohol abuse*, page 144.)

Complications of alcohol abuse

Alcohol can damage body tissues by its direct irritating effects, changes that take place in the body during its metabolism, aggravation of existing disease, accidents occurring during intoxication, and interactions between the alcohol and drugs. Such tissue damage can lead to a range of complications, including those listed below.

Cardiopulmonary complications
- Cardiac arrhythmias
- Cardiomyopathy
- Chronic obstructive pulmonary disease
- Essential hypertension
- Increased risk of tuberculosis
- Pneumonia

Hepatic complications
- Alcoholic hepatitis
- Cirrhosis
- Fatty liver

Gastrointestinal complications
- Chronic diarrhea
- Esophageal cancer
- Esophageal varices
- Esophagitis
- Gastric ulcers
- Gastritis
- Gastrointestinal (GI) bleeding
- Malabsorption
- Pancreatitis

Neurologic complications
- Alcoholic dementia
- Alcoholic hallucinosis
- Alcohol withdrawal delirium
- Korsakoff's syndrome
- Peripheral neuropathy
- Seizure disorders
- Subdural hematoma
- Wernicke's encephalopathy

Psychiatric complications
- Amotivational syndrome
- Depression
- Impaired social and occupational functioning
- Abuse of multiple substances
- Suicide

Other complications
- Beriberi
- Hypoglycemia
- Leg and foot ulcers
- Prostatitis
- Fetal alcohol syndrome (from alcoholism while pregnant)

Chronic drug abuse, especially intravenous (I.V.) use, can lead to life-threatening complications, including:
- cardiac and respiratory arrest, subacute bacterial endocarditis, pulmonary emboli, and respiratory infections
- intracranial hemorrhage
- vasculitis, thrombophlebitis, and gangrene
- musculoskeletal dysfunction
- acquired immunodeficiency syndrome (AIDS) and hepatitis
- tetanus, septicemia, and malaria
- malnutrition
- trauma
- depression, psychosis, and increased risk of suicide.

How it's treated

Treatment for alcoholism and drug abuse must be long-term and requires the support of the child's parents and other significant people in his life.

Alcohol abuse

Total abstinence from alcohol is the only effective treatment for alcoholism. Participation in supportive programs, including Alcoholics Anonymous and Ala-Teen, may produce favorable long-term results, although failure and relapse rates are high. The recovering individual must also be able to fill the niche once occupied by alcohol with something constructive.

Symptom support

Acute intoxication is treated symptomatically by:
• supporting respiration
• preventing aspiration of vomitus
• replacing fluids
• initiating emergency treatment for trauma, infection, and GI bleeding.

Drug abuse

Treatment of drug dependence commonly involves a triad of care: detoxification, short- and long-term rehabilitation, and aftercare (meaning a lifetime of abstinence). Aftercare is usually aided by participation in Narcotics Anonymous or a similar self-help group.

Slowly but surely

The teen with acute drug intoxication should receive symptomatic treatment based on the drug ingested. Detoxification with the same drug or a pharmacologically similar drug may be necessary. Depending on the dosage and the time elapsed since ingestion, additional treatment may include gastric lavage, induced emesis, activated charcoal, or forced diuresis.

What to do

• Be alert for potential alcohol and drug abuse problems. Ask the teen about his own use of substances and about his friends' usage. Ensure confidentiality, and ask questions and provide information in a straightforward manner to promote an open discussion.
• Be aware of signs and symptoms of intoxication with alcohol and commonly used drugs so you'll be prepared to identify them if seen in a patient.
   During an acute intoxication:
• Continuously monitor the patient's vital signs.
• Observe for complications of overdose and withdrawal, such as cardiopulmonary arrest, seizures, and aspiration.

When the party's over

After an acute intoxication:
• Refer the patient for detoxification and rehabilitation as appropriate, and provide a list of available community resources, including meeting times and places for Alcoholics Anonymous and Narcotics Anonymous.
• Refer parents of a child in crisis to an organization such as Parents Anonymous.

• Monitor the patient for signs of depression or impending suicide.
• Encourage family members to seek professional help whether or not the patient does so.

> It doesn't matter how thin they say I am. There's always a fat person in my mirror.

Anorexia nervosa

Anorexia nervosa is a disorder that involves voluntary refusal to eat, accompanied by a severe loss of body weight without an organic cause. It results from a distorted, unrealistic perception of body size, weight, and food intake. It may coexist with bulimia. (See *Bulimia*.)

The skinny on being skinny

These perceptions override feelings of hunger, family members' threats or pleas to eat, and an intellectual (but not emotional) acknowledgement of the problem.

Girl power?

Although more than 90% of those with anorexia nervosa are adolescent girls and young women, the condition is

Bulimia

Bulimia is defined as regular episodes of binge eating, followed by self-induced vomiting, strict dieting or fasting, vigorous exercise, or taking laxatives or diuretics. The condition usually begins in adolescence or early childhood and may coexist with anorexia nervosa. The exact cause of bulimia is unknown.

Signs and symptoms
• Alternating episodes of binge eating and purging
• Thin or slightly overweight build
• Use of diuretics or laxatives
• Vomiting
• Reports of abdominal and epigastric pain, amenorrhea, and painless swelling of the salivary glands
• Hoarse and irritated voice
• Calluses on the knuckles from vomiting (Russell's sign)

• Anxiety and avoidance of conflict
• Extreme need for approval
• Guilt and self-disgust
• Constant preoccupation with food
• Preoccupation with exercise (and excessive exercise)

Key test findings
The Beck Depression Inventory may reveal depression; an Eating Attitudes Test (EAT) may suggest an eating disorder. Metabolic acidosis may

occur from diarrhea caused by enemas and excessive laxative use. Metabolic alkalosis (the most common metabolic complication) may occur from frequent vomiting. Laboratory tests reveal elevated bicarbonate, decreased potassium, and decreased sodium levels.

Bulimia complications
• Dental caries
• Erosion of tooth enamel and gum infections

• Increased risk of esophageal tears, gastric rupture, and mucosal damage to the intestines
• Life-threatening cardiac arrhythmias, cardiac failure, or sudden death

Treating bulimia
• Inpatient or outpatient therapy
• Self-help groups
• Selective serotonin reuptake inhibitors, such as paroxetine and fluoxetine

increasingly appearing in males and has been diagnosed in children as young as age 7.

By conservative estimates, 0.5% to 1% of females in late adolescence and early adulthood meet the diagnostic criteria. Over their entire lifetime, an estimated 0.5% to 3.75% of females will suffer from anorexia.

What causes it

The exact cause of anorexia nervosa is unknown; however, a number of external and internal influences are thought to contribute to the disorder. These influences include:
- societal attitudes that equate slimness with beauty
- excessive pressure to achieve
- dependence and independence issues
- control issues
- stress due to multiple responsibilities.

Related risks

Anorexia nervosa is a subconscious effort to exert personal control over life or to protect oneself from dealing with issues surrounding sexuality. Several risk factors have been identified, including:
- low self-esteem
- compulsive personality
- history of sexual abuse
- high, sometimes unrealistic, achievement goals (set by the person at risk or by parents or other authority figures).

How it happens

Decreased caloric intake depletes body fat and protein stores. In adolescent girls and women, estrogen deficiency occurs because the stress on the body diminishes the production of LH and FSH, resulting in amenorrhea.

In adolescent boys and in men, testosterone levels fluctuate, resulting in reduced erectile function and a reduction in sperm count. Ketoacidosis occurs from increased use of body fat as energy.

What to look for

When anorexia nervosa is suspected, look for:
- emaciated or skeleton-like appearance, not regarded by the teen as being abnormal or undesirable
- evidence of secret dieting
- lack of satisfaction with weight loss (constantly setting new, lower weight goals)
- body image distortion (weight, size, shape)

Cold, constipated, weak, and absent

• possible reported symptoms, including cold intolerance, low blood pressure, low pulse rate, and abdominal pain
• GI symptoms such as constipation or laxative dependence
• muscle weakness, seizures, or cardiac arrhythmias
• emaciated appearance with dry skin and lanugo hair over back and extremities
• amenorrhea (absence of at least three consecutive menstrual cycles when otherwise expected to occur), fatigue, loss of libido, and infertility
• cognitive distortions, such as overgeneralization, or *dichotomous thinking* (black or white, good or bad, all or nothing)
• compulsive behavior such as excessive exercising
• dependency on others for self-worth

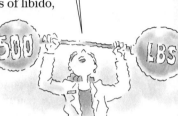

A child or teen with anorexia nervosa may exercise to excess.

Guilty, impaired, and needing to please

• guilt associated with eating
• impaired decision-making
• need to achieve and please others
• overly compliant attitude
• perfectionist attitude
• obsessive rituals concerning food and a preoccupation with food preparation
• refusal to eat and to maintain or achieve normal weight for age and height
• intense fear of gaining weight or becoming fat, even though underweight.

What tests tell you

All criteria described in the *Diagnostic and Statistical Manual of Mental Disorders*, Fifth Edition, Text Revision must be met for a diagnosis of anorexia nervosa. (See *Diagnosing anorexia nervosa*.)

In addition, findings from an EAT performed on a patient with anorexia nervosa suggest an eating disorder, and an electrocardiogram (ECG) reveals nonspecific ST interval, prolonged PR interval, and T wave changes. Other findings include:
• low estrogen levels in female patients
• low testosterone levels in male patients
• low hemoglobin levels and low platelet and white blood cell counts
• elevated blood urea nitrogen
• electrolyte imbalances.

Diagnosing anorexia nervosa

According to the *Diagnostic and Statistical Manual of Mental Disorders*, Fifth Edition criteria, to be diagnosed as having anorexia nervosa, a person must display:
• persistent restriction of energy intake leading to significantly low body weight (in context of what is minimally expected for age, sex, developmental trajectory, and physical health)
• either an intense fear of gaining weight or of becoming fat or persistent behavior that interferes with weight gain (even though significantly low weight)
• disturbance in the way one's body weight or shape is experienced, undue influence of body shape and weight

on self-evaluation, or persistent lack of recognition of the seriousness of the current low body weight.

Subtypes of anorexia nervosa
There are two subtypes of anorexia nervosa:

    restricting, in which a patient hasn't regularly engaged in binge-eating or purging (self-induced vomiting or misuse of laxatives, diuretics, or enemas) during the current episode of the disorder

    binge-eating or purging, in which the patient has regularly engaged in binge-eating or purging during the current episode.

Complications

Complications of anorexia nervosa include:
• electrolyte imbalances
• chronic malnutrition
• acute dehydration
• esophageal erosion, ulcers, tears, and bleeding
• tooth and gum erosion and dental caries
• decreased left ventricular muscle mass and chamber size
• decreased cardiac output and hypotension
• ECG changes
• increased susceptibility to infection
• anemia.

How it's treated

Medical management includes behavior modification and group, family, or individual psychotherapy with a clinician who specializes in disordered eating. Teens should be placed on a well-balanced diet with a normal eating pattern and vitamin supplements. However, a rapid weight gain should be avoided due to the potential for severe metabolic abnormalities.

Bring out the troops

Drug therapy may include antianxiety agents, such as lorazepam and alprazolam; antidepressants, such as amitriptyline and imipramine; and selective serotonin reuptake inhibitors, such as paroxetine and fluoxetine.

Hospitalization may be as brief as 2 weeks or more than 2 years. Many clinical centers now have inpatient and outpatient programs designed specifically to manage eating disorders.

What to do

Early recognition is key. Young people need to be aware of the seriousness of this type of self-imposed disease. Positive, early interventions include:
• teaching coaches, teachers, and parents to recognize early signs
• supporting the teen's efforts to achieve her target weight and helping to negotiate adequate food intake in a relaxed, nonpunitive treatment atmosphere.

Express for success

Long-term success involves helping the teen identify coping mechanisms for dealing with anxiety and encouraging the teen to express her feelings without fear of reprisal or judgment.

In addition, the nurse should:
• Provide a specific goal-oriented plan that can be followed consistently.
• Encourage early family therapy, which is most effective when it's started soon after the diagnosis is made.
• Foster an open, honest therapeutic relationship with the adolescent, yet be firm to counteract manipulative behavior; behavior modification therapy may be helpful to decrease the adolescent's manipulative behavior.

Attention deficit hyperactivity disorder

Attention deficit hyperactivity disorder (ADHD) is a behavior problem characterized by difficulty in focusing attention; difficulty engaging in quiet, passive activities; or both. It's possible to have attention deficit without hyperactivity.

One in every classroom . . .

ADHD affects roughly 3% to 5% of school-age children in the United States. This amounts to as many as 2 million children— an average of one in every classroom. It affects at least twice as many boys as girls.

. . . and in the office, too

Until recently, experts thought that children outgrew ADHD by adolescence. We now know that many symptoms continue into adulthood. In fact, the disorder affects approximately 2% to 4% of adults.

To be diagnosed with ADHD, a child's behaviors must:
• be present in two or more settings
• begin before age 12
• result in significant impairment in social or academic functioning.

What causes it

The underlying causes are unknown. There's limited evidence of a genetic component, and some studies suggest that it may result from altered neurotransmitter levels in the brain. Other theories point to a deficit within the right hemisphere of the brain or an alteration of the reticular activating system of the midbrain that causes the child to react to all stimulation, not just selected stimuli.

How it happens

Alleles of dopamine genes may alter dopamine transmission in the neural networks. During fetal development, bouts of hypoxia and hypotension could selectively damage neurons located in some of the critical regions of the anatomic networks.

What to look for

A child or adolescent with ADHD may exhibit several behaviors and difficulties, including:
- climbing, running, or talking excessively
- decreased attention span
- difficulty organizing tasks and activities
- difficulty waiting for turns or playing quietly
- being easily distracted; failing to give close attention to school-work or to finish an activity
- failing to listen when spoken to directly

So many things to do . . .

- fidgeting or squirming in his seat (being disruptive in the classroom)
- frequent periods of forgetfulness (frequently losing things needed for tasks)
- impulsive behavior
- losing his temper easily
- inability to follow directions.

What tests tell you

Complete psychological, medical, and neurologic evaluations must rule out other problems before an ADHD diagnosis can be made. To make the diagnosis, the findings are combined with data from several sources, including parents, teachers, and the child. (See *Diagnosing ADHD*, page 152.)

Complications

Complications of ADHD include emotional and social difficulties (which may be extreme) and poor nutrition. Children with ADHD may also be at increased risk of abuse because parents may become exasperated with the child's behavior and may become abusive out of frustration and exhaustion.

Diagnosing ADHD

The *Diagnostic and Statistical Manual of Mental Disorders*, Fifth Edition groups a selection of symptoms into inattention and hyperactivity-impulsivity categories.

People with ADHD show a persistent pattern of inattention and/or hyperactivity-impulsivity that interferes with functioning or development:

Inattention: Six or more symptoms of inattention for children up to age 16, or five or more for adolescents age 17 and older and adults; symptoms of inattention have been present for at least 6 months, and they are inappropriate for developmental level:

• often fails to give close attention to details or makes careless mistakes in schoolwork, at work, or with other activities
• often has trouble holding attention on tasks or play activities
• often does not seem to listen when spoken to directly
• often does not follow through on instructions and fails to finish schoolwork, chores, or duties in the workplace (e.g., loses focus, sidetracked)
• often has trouble organizing tasks and activities
• often avoids, dislikes, or is reluctant to do tasks that require mental effort over a long period of time (such as schoolwork or homework)
• often loses things necessary for tasks and activities (for example, school materials, pencils, books, tools, wallets, keys, paperwork, eyeglasses, mobile telephones)
• is often easily distracted
• is often forgetful in daily activities.

Hyperactivity and impulsivity: Six or more symptoms of hyperactivity-impulsivity for children up to age 16, or five or more for adolescents age 17 and older and adults; symptoms of hyperactivity-impulsivity have been present for at least 6 months to an extent that is disruptive and inappropriate for the person's developmental level:

• often fidgets with or taps hands or feet, or squirms in seat
• often leaves seat in situations when remaining seated is expected
• often runs about or climbs in situations where it is not appropriate (adolescents or adults may be limited to feeling restless)

• often unable to play or take part in leisure activities quietly
• is often "on the go" acting as if "driven by a motor"
• often talks excessively
• often blurts out an answer before a question has been completed
• often has trouble waiting his or her turn
• often interrupts or intrudes on others (e.g., butts into conversations or games).

In addition, the following conditions must be met:
• Several inattentive or hyperactive-impulsive symptoms were present before age 12 years.
• Several symptoms are present in two or more setting (e.g., at home, school, or work; with friends or relatives; in other activities).
• There is clear evidence that the symptoms interfere with, or reduce the quality of, social, school, or work functioning.
• The symptoms do not happen only during the course of schizophrenia or another psychotic disorder. The symptoms are not better explained by another mental disorder (e.g., mood disorder, anxiety disorder, dissociative disorder, or a personality disorder).

Based on the types of symptoms, three kinds (presentations) of ADHD can occur:

Combined presentation: if enough symptoms of both criteria, inattention and hyperactivity-impulsivity, were present for the past 6 months

Predominantly inattentive presentation: if enough symptoms of inattention, but not hyperactivity-impulsivity, were present for the past 6 months

Predominantly hyperactive-impulsive presentation: if enough symptoms of hyperactivity-impulsivity but not inattention were present for the past 6 months.

Because symptoms can change over time, the presentation may change over time as well.

In addition, the child may experience long-term difficulties at school because of being "labeled" with an ADHD diagnosis. Children with ADHD may also have adverse reactions to medications used to treat the disorder.

How it's treated

Medical management starts with behavior modification and psychological therapy. Interdisciplinary interventions include vision screening, hearing tests, and an assessment of specific learning needs.

Pharmacologic therapy may include amphetamines, such as methylphenidate or dextroamphetamine, to help the child concentrate.

What to do

The child with ADHD and his parents need information and ongoing support:
• Monitor the child's growth, especially if he's receiving methylphenidate (as growth may be slowed).
• Give one simple instruction at a time so the child can successfully complete the task (which promotes self-esteem).

• Because some ADHD medications may decrease children's appetite, educate parents to give medications before breakfast in the morning to ensure that children are receiving adequate calories.
• Encourage adequate nutrition as medications and hyperactivity may increase nutrient needs.
• Suggest that parents reduce environmental stimuli to decrease distraction, and formulate a schedule for the child to provide consistency and routine.

• Suggest that teachers and coaches provide a daily report on the child's progress to ensure that rules given at the home are being reinforced in other environments.
• Provide parents with information about support groups, such as local organizations and online groups.

Obesity

Obesity is an excess of body fat that's generally 20% or more above ideal body weight for a person's age and height. Obese adolescents increased from 5% in 1980 to 18% in 2010.

Cultured pearls

Obesity and minorities

Although obesity seems to affect school-age and adolescent girls and boys equally, one recent study found rates of obesity in minorities to be significantly greater than in nonminority populations.

School-age children
In school-age children, the study found that Hispanic children (24%) were twice as likely as White children (12%) to be overweight. Black children had a slightly lower rate of obesity than Hispanic children (20%).

Adolescents
In adolescents, the rates remain higher for Blacks and Hispanics. About 24% in both groups were more likely to be overweight than White adolescents (13%).

It starts early
The study also found that preschool-age Black, Hispanic, and White children were more equal in their tendency to be overweight (8%, 11%, and 10%, respectively), which suggests that early teaching about healthy eating and exercise habits could be beneficial.

Equality of the sexes

In addition, boys and girls seem equally at risk for obesity in both age-groups (school-age boys, 16%; school-age girls, 14.5%; adolescent girls and boys, 15.5%). (See *Obesity and minorities*.)

What causes it

Obesity results when a person takes in or consumes more calories than he expends. Simply put, the child eats more calories than his body burns.

Obesity in childhood and adolescence can be related to these factors:
• sedentary lifestyle (couch-potato children due to increased television viewing and decreased physical activity)
• overeating
• poor eating habits
• stressful changes or life events, such as divorce, death, moving, or abuse
• low self-esteem
• depression
• family problems or problems with peers.

How it happens

The etiology of obesity is complex and usually multifactorial. Theories to explain this condition include:
• genetic predisposition
• biological factors
• psychological factors.

Genetic predisposition

Obesity in parents increases the probability of obesity in children. In fact, a child of parents with obesity has an 80% chance of having obesity as a child. A child who's obese between the ages of 10 and 13 has an 80% chance of becoming obese as an adult.

Some contributors to the genetic disposition toward obesity include:
• a body type that's predisposed to the accumulation of subcutaneous fat (such as those with a rounded, soft body shape)
• an inherited defect that interferes with the metabolic breakdown of fat
• familial and cultural eating patterns and behaviors.

Biological factors

Certain diseases and endocrine and metabolic problems can contribute to childhood obesity. Underlying disease is attributed to only 5% of cases of childhood obesity. Such conditions as hypothyroidism, muscular dystrophy, Down syndrome, and spina bifida can cause accumulation of fat due to decreased metabolism or limited mobility.

Endocrine and metabolic factors are complex. The relationships between feelings of hunger and satiety, the central nervous system, and the body's ability to metabolize carbohydrates, protein, and fat are still under investigation.

Psychological factors

Many children, as well as adults, eat in response to how they're feeling. Eating gives older children and adolescents a sense of well-being, satiety, and security—feelings that were developed when they ate during infancy.

However, for a child who's bored, tired, depressed, sad, or lonely, eating is his way of obtaining those warm, nurturing feelings; it becomes a comfort for him. In addition, parents may use food as a reward, or withhold it as punishment, furthering the child's misuse of food.

What to look for

Observation and comparison of height and weight to a standard table indicate obesity. A waist to hip ratio may be measured.

Measurement of the thickness of subcutaneous fat folds with calipers provides an approximation of total body fat.

What tests tell you

Body mass index can be calculated by dividing a person's weight by the square of his height. This number can be compared to normal values on standardized graphs to diagnose progressive levels of obesity.

Complications

Obesity may lead to serious complications, such as respiratory difficulties, hypertension, cardiovascular disease, diabetes mellitus, and renal disease as well as psychosocial difficulties, including emotional taunts from peers.

How it's treated

Weight-loss diets may not be the answer for children and adolescents because of their nutritional needs during a time of rapid growth. Instead, it's recommended that the child be helped to maintain his current weight while allowing for his stature to continue growing. The child, in effect, outgrows his obesity (this isn't necessarily the case with adolescents).

Although restrictive diets aren't the normal treatment, dietary changes can have significant results. Suggestions include:
- avoiding fast-food establishments
- providing low-fat alternatives for after-school snacks
- switching from whole milk to skim milk
- exchanging fresh vegetables for fried snack foods
- offering a variety of fresh and dried fruits.

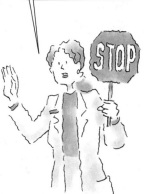

Weight-loss diets and children aren't a good mix. Instead, the emphasis needs to be on maintaining current weight because they'll "grow into it."

What to do

When providing care to a child or adolescent with obesity:
- Obtain an accurate dietary history to identify the child's eating patterns and determine the importance of food to his lifestyle.
- Encourage the child and parents to adhere to the prescribed dietary meal plan to help ensure a successful outcome.
- Suggest low-calorie, low-fat snacks such as fresh fruits and vegetables.
- Encourage parents to avoid overfeeding their children and discourage the use of food as a reward for good behavior.

- Promote physical activities, such as involvement in organized sports teams and individual events, and a personalized exercise program.

Vim and vigor

Children with obesity or normal weight should be encouraged to participate in some type of daily, vigorous, aerobic activity to help reduce or prevent childhood obesity and to promote a habit of daily exercise that will last a lifetime.

Sexually transmitted infections

An important group of sex-related disorders results from infection that are transmitted through sexual contact include:
- HIV or HIV/AIDS
- chancroid
- chlamydial infections
- genital herpes
- genital warts
- gonorrhea
- lymphogranuloma venereum
- syphilis
- trichomoniasis.

They're everywhere

Sexually transmitted infections (STIs) are among the most prevalent infections around the world. Gonorrhea, chlamydial infections, and genital warts are approaching epidemic proportions in the United States. In the past 10 years, between one-fifth and one-third of all reported cases of chlamydia, gonorrhea, and syphilis affect adolescents and young adults up to age 24.

What causes it

The cause of an STI may be bacterial, viral, or parasitic. (See *Common STIs*, page 158.)

How it happens

STIs are passed from one person to another through anal, oral, or vaginal sexual contact. The rate of transmission and, therefore, the incidence of these diseases, is rising because of societal attitudes toward sex (such as those that condone multiple sexual partners), a lack of health promotion (for condom use or abstinence), and increased reporting of new cases.

When STIs are diagnosed in children who are school-age or younger, child abuse must be investigated.

Common STIs

This chart lists several STIs along with their causative organisms, assessment findings, and appropriate treatments (including those used in pregnant patients).

STI	Assessment findings	Treatment
Chlamydia *Chlamydia trachomatis*	• Asymptomatic (commonly); suspicion should be raised if partner has been treated for nongonococcal urethritis • Heavy, gray-white vaginal discharge • Painful urination • Positive chlamydial urine test or vaginal culture using special chlamydial test kit	• Macrolides (azithromycin, clarithromycin), tetracyclines (doxycycline; tetracycline)
Syphilis *Treponema pallidum*	• Painless ulcer on vulva or vagina (primary syphilis) • Hepatic and splenic enlargement, headache, anorexia, and maculopapular rash on the palms of the hands and soles of the feet (secondary syphilis; occurring about 2 months after initial infection) • Cardiac, vascular, and central nervous system changes (tertiary syphilis; occurring after an undetermined latent phase) • Positive Venereal Disease Research Laboratory serum test; confirmed with positive rapid plasma reagin and fluorescent treponemal antibody absorption tests • Dark-field microscopy positive for spirochete	• Penicillin G benzathine (Bicillin L-A) intramuscularly (I.M.) (single dose) or a single dose of oral azithromycin
Genital herpes Herpes simplex virus, type 2	• Painful, small vesicles with erythematous base on vulva or vagina, rupturing within 1 to 7 days to form ulcers • Low-grade fever • Dyspareunia • Positive viral culture of vesicular fluid • Positive enzyme-linked immunosorbent assay	• Acyclovir (Zovirax) orally or in ointment form
Gonorrhea *Neisseria gonorrhoeae*	• May not produce symptoms • Yellow-green vaginal discharge • Male partner who experiences severe pain on urination and purulent yellow penile discharge • Positive gonorrheal urine test or culture of vaginal, rectal, or urethral secretions	• Ceftriaxone (Rocephin) as a one-time I.M. injection
Condyloma acuminata Human papillomavirus	• Discrete papillary structures that spread, enlarge, and coalesce to form large lesions; increasing in size during pregnancy • Possible secondary ulceration and infection with foul odor	• Topical application of trichloroacetic acid or bichloracetic acid to lesions • Lesion removal with laser therapy, cryocautery, or knife excision

What to look for

Symptoms vary depending on the infectious organism, and symptoms of a particular STI may vary by gender. Some classic symptoms of STIs include:
• pain during urination
• vaginal or penile discharge
• growths that appear on the genitalia and sores on the mouth or genitalia
• evidence of sexual abuse, such as vaginal tears, vaginal bruising, blood in the child's underwear, and difficulties void-ing. (Never assume that a child of any age, including a teen, has acquired an STI by consensual sexual contact.)

What tests tell you

A sexual history provides the basis for prevention, diagnosis, and treatment of an STI. The physical assessment, primarily a diagnostic tool, can also serve as an excellent opportunity for patient teaching.

I.D. the STI

To help identify the infectious organism, an appropriate urine test may be ordered (for gonorrhea and chlamydia) or the sus-pected lesion is cultured with the appropriate culture method:
• A genital tract specimen from a male should contain urethral discharge or prostatic fluid.
• From a female, the specimen should contain urethral or cervical specimens.
• Two swabs should always be collected simultaneously.

Privacy is paramount

Keep in mind that examinations of this kind can be extremely difficult and embarrassing for school-age children and teens. Procedures should be explained thoroughly and as much privacy as possible should be provided.

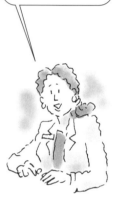

Reassure the child that you're there to help and that nothing that has happened is his fault.

Complications

Complications that are common to all STIs include emotional stress, male or female infertility, ectopic pregnancies, and even death.

How it's treated

STIs may be treated with oral or I.M. antibiotics and antiviral medications. They're also treated symptomatically with analgesics and antipyretics. Some infections, such as herpes and HIV/AIDS, have no known cure.

What to do

Protection against and prevention of STIs should be the focus of nursing education. This information should be kept in mind when educating about STIs:

• Abstinence is the safest way to ensure that teens stay healthy.

• Although sex education and handing out condoms in public schools remain controversial, the use of latex condoms for those who are sexually active could protect a teen from acquiring an STI.

• Teens should be strongly encouraged to seek medical treatment immediately if they suspect that they have contracted an STI.

• If approached by a teen about treatment, remain nonjudgmental and try to address all of his concerns.

• Urge the teen to inform sexual contacts of his or her infection so he or she can receive medical treatment, and stress the importance of remaining abstinent until the completion of treatment.

Suicide and attempted suicide

Suicide is the third leading cause of death among 15- to 24-year-olds and is commonly committed with a firearm. The rate of attempted suicides is higher in females, but males are three times as successful as females in their attempts. The highest suicide rate is in Native American males and Black females.

What causes it

One-third of those attempting suicide wish to die, whereas others seek to gain attention, communicate love or anger, or escape a difficult or painful situation.

What to look for

Risk factors include:
• interpersonal conflict or loss
• family discord
• legal or disciplinary problems
• chronic drug or alcohol abuse
• history of physical or sexual abuse
• recent failure or disappointment
• preoccupation with death
• previous suicide attempt. (See *Suicide warning signs.*)

Complications

After an adolescent or school-age child attempts suicide, he's at risk for another attempt. Existing emotional problems may be

Advice from the experts

Suicide warning signs

During the patient interview, be alert for these signs of suicidal behavior:

• overwhelming anxiety (the most frequent precipitant of a suicide attempt)
• withdrawal and social isolation
• signs and symptoms of depression, including crying, fatigue, helplessness, poor concentration, reduced interest in previously enjoyable activities, sadness, constipation, and weight loss
• good-byes expressed to friends and family members
• giving away prized possessions
• covert suicide messages and death wishes
• obvious suicide messages such as "I'd be better off dead."

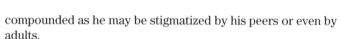

compounded as he may be stigmatized by his peers or even by adults.

The parents of an adolescent or child who commits suicide must deal with a range of emotions, including intense grief and guilt. Parents are also likely to feel guilty when an attempt is unsuccessful. They may become excessively protective of the child who made the attempt and of their other children.

How it's treated

Treatment for a suicide attempt is based on the underlying psychiatric, emotional, or physical difficulty that led the child or adolescent to feel suicide was the only option.

Immediate hospitalization without the adolescent's consent is warranted if threat of self-harm still exists. Treatment might also involve therapy (both group and individual), medications (such as tricyclic antidepressants), remediation of social and problem-solving deficits, and family conflict resolution.

What to do

To help deter potential suicide in the child or adolescent with major depression, the nurse should keep certain guidelines in mind. (See *Suicide prevention guidelines*, page 162.)

Advice from the experts

Suicide prevention guidelines

To help deter potential suicide in the patient with major depression, keep the following guidelines in mind.

Assess for clues
Watch for such clues as:
- communicating suicidal thoughts, threats, and messages and talking about death and feelings of futility
- hoarding medication
- giving away prized possessions
- describing a suicide plan
- changing behavior, especially as depression begins to lift.

Provide a safe environment
Check patient areas and correct dangerous conditions, such as:
- exposed pipes
- windows without safety glass
- access to the roof or open balconies.

Remove dangerous objects
Remove potentially dangerous objects from the patient's environment, such as:
- belts
- razors
- suspenders
- light and window blind cords
- glass
- knives or guns
- nail files and clippers.

Consult with staff
Include the health care team in aspects of care and be sure to:
- recognize and document both verbal and nonverbal suicidal behaviors
- keep the doctor informed and share data with all staff
- clarify the patient's specific restrictions
- assess the patient's risk and plan for observation
- clarify day and night staff responsibilities and frequency of consultation.

Observe the suicidal patient
Take some steps for easy observation of a suicidal patient, including:
- being alert when the patient is using a sharp object (shaving), taking medication, or using the bathroom (to prevent hanging or other injury)
- assigning the patient to a room near the nurses' station and with another patient
- continuously monitoring the acutely suicidal patient.

Maintain personal contact
Help the patient remain in contact with his environment by:
- reassuring the suicidal patient that he's not alone or without resources or hope
- encouraging continuity of care and consistency of primary nurses
- helping the patient build emotional ties to others (the ultimate technique for preventing suicide).

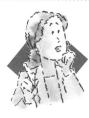

Quick quiz

1. What's the first area of the body that's easily recognized as the beginning of the growth spurt in puberty?
  A. Hands, followed by lengthening of the arms
  B. Feet, followed by lengthening of the legs
  C. Shoulder width
  D. Abdominal girth

Answer: B. Different areas of the body reach their peak growth at different times. Changes are easily recognized in the feet, which are the first part of the body to experience a growth spurt. Increased foot size is followed by a rapid increase in leg length and then trunk growth.

2. Which statement by your female adolescent patient reveals an early sign of anorexia nervosa?
  A. "I have my menstrual period every 28 days."
  B. "I go out to eat with my friends at least 3 times per week."
  C. "I jog three times a day for a total of 5 hours per day."
  D. "I try to maintain my weight around 115 lb for my height of 5′."

Answer: C. Excessive exercise, consumption of very small amounts of food, and food rituals are all signs of anorexia nervosa. Menstruation commonly stops, and the patient's weight is below normal.

3. Which statement is true about physical growth during adolescence?
  A. Boys will typically grow much faster than girls.
  B. Girls will typically continue their growth in height until age 21.
  C. Most major organs will double in size.
  D. Motor coordination is even with growth in stature and musculature.

Answer: C. Major organs double in size during adolescence; the exception is the lymphoid tissue, which decreases in mass.

4. Because of the effects of menstruation, a girl should increase her dietary intake of:

    A.   calcium.

    B.   iron.

    C.   carbohydrates.

    D.   fats.

Answer: B. Iron is needed in the production of the protein hemoglobin, which is vital to carrying oxygen in the blood and is lost during menses.

5. Russell's sign is one way to assess for:

    A.   anorexia nervosa.

    B.   bulimia.

    C.   obesity.

    D.   attempted suicide.

Answer: B. Russell's sign includes calluses on the knuckles or abrasions and scars on the dorsum of the hand due to induced vomiting with bulimia.

Scoring

★★★ If you answered all five items correctly, call your parents! They'll be proud of the abstract thinking and formal operational thought it took to master the tasks in this chapter.

★★ If you answered three or four items correctly, tell your peers! They'll say your understanding of middle childhood and adolescence is "way cool."

★ If you answered fewer than three items correctly, don't get depressed! Your knowledge of middle childhood and adolescence is due for a growth spurt.

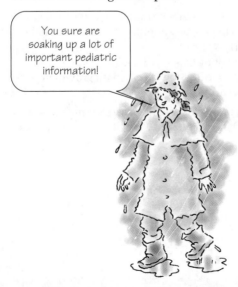

You sure are soaking up a lot of important pediatric information!

6

Infectious diseases and immunizations

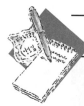

Just the facts

In this chapter, you'll learn:

♦ the chain of infection

♦ recommended immunization practices for infants and children

♦ common childhood infectious diseases of viral and bacterial etiology

♦ nursing interventions for the care of children with viral and bacterial illnesses.

Infection

Infection is the invasion and multiplication of micro-organisms in the body. Infection can cause numerous illnesses during childhood, most of which are common, but some of which are less common or even rare.

The severity of illness caused by infection can range from subclinical to life-threatening. A thorough understanding of the etiology and symptoms of infectious diseases as well as the appropriate diagnostic and therapeutic interventions will help the nurse provide optimal care.

Chain of infection

Chain of infection is a term used to describe the circle of links needed for the transmission of infectious diseases

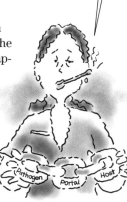

Unfortunately, I'm the weakest link in this chain of infection.

in humans. All links must be present and in order for an infection to occur.

The chain begins with a pathogen that's capable of producing disease in humans, that is, bacteria, virus, fungi, or parasite.

The reservoir of an infectious agent. This is where the infectious agent will grow. Humans are the most common reservoir. Other reservoirs include the environment, hospital settings, water supply, and rodents or animals.

The third link in the chain is the portal of exit. The pathogen leaves the reservoir via mucus, blood, or feces.

The organism is transmitted from one host to another.

The fifth link in the chain is the *portal of entry* (the site where disease transmission occurs), through which a pathogen can enter the body by penetrating the skin or a mucous membrane barrier by direct contact or ingestion.

The last link is the *host*; a susceptible host is necessary for an infectious disease to be transmitted.

Immature immunity

Infants and children are susceptible to infectious diseases because their immune systems are immature. As children mature and grow, their exposure to infectious agents increases and they develop antibodies naturally. Subsequent infections with the same pathogen may be less severe or avoided completely.

Stages of infection

Infections follow a predictable sequence of events during transmission that results in five distinct stages of disease.

The *incubation period* is the phase during which the pathogenic organism begins active reproduction in the host; the child has no clinical symptoms but may be contagious to others during this time.

The *prodromal phase* is the initial appearance of clinical symptoms in the host; common symptoms include fever, malaise, headache, sore throat, cough, and rhinitis.

During the *acute stage*, maximum symptoms are experienced by the host; toxins deposited by the pathogenic organism can produce tissue damage. (Inflammatory changes and tissue damage can also occur as a result of the immune response of the host.)

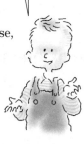

I may look healthy during the incubation period, but I'm already giving my infection to my mom, my brother, and my bratty little sister.

The *convalescent stage* is characterized by progressive elimination of the infection (or elimination of the pathogen), healing of damaged tissue, and symptom resolution.

The *resolution stage* is the host's recovery from the infection without residual signs or symptoms of disease.

Cover your mouth, please

The *period of communicability* is the time when the infectious organism may move from the infected host to another person. It varies with different disease states but usually begins during the incubation phase.

Immune protection

Children receive protection from infectious diseases naturally and artificially.

Methods of obtaining immune protection

There are five different methods in which immune protection can be obtained: natural immunity, naturally acquired active immunity, naturally acquired passive immunity, artificially acquired active immunity, and artificially acquired passive immunity.

Natural (innate) immunity

Innate immunity is a combination of natural and nonspecific immunity that can protect the human body from pathogens and foreign agents. For example, the phagocytic action of white blood cells (macrophages) may be triggered by the body's innate ability to recognize and distinguish normal cells from foreign cells. The body's ability to distinguish self from non-self is natural, or innate, immunity.

Naturally acquired active immunity

Naturally acquired active immunity is obtained when the body's immune system responds to a specific pathogen. Antibodies and memory cells prevent or reduce the severity of subsequent infection with that specific pathogen. Naturally acquired active immunity persists for many years.

Naturally acquired passive immunity

Naturally acquired passive immunity involves mother-to-fetus transmission of maternal antibodies.

A gift that keeps on giving . . .

The mother's immunoglobulin G crosses the placenta and is transmitted to the fetus. After birth, the infant can receive passive immunity through maternal antibodies in breast milk.

. . . for up to 2 months

Naturally acquired passive immunity differs from active immunity. Although active immunity lasts many years, or even a lifetime, passive immunity lasts only as long as the antibodies remain in the blood of the fetus or infant (usually from a few weeks to about 2 months). Even so, some antibodies transferred across the placenta have been isolated up to age 1 year, which is why measles immunization must be delayed until age 15 months.

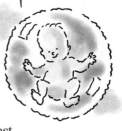

Hey, Mom—got milk? If you do, I'll have at least a few more weeks of passive immunity once I get out of here.

Artificially acquired active immunity

Artificially acquired active immunity is achieved by deliberate administration of a vaccine or toxoid. The vaccine or toxoid stimulates the immune system's production of antibodies against a specific antigen, but symptoms of the disease aren't produced in the person receiving the vaccine.

Artificially acquired passive immunity

Artificially acquired passive immunity is conferred when antibodies developed in another person or animal donor are injected into an individual. In pediatric patients, this transfer usually involves intravenous (I.V.) administration of a specific immunoglobulin, or *antisera*. Examples include:
• gamma globulin (a mixture of antibodies against prevalent community diseases, pooled from 1,000 human plasma donors)
• hyperimmune or convalescent serum globulin (such as tetanus antitoxin, hepatitis B immune globulin, and varicella-zoster immune globulin).

Types of immunizations

Various immunizations are given at specific times to protect pediatric patients from certain diseases. These vaccines fall into two general categories:
• live, attenuated vaccines
• inactivated vaccines.

Live, attenuated

Live, attenuated vaccines are created from a live organism that's grown under suboptimal conditions to produce a live vaccine with reduced virulence.

Weak but stimulating

Thus, an attenuated immunization contains weakened micro-organisms and stimulates immune response and production of antibodies in the host. The vaccine confers 90% to 95% protection for more than 20 years with a single dose.

Measles, mumps, and rubella—itch, ouch

Examples of live, attenuated vaccines include the measles, mumps, and rubella (MMR) vaccine; the rotavirus vaccine; and the varicella vaccine.

Inactivated

- An inactivated, or *killed*, vaccine confers a weaker response than a live vaccine, necessitating frequent boosters.
- An inactivated vaccine doesn't promote replication and provides 40% to 70% protection.

Toxoids

Some bacteria, such as diphtheria, produce toxins, which cause disease. The vaccine to prevent a disease caused by a toxin is called a *toxoid*. A toxoid:
- is another form of an inactivated vaccine
- is a toxin that has been specially treated with formalin or heat to weaken its toxic effect but retain its antigenicity
- provides 90% to 100% protection by stimulating the production of antibodies.

Inactive but popular

Examples of inactivated vaccines include:
- diphtheria and tetanus toxoids
- inactivated poliovirus vaccine (IPV)
- pertussis vaccine
- hepatitis B vaccine.

Immunization schedule

Childhood immunizations include the hepatitis A and B vaccines, diphtheria and tetanus toxoids and acellular pertussis (DTaP) vaccine, *Haemophilus influenzae* type B (Hib) vaccine, human papillomavirus (HPV) vaccine, influenza vaccine, IPV vaccine, meningococcal vaccine, MMR vaccine, rotavirus vaccine, varicella virus vaccine, and pneumococcal 13-valent conjugate vaccine (PCV). These immunizations are usually given according to a predetermined schedule. (See *Recommended immunization schedule for children*, page 170.)

Advice from the experts

Recommended immunization schedule for children

In addition to following the recommended immunization schedule for children in the following table, considering these simple steps will help ensure the child's safety.

Before immunization
• Obtain a history of allergic responses, especially life-threatening anaphylactic reactions to antibiotics or past vaccinations (certain vaccinations may be contraindicated in these children).
• Assess the child for moderate or severe illness. Vaccinations may be delayed in these children until they recover. However, a child with a minor illness, such as a cold, may receive immunizations.
• Keep in mind that children receiving corticosteroids for longer than 2 weeks, chemotherapy, or radiation therapy; those with human immunodeficiency virus infection, acquired immunodeficiency syndrome, or another disease that affects the immune system; and those with cancer will need special consideration for vaccination. (They may not be able to receive live virus vaccines, such as MMR, rotavirus, or varicella vaccines.)

After immunization
• Tell the parents to watch for and report reactions other than local swelling and pain and mild temperature elevation.
• Give parents the child's immunization record.

2013 general vaccine recommendations
At right are the 2013 general vaccine recommendations approved by the Advisory Committee on Immunization Practices, the American Academy of Pediatrics, and the American Academy of Family Physicians.

Age	Immunization
Birth	Hepatitis B #1
1 to 4 months	Hepatitis B #2
2 months	DTaP #1, Hib #1, IPV #1, PCV #1, rotavirus #1
4 months	DTaP #2, Hib #2, IPV #2, PCV #2, rotavirus #2
6 months	DTaP #3, Hib #3 (if needed), PCV #3
6 to 18 months	Hepatitis B #3, IPV #3
12 to 15 months	Hepatitis A #1, Hib #4, MMR #1, PCV #4
12 to 18 months	Varicella #1
15 to 18 months	DTaP #4, Hepatitis A #2 (6 months after first dose)
4 to 6 years	DTaP #5, IPV #4, MMR #2, varicella #2
11 to 12 years	HPV #1, MCV #1, Tdap HPV #2 (2 months after first dose) HPV #3 (6 months after first dose) MCV #2 if first dose between 13 and 15 years Influenza annual starting at 6 months of age Td every 10 years starting after last Tdap

Key:
DTaP: Diphtheria and tetanus toxoids and acellular pertussis
Hib: *Haemophilus influenzae* type B
HPV: Human papillomavirus
IPV: Inactivated poliovirus vaccine
MCV: Meningococcal conjugate vaccine
MMR: Measles, mumps, rubella
PCV: Pneumococcal conjugate vaccine
Td: Tetanus and diphtheria toxoids
Tdap: Tetanus and diphtheria toxoids and acellular pertussis

In the United States, immunization recommendations are governed by the Advisory Committee on Immunization Practices, the American Academy of Pediatrics, and the American Academy of Family Physicians.

Hepatitis A vaccine

Hepatitis A is recommended for all children starting at 12 months of age. It is also recommended for people at risk for acquiring hepatitis A. These people include:
• people who live in endemic areas
• military personnel or others traveling to high-risk areas of the world
• persons at high risk (Native Americans, Alaskan natives, those with chronic liver disease, homosexual or bisexual adolescent males, or users of injectable and illicit drugs).

Dosing

This vaccine is a series of two doses given starting at age 12 months; the two doses should be administered at least 6 months apart. Children 12 months to 18 years of age receive two doses of 0.5 ml (given at least 6 months apart). Those 19 years and older receive 1 ml given intramuscularly (I.M.) (at least 6 months apart). (See *Tips for pediatric injections*, page 172.)

Adverse reactions

Adverse reactions to the hepatitis A vaccine are rare. Administration is contraindicated for those with febrile illness or bleeding disorders.

Hepatitis B vaccine

Acquired during childhood or adolescence, hepatitis B can cause acute illness, with anorexia, jaundice, diarrhea, vomiting, and fatigue. It can also have fatal long-term consequences from cirrhosis or liver cancer. The virus that causes hepatitis B can be spread by:
• passing of the virus from an infected mother to her infant during birth
• having unprotected sexual intercourse with an infected person
• I.V. drug abuse or accidental needle-stick injuries
• exposure to infected blood or body fluids.
    Hepatitis B vaccine is indicated for infants, children, and adolescents to prevent hepatitis B.

Dosing

Various vaccine formulations are available in different strengths. Read the label carefully to determine the proper dosage for pediatric use.

Advice from the experts

Tips for pediatric injections

When giving a child an injection, the major goals should be minimizing trauma and discomfort while providing safe, efficient administration of a necessary medicine or vaccination.

Minimizing trauma

To most toddlers and preschoolers, and to many older children, the prospect of getting an injection is the most frightening part of a doctor's visit or even a hospitalization.

Many strategies, including those outlined in the following texts, can be used to reduce the trauma of receiving an injection, while establishing trust between the child and the health care team and making future injections easier for the child (and for the nurse who's giving the injection).

Medicine to keep you healthy
• Give the child a simple, age-appropriate explanation for why the injection is being given. When a child is being vaccinated, that explanation might be, "This shot will give you medicine to keep you from getting sick." (Young children may think an injection is being given as a punishment and may not even realize that medication is being given.)
• Allow the child to give a "shot" to a doll or stuffed animal; this gives him a sense of control, lets him see that the injection has a beginning and an end, and gives him a concrete understanding of what will happen.

The best policy
• Be honest; tell the child that it will hurt for a moment but that it will be over quickly. (Honesty promotes trust; if a nurse is honest about the potential for pain, the child will believe her when she tells him something won't hurt.)

Coping and comfort
• Give the child a coping strategy, such as squeezing his mother's hand, counting to five, singing a song, and looking away.

• Have a parent hold and comfort the child while the injection is being given. A parent's presence reassures the child that nothing truly bad will happen. (The child may actually cry more when a parent is present, but this is because he feels safe enough to do so.)

Praise and cover
• When the injection has been given, tell the child that "the hurting part" is over, and praise him for what a good job he did (regardless of how he reacted). Never tell a child to "be brave," to "be a big boy," or not to cry, as these requests will set the child up for failure.
• Give the child a bandage. (A young child may not believe the "hurting part" is over until a bandage has been applied.)
• Always give injections in a designated treatment area. Avoid performing painful procedures in a playroom or, if possible, in the child's hospital room, because he needs to know there are places where he can feel completely safe.

Giving the injection
• Apply firm pressure at the site for 10 to 15 seconds immediately before giving the injection to decrease discomfort (a numbing patch may be used).
• When two or more injections are needed, give them simultaneously in different extremities; have two or more nurses to assist (and provide manual restraint, if needed) during the procedures. (The child has only one painful experience when multiple injections are given simultaneously; this is believed to be less traumatic than receiving painful injections one after the other.)
• Apply bandages to each site, and immediately comfort and console the child following the injections.
• Always keep resuscitation equipment and epinephrine readily available in case of an anaphylactic response to an immunization.

Baby's first ouch

The vaccine is given I.M. at birth (or before hospital discharge) and again at ages 1 to 4 months and ages 6 to 18 months, for a total of three doses. For older children and adolescents, the initial I.M. dose should be given as early as possible, with the second dose given 1 month later and the third dose given 6 months after the first dose.

Positive mom, extra ouch

Before immunizing a neonate, check the results of the mother's hepatitis B surface antigen (HBsAg) test. If the mother is HBsAg-positive or her HBsAg status is unknown, the vaccine must be given within 12 hours of birth, along with hepatitis B immune globulin (also within 12 hours of birth) administered in two different sites.

Adverse reactions

Common reactions are pain and redness at the site of injection and elevated liver enzymes. Mild to moderate fever may occur (more common in children and adolescents than in adults). Anaphylaxis is rare.

DTaP vaccine

The DTaP vaccine is given to protect infants and young children from acquiring diphtheria, tetanus, and pertussis. The bacterium that causes diphtheria can create a toxin that damages tissue and attacks the heart and nerves. Such an attack can be fatal. Tetanus can cause muscle spasms that can interfere with breathing, which can lead to death. Pertussis is particularly dangerous for young children, especially infants younger than age 1 year, who are most at risk for complications and death.

Dosing

The dosage for the DTaP vaccine is 0.5 ml given I.M. at ages 2 months, 4 months, 6 months, 15 to 18 months, and 4 to 6 years, for a total of five doses. The tetanus and diphtheria toxoids and acellular pertussis (Tdap) vaccine is given as a booster between ages 11 and 12 years and a tetanus and diphtheria toxoids (Td) booster is then given at 10-year intervals.

Adverse reactions

Fever, fussiness, and anorexia are common adverse reactions as well as redness, pain, and swelling at the injection site. Redness, pain, and swelling at the injection site occur more commonly after the fourth or fifth dose in the DTaP series. Anaphylaxis, fever above 102° F (38.9° C), persistent crying for 3 hours or longer, and seizures are rare but severe reactions that require emergency treatment.

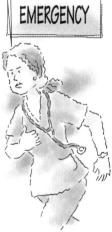

Some adverse reactions to the DTaP vaccine require emergency treatment.

EMERGENCY

Hib vaccine

The Hib vaccine is used to prevent infection with *H. influenzae* type B. This infection can lead to severe invasive illnesses, including meningitis, epiglottitis, and pneumonia. Until recently, *H. influenzae* type B was the most common cause of meningitis in children older than age 1 month, but vaccination with the Hib vaccine has drastically reduced the incidence.

Dosing

The Hib vaccine dosage is 0.5 ml given I.M. for three or four doses. Schedules for different product preparations vary. (Refer to the manufacturer's guidelines and package inserts.)

Three for PedvaxHIB . . .

For the PedvaxHIB preparation, three total doses are recommended, with the first given at age 2 months, the second at age 4 months, and the third at ages 12 to 15 months.

. . . Omni, Act get one dose more

For other preparations, such as OmniHIB and ActHIB, four total doses are recommended, with the first given at age 2 months, the second at age 4 months, the third at age 6 months, and the fourth at ages 12 to 15 months.

Adverse reactions

Hib is one of the safest vaccines available because it causes only mild reactions, if any. Common adverse reactions are low-grade fever, localized pain, redness, and swelling at the injection site. Anaphylaxis is rare.

Human papillomavirus vaccine

The HPV vaccine is available for boys and girls age 9 and older to protect against HPV, which is associated with increased risk for developing certain cancers.

Dosing

HPV vaccine is 0.5 ml administered in three doses I.M. The vaccine series is usually offered around 11 to 12 years of age on a 0, 2-month, and 6-month schedule.

Adverse reactions

Side effects associated with the HPV vaccine include fainting and injuries associated with falling, dizziness, pain at site, fever, and nausea. The Centers for Disease Control and Prevention (CDC) and U.S. Food and Drug Administration (FDA) recommend that patients sit or lie down for 15 minutes after the injection.

IPV

The IPV is recommended to prevent infection with the poliovirus. The live oral trivalent polio vaccine (OPV) is no longer used in the United States.

Dosing

The IPV dose is 0.5 ml administered subcutaneously (S.C.) at ages 2 months, 4 months, 6 to 18 months, and 4 to 6 years, for a total of four doses.

Adverse reactions

Localized pain, redness, and swelling at the injection site are common adverse reactions, although IPV is safe and usually well tolerated. Anaphylaxis is rare.

MMR vaccine

The MMR vaccine stimulates immunity against measles, mumps, and rubella. Because the vaccine contains live virus, it's contra-indicated during pregnancy. Females shouldn't become pregnant within 1 month of immunization.

Intact immunity required

Live virus shouldn't be administered to anyone receiving immunosuppressive therapy or to those with immunodeficiency diseases.

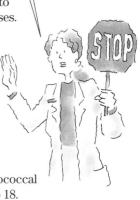

Immunization with live vaccines is contraindicated in children with any type of immune deficiency.

Dosing

The MMR vaccine dose is 0.5 ml administered S.C. at ages 12 to 15 months and again at ages 4 to 6 years, for a total of two doses.

Adverse reactions

Common adverse reactions to the MMR vaccine are low-grade fever for 1 week after immunization; localized pain, redness, and swelling at the injection site; rash; and joint pain. Severe reactions are rare but include viral encepha-lopathy and anaphylaxis.

Meningococcal vaccine

The meningococcal vaccine prevents most types of meningococcal infections and is recommended for all adolescents age 11 to 18.

Dosing

The dose of meningococcal vaccine is given I.M. at ages 11 to 12 years and a booster should be given at 16 years of age. Patients receiving their first dose between the ages of 13 and 15 need a booster between 16 and 18 years of age. Adolescents receiving their first dose after age 16 do not require a booster dose.

Adverse reactions

Side effects associated with meningococcal vaccine include redness and pain at the site; fever and dizziness have been reported. It has been recommended that patients sit or lie down 15 minutes after the vaccine.

Pneumococcal 13-valent conjugate vaccine

Pneumococcal 13-valent conjugate vaccine (PCV13) is recommended for preventing and decreasing the severity of pneumococcal infections caused by *Streptococcus pneumoniae*. These invasive infections can result in otitis media, pneumonia, meningitis, and sepsis, with the most serious illness occurring in children younger than age 2 years.

Dosing

The 0.5-ml dose of PCV13 is administered I.M. A total of four doses are recommended, with one dose each at ages 2 months, 4 months, 6 months, and 12 to 15 months.

Adverse reactions

Common adverse reactions from PCV are drowsiness, irritability, restless sleep, diarrhea, vomiting, decreased appetite, and injection site reactions (including swelling, redness, induration, inflammation, skin discoloration, and tenderness).

Rotavirus vaccine

The rotavirus is the leading cause of gastroenteritis in children younger than the age of 5 causing severe vomiting and watery diarrhea. Currently, there are two vaccines licensed in the United States to protect against rotavirus.

Dosing

The two vaccines RotaTeq and Rotarix are administered by mouth. RotaTeq is given in three doses at age 2 months, 4 months, and 6 months. Rotarix is administered at 2 and 4 months of age. The maximum age for the first dose is 14 weeks and 6 days, with the maximum age for the last dose in 8 months 0 days.

Adverse reactions

Common side effects from the rotavirus include irritability, mild diarrhea, or vomiting. A small but increased risk for developing intussusception has been noted after receiving the first dose of rotavirus vaccine.

Varicella virus vaccine

Varicella virus vaccine is used to stimulate immunity to varicella (chickenpox). The vaccine contains a live virus and is contraindicated during pregnancy. It's also contraindicated in individuals receiving immunosuppressive therapy and in those with immunodeficiency diseases.

Dosing

Two 0.5-ml doses of varicella virus vaccine (Varivax) are given S.C. between ages 12 and 18 months and between 4 and 6 years of age.

Two for teens and teens for two . . .

If patients did not receive varicella vaccine as a child, adolescents age 13 and older receive two doses; each dose is separated by a 4- to 8-week interval.

Adverse reactions

Common adverse reactions to the varicella virus vaccine are pain, redness, localized swelling, and varicella-like rash at the injection site. Low-grade fever and irritability for 1 week after vaccine administration are also common. Anaphylaxis is rare.

Influenza vaccine

Also known as the *flu shot*, the influenza vaccine is either an inactivated or killed vaccine or live, attenuated vaccine. Because the influenza virus changes each year, the vaccine gets updated every year in an attempt to prevent the most common strains that are circulating at that time. Therefore, the influenza vaccine needs to be given yearly.

Protection from the influenza virus should begin 2 weeks after the vaccination and may last for up to 1 year.

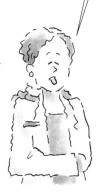

The influenza virus changes every year . . . which is why you need to get a flu shot every year!

Who gets it?

The influenza vaccine is recommended for all children 6 months of age or older. Household contacts and caretakers of children younger than age 6 months or with a chronic health condition are encouraged to get the vaccine.

Dosing

The inactivated vaccine is administered I.M. once per year and is most effective when given early in the flu season, typically in October or November. For children younger than age 9 who are receiving the influenza vaccine for the first time, two doses are necessary and should be given 1 month apart. Children 6 to 35 months receive a dose of 0.25 ml and those 36 months and older receive a dose of 0.5 ml.

There is an intranasal form of the influenza vaccine, which is a live, attenuated vaccine acceptable for healthy children ages 2 years and older.

Adverse reactions

The influenza vaccine typically produces only mild adverse reactions, such as soreness, redness, or swelling at the injection site; fever; or body aches. Such severe adverse effects as a life-threatening allergic reaction rarely occur.

Contraindications to vaccine administration

Mild illnesses and low-grade fevers that are common in children aren't contraindications to vaccine administration. However, there are several reasons to withhold or delay vaccine administration:
• Vaccination is contraindicated in patients with moderate to severe illness or a history of allergic response or anaphylaxis to the vaccine or certain antibiotics.
• Vaccination with preparations containing live or attenuated viruses shouldn't be performed in patients who are pregnant, have an immunodeficiency disease, or are receiving immunosuppressive therapy.
• The DTaP vaccine shouldn't be given to a child who has a progressive and active central nervous system (CNS) problem. However, a child with cerebral palsy can receive immunizations.
• The measles vaccine shouldn't be given at the same time as a tuberculin purified protein derivative test. The measles vaccine can make a person who's positive for tuberculosis (TB) appear to be TB negative.

Bacterial infections

Bacteria are single-celled microorganisms that break down dead tissue. They have no true nucleus and reproduce by cell division. Pathogenic bacteria contain cell-damaging proteins that cause infection. These proteins come in two forms:
• exotoxins—released during cell growth
• endotoxins—released when the bacterial cell wall decomposes. These endotoxins cause fever and aren't affected by antibiotics. (See *How bacteria damage tissue*.)

A class by any other class

Bacteria are classified several other ways, such as by their shape, growth requirements, motility, and whether they're aerobic (requiring oxygen) or anaerobic (not requiring oxygen).

The young and the susceptible

Bacterial infections are common in infants and young children who haven't achieved active immunity because their immune systems haven't been challenged by many pathogens. Such infections in

How bacteria damage tissue

The human body is constantly infected by bacteria and other infectious organisms. Some are beneficial, such as the intestinal bacteria that produce vitamins, and others are harmful, causing illnesses ranging from the common cold to life-threatening septic shock.

Invading forces

To infect a host, bacteria must first enter it. They do this by adhering to the mucosal surface and directly invading the host cell or attaching to epithelial cells and producing toxins, which invade host cells.

I will survive

To survive and multiply within a host, bacteria or their toxins adversely affect biochemical reactions in cells. The

result is a disruption of normal cell function, or cell death (shown below left). For example, the diphtheria toxin damages heart muscle by inhibiting protein synthesis. In addition, as some organisms multiply, they extend into deeper tissue and eventually gain access to the bloodstream.

Clot and deprive

Some toxins cause blood to clot in small blood vessels. The tissues supplied by

these vessels may be deprived of blood and may be damaged (shown below center).

Bring down the walls

Other toxins can damage the cell walls of small blood vessels, causing leakage. This fluid loss results in decreased blood pressure, which, in turn, impairs the heart's ability to pump enough blood to vital organs (shown below right).

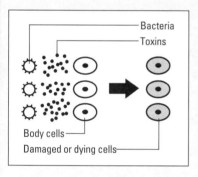

Bacteria
Toxins
Body cells
Damaged or dying cells

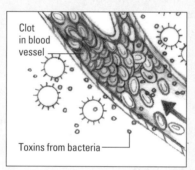

Clot in blood vessel
Toxins from bacteria

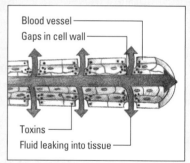

Blood vessel
Gaps in cell wall
Toxins
Fluid leaking into tissue

infants include diphtheria, tetanus, pertussis, Hib, and Lyme disease. Antibiotic therapy is the treatment for bacterial infection.

Diphtheria

Diphtheria is an acute, highly contagious, toxin-mediated infection that's preventable by vaccine. Diphtheria is rare in the United States but remains a serious problem in some other parts of the world.

What causes it

Diphtheria is caused by an infection of *Corynebacterium diphtheriae*, a gram-positive rod that usually infects the respiratory tract (primarily the tonsils, nasopharynx, and larynx). It's more serious when it occurs in infants because they have smaller airways, which are more susceptible to obstruction because of their size.

How it happens

The infection is transmitted by:
• contact with an infected patient's or carrier's nasal, pharyngeal, eye, or skin lesion discharge
• contact with articles contaminated with the bacteria
• ingestion of unpasteurized milk.

Incubation and communicability

The diphtheria incubation period is 2 to 7 days. The period of communicability is 2 to 4 weeks after the onset of symptoms, or until 4 days after the initiation of antibiotic therapy.

What to look for

Symptoms of diphtheria include:
• fever
• malaise
• purulent rhinitis
• cough, hoarseness, and stridor
• cervical lymphadenopathy
• pharyngitis.

Obstruction production

The infection, localized to the tonsils and posterior pharynx, is characterized by a thick, patchy, grayish green, membranous lesion that can lead to airway obstruction. Some children also exhibit infectious, ulcerated skin lesions as a manifestation of the disease.

What tests tell you

• Culture specimens from the nose, throat, and skin lesions reveal the presence of coryneform organisms.
• Sensitivity tests determine the optimal antibiotic therapy.
• Serologic testing will identify the presence of diphtheria toxin.

Complications

Infection with the toxin can result in myocarditis, thrombocytopenia, peripheral neuropathy, or an ascending paralysis with symptoms similar to Guillain-Barré syndrome. Renal, cardiac, and peripheral CNS damage may also occur.

It's a cover-up

The membranous lesion that covers the tonsils can spread to cover the posterior pharynx, which can result in airway obstruction. Removal of the membrane may be indicated, but attempting to do so can cause bleeding. Left untreated, however, it can result in death.

How it's treated

Diphtheria is treated with antitoxin and antibiotics.

No time to waste

I.V. administration of diphtheria antitoxin and antibiotic therapy must begin within 3 days of the onset of symptoms. The patient should be tested for allergy to horse serum before administering the antitoxin. The antibiotic of choice is usually penicillin G or erythromycin for those allergic to penicillin.

Too close for comfort

Close contacts of the infected child should be identified, monitored for signs of illness, and treated with prophylactic antibiotic therapy (oral erythromycin for 7 to 10 days). Cultures of the nose, the throat, and skin lesions should be obtained.

What to do

Diphtheria is a preventable disease. The immunization series is designed to begin at age 2 months. The vaccine confers immunity for 10 years, after which boosters should be given every 10 years throughout the life span. Passive immunity conferred from the presence of maternal antibodies lasts as long as 6 months after birth.

To avoid frightening a child, explain why masks and gowns are worn, and tell the child your name every time you enter the room (because he might not recognize you).

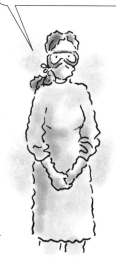

Diagnose, then act

When the disease is diagnosed, follow these steps:
• Report the infection to public health officials.
• Place the infected child in droplet isolation to prevent respiratory transmission. (Show the child isolation gowns, masks, and gloves that will be worn, and provide a simple explanation such as, "Your parents and nurses and doctors are going to wear these so everyone stays healthy.")
• Institute contact isolation precautions if skin lesions are present.
• Maintain infection precautions until after two consecutive negative nasopharyngeal cultures to prevent spread of the disease.
• Closely monitor the patient for signs of airway obstruction. Provide humidified oxygen, if oxygen is ordered, to reduce airway inflammation.
• Administer antitoxin and antibiotics as ordered. Monitor for allergic or anaphylactic reaction.
• Maintain the child on complete bed rest to prevent myocarditis. Provide age-appropriate activities to prevent boredom.

Haemophilus influenzae type B

H. influenzae is a bacterium with several serotypes, but type B is the particularly virulent one. Bacterial infection can result in invasive and devastating illnesses in the pediatric population.

What causes it

Infection is caused by the coccobacillus *H. influenzae*, which is a gram-negative, pleomorphic, aerobic bacillus.

How it happens

Hib can be isolated as part of normal upper respiratory flora in healthy children and adults. However, in some instances, it breaks through the body's natural defense system and causes infection. Infectious symptoms typically begin with a viral upper respiratory infection.

The invasion begins

The pathogenic organisms can invade mucosal tissues and reach the bloodstream, resulting in bacteremia.

All systems aren't go

Systemic bacteremia can cause:
- meningitis
- cellulitis
- epiglottitis
- pneumonia
- septic arthritis
- sepsis.

> Sometimes there's more to an earache than meets the eye. Otitis media can be secondary to *H. influenzae*.

Not-so-honorable mention

Otitis media, sinusitis, and conjunctivitis are examples of localized, noninvasive diseases secondary to *H. influenzae* infection.

Incubation and communicability

The incubation period of *H. influenzae* infection isn't known. The period of communicability begins 3 days after transmission and lasts until the development of symptoms.

What to look for

H. influenzae infections are a common cause of epiglottitis, laryngotracheobronchitis, pneumonia, bronchiolitis, otitis media, and meningitis.

You'd be irritable too

Symptoms vary according to the disease state and whether it's localized (noninvasive) or invasive. For example, a child with *H. influenzae* meningitis might complain of headache, fever, neck stiffness, and photophobia. Infants may be irritable and demonstrate signs of increased intracranial pressure (ICP), such as a bulging fontanel and a high-pitched cry.

Tender to the touch

When cellulitis develops as a complication of *H. influenzae*, there's usually no history of trauma. A localized area of soft tissue edema and erythema with indistinct margins is present. The area is tender to touch, and the patient usually has a fever.

What tests tell you

• Culture and sensitivity tests positively identify *H. influenzae*.
• Peripheral blood smear may reveal leukocytosis as the body responds to the bacterial infection.

Complications

Potential complications of Hib include:
• permanent neurologic sequelae from meningitis
• complete upper airway obstruction from epiglottitis
• cellulitis
• pericarditis
• pleural effusion
• respiratory failure from pneumonia.

Not the time to procrastinate

Complications are rare with noninvasive disease. In invasive disease, complications are less likely when the disease is diagnosed promptly and appropriate antibiotic therapy is begun early. How complications develop also depends on the disease caused by the infecting organism; for example, hearing impairment can result from meningitis. When appropriate treatment is delayed, the potential for serious and life-threatening complications is greater.

How it's treated

I.V. administration of broad-spectrum antibiotics (in particular, antibiotics that are effective against penicillin-resistant strains) is indicated for invasive disease. Cephalosporins, such as ceftriaxone (Rocephin), cefotaxime (Claforan), and chloramphenicol (Chloromycetin) are effective.

Noninvasive disease, such as sinusitis and otitis media, can be treated effectively with oral antibiotics.

Stamp out colonization

Rifampin (Rifadin) may be given prophylactically to close contacts of the infected child. Rifampin is effective in eliminating colonization of the organism.

What to do

• Use droplet isolation precautions with the infected patient until 24 hours after antibiotic therapy has been initiated.
• Maintain adequate respiratory function through cool humidification, oxygen as needed, and a croup or face tent.
• In patients with meningitis, continually monitor level of consciousness.
• Advocate active immunization at ages 2, 4, 6, and 12 to 15 months to prevent both noninvasive disease and severe invasive diseases.

Lyme disease

In the United States, Lyme disease is the most common vector-borne disorder. Although Lyme disease occurs year-round, most infections occur during warm seasons (late spring and summer). Infection with Lyme disease doesn't produce active immunity so a patient may be reinfected upon reexposure.

What causes it

Lyme disease is caused by a spirochete, *Borrelia burgdorferi*, which is transmitted to humans through the bite of an infected deer tick.

How it happens

The spirochete enters the bloodstream via the tick's saliva as its bite penetrates the skin barrier.

Tick tock

The tick must feed for 36 to 72 hours or longer to transmit the infection. Most people who realize they have been bitten will remove the tick before the infection can be transmitted.

What to look for

Once infected, the skin's inflammatory response causes a localized, red, "bull's-eye" rash (*erythema migrans*) at the site of the tick bite. The rash may itch and be painful.

The rash that knows no bounds

Without treatment, the rash will expand to 6″ (15 cm) in diameter or larger. Fever, headache, malaise, and lymphadenopathy are systemic symptoms of the disease.

More reasons to treat

If the infection is left untreated, arthritic pain and swelling of the joints (Lyme arthritis), facial palsy, meningitis, and carditis may result.

What tests tell you

Diagnosis of Lyme disease is based on signs and symptoms and history of exposure. The CDC recommends a two-step process confirmed by the presence of antibodies to *B. burgdorferi* in the blood. The first step is enzyme immunoassay (EIA). If the EIA is negative, no further testing is needed. If the EIA is positive, a Western blot test is performed. If both the EIA and Western blot are positive, the patient has Lyme disease.

Complications

Symptoms of arthritis, including painful joint swelling and stiffness, are the most common complications of untreated disease. Meningitis, focal neurologic problems, and carditis are rare.

How it's treated

Amoxicillin (Amoxil) and cefuroxime (Ceftin) may be used in children younger than age 8 years. Amoxicillin and doxycycline are used for children older than age 8, but doxycycline shouldn't be used in younger children because it can cause permanent discoloration of the teeth. A full course of antibiotic therapy is administered and is continued for 14 to 21 days.

What to do

• Teach parents that tick-infested areas should be avoided to help prevent Lyme disease. If children must be in such areas, protective clothing should be worn, and ticks that do attach must be removed immediately. (See *Preventing tick-borne illnesses*, page 186.)
• Teach parents how to recognize the characteristic bull's-eye rash of Lyme disease to promote early diagnosis and treatment.

It's all relative

Preventing tick-borne illnesses

The following are measures to prevent tick-borne illnesses.

Keep 'em off

It's always preferable to stay out of tick-infested areas. Follow these tips to avoid such areas or, if unavoidable, protect yourself and others from acquiring a tick bite:

• Treat household pets that may harbor ticks (such as cats and dogs) to eliminate the ticks.

• Avoid grassy and wooded areas where ticks are abundant.

• If children must be in such areas, dress them in appropriate protective clothing (such as long-sleeved shirts and long pants).

• Consider using insect repellents. However, repellents containing diethyltoluamide (DEET) shouldn't be used in children younger than age 1 year. DEET is absorbed through the skin and may cause toxicity in this population.

• Check the child for ticks frequently.

Take 'em off

If a tick attaches to the skin:

• Remove it immediately using tweezers or forceps, making sure to remove the entire tick, including the mouth parts.

• Don't crush or squeeze the tick to avoid causing more organisms from the tick to enter the bite.

• Clean the site.

• Wash your hands thoroughly after cleaning the site.

• Seek prompt medical attention for initiation of antibiotic therapy if symptoms develop, such as fever, erythema, or a rash in the area of the bite.

Pertussis

Pertussis, also known as *whooping cough*, is an extremely contagious acute respiratory tract infection. It typically produces an irritating cough that becomes paroxysmal and commonly ends in a high-pitched inspiratory whoop.

Approximately 5,000 to 7,000 cases occur in the United States every year. Children who are too young to have been fully immunized and those who haven't completed the immunization series are at highest risk for serious illness.

What causes it

The pertussis infection is usually caused by the nonmotile, gram-negative coccobacillus *Bordetella pertussis*.

How it happens

The disease is transmitted through inhalation of contaminated respiratory droplets or by direct contact with contaminated articles such as soiled bed linens.

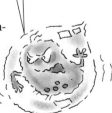

Go ahead, make my day . . . and inhale me!

Incubation and communicability

The incubation period ranges from 3 to 12 days. The period of communicability begins about 1 week after exposure and lasts for 5 to 7 days after antibiotic therapy has begun.

What to look for

Symptoms of rhinorrhea and nasal congestion begin insidiously, followed by a nonproductive cough. These symptoms are commonly accompanied by a low-grade fever, sneezing, and watery eyes.

The cough of the giant crane

The coughing becomes increasingly more severe. Spasms of paroxysmal coughing followed by stridor on inspiration produce the characteristic "whooping" sound.

Flushing and draining

Flushing; cyanosis; and watery drainage from the nose, eyes, and mouth may accompany the coughing. Infants can have symptoms of choking and gasping for air, and vomiting may occur if the patient chokes on mucus.

What tests tell you

Isolation of *B. pertussis* in laboratory culture of respiratory secretions remains the gold standard for confirming pertussis infection. A peripheral blood smear may demonstrate leukocytosis caused by the body's response to the bacterial infection.

Complications

Complications from pertussis infection are most severe, and death rates are highest in infants younger than age 6 months. Complications include:

- secondary infection, such as pneumonia and otitis media
- increased venous pressure
- anterior eye chamber hemorrhage, detached retina, and blindness
- rectal prolapse
- inguinal or umbilical hernia
- encephalopathy
- seizures.

How it's treated

Erythromycin, azithromycin, or clarithromycin given orally for 14 days is standard treatment for pertussis infection. Co-trimoxazole (Bactrim) may be used in patients who can't tolerate erythromycin.

> **Memory jogger**
>
> To remember the complications from pertussis, just remember that the disease is highly contagious, so it IS SHARED:
>
> Increased venous pressure
> Seizures
> Secondary infection
> Hernia
> Anterior eye chamber hemorrhage
> Rectal prolapse
> Encephalopathy
> Death

What to do

To prevent pertussis, nurses should advocate active immunization beginning at age 2 months and continuing at ages 4 months, 6 months, 15 to 18 months, and 4 to 6 years, for a total of five doses. When providing care to a child with pertussis, follow these steps:
• Use droplet isolation for those with suspected or documented infection, until 5 to 7 days after antibiotic therapy has been initiated.
• Closely monitor cardiorespiratory function and oxygen saturation. Maintain a patent airway; keep suctioning equipment readily available.
• Create a quiet environment to decrease coughing stimulation.
• Offer the child a small amount of fluids frequently to prevent dehydration.
• Report diagnosed disease to public health officials.
• Treat close contacts of the infected child prophylactically with oral erythromycin.

Tetanus

Tetanus is a vaccine-preventable disease caused by an acute exotoxin-mediated infection that's usually systemic but may also be localized.

Tetanus causes painful muscle rigidity and spasms all over the body, tightening the muscles of the jaw (*lockjaw*), which makes opening the mouth for breathing or swallowing impossible. It leads to death in 1 of 10 cases.

What causes it

Tetanus is caused by *Clostridium tetani*, a spore-forming anaerobic bacterium. Because *C. tetani* spores exist everywhere, tetanus is a global health problem. However, the disease occurs primarily in those who are unvaccinated or inadequately immunized.

How it happens

The tetanus bacterium is transmitted through penetrating wounds; burns; open wounds in the skin; or contact with contaminated soil, dust, animal excreta, or surgical instruments.

No room at the inn

C. tetani can infect neonates who are born in a contaminated environment or when a contaminated instrument is used to cut the umbilical cord.

Axon reaction

The infection reaches the axons of the nerves, causing involuntary muscle contraction, muscle rigidity, and painful paroxysmal seizures.

Incubation and communicability

The incubation period averages 2 to 14 days. The disease isn't communicable, except through contact with infected skin wounds.

What to look for

History will reveal birth in unclean conditions (for neonatal tetanus) or an injury or wound in an unimmunized child. Clinical manifestations of the disease include:
- stiffness of the neck and jaw
- dysphagia
- painful facial muscle spasms that progress to involve the respiratory muscles as well as the muscles of the abdomen, hips, and thighs
- irregular heartbeat and tachycardia
- hyperactive deep tendon reflexes
- high sensitivity to external stimuli
- profuse sweating
- low-grade fever.

The child remains alert throughout the disease process because mentation is unaffected.

What tests tell you

Diagnosis is based on the history and symptoms of muscle rigidity in a neurologically intact patient. There's also no history of previous tetanus immunization. Serum laboratory studies are usually normal. An increase in leukocytes on the peripheral blood smear may be noted from a wound infection or from the stress of tetanic muscle contractions.

Complications

Tetanic seizures and severe, sustained tetanic contractions as well as rigid muscle paralysis produce many complications. Laryngospasm, respiratory muscle spasms, and respiratory distress can lead to asphyxia and death. Autonomic instability, unstable blood pressure, and cardiac arrhythmias may also occur.

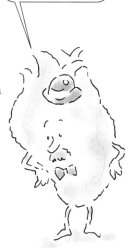

I do believe that cardiac arrhythmias can occur with tetanus. Interesting . . .

How it's treated

Treatment of tetanus is multifaceted and includes:
• tetanus immune globulin (used to neutralize tetanus toxin) administered simultaneously with tetanus toxoid (Td) injected at a different site
• penicillin G, the antibiotic of choice, administered I.V. (or metronidazole, erythromycin, or tetracycline for patients with penicillin allergy)
• surgical wound excision or debridement, if needed
• muscle relaxants and sedatives, if necessary, to treat muscle spasms
• intensive care and careful monitoring of cardiorespiratory status, if needed.

What to do

Active immunization begins at age 2 months with DTaP. The series continues with immunizations at ages 4 months, 6 months, 15 to 18 months, and 4 to 6 years, for a total of five doses.

Ten-year reunion

After the completion of the series, the Tdap vaccine should be administered between the age of 11 and 12 and then Td at 10-year intervals and should continue throughout adulthood.

It is recommended that adolescents and adults (e.g., parents, siblings, grandparents, child-care providers, and health care personnel) who have or anticipate having close contact with an infant aged younger than 12 months should receive a single dose of Tdap to protect against pertussis if they have not previously received Tdap. Ideally, these adolescents and adults should receive Tdap at least 2 weeks before beginning close contact with the infant. This process is known as "cocooning."

Close encounter with a rusty nail

Td vaccine is given to any person with any potentially contaminated wound if his tetanus immunization status isn't known or if it has been more than 5 years since the last immunization.

Child care essentials

For the child with tetanus, follow these steps:
• Maintain a patent airway and adequate ventilation; keep emergency airway equipment readily available. Closely monitor vital signs.
• Maintain a quiet environment, reducing external stimuli from light, sound, and touch. Schedule care to reduce handling of the child and allow for extended periods of rest.
• Remember that the child's mentation is unaffected and that he may be fearful of the muscle spasms and rigidity. If potent muscle

Make sure you create a quiet environment for the child with tetanus.

relaxants are used, the resulting paralysis can make it impossible for the child to communicate clearly. Thoroughly explain procedures to the child, and observe closely for changes in vital signs, which can indicate pain or anxiety, particularly if the child can't communicate. Stay with the child as much as possible, and use a calm and reassuring tone to reduce the child's fear and anxiety.

Viral infections

Viruses are the smallest known organisms; they're visible only with an electron microscope. Independent of host cells, viruses can't replicate; instead, they invade a host cell and stimulate it to participate in forming additional virus particles.

Supportive therapy is the treatment for viral infections. Antiviral medications are sometimes used. Antibiotic therapy isn't indicated for illnesses caused by viral infection but may be appropriate if a secondary bacterial infection has complicated the clinical course of the viral illness.

Rash of rashes

Common childhood rash-producing viruses include:
• fifth disease
• roseola infantum
• rubella
• rubeola
• varicella. (See *Common rash-producing infections.*)

Not so rash

Common viral infections without rash include:
• mumps
• poliomyelitis.

Common rash-producing infections

Infection	Incubation (days)	Duration (days)
Fifth disease	6 to 14	7 to 21
Roseola infantum	10 to 15	3 to 6
Rubella	14 to 21	3
Rubeola	8 to 14	5
Varicella	14 to 17	7 to 14

Fifth disease

Fifth disease is a contagious viral disease characterized by rose-colored eruptions diffused over the skin, usually starting on the cheeks.

The fifth dimension

Fifth disease got its unusual name when it was counted as the fifth of the classic, rash-producing infections of children. The other rash-producing infections referred to in this chronology were measles, scarlet fever, rubella, and another rash that's unknown to doctors today but was referred to as "the fourth disease."

What causes it

Fifth disease is caused by human parvovirus B19.

How it happens

The virus is transmitted through infected respiratory droplet secretions and through infected blood.

Incubation and communicability

The incubation period for fifth disease is 6 to 14 days. The period of communicability lasts from several days before the appearance of a rash until the appearance of the rash.

What to look for

Clinical manifestations in the prodromal phase are mild, including low-grade fever, headache, and symptoms of upper respiratory infection.

A slap in the face

The typical rash in the initial stage is described as a red facial flushing, or a "slapped-cheek" appearance. The macular rash spreads rapidly to the truck and proximal extremities. The centers of the macules fade, which gives the rash a lacy appearance.

Spare the hands, spoil the feet

The rash isn't present on the palms or soles. It resolves spontaneously in 1 to 3 weeks. (See *Fifth disease rash.*)

What tests tell you

Diagnosis of fifth disease is usually based on reviewing the clinical presentation of the child, observing the rash, and excluding other differential diagnoses. Methods to detect the virus in laboratory studies are available, though not routinely ordered.

Fifth disease rash

The rash that appears on the face of a child with fifth disease makes it look as if the child has been slapped.

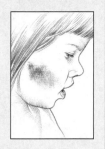

Complications

Complications of fifth disease are rare. Children with chronic hematologic conditions may experience transient anemias. Arthritis and joint symptoms may occur in adults but are rare in children.

Pregnant? Watch out!

Infection of a pregnant woman is associated with fetal disease and may result in fetal death. Even so, risk of infection is minimal in pregnant women who come into contact with affected children.

How it's treated

No specific treatment or cure for fifth disease exists. Nursing care is supportive. No vaccine is available to prevent the illness.

What to do

Treatment is supportive and directed toward relief of symptoms:
- Antipyretics, such as acetaminophen, are given to relieve fever.
- Soothing baths or antipruritics can be used to alleviate itching.

Don't fence me in

Fifth disease is benign and self-limiting. Because the child isn't infectious to others when the rash appears, there's no reason to isolate the child.

Mumps

Mumps, also called *parotitis*, is an acute inflammation of one or both parotid glands and sometimes the sublingual or submaxillary glands. Painful swelling of the salivary glands is a common presenting symptom.

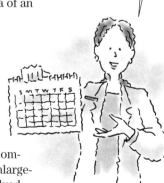

Mark your calendars! The incubation period for mumps is 12 to 25 days.

What causes it

Mumps is caused by paramyxovirus found in the saliva of an infected person.

How it happens

Mumps is spread by contaminated airborne respiratory droplets or by direct contact with the saliva of an infected person.

Incubation and communicability

The incubation period is 12 to 25 days. The period of communicability is from 7 days before the parotid gland enlargement until 9 days after the glandular swelling has resolved.

What to look for

During the prodromal phase of the illness, symptoms include:
- headache
- neck pain
- fever
- malaise
- painful chewing
- anorexia.

   These symptoms are followed by acute and painful swelling of the parotid glands.

What tests tell you

- Peripheral blood smear may reveal leukocytosis and lymphocytosis.
- Serum amylase may be elevated when the parotid glands are enlarged.

Complications

Complications of mumps include:
- epididymitis
- oophoritis
- pancreatitis
- meningoencephalitis
- deafness
- orchitis (most common in adolescent boys and rare in prepubescent boys).

How it's treated

Mumps is treated symptomatically. The child should be on bed rest during the acute phase of the illness, and his diet should be adjusted according to his ability to chew.

   Orchitis should be treated with scrotal support and bed rest. Corticosteroids or nonsteroidal anti-inflammatory drugs (NSAIDs) may be given for arthritis symptoms.

What to do

Most children with mumps are uncomfortable but not seriously ill and are usually cared for at home.
- If a child with mumps is hospitalized, droplet precautions should be maintained until the period of communicability has passed.

- Acetaminophen (Tylenol) and NSAIDs, such as ibuprofen (Advil) or naproxen sodium (Aleve), may be administered to control pain and fever.
- A soft or puréed diet may be needed.
- Warm, moist, or cool compresses may be offered to place on the swollen areas.
- The child should be monitored for such signs of complications as meningeal signs (positive Kernig's and Brudzinski's signs) and testicular swelling in males.
- Confirmed cases should be reported to local and state health officials.

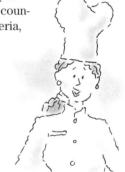

Tell parents to be creative! Just about any food a child craves can go in a blender—and makes mumps a little easier to stomach.

Poliomyelitis

Poliomyelitis, or *polio*, is a viral illness. Eradication is an important priority of the CDC and other organizations. Only three countries continue to have an endemic of polio: Afghanistan, Nigeria, and Pakistan.

In the United States, the last case of "wild" polio (polio occurring directly from infection with the poliovirus) was reported in 1979. Since then, the only cases in the United States have been those resulting from the oral polio vaccine (vaccine-associated paralytic polio [VAPP]), at a rate of 8 to 10 cases per year.

Oral is ousted

For that reason, oral polio vaccine is no longer used in the United States; it was replaced with IPV in 2000. With this change, no cases of VAPP have occurred in the United States since 1999.

Poliomyelitis may range in severity from minor symptoms to fatal paralytic illness.

What causes it

Polio is caused by polioviruses type 1, type 2, and type 3.

What's in a name?

The three types of poliovirus were named for the first people known to have the disease:

 Type 1 is also called *Brunhilde.*

 Type 2 is also called *Lansing.*

 Type 3 is also called *Leon.*

How it happens

Transmission of the virus occurs by direct contact with infected oropharyngeal secretions or stool, infecting the gastrointestinal (GI) tract. When a susceptible person is infected with the poliovirus, the responses may range from a brief, febrile, minor illness to a major illness with CNS involvement and paralysis.

Incubation and communicability

The incubation period is usually 7 to 10 days. The period of communicability isn't completely understood. The infected child can infect others for weeks before the development of symptoms. The virus is shed in respiratory secretions for a few days and in stool for several weeks.

What to look for

Children with poliomyelitis have a wide range of symptoms. In subclinical cases, the child may report or show no symptoms at all. Clinical manifestations of a mild infection include fever, headache, nausea, vomiting, and pharyngitis. Major infections may be nonparalytic or paralytic.

Nonparalytic

Clinical manifestations of nonparalytic poliomyelitis include:
• irritability
• moderate fever
• headache
• vomiting
• lethargy
• pains in the neck, back, arms, and legs; abdominal muscle tenderness and weakness; and spasms in the extensors of the neck and back.

Paralytic

Clinical manifestations of paralytic poliomyelitis are similar to those of nonparalytic poliomyelitis. In addition, patients may have:
• asymmetric weakness of various muscles
• loss of superficial and deep reflexes
• paresthesia
• hypersensitivity to touch
• urine retention
• constipation
• abdominal distention.

What tests tell you

Diagnosis is usually based on the patient's clinical history and presentation. The virus can be detected in specimens from the pharynx and stool. Rising antibody titers in the blood can also indicate recent infection.

Complications

Complications include hypertension, urinary tract infection, urolithiasis, atelectasis, pneumonia, myocarditis, skeletal and soft-tissue deformities, paralytic ileus, permanent paralysis, respiratory arrest, and death.

How it's treated

No cure for polio exists. Treatment is supportive and is directed at symptom relief. Lifesaving measures may be necessary in cases of respiratory distress or failure. In general, the more extensive the paralysis, the greater the resulting disability.

What to do

Passive antibodies transferred across the placenta from mother to fetus persist for about 6 months. Vaccination is the only effective method of disease prevention.

Children should be vaccinated with the IPV according to the recommended schedule (at ages 2 months, 4 months, 6 to 18 months, and 4 to 6 years). The vaccine provides lifelong immunity to polio. When providing care to a child who's hospitalized with polio, follow these steps:

• Consider the child infectious and institute droplet precautions.
• Allow direct patient contact with only his family members and facility personnel who have been vaccinated against poliomyelitis.
• Ensure good body positioning and range of motion to prevent contractures. Apply high-top sneakers or use a footboard to prevent footdrop.
• Provide continuous, vigilant monitoring of respiratory function.
• Monitor for all complications of immobility, including skin breakdown, bone demineralization, and pneumonia.
• Report confirmed cases to local and state public health officials.

Roseola infantum

Roseola is a common, acute, benign, presumably viral illness characterized by fever with subsequent rash. Children with roseola usually present with a high fever of an unknown origin.

What causes it

Roseola is caused by the human herpes virus 6.

How it happens

Transmission of roseola isn't completely understood. The virus is detected in human saliva and is believed to be passed by oral viral shedding.

Incubation and communicability

The incubation period for roseola is 5 to 15 days. The period of communicability is unknown.

What to look for

The onset of symptoms occurs with a sudden, high fever. Children can have fevers of 103° to 106° F (39.4° to 41.1° C). Other than the unexplained fever, the child appears well, behaving normally. Most cases occur in infants and children younger than age 2 years, with peak incidence in children ages 6 to 12 months. The fever resolves on the third or fourth day of the illness.

Don't be rash

The febrile phase is typically followed by the development of a body rash that begins on the trunk and spreads to the neck, face, arms, and legs. The rash fades within 3 days. Some children, however, don't develop a rash.

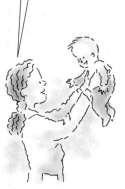

At the onset of roseola, appearances can be deceiving. Aside from a sudden, high fever, the child can appear perfectly well.

What tests tell you

Diagnostic laboratory tests aren't usually performed. It's possible to perform antibody titers to detect the virus.

Complications

Complications of roseola are rare but include extreme hyperthermia, persistent seizures, encephalitis, and hepatitis.

How it's treated

Treatment is supportive and directed at relief of symptoms. Non-aspirin antipyretics, such as acetaminophen, are given to relieve fever. Treating fever is important to prevent febrile seizures.

What to do

Roseola is benign and self-limiting. In addition to treatment for fever, care of a child with roseola should include:
• observation for the development of complications
• replacement of fluids and electrolytes as needed
• investigation of other common causes of high fever in young children such as otitis media.

Rubella

Rubella, also known as *German measles* or *3-day measles*, causes a distinctive maculopapular rash (resembling that of rubeola or scarlet fever) and lymphadenopathy.

What causes it

Rubella is caused by a viral infection with rubella virus (a togavirus).

How it happens

Rubella is a mild viral illness transmitted by airborne respiratory droplets, direct contact with an infected person, or direct contact with contaminated articles. The virus then enters the bloodstream.

Incubation and communicability

The incubation period of rubella is 14 to 21 days. The period of communicability is from 1 week before the onset of the rash until about 4 days after the appearance of the rash.

What to look for

Prodromal symptoms include:
- fever
- malaise
- headache
- purulent nasal drainage
- sore throat
- lymphadenopathy
- anorexia.

Not so pretty in pink

Prodromal symptoms occur for about 1 to 5 days before the onset of a pink rash. The exanthematous, maculopapular, mildly pruritic rash appears first on the face and then spreads to the neck, trunk, and legs. Small, red, petechial macules on the soft palate (Forchheimer spots) usually precede or accompany the rash.

What tests tell you

- Clinical presentation usually confirms diagnosis of rubella. The presence of lymphadenopathy helps to distinguish rubella from other illnesses involving rashes.
- Cell cultures of the throat, blood, urine, and cerebrospinal fluid, as well as convalescent serum that shows a fourfold rise in antibody titers, also confirms the diagnosis.

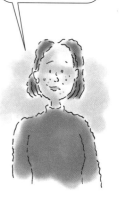

I hope they named it 3-day measles for a reason! Of course, 1-day measles would have been even better.

Complications

Complications of rubella are rare but can occur. Neuritis, arthritis, encephalitis, and thrombocytopenic purpura can complicate the disease. In fetal infection (rare after 20 weeks' gestation), intrauterine death, spontaneous abortion, and congenital malformations of major organ systems can occur.

How it's treated

Rubella is a mild, self-limiting illness. Treatment is supportive and directed at relief of symptoms. Antipyretic medications, such as acetaminophen, are used to control fever, and fluid intake is encouraged to promote and maintain adequate hydration.

What to do

Children with rubella are rarely hospitalized; they're usually treated at home because rubella is generally a mild, self-limiting viral illness:
• During the period of communicability, the child shouldn't attend school or day care and should be isolated from pregnant women.
• If the child is hospitalized, droplet precautions should be instituted until 5 days after the rash disappears.

Pregnant women, beware

Rubella in early pregnancy may cause severe congenital anomalies of the fetus. All females of childbearing age should be immunized to prevent rubella and the potential for congenital rubella syndrome in their offspring. When caring for a patient with rubella:
• Make sure that the patient receives care only from nonpregnant hospital workers who aren't at risk for contracting rubella.
• Make sure that all health care providers have documented immunity to rubella through a positive rubella titer.
• Report confirmed rubella cases to local public health officials.

> Better safe than sorry. Pregnant health care workers at risk for rubella should leave the care of children with the virus to someone else.

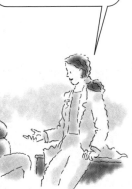

Rubeola

Rubeola, also known as *measles*, is a highly contagious viral disease that causes a characteristic maculopapular rash.

What causes it

Rubeola infection is caused by the rubeola virus. Outbreaks of illness occur mostly in unimmunized children or in those with compromised immune systems.

How it happens

Rubeola is transmitted by airborne respiratory droplets or by direct contact with contaminated articles.

Incubation and communicability

The incubation period for rubeola is 8 to 12 days. The period of communicability begins several days before the appearance of the red rash and continues until 5 days after the rash has resolved.

What to look for

Symptoms of the prodromal phase include:
• fever
• malaise
• lethargy
• cough
• periorbital edema
• conjunctivitis
• profuse drainage from the nose
• Koplik's spots, which are tiny gray-white specks surrounded by red halos that may be noted on the buccal mucosa opposite the molars about 2 days before the appearance of the body rash. (See *Spotting Koplik's spots*.)

You look acute

During the acute phase of the illness, a red, blotchy, flat rash begins on the face and spreads to the trunk and extremities. The rash and other symptoms (severe cough, rhinorrhea, and lymphadenopathy) gradually subside in 5 to 7 days.

What tests tell you

Diagnosis of rubeola is usually based on clinical presentation. Laboratory tests are rarely needed.

Complications

Potential complications include:
• pneumonia
• otitis media

Spotting Koplik's spots

Koplik's spots differentiate rubeola from other rash-producing viruses. The spots appear on the buccal mucosa opposite the molars and then extend to the entire buccal surface. The raised base of the spots may join together so that the blue-white centers stand out (looking like grains of salt) on the erythematous membrane.

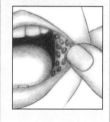

- encephalitis
- seizures
- secondary bacterial infections
- autoimmune reactions.

The infection can be severe or fatal in patients with impaired cell-mediated immunity; mortality is highest in children younger than age 2 years and in adults, who can contract pneumonia secondary to the disease.

How it's treated

Maternal immunity to rubeola is active in the infant for about 1 year after birth. Immunization with MMR vaccine induces active immunity. The first vaccine is given at age 12 to 15 months, and the second is given between ages 4 and 6 years. After the disease is diagnosed, treatment is supportive and is directed at the relief of symptoms:

- Antipyretic medications, such as acetaminophen, are used to control fever.
- Antipruritic medications may be administered for itching.
- A cool mist vaporizer may be soothing to inflamed mucous membranes.
- Gentle suctioning with a bulb syringe may be needed to remove accumulated nasal secretions.

What to do

In addition to providing supportive treatment:
- Monitor breath sounds to detect adventitious sounds.
- Encourage fluid intake to promote hydration and decrease the viscosity of secretions.
- In the hospitalized child, maintain droplet precautions during the period of communicability.
- Report measles cases to local public health officials.

Varicella

Varicella, also called *chickenpox*, is an acute, highly contagious viral infection that can occur at any age.

What causes it

Infection with varicella-zoster virus (VZV) causes chickenpox. The virus remains latent in dorsal root ganglia. Reactivation of the virus can cause herpes zoster infection (shingles) later in life.

How it happens

Airborne spread of respiratory secretions or, less commonly, direct contact with lesions of an infected person can cause infection in a susceptible child.

Incubation and communicability

The incubation period for chickenpox is 10 to 21 days. The period of communicability begins up to 5 days before the appearance of the body rash and continues until all lesions on the skin are crusted over.

What to look for

The onset of symptoms usually occurs 14 to 16 days after exposure. Prodromal symptoms of fever, malaise, and anorexia occur 24 to 48 hours before the development of the rash.

The clinical picture is one of a child with lesions in all stages of evolution present on the skin. The rash is pruritic. In addition:
• The rash begins as itchy red macules on the face, scalp, or trunk that progress to papules.
• Papules develop into clear vesicles on an erythematous base (called "dewdrops on rose petals").
• Vesicles become cloudy and break easily; then scabs form.
• As initial lesions are crusting over, new lesions form on the trunk and extremities.

What tests tell you

VZV antibody tests and titers may be useful in establishing a diagnosis. Most commonly, diagnosis is based on the clinical history and presentation of a child with the characteristic vesicular rash.

Vaccination

To prevent varicella, a vaccine is given at 12 to 15 months, with a booster between 4 and 6 years of age.

Complications

Complications of varicella are rare. The disease can have significant, life-threatening complications in children who are immunocompromised.

Complications of varicella include secondary bacterial infections, such as cellulitis, lymphadenitis, abscesses, and sepsis. Other potential complications include encephalitis and meningoencephalitis, hepatitis, acute thrombocytopenia, and pneumonia.

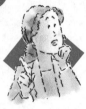

Quick quiz

1. Which statement about Lyme disease is true?
 A. Lyme disease is vaccine-preventable.
 B. Lyme disease is caused by a spirochete that enters the body through a tick bite.
 C. Lyme disease is common in tropical areas where spores are found in the soil.
 D. Children with Lyme disease should be isolated from others because of the risk of disease transmission.

Answer: B. Lyme disease is caused by a spirochete, *Borrelia burgdorferi*, which is transmitted to humans through the bite of an infected deer tick.

2. Which sexually transmitted disease is preventable through vaccination?
 A. Syphilis
 B. Gonorrhea
 C. Hepatitis A
 D. Hepatitis B

Answer: D. The hepatitis B vaccine is given I.M. at birth (or before hospital discharge), at ages 1 to 4 months, and again at ages 6 to 18 months, for a total of three doses. For older children and adolescents, the initial I.M. dose is given, the second dose is given 1 month later, and the third dose is given 6 months after the first dose.

3. The mother of a child with varicella asks the nurse when the child may return to day care. The nurse correctly responds by telling the mother that the child can return:
 A. when the fever is resolved.
 B. 24 hours after the appearance of the rash.
 C. when all lesions are crusted over.
 D. after receiving the first dose of diphenhydramine (Benadryl).

Answer: C. The period of communicability for varicella (chickenpox) begins up to 5 days before the appearance of the body rash. The period of communicability continues until all lesions on the skin are crusted over.

4. What's an early symptom of roseola infantum?
A. High, unexplained fever
B. Vomiting
C. Development of a body rash
D. Behavioral changes and anorexia

Answer: A. The onset of symptoms of illness occurs with sudden, high fever. Fevers of 103° to 106° F (39.4° to 41.1° C) can occur. Other than the unexplained fever, the child appears well, with normal behaviors.

Scoring

☆☆☆ If you answered all four items correctly, bravo! Go forth and spread your understanding of viral and bacterial illnesses.

☆☆ If you answered three items correctly, excellent work! Your knowledge of communicable disease is infectious.

☆ If you answered fewer than three items correctly, don't go into isolation! Take another look at the chapter, and forge ahead.

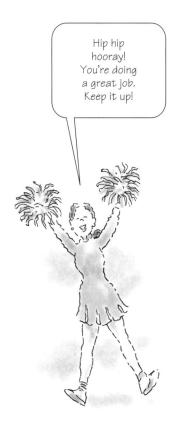

Neurologic problems

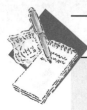

Just the facts

In this chapter, you'll learn:

♦ structures of the neurologic system

♦ assessment of patients with problems involving the neurologic system

♦ diagnostic tests for neurologic problems

♦ treatments and nursing interventions for children with neurologic disorders.

Anatomy and physiology

The neurologic system consists of the central nervous system (CNS), the peripheral nervous system, and the autonomic (involuntary) nervous system (ANS). Through complex and coordinated interactions, these three parts integrate all physical, intellectual, and emotional activities. Understanding how each part works is essential to conducting an accurate neurologic assessment.

Central nervous system

The CNS is composed of the brain and all its component parts and the spinal cord. Structurally, the CNS is contained within the skull and the vertebral column.

Central command

Integration among all parts of the nervous system enables normal functioning of body parts, both voluntary and involuntary. A person's perception of himself and his environment, his reactions and interactions with the environment, and his adjustment to development and environmental changes are greatly influenced by the proper integration and functioning of the nervous system.

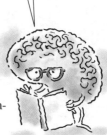

I like to think of myself as an intellectual. Seems like I'm the brains in this operation.

Brain

The brain, the center of the CNS, collects, integrates, and interprets stimuli and initiates and monitors voluntary and involuntary motor activity.

The incredible expanding brain

Head circumference, which is measured in children up to age 3 years, averages 13″ to 14″ (33 to 35.5 cm) and should be ½″ to 1″ (2 to 3 cm) larger than chest circumference at birth. Fifty percent of brain growth is achieved in the first year of life, 75% by age 3, and 90% by age 6. The brain comprises 12% of body weight at birth, doubles in weight in the first year, and triples by age 5 or 6.

I'm the body's go-to organ. When the body needs a stimulus interpreted or a motor activity initiated, I'm the only guy for the job.

Separated at birth

Since the skull protects the brain, the anterior and posterior fontanels are separated at birth to allow for brain expansion. The posterior fontanel closes between ages 4 and 8 weeks, and the anterior fontanel closes between ages 12 and 18 months.

A mass of nerves in a house of bones

Physiologically, the brain is the large, soft mass of nervous tissue housed in the cranium and protected and supported by the meninges and the skull bones. It consists of the:
- cerebrum
- cerebellum
- brain stem.

Other noteworthy figures

Other structures and elements of the brain include the:
- neurons
- meninges
- cerebrospinal fluid (CSF)
- ventricles.

Cerebrum

The cerebrum, the largest portion of the brain, is the nerve center that controls sensory and motor activities and intelligence.

The outer layer of the cerebrum, the *cerebral cortex*, consists of neuron cell bodies (gray matter); the inner layers consist of axons (white matter) and basal ganglia, which control motor coordination and steadiness.

Bridging the hemispheres

A longitudinal fissure divides the cerebrum into two hemispheres connected by a wide band of nerve fibers called the *corpus callosum*. These hemispheres share information through the corpus callosum. Because motor impulses descending from the brain cross in the medulla, the right hemisphere controls the left side of the body and the left hemisphere controls the right side of the body.

Not the piercing kind

Several fissures divide the cerebrum into lobes, each of which is associated with specific functions. (See *A look at the lobes.*)

Passing the baton

The thalamus, a relay center below the corpus callosum, further organizes cerebral function by transmitting impulses to and from appropriate areas of the cerebrum.

The body's thermostat

The hypothalamus, which lies beneath the thalamus, is an autonomic center that regulates temperature control, appetite, blood pressure, breathing, sleep patterns, and peripheral nerve discharges that occur with behavioral and emotional expression.

Cerebellum

Beneath the cerebrum, at the base of the brain, is the cerebellum. It's responsible for smooth-muscle movements, coordinating sensory impulses with muscle activity, and maintaining muscle tone and equilibrium.

Brain stem

The brain stem relays nerve impulses between the spinal cord and other parts of the brain. It houses cell bodies from most of the cranial nerves (CNs) and includes the:
• *midbrain,* which is the reflex center for the third and fourth CNs and mediates pupillary reflexes and eye movements
• *pons,* which helps regulate respirations and mediate chewing, taste, saliva secretion, hearing, and equilibrium
• *medulla oblongata,* which affects cardiac, respiratory, and vasomotor functions.

Neurons

The fundamental unit of the nervous system is the neuron, a highly specialized conductor cell that receives and transmits electrochemical nerve impulses. Neurons develop at between 15 and 30 weeks' gestation.

Delicate and impulsive

Its structure contains delicate, threadlike nerve fibers that extend from the central cell body and transmit signals, or

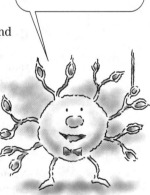

Conducting the nervous system's electrochemical impulses is music to my ears!

A look at the lobes

Several fissures divide the cerebrum into hemi-spheres and lobes; each lobe has a specific function.

The great dividers

The *fissure of Sylvius* (lateral sulcus) separates the temporal lobe from the frontal and parietal lobes. The *fissure of Rolando* (central sulcus) separates the frontal lobes from the parietal lobe. The *parieto-occipital fissure* separates the occipital lobe from the two parietal lobes.

Lovely lobes

Each lobe controls specific body functions:
• The *frontal lobe* controls voluntary muscle movements and contains motor areas (including the motor area for speech, or *Broca's area*). It's the center for personality, behavioral, and intellectual functions, such as judgment, memory, and problem solving; for autonomic functions; and for cardiac and emotional responses.
• The *temporal lobe* is the center for taste, hearing, and smell. Also, in the brain's dominant hemisphere, it interprets spoken language.
• The *parietal lobe* coordinates and interprets sensory information from the opposite side of the body.
• The *occipital lobe* interprets visual stimuli.

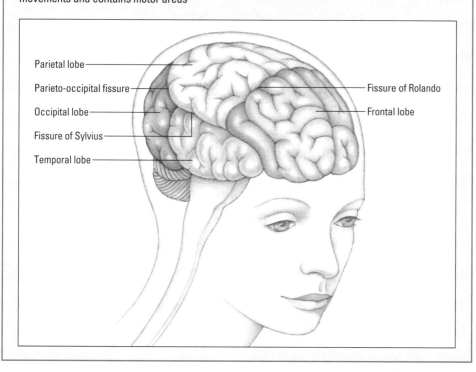

Parietal lobe

Parieto-occipital fissure

Occipital lobe

Fissure of Sylvius

Temporal lobe

Fissure of Rolando

Frontal lobe

axons, which carry impulses away from the cell body, and *dendrites*, which carry impulses to the cell body.

Meninges

The brain is covered with three thin membranes called *meninges*:

The outer membrane is the *dura mater*, or "hard mother"; it has various folds that separate the brain into compartments.

The second structure is the *arachnoid*; it has two layers of fibrous and elastic tissue and, between the layers, a spongy, cobweblike structure containing subarachnoid fluid.

The third structure is the *pia mater*, or "tender mother," a very fine membrane that's rich in minute blood plexuses and follows the brain in all its folds. (See *Meningeal layers of the brain.*)

CSF

The ventricles of the brain and the entire subarachnoid space around the brain and spinal cord contain CSF.

Clear liquid with a protein chaser

CSF is a clear liquid containing water and traces of organic materials (especially protein), glucose, and minerals. CSF is formed from blood in capillary networks called *choroid plexuses*, which are located primarily in the brain's lateral ventricles. The fluid is eventually reabsorbed into the venous blood through the arachnoid villi, located in dural sinuses on the brain's surface.

Better than a bubble bath

The brain floats in, and is bathed by, CSF. It acts as a shock absorber and helps reduce forces that jar or shake the brain. CSF is in contact with the entire brain and spinal cord surface as well as the surfaces of the ventricles.

> There's nothing like a soothing bath to protect me from the jarring forces of the outside world. Not bad for the ole' noggin either!

Ventricles

The four ventricles are large, CSF-filled cavities within the brain. There are two lateral ventricles, one in each cerebral hemisphere. A third ventricle (located directly above the midbrain of the brainstem) communicates with both the lateral ventricles and the fourth ventricle (located in the posterior brain fossa).

Meningeal layers of the brain

Three primary membranes, or meninges, help protect the CNS: the dura mater, the arachnoid membrane, and the pia mater.

Dura mater

The dura mater is a fibrous membrane that lines the skull and forms folds (reflections) that descend into the brain's fissures and provide stability. The dural folds include the:
• falx cerebri, which lies in the longitudinal fissure and separates the hemispheres of the cerebrum
• tentorium cerebelli, which separates the cerebrum from the cerebellum
• falx cerebelli, which separates the two cerebellar lobes.

The arachnoid villi (projections of the dura mater into the superior sagittal and transverse sinuses) serve as the exit points for CSF drainage into venous circulation.

Arachnoid membrane

A fragile, fibrous layer with moderate vascularity, the arachnoid membrane lies between the dura mater and the pia mater. Injury to its blood vessels during head trauma, lumbar puncture, or cisternal puncture may cause hemorrhage.

Pia mater

An extremely thin and highly vascular membrane, the *pia mater* closely covers the brain's surface and extends into its fissures. It contains minute arteries and veins that supply the brain.

Additional layers

Three layers of space further cushion the brain and spinal cord against injury:
• The *epidural space* (a potential space) lies over the dura mater.

• The *subdural space* lies between the dura mater and the arachnoid membrane and is commonly the site of hemorrhage after head trauma.
• The *subarachnoid space*, which is filled with CSF, lies between the arachnoid membrane and the pia mater.

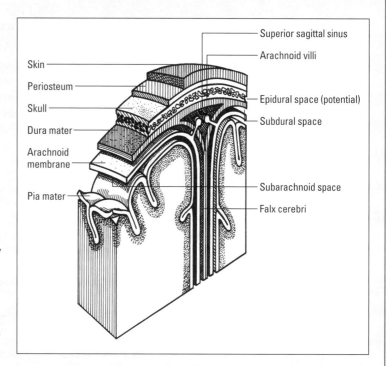

Skin
Periosteum
Skull
Dura mater
Arachnoid membrane
Pia mater

Superior sagittal sinus
Arachnoid villi
Epidural space (potential)
Subdural space
Subarachnoid space
Falx cerebri

Spinal cord

The spinal cord extends downward from the brain, through the vertebrae, to the level of approximately the second lumbar vertebra. It functions as a conductive pathway to and from the brain. It's also the reflex center for activities that don't require brain control such as deep tendon reflexes (the jerking reaction elicited by tapping with a reflex hammer).

Can you hear me now?

Within the spinal cord, connections are made between incoming and outgoing nerve fibers. Thirty-one pairs of spinal nerves are connected to the cord. The sensory, or ascending, tracts carry sensory impulses up the spinal cord to the brain; the motor, or descending, tracts carry motor impulses down the spinal cord and out to the peripheral nervous system.

Peripheral nervous system

The part of the nervous system outside of the skull and vertebral column is considered the peripheral nervous system. It's composed of 31 spinal nerves and 12 CNs and is divided into two functional systems: the somatic nervous system and the ANS.

Spinal nerves

Messages transmitted through the spinal cord reach outlying areas through 31 pairs of segmentally arranged spinal nerves attached to the spinal cord. Spinal nerves are numbered according to their point of origin in the cord:
- eight cervical nerves—C1 to C8
- 12 thoracic nerves—T1 to T12
- five lumbar nerves—L1 to L5
- one coccygeal nerve.

It's rude to interrupt

After leaving the vertebral column, each spinal nerve separates into *rami* (branches), distributed peripherally, with extensive but organized overlapping. This overlapping reduces the risk of lost sensory or motor function from interruption of a single spinal nerve.

Cranial nerves

The 12 pairs of CNs transmit motor or sensory messages (or both) primarily between the brain or brain stem and the head and neck. All CNs except the olfactory and optic nerves exit from the midbrain, pons, or medulla oblongata of the brain stem. (See *Exit points of the cranial nerves.*)

Somatic nervous system

The somatic (voluntary) nervous system is activated by will but can function independently. It's responsible for all conscious and

Exit points of the cranial nerves

As this illustration reveals, 10 of the 12 pairs of CNs exit from the brain stem. The remaining two pairs—the olfactory and optic nerves—exit from the forebrain.

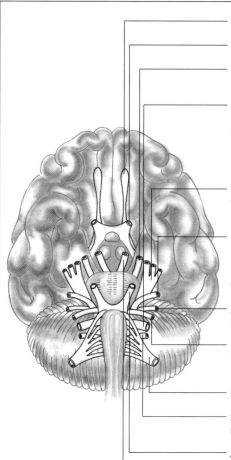

Olfactory (CN I). *Sensory:* smell

Optic (CN II). *Sensory:* visual

Trochlear (CN IV). *Motor:* extraocular eye movement (inferior medial)

Vagus (CN X). *Motor:* movement of palate, swallowing, gag reflex, activity of the thoracic and abdominal viscera, such as heart rate and peristalsis. *Sensory:* sensations of throat, larynx, and thoracic and abdominal viscera (heart, lungs, bronchi, and GI tract)

Trigeminal (CN V). *Sensory:* transmitting stimuli from face and head, corneal reflex. *Motor:* chewing, biting, and lateral jaw movements

Facial (CN VII). *Sensory:* taste receptors (anterior two-thirds of tongue). *Motor:* facial muscle movement, including muscles of expression (those in the forehead and around the eyes and mouth)

Acoustic (CN VIII). *Sensory:* hearing, sense of balance

Glossopharyngeal (CN IX). *Motor:* swallowing movements. *Sensory:* sensations of throat, taste receptors (posterior one-third of tongue)

Hypoglossal (CN XII). *Motor:* tongue movement

Spinal accessory (CN XI). *Motor:* shoulder movement, head rotation

Abducens (CN VI). *Motor:* extraocular eye movement (lateral)

Oculomotor (CN III). *Motor:* extraocular eye movement (superior, medial, and inferior lateral), pupillary constriction, upper eyelid elevation

higher mental processes as well as subconscious and reflex actions such as shivering.

Autonomic nervous system

The ANS regulates unconscious processes to control involuntary body functions, such as digestion, respiration, and cardiovascular function. It's usually divided into two antagonistic systems that balance each other's activities to support homeostasis under normal conditions:
• The *sympathetic nervous system* controls energy expenditure, especially in stressful situations, by releasing adrenergic catecholamines.
• The *parasympathetic nervous system* helps conserve energy by releasing the cholinergic neurohormone acetylcholine.

Neurologic assessment

A complete assessment of the neurologic system includes evaluation of:
• mental and emotional status
• CN function
• sensory function
• motor function
• reflexes.

Knowledge of the pediatric patient's physical, psychomotor, and cognitive developmental milestones is an essential assessment tool for detecting significant deviations. For toddlers and preschoolers, make a game of the assessment process when possible. Have older children assist with the assessment.

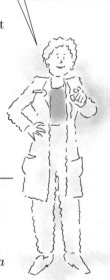

Could you recognize a developmental lag? If you know the milestones, you can tell if a child is falling behind.

Mini-assessment

Because there isn't always enough time to completely assess neurologic function, a bedside assessment might focus on level of consciousness (LOC), pupillary response, motor function, reflexes, sensory functions, and vital signs.

Glasgow Coma Scale

The Glasgow Coma Scale (GCS), which assesses eye opening as well as verbal and motor responses, provides a quick, standardized account of neurologic status. A pediatric version of the scale considers the preverbal child. (See *Pediatric coma scale*.)

Pediatric coma scale

To quickly assess a patient's LOC and to uncover changes from baseline, use the pediatric coma scale. This assessment tool grades consciousness in relation to eye opening and motor response, and responses to auditory or visual stimuli. A decreased reaction score in one or more categories warns of an impending neurologic crisis. A patient scoring 7 or lower is comatose and probably has severe neurologic damage.

Test	Patient's reaction	Score
Best eye opening response	Open spontaneously	4
	Open to verbal command	3
	Open to pain	2
	No response	1
Best motor response	Obeys verbal command	6
	Localizes painful stimuli	5
	Flexion-withdrawal	4
	Flexion-abnormal (decorticate rigidity)	3
	Extension (decerebrate rigidity)	2
	No response	1

Test	Patient's reaction	Score
Best response to auditory and/or visual stimulus	For the child older than age 2 years:	
	Oriented	5
	Confused	4
	Inappropriate words	3
	Incomprehensible sounds	2
	No response	1
	OR For the child younger than age 2 years: Smiles, listens, follows	5
	Cries, consolable	4
	Inappropriate persistent cry	3
	Agitated, restless	2
	No response	1

Total possible score	*3 to 15*

In this exam, each response receives a numerical value; the final score is the sum total of the values.
- A total score of 15 for all three parts is normal.
- A score of 7 or lower indicates coma.
- A score of 3, the lowest possible score, usually (but not always) indicates brain death.

Motor function

Motor function is also a good indicator of LOC and can point to central or peripheral nervous system damage.

Myelination mastery

The mastery of gross and fine motor skills is related to the myelination of the nervous system and follows the concept of cephalocaudal-proximodistal development. *Cephalocaudal development* is the sequence in which the greatest growth always occurs at the head and gradually works its way toward the "tail." *Proximodistal development* proceeds from the center toward the extremities.

Reflex rules

Infant activities are primarily driven by reflex but, with myelination and development, a growing child progressively performs complex tasks requiring coordinated movements.

How strong are you?

To evaluate muscle strength, follow these steps:
- Have the patient grip your hands and squeeze.
- Ask him to push against your palm with his foot.
- Compare muscle strength on each side to ensure the results are the same bilaterally.

> Assess pupillary response at the bedside.

Pupillary response

Brain damage is indicated by a lack of change in pupil size in response to light. Use a flashlight to assess pupillary response at the bedside. While shining the outer edge of the light into the patient's eye, observe the initial size of the pupil and the speed of the pupil's response to the light. Compare both eyes to ensure an equal bilateral response.

Diagnostic tests

Several invasive and noninvasive tests are used to diagnose neurologic disorders.

Minimizing emotional trauma

Tests performed to diagnose neurologic disorders can be extremely frightening to a child. Children may have misconceptions related to what will happen and why a test is being performed. Preparing a child helps allay fears and misconceptions and gives him the tools to cope effectively with a frightening experience. The timing of the preparation depends on the age/developmental level of the child. For the younger child, the preparation should be closer to the occurrence of the procedure, sometimes just prior to. The older child can be given information about a procedure more in advance.

Before a test is performed, follow these steps:
• Tell the child what to expect in simple, age-appropriate terms (what he'll see, hear, and feel) and explain why the test is being performed.
• Be honest about pain or discomfort the child might experience and suggest coping strategies (for example, "Count to 5 and the hurting part will be over").

Big boys do cry

• Tell the child that it's OK to be afraid, and reassure him that everyone involved is there to help him and keep him safe.
• Whenever possible, allow the child to see the equipment (for example, the scanning machine) before the test. Pictures may be used, if necessary.
• Encourage the child to ask questions and express his concerns.
• Allow the parents to remain with the child during testing whenever possible; when this isn't possible, tell the child where his parents will be waiting for him.

A job well done

• Give the child a "job" to do during the test (for example, "Your job is to hold very still.") to give him a sense of control.
• After the test, praise the child for doing a good job, and encourage him to talk about the test or draw a picture that depicts his experience (to help the child master the experience and put it in perspective).

Specialist to the rescue

Most hospitals have one or more child life specialists who will meet with the child and his parents before a test, explain the procedure, and accompany and support the child and his parents during the test.

CT scan

Computed tomography (CT) scan is indicated when CNS disease is suspected. The scan produces three-dimensional images that can identify congenital abnormalities, fractures, brain tumors, infarction, bleeding, and hematomas as well as provide information about the ventricular system of the brain. CT scan may be done with or without contrast.

Nursing considerations

A child who knows what to expect will be less fearful and more cooperative during a CT scan. To help the child know what to expect, consider these steps:
• Explain the procedure to the child. Cooperation is necessary because the patient must lie still during the procedure.
• Show the child a picture of the CT machine to help alleviate fears. (It may be necessary to premedicate the patient.)
• Tell the child that he may hear a clicking noise as the scanner moves around his head but that the machine won't touch him.
• Explain that the child won't be able to eat or drink for 4 hours before the scan (depending on age); contrast dye may cause nausea.
• Assess the patient for allergy to iodinated dye or shellfish.
• Encourage the child to drink fluids after the scan (because dye is excreted by the kidneys).

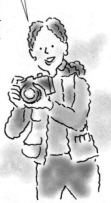

Seeing is believing. Show the child a picture of the imaging machine (or the machine itself) to help allay his fear of the unknown.

EEG

Electroencephalogram (EEG) is a graphic recording of the electrical activity of the brain. It's performed to identify and evaluate patients with seizures. Pathologic conditions involving the brain cortex (such as tumors and infarctions) can also be detected. EEG is also used to confirm brain death.

Nursing considerations

After explaining the procedure to the child and his parents:
• Reassure the child that he won't feel anything during the test.
• Make sure the child continues to eat and drink before the test because fasting may cause hypoglycemia, which could alter the test results.
• Make sure the child doesn't drink anything with caffeine on the morning of the test because of caffeine's stimulating effect.
• Tell the patient that he needs to remain still during the test; any movement will create interference and alter the EEG recording.

Lumbar puncture

By placing a needle in the subarachnoid space of the spinal column, one can measure the pressure of that space and obtain CSF for examination and diagnosis. The needle is commonly placed between L3 and L4 (or L4 and L5). This examination may assist in the diagnosis of metastatic brain or spinal cord neoplasm, meningitis, cerebral hemorrhage, and encephalitis.

Nursing considerations

The procedure should be explained, and written informed consent should be obtained. In addition, follow these steps:
• Apply eutectic mixture of local anesthetics (EMLA) cream to puncture site 30 to 60 minutes before procedure to reduce pain if ordered.
• Instruct the child to empty his bladder and bowels before the procedure.
• Monitor the child's vital signs during and after the procedure because sedation is used to complete the procedure.
• Explain the importance of remaining still throughout the procedure in the side-lying knee-chest position. (See *Lumbar puncture positioning*, page 220.)
• Gently hold even a cooperative child during the procedure to prevent injury from unexpected or involuntary movement.

Maintain, encourage, assess

• Keep the child flat for 1 hour after procedure.
• Keep the child in a reclining position for up to 12 hours after the procedure to avoid the discomfort of potential postprocedure spinal headache.
• Encourage the child to drink increased amounts of fluid with a straw to replace the CSF removed during the puncture. (Drinking with a straw allows the patient to keep his head flat.)
• Assess the child for numbness, tingling, and decreased movement of the extremities; pain at the injection site; drainage of blood or CSF at the injection site; and inability to void.

MRI

Magnetic resonance imaging (MRI) is a noninvasive diagnostic procedure that provides valuable information about the body's anatomy in greater detail than a CT scan does. It doesn't require exposure to ionizing radiation. MRI is indicated for the evaluation of headache or neurologic signs of CNS lesions; it's also used to assess neck and back pain as well as lesions of the bones and joints.

Advice from the experts

Lumbar puncture positioning

When positioning a child for a lumbar puncture, follow these steps:

1.   Have the child lie on his side at the edge of the bed, with his chin tucked to his chest and his knees drawn up to his abdomen.

2.   Make sure the child's spine is curved and his back is at the edge of the bed (as shown below); this position widens the spaces between the vertebrae, easing insertion of the needle.

3.   To help the child maintain this position, place one of your hands behind his neck; place the other hand behind his knees, and pull gently.

4.   Hold the child firmly in this position throughout the procedure to prevent accidental needle displacement. (Typically, the doctor inserts the needle between the third and fourth lumbar vertebrae.)

The sitting position may be used for infants. However, because the flexed position may interfere with the infant's breathing, monitor his color and respiratory status closely during the procedure.

Positioning a young child

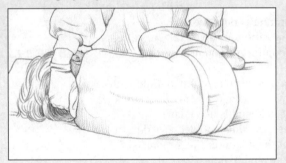

Positioning an infant

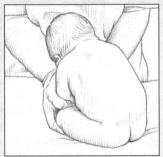

Nursing considerations

Begin by explaining the procedure to the patient and his family and telling them that there's no exposure to radiation during MRI. In addition, follow these steps:
• Tell the parents that, because no radiation is used, they may read or talk to their child in the imaging room during the procedure.
• Inform the parents that young children may need to be sedated because of the need to remain motionless during the procedure.
• Tell the child that he may eat or drink as usual before and after the procedure. (No food or fluid restrictions are necessary before MRI, unless sedation is given.)

PET scan

In positron emission tomography (PET) scanning, radioactive chemicals are administered to the patient. These chemicals are used in the normal metabolic process of the particular organ being studied. Positrons emitted from the radioactive chemicals in the organ are sensed by a series of detectors positioned around the patient.

PET scanning can help detect cerebral dysfunction caused by tumors, seizures, head trauma, and some mental illnesses. It's most commonly used for evaluation of the heart and brain and in many aspects of oncology.

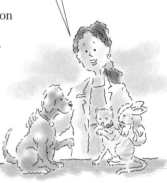

It may not be cute and cuddly, but a PET scan is the best thing going for detecting cerebral dysfunction.

Nursing considerations

Keep in mind that many people haven't heard of PET scanning; the child and his parents may be anxious about what they perceive to be a new procedure. To prepare the child and parents for the procedure, follow these steps:
• Explain the procedure to the child and his family.
• Explain to the child that an intravenous (I.V.) injection will be inserted and that this is the only "hurting part" of the procedure.
• Explain that food or fluids may need to be restricted for 4 hours on the day of the test.
• Don't sedate the child; he may need to perform certain mental activities during a brain PET scan.
• After the scan, encourage the child to drink fluids and urinate frequently to aid removal of the radioisotope from the bladder.

Ventricular tap

A ventricular tap may be performed if an infant has unexplained, excessive head growth or a bulging fontanel caused by increased intracranial pressure (ICP), associated with an increased accumulation of CSF that has been confirmed by ultrasound or CT scan.

Going in

When performing a ventricular tap:
• The needle is inserted into the subdural space or the ventricle through the open anterior fontanel or the coronal suture.
• The fluid is removed slowly to prevent intracranial hemorrhage caused by pressure shifts.

Nursing considerations

Parents are likely to feel anxious when their infant must undergo a procedure that involves pain, discomfort, or stress. The nurse should encourage the parents to ask questions and express concerns.
• Explain the procedure to the parents.
• Hold the infant's head securely in the correct position to prevent meningeal laceration.
• Number and label the tubes of fluid in the order in which they're collected.
• Maintain the infant in a semi-erect position (an infant seat may be used) to reduce the possibility of further leakage of fluid from the site of the puncture.
• Assess the pressure dressing for leakage of fluid and bleeding.
• Keep the infant as quiet and comfortable as possible; crying increases ICP.

Procedures and treatments

The care of a child with suspected or diagnosed neurologic problems may involve invasive procedures to monitor or treat the child's condition.

ICP monitoring

ICP monitoring allows assessment of the pressure exerted by the blood, brain, CSF, and any other space-occupying fluid or mass; increased ICP is defined as pressure sustained at 20 mm Hg or higher.

Look closely . . .

Assessment of the child with increased ICP requires close observation because the common signs and symptoms may not appear until ICP is significantly elevated, placing the child in grave danger. The subarachnoid bolt and the intraventricular catheter (gold standard of ICP monitoring) are the two major instruments used for monitoring ICP in a child:
• The end of the bolt is placed in the subarachnoid space. The top of the bolt is attached to a transducer to conduct a waveform to the monitor.
• The catheter is placed in the lateral ventricle or subarachnoid space. (The catheter provides a method for measuring pressure as well as a conduit to drain off extra fluid into a drainage bag.) The drainage bag and the manometer are part of a sterile closed system. (The manometer is used to measure the ICP within the closed system.)

Less invasive

In an infant, ICP monitoring can be performed without penetrating the scalp. In this external method, a photoelectric transducer with a pressure-sensitive membrane is taped to the infant's anterior fontanel. The transducer responds to pressure at the site and transmits readings to a bedside monitor and recording system.

Sorry, not for everyone

The external method is restricted to infants because pressure readings can be obtained only at the fontanels (the incompletely ossified areas of the skull). ICP monitoring from the fontanels can be inaccurate if the equipment is poorly placed or inconsistently calibrated.

Nursing considerations

Before ICP monitoring is performed, thoroughly explain the procedure to the child and his parents. In addition, follow these steps:
• Be thoroughly familiar with the monitoring system being used, and prepare the child and his family for what they can expect after placement of the selected monitoring device.
• Explain that the procedure doesn't hurt the child and that he may have sand bags placed on either side of his head to prevent head movement.
  • Head of bed is usually elevated 15 to 30 degrees.
• Assess whether the child has an allergy to iodine preparations.
• Maintain the sterility of the system.
  • Monitor the child closely for signs of infection.
• Monitor the amount of fluid in the drainage bag.
• Constantly monitor the child for signs of increased ICP.
  • Minimize activities that may elevate ICP, such as those that may cause stress, pain, or crying; bright lights, noise, and other environmental stimuli, and vigorous range-of-motion (ROM) exercises. Remember that suctioning and percussion are contraindicated because they acutely elevate ICP. Suctioning may be performed if absolutely necessary by hyperoxygenating the patient with 100% oxygen before the procedure. Vibration may be used instead of percussion because it doesn't increase ICP.

VP shunt insertion

A ventriculoperitoneal (VP) shunt is implanted in the child with hydrocephalus to prevent excess accumulation of CSF in the ventricles. The tubing diverts the CSF from the ventricles into the peritoneal cavity, where it's reabsorbed. The procedure is performed under general anesthesia.

Nursing considerations

Young children may have misconceptions about procedures involving general anesthesia. When explaining this procedure (and all procedures involving general anesthesia), make sure the child understands that he will be given "a special medicine" to make sure he doesn't feel anything during the procedure.

A special sleep

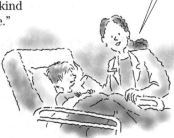

Explain that sleeping at night is different from sleeping during general anesthesia so that the child isn't scared to close his eyes at night or nap time.

Rather than telling a child he'll be asleep (which may make him afraid to go to sleep at night or nap time or cause him to worry that he'll wake up during the procedure), tell him, "The medicine gives you a special kind of sleep that isn't like sleeping at night or nap time."

Monitor and measure

In addition to preparing the child for the procedure, follow these care measures:

Preoperatively

Frequent neurologic assessments:
• Monitor the patient for signs of increased ICP.
• Measure head circumference daily at the occipital frontal circumference; place the tape measure just above the top of the ears, around the midforehead, and around the most prominent part of the occiput.
• Gently palpate fontanels and suture lines for signs of bulging, tenseness, and separation, which may indicate increased ICP or increasing ventricular size.

Postoperatively

Continue frequent neurologic assessments:
• Monitor the patient for pain, and administer pain medications as ordered.
• Check orders regarding allowable activities.
• Observe the child for signs of increased ICP, which may indicate an obstructed shunt.
• Monitor the child for abdominal distention, which may indicate distal catheter displacement.
• Be alert for signs of shunt infection (fever, lethargy, irritability, redness along shunt device, abdominal discomfort or apnea), which is the greatest postoperative risk.
• Monitor for fluid leak from the incision.
• Administer antibiotics as ordered.
• Teach parents to be aware of bowel patterns and recommend use of laxatives and diet to prevent constipation, which has been associated with shunt malfunction.

• Teach parents signs and symptoms of shunt failure (persistent headache, emesis, lethargy, visual changes, or swelling or redness along the device).

Neurologic disorders

A diagnosis of a neurologic disorder, whether acute, chronic, or progressive, can be terrifying to a child and his parents. They'll look to their nurses to help allay fears and concerns, answer questions, and provide ongoing support.

Bacterial meningitis

Meningitis, an inflammation of the meninges, is the most common infectious process of the CNS. It can be bacterial or viral and can occur as a primary disease or as a result of complications of neurosurgery, trauma, systemic infection, or sinus or ear infections.

What causes it

Prior to the addition of the *Haemophilus influenzae* vaccine (HiB vaccine), *H. influenzae* type B was the most common cause of meningitis in children older than age 1 month, but vaccination has drastically reduced its incidence. *Neisseria meningitidis* (meningococcal meningitis) and *Streptococcus pneumoniae* (pneumococcal meningitis) took the lead as the most common bacterial causes of meningitis beyond infancy. In 2001, a pneumococcal vaccine (PCV-7 [later PCV-13]) was added to the vaccine schedule, and since then, the incidence of meningitis caused by *S. pneumoniae* has decreased. By the end of the decade, meningococcal vaccines (MCV4) were widely available and added to the recommended vaccines for adolescents. The incidence of bacterial meningitis dropped by 31% between 1998 and 2007.

Still strong

The incidence of *Escherichia coli* and beta-hemolytic streptococcus meningitis is higher during the first 2 years of life, especially during the first month of life.

How it happens

• Bacteria reach the meninges via the bloodstream from nearby infections (for example, sinusitis, mastoiditis, otitis media) or by communication of CSF with the exterior (for example, myelomeningocele, penetrating injuries, or neurosurgical procedures).

• The organism becomes implanted in CSF and throughout the arachnoid space. Because CSF has relatively low levels of antibodies, complement, and white blood cells (WBCs), the infection flourishes.

• As the process continues, increased ICP develops, along with empyema.

• If the infection spreads to the ventricles, edema and tissue scarring around the ventricle cause obstruction of the CSF and subsequent hydrocephalus. Because CSF contains such nutrients as protein and glucose, it's an excellent medium for bacterial growth. Thus, the process of infection, edema, obstruction, and hydrocephalus can occur rapidly.

What to look for

Symptoms of bacterial meningitis are variable and depend on the child's age, pathogen, and duration of the illness before diagnosis. Findings in young infants and toddlers (between ages 3 months and 2 years) may include:

• fever
• change in feeding pattern
• vomiting or diarrhea
• bulging anterior fontanel
• irritability (becoming more so with rocking and cuddling)
• high-pitched cry
• seizures.

A high-pitched cry is one symptom of bacterial meningitis in infants.

Bigger kids

In older children, look for:

• fever
• irritability
• lethargy
• confusion
• vomiting
• muscle or joint pain
• headache
• photophobia
• nuchal rigidity (resistance to neck flexion)
• opisthotonos (hyperextension of the head and neck to relieve discomfort)
• seizures
• coma
• positive Kernig's or Brudzinski's sign, or both. (See *Two telltale signs of meningitis.*)

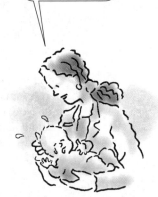

Two telltale signs of meningitis

A positive response to these tests helps to establish a diagnosis of meningitis.

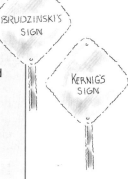

Brudzinski's sign

To test for Brudzinski's sign, place the patient in a dorsal recumbent position and put your hands behind his neck and bend it forward. Pain and resistance may indicate meningeal inflammation, neck injury, or arthritis. However, if the patient also flexes his hips and knees in response to the manipulation, chances are he has meningitis.

Kernig's sign

To test for Kernig's sign, place the patient in a supine position. Flex his leg at the hip and knee and then straighten the knee. Pain or resistance points to meningitis.

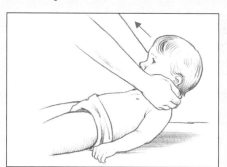

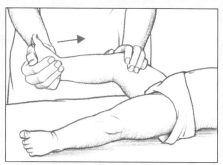

Children with a hemorrhagic rash, first appearing as petechiae and changing to purpura or large necrotic patches, may have meningococcal meningitis.

What tests tell you

Lumbar puncture is performed to evaluate the CSF for protein and glucose levels and the number of WBCs. The fluid may appear cloudy or milky white. CSF protein levels tend to be high; glucose levels may be low. Polymerase chain reaction techniques are useful when the cultures are negative because of partially treated meningitis.

A CT scan or MRI can rule out cerebral hematoma, hemorrhage, or tumor and identify an abscess. Other tests performed to aid in diagnosis include:

- blood cultures
- complete blood count (CBC)

- serum electrolytes and osmolality
- clotting factors
- nose and throat cultures.

Complications

The most common neurologic complications of meningitis are hearing loss, neurologic deficit, seizures, visual impairment, and behavioral problems. Other complications include CN dysfunction, brain abscess, and syndrome of inappropriate antidiuretic hormone (SIADH). Death occurs in 10% to 15% of cases (especially neonatal meningitis).

How it's treated

Treatment should begin before the causative organism is identified because it may take up to 2 days to obtain culture results and delays could be fatal. Treatment includes the following:
- Two broad spectrum antibiotics should be started as an initial treatment regimen.
- Antibiotics may be changed when culture and sensitivity results are known.
- Adjunctive therapy with dexamethasone (Decadron) may be provided to reduce the risk of sequelae such as hearing loss and neurologic complications.
- Isolation of the child is necessary for the first 24 hours of therapy to prevent spreading the infection.
- Medications to control fever and pain/discomfort should be administered as needed.

No antibiotics needed if culture results come back negative

Treatment for viral (aseptic) meningitis is supportive; medications such as analgesics may be used to keep the child comfortable. (See *Aseptic meningitis.*) The initial symptoms of viral and bacterial meningitis are similar, so children with signs of meningitis should be treated as if it is bacterial until the culture proves otherwise.

What to do

Nursing interventions include a thorough history and careful assessment:
- Review the medical history with the patient and his family for recent illnesses, such as upper respiratory infection, head injury, otitis media, and sinusitis (or a previous lumbar puncture).
- Assess the patient for the presence or absence of headaches, hearing loss, seizure activity, change in food and fluid intake, changes in LOC, pupil reaction and size, and nuchal rigidity.

Aseptic meningitis

Aseptic meningitis is a benign syndrome characterized by headache, fever, vomiting, and meningeal symptoms. It results from some form of viral infection, including enteroviruses (most common), arboviruses, herpes simplex virus, mumps virus, or lymphocytic choriomeningitis virus.

Signs and symptoms

Aseptic meningitis begins suddenly with a fever up to 104° F (40° C), alterations in consciousness (drowsiness, confusion, stupor), and neck or spine stiffness, which is slight at first. (The patient experiences such stiffness when bending forward.) Other signs and symptoms include headaches, nausea, vomiting, abdominal pain, poorly defined chest pain, and sore throat.

Diagnostic tests

Patient history of recent illness and knowledge of seasonal epidemics are essential in differentiating among the many forms of aseptic meningitis. Negative bacteriologic cultures and CSF analysis showing pleocytosis and increased protein levels suggest the diagnosis. Isolation of the virus from CSF confirms it.

Treatment

Treatment is supportive and includes:
• bed rest
• maintenance of fluid and electrolyte balance
• analgesics for pain
• exercises to combat residual weakness
• careful handling of excretions and good hand-washing technique to prevent spreading the disease (isolation isn't necessary).

• Assess peaks and troughs of antibiotic levels to ensure adequate treatment and prevent ototoxicity.
• Ongoing assessment of LOC is the priority nursing assessment.
• Teach the parents about the possible complications of meningitis and about the prescribed medications.
• Question the parents about the child's close contacts because they will need prophylactic treatment. (Close contacts shouldn't wait for signs of meningitis to develop but should seek medical attention promptly because they could be incubating the infection.)

Brain tumors

CNS tumors are the most common solid tumors in children and cause more deaths in children than any other form of malignancy. Most brain tumors in children are *supratentorial* (above the roofline of the cerebellum); the remaining tumors are *infratentorial* (below the roofline of the cerebellum).

What causes it

The cause of brain tumors is unknown, but heredity and environment have been associated with their development.

How it happens

Brain tumors are generally classified according to the tissue from which they arise: those arising inside the brain substance (such as gliomas and vascular tumors) or those arising outside the brain substance (such as meningiomas and CN tumors).

Common in kids

The most common brain tumors in children are:
- cerebellar astrocytoma
- medulloblastoma
- ependymoma
- brain stem glioma. (See *Locations of brain tumors in children.*)

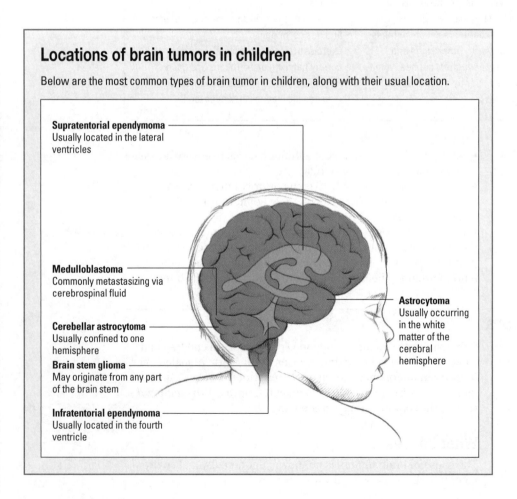

Locations of brain tumors in children

Below are the most common types of brain tumor in children, along with their usual location.

Supratentorial ependymoma
Usually located in the lateral ventricles

Medulloblastoma
Commonly metastasizing via cerebrospinal fluid

Cerebellar astrocytoma
Usually confined to one hemisphere

Brain stem glioma
May originate from any part of the brain stem

Infratentorial ependymoma
Usually located in the fourth ventricle

Astrocytoma
Usually occurring in the white matter of the cerebral hemisphere

What to look for

Signs and symptoms are directly related to the anatomic location and size of the tumor and, to some extent, the age of the child:
- The hallmark symptoms of a brain tumor are morning headache and early morning vomiting related to the child getting out of bed.
- The child may experience vision changes, such as diplopia, strabismus, and nystagmus, which may manifest as difficulties with schoolwork.
- *Papilledema* (edema of the optic disc) may be a late sign; this may be hard to evaluate in children because ophthalmic examinations require the child's cooperation.
- Enlargement of the head or bulging fontanels may be present in children before the closure of cranial sutures (at ages 12 to 18 months).
- Personality changes may be most critical and easily observable (such as crying, irritability, and not wanting to play).
- *Ataxia*, or uncoordinated gait, may be mistaken for clumsiness and is the most common sign of cerebellar involvement.

What tests tell you

History and physical and neurologic examinations provide the most important information. Diagnostic studies include:
- MRI (most common), CT scan, and PET scan showing the location and extent of the tumor
- lumbar puncture and serology of CSF to assess for the presence of tumor cells.

Complications

Some children with brain tumors experience some permanent sequelae, especially if they receive radiation therapy. They may have slowed development, incoordination, learning disabilities, or other effects. In some instances, brain tumors result in death.

How it's treated

Treatment includes:
- removing a resectable tumor
- reducing a nonresectable tumor
- relieving cerebral edema, increased ICP, and other symptoms
- preventing further neurologic damage.

The mode of therapy depends on the tumor's histologic type, radiosensitivity, and location; it may include surgery, radiation, chemotherapy, or decompression of increased ICP with diuretics, corticosteroids or, possibly, VP shunting of CSF.

Treatment of choice

Surgical excision is usually performed when possible. However, combination therapy (surgery and radiation with or without chemotherapy) has been proven to improve outcomes.

What to do

During your first contact with the child, perform a comprehensive assessment (including a complete neurologic evaluation) to provide baseline data and help develop your care plan. In addition, follow these steps:

• Continually assess for signs of increased ICP, including decreasing pulse and respirations, increasing systolic blood pressure, and a widening pulse pressure.

• Monitor for changes in the child's LOC. (A change in behavior is most significant in young children. A change in sleeping and waking patterns may also be significant.)

• Report changes in ocular signs, such as pupil response, shape, and size.

• Measure head circumference daily in children younger than age 2 years.

Better safe than sorry

• Observe seizure precautions; seizures are always a possibility in a child with brain tumor.

• Always keep the bed's side rails up and assist with ambulation because CN dysfunction may lead to ataxia and weakness.

• Provide emotional support for the child, his parents, and other family members; referral to a social worker, psychologist, or other health care professional may be needed to help the child and his family cope with the diagnosis.

> It may take the whole team—a social worker, a psychologist, and other health care workers—to help the family cope.

Postoperative care

Children who undergo surgery for a brain tumor require specialized care. Positioning is important and varies with the type of surgery performed, and diligent monitoring of vital signs, neurologic status, and pain is essential. In addition, follow these steps:

• The child may be kept flat at first; positioning may be limited to a 10- to 20-degree elevation for the first 24 to 48 hours. (The doctor will prescribe the patient's position.)

• Never place the child in Trendelenburg's position because it increases ICP and the risk of bleeding.

- Assess vital signs, mental status, and neurologic status frequently because the child is at risk for increased ICP related to cerebral edema, hydrocephalus, or hemorrhage.

High temp, cool blanket

- The child's temperature may be labile (usually elevated) because of edema of the brain stem; a hypothermia blanket may be used if the child becomes hyperthermic.
- Be careful not to place tension on the suture line when turning the child.
- Assess the child frequently for pain. (Analgesics should be provided according to the doctor's orders.)

Hair today, gone tomorrow

- Body image issues (shaven head, edema, or fear of disfigurement) may be a problem for older children; help them to work through these feelings.
- Provide emotional support to the parents; help them to work through their feelings regarding diagnosis, treatment, and prognosis (refer them to appropriate agencies and support groups for further assistance).

> Hair loss from treatment may be more difficult for a child or teen. Suggest using hats, scarves, and wigs, and reassure the child that her hair will grow back.

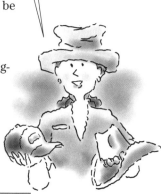

Cerebral palsy

Cerebral palsy (CP) is a nonprogressive, neuromuscular disorder of varying degrees resulting from damage or developmental defects in the part of the brain that controls motor function.

Children with CP can't control movements in certain parts of their bodies and may be partially paralyzed. They may have completely normal intelligence and may feel as if they're trapped in a body they can't control.

What causes it

Conditions that result in cerebral anoxia, hemorrhage, or other damage are probably responsible for CP.

In the womb

Prenatal conditions that may increase the risk of CP include maternal infection (especially rubella), maternal drug ingestion, radiation, anoxia, toxemia, maternal diabetes, abnormal placental attachment, malnutrition, and isoimmunization.

A shaky start

Perinatal and birth difficulties that increase the risk of CP include forceps delivery, breech presentation, placenta previa, abruptio placentae, metabolic or electrolyte disturbances, abnormal maternal vital signs from general or spinal anesthetic, prolapsed cord with delay in delivery of the head, premature birth, prolonged or unusually rapid labor, and multiple birth (especially infants born last in a multiple birth).

A traumatic legacy

Infection or trauma during infancy that increases the risk of CP includes poisoning, severe kernicterus resulting from erythroblastosis fetalis, brain infection, head trauma, prolonged anoxia, brain tumor, cerebral circulatory anomalies causing blood vessel rupture, and systemic disease resulting in cerebral thrombosis or embolus.

How it happens

A perinatal anoxic episode plays the largest role in the pathologic state of brain damage. Structural or functional defects occur, impairing motor or cognitive function. Defects may not be distinguishable until several months after birth or when the child fails to meet developmental milestones.

What to look for

There are three distinct types of CP:

 spastic

 athetoid

 ataxic.

Spastic

Spastic CP is the most common type, affecting about 70% of CP patients. The affected area of the brain is the cortex. Typically, the child with spastic CP walks on his toes with a scissor gait, crossing one foot in front of the other. Spastic CP is characterized by:

- increased deep tendon reflexes
- hypertonia
- flexion
- tendency to have contractures
- rapid involuntary muscle contraction and relaxation
- underdevelopment of affected limbs.

Athetoid

In athetoid CP, which affects about 20% of CP patients, involuntary, uncoordinated motion occurs with varying degrees of muscle tension. The area of injury is the basal ganglia. The child exhibits slow, writhing, uncontrolled movements involving all extremities whenever voluntary movement is attempted. Facial grimacing, poor swallowing, and drooling make speech difficult.

Ataxic

Ataxic CP accounts for about 10% of CP patients. The affected area of the brain is the cerebellum. Its characteristics include poor balance and muscle coordination caused by disturbances in movement and balance. An unsteady, wide-based gait appears as the child begins to learn to walk; overall, the child appears clumsy.

Mixed together

Some children with CP display a combination of these clinical features:
• In most, delayed gross motor development makes eating, especially swallowing, difficult.
• Abnormal motor performance and coordination can manifest early in life as poor sucking and feeding difficulty.
• Spasticity of hip muscles and lower extremities makes diapering difficult.
• Posture abnormalities occur at rest or when changing position.
• Cognitive impairment occurs in varying degrees in 18% to 50% of patients (most children with CP have an IQ that's normal or higher, but they can't demonstrate it on standardized tests).
• Seizures occur in 25% of CP patients.
• Many children have sensory deficits related to vision (strabismus), hearing, and speech.

What tests tell you

• Developmental screening reveals delay in achieving milestones.
• EEG may identify the source of seizure activity.
• Neuroimaging studies (CT scan, MRI) determine the site of brain impairment.
• Cytogenic studies (genetic evaluation of the child and other family members) and metabolic studies are performed to rule out other potential causes.

Complications

Children with CP may also have associated disorders, such as impaired intellectual development, seizures, failure to grow and thrive, and problems with vision and sense of touch.

MRI shows the part of the brain that's impaired.

How it's treated

CP can't be cured, but proper treatment can help affected children reach their full potential within the limitations set by this disorder. Treatment includes the following:

• A baclofen (Lioresal) pump may be inserted to treat spasticity by delivering the skeletal muscle relaxant directly to the intrathecal space around the spinal cord (the pump lasts for 3 to 5 years, after which a new pump must be implanted).
• Botulinum toxin A (Botox) may be used, especially for spasticity in lower extremities.
• Oral muscle relaxants may be used or neurosurgery may be required to decrease spasticity.
• Braces or splints and special appliances, such as adapted eating utensils and a low toilet seat with arms, can help the child perform activities independently.
• ROM exercises minimize contractures.
• An artificial urinary sphincter may be indicated for the incontinent child who's able to use hand controls.

Correct those contractures

• Orthopedic surgery may be indicated to correct contractures.
• Antiepileptics may be used to control seizures.

What to do

Care of the child with CP involves attention to diet and physical activity:

• Institute a high-calorie diet for the child with increased motor function to help him keep up with increased metabolic demands.
• Assist with locomotion, communication, and educational opportunities to enable the child to attain an optimal developmental level.
• Perform ROM exercises to minimize contractures.
• Plan activities that involve gross and fine motor skills (such as holding toys or eating utensils and positioning items to encourage reaching and rolling over).
• Provide a safe environment; have the child use protective headgear or bed pads to prevent injury.

Skilled labor of love

The nurse should also teach the family the skills needed to manage the child's care (such as medication administration, physical rehabilitation, and seizure management). Siblings should be involved in the child's care to prevent feelings of being left out.

Family members need help in setting realistic goals and managing stress. They should be referred to community agencies that will enhance the child's quality of life (early childhood stimulation programs, recreational programs for children with disabilities) and provide caregiver support.

Down syndrome

Down syndrome, also known as *trisomy 21*, is the most common genetic disorder, causing moderate to severe retardation.

What causes it

Down syndrome is the result of abnormal cell division involving chromosome 21.

There is an increased incidence in advanced parental age (when the mother is age 35 or older at delivery or the father is age 42 or older).

How it happens

A spontaneous extra chromosome causes Down syndrome; the child has 47, rather than 46, chromosomes. The most common chromosome affected is chromosome 21. The child has three copies of chromosome 21 rather than the usual two—hence, the name "trisomy."

What to look for

The physical signs of Down syndrome may be apparent at birth, especially hypotonia as well as some dysmorphic facial features and heart defects. The degree of mental retardation may not become apparent until the infant grows older.

Facial features

Facial features common in children with Down syndrome include:
- flat, broad forehead
- flat nasal bridge
- protruding tongue (due to the small oral cavity)
- small head (with slow brain growth)
- upward slanting eyes
- small, short ears (which may be low-set).

Body features

Body features associated with Down syndrome include:
- hypotonia
- short stature
- simian crease (a single crease along the palm with an in-curved little finger)
- short, broad hands and neck
- genital abnormalities.

Level of functioning

Intellectual dysfunction associated with Down syndrome includes mild to severe retardation, with intellectual abilities declining with age, and the onset of Alzheimer's-type dementia with increasing age.

Level of functioning varies markedly among children (and adults) with Down syndrome. Some children remain entirely dependent on their parents or caregivers throughout their lives. Other, higher functioning children communicate well, develop relationships outside the home, attend school, and even live independently at some point (although this process takes longer than it does in children without Down syndrome).

A special gift

Many parents describe their child with Down syndrome as extraordinarily loving, gentle, affectionate, and extremely demonstrative.

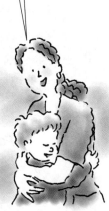

Children with Down syndrome can be extremely engaging, affectionate, and loving.

What tests tell you

Physical findings at birth, especially hypotonia, may suggest Down syndrome, but no physical feature is diagnostic by itself. A karyotype showing the specific chromosomal abnormality provides a definitive diagnosis.

Amnio alert

Amniocentesis allows prenatal diagnosis and is recommended for pregnant women older than age 34, even if the family history is negative. Amniocentesis is also recommended for a pregnant woman of any age when either she or the father carries a translocated chromosome.

Complications

In approximately 60% of patients, early death usually results from complications precipitated by associated congenital heart defects; up to 44% die before age 1 year. An increased incidence of upper respiratory infections, aspiration, leukemia, and hypothyroidism is common.

How it's treated

Because there's no cure for the disorder, management of Down syndrome is manifestation-specific and includes surgery to correct cardiac, gastrointestinal (GI), and other congenital problems. Skeletal, immunologic, metabolic, biochemical, and oncologic problems are treated according to the specific problem.

Atlantoaxial instability (a spinal deformity resulting in instability of the upper cervical spine) should be assessed frequently. Growth and development should be monitored using specific growth charts.

What to do

• Offer assistance and support to the parents; give clear explanations to promote understanding and compliance.

Just the way you are

• Assist in identifying positive features and behaviors in the child to alleviate anxiety and promote parental acceptance of the child's disabilities.
• Plan activities based on the child's cognitive and motor abilities, rather than chronological age, to promote a healthy emotional and physical environment.
• Provide activities and toys appropriate for the child to support optimal development.
• Refer the parents for nutritional counseling as needed.

Sherlock Mom

• Teach parents to recognize symptoms of problems, such as upper respiratory infections and constipation, and to administer thyroid medication if needed.
• Keep the environment as routine as possible; a change in routine commonly results in frustration and decreased coping abilities.
• Refer the parents for genetic counseling to explore the cause of the disorder and to discuss the risk of recurrence in a future pregnancy.

The thrill of success

• Encourage participation in success-oriented activities such as Special Olympics.
• Refer the parents to a social worker or grief counselor, if needed; many parents grieve for the "normal" child they had expected.

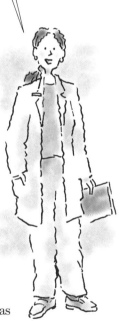

Parents of a child with Down syndrome may need counseling to help them grieve the loss of the healthy child they had hoped for.

Duchenne's muscular dystrophy

Muscular dystrophy is a group of inherited, progressively degenerative diseases that cause muscle fiber degeneration and muscle weakness and atrophy. The most common type of muscular dystrophy is Duchenne's muscular dystrophy (DMD).

What causes it

DMD is an X-linked recessive disorder and affects mostly males; it occurs in 1 in 3,000 male children. Females are usually carriers and pass the defect on to their male offspring.

How it happens

In DMD, there's an absence of the muscle protein dystrophin, which helps support the structure of muscle fibers. This results in degeneration of skeletal or voluntary muscles that control movement. Fat and connective tissue replace the degenerated muscle fibers.

What to look for

Muscular dystrophy affects the upper arms, legs, and trunk muscles first. Pelvic muscles begin to weaken between ages 3 and 5 years. Signs include the following:
• Calves appear large and strong but are weak because of infiltration of the muscles with fat and connective tissue.
• Children have difficulty climbing stairs, running, and riding a bicycle.
• The child has a wide stance and a waddling gait.
• Gowers' sign may be displayed when rising from a sitting or supine position. (See *Observing Gowers' sign.*)

Rapid changes

The disease progresses rapidly; by age 12, the child usually can't walk. Signs include the following:
• Posture changes occur as abdominal and paravertebral muscles weaken.
• Weakened thoracic muscles may cause scapular "winging" or flaring when the child raises his arms.
• Bone outlines become prominent as surrounding muscles atrophy.
• In later stages, contractures and pulmonary signs, such as tachycardia and shortness of breath, become noticeable.

What tests tell you

• Muscle biopsy reveals replacement of normal muscle with connective and fatty tissue. It also shows degeneration and necrosis of muscle fibers and a deficiency of the muscle protein dystrophin.
• Electromyography (EMG) shows decreased and weakened electrical impulses in the child with DMD.
• Nerve conduction velocity, in which electrical impulses are sent down the nerves of the arms and legs, reveals abnormal nerve function.

Observing Gowers' sign

Because DMD weakens pelvic and lower extremity muscles, the child must use his upper body to maneuver from a prone to an upright position. This maneuver is called *Gowers' sign*. Lying on his stomach with his arms stretched in front of him, the child raises his head, backs into a crawling position, and then into a half-kneel. Then stopping, he braces his legs with his hands at the ankles and walks his hands (one after the other) up his legs until he pushes himself upright.

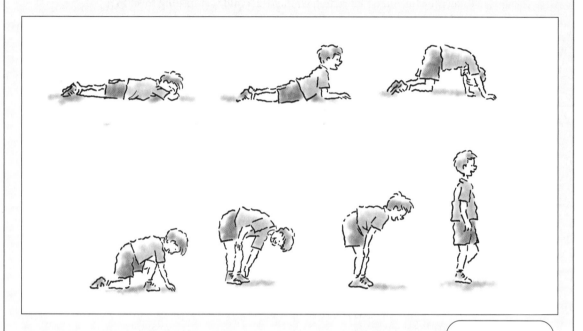

• Creatine kinase levels increase before muscle weakness becomes severe, providing an early indicator of muscular dystrophy.

Complications

Respiratory infections become common as the muscles of the diaphragm weaken. Cardiomyopathy occurs as the heart deteriorates and weakens. Death occurs in the 20s from respiratory failure, heart failure, or pneumonia.

How it's treated

Because there's no cure, treatment is supportive and aimed at maintaining ambulation and independence for as long as possible. Physical and occupational therapies help

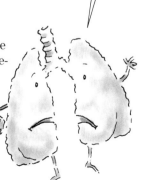

DMD can cause respiratory failure and ultimately death.

the child maximize his level of functioning. The goal of occupational therapy is to help the child compensate for physical limitations and to achieve a level of success in performing activities of daily living.

Heels, hips, and knees

Surgery may be done to release the heel cord as contractures develop in this area. Surgery is also performed on the hips and knees as they become contracted, so that the child will be able to sit in a chair with some degree of comfort.

What to do

Care of a child with DMD is multidisciplinary:
• Monitor respiratory and cardiac status regularly.
• When respiratory involvement occurs, encourage coughing, deep-breathing exercises, and diaphragmatic breathing.
• Ensure proper nutrition, and emphasize the importance of preventing obesity.
• Assess the family's ability to cope with the diagnosis and poor prognosis.
• Protect the child from others with respiratory and contagious diseases.
• Encourage and assist with active and passive ROM exercises to preserve joint mobility and prevent muscular atrophy.

Bring in the troops

• Coordinate other health services that would be beneficial to the child—for example, physical therapy, occupational therapy, and nutritional services.
• As movement becomes more difficult, assist the child with position changes every 2 hours to prevent pressure ulcers.
• Encourage genetic screening and counseling, which are indicated for parents and siblings of children with DMD.
• Refer the parents to agencies that can assist them with the child's home needs and provide emotional support.

Guillain-Barré syndrome

Guillain-Barré syndrome is an acute, rapidly progressing, potentially fatal form of polyneuritis. It leads to deteriorating motor function and paralysis that progress in an ascending pattern. The condition affects the peripheral nervous system, resulting in edema and inflammation of the affected nerves and a loss of myelin.

What's myelin is your-e-lin

Myelin is the phospholipid protein of the cell membranes that forms the myelin sheath of neurons. It acts as an electrical insulator and increases the velocity of impulse transmission.

What causes it

Guillain-Barré syndrome is caused by an autoimmune response to an infectious organism, usually from a GI or respiratory illness 1 to 3 weeks before onset. It has also been linked to viral immunizations (such as the swine flu vaccine) and cytomegalovirus.

How it happens

The syndrome is commonly preceded by immune system stimulation from a viral illness, trauma, surgery, immunizations, or human immunodeficiency virus. These stimuli are thought to alter the immune system, resulting in sensitization of lymphocytes to the patient's myelin, and subsequent myelin damage. Demyelination occurs, and the transmission of motor and sensory nerve impulses is stopped or slowed down.

What to look for

Symptoms usually develop 1 to 3 weeks after an upper respiratory or GI infection. Infants have an onset of rapidly progressive and severe hypotonia, possible respiratory distress, and feeding difficulties.

Weak from the legs up

Older children have rapidly progressive symmetric weakness and muscle pain with varying degrees of distal paresthesia and numbness of the legs. The weakness spreads to the upper extremities, trunk, chest, neck, face, and head, and there's an ascending loss of deep tendon reflexes with flaccid paralysis. Unexplained autonomic instability may result in hypertension, orthostatic hypotension, and sinus tachycardia.

From dysfunction to failure

Other clinical features include urinary and bowel incontinence, CN dysfunction resulting in Bell's palsy, difficulty swallowing, and respiratory failure.

What tests tell you

Diagnosis is based primarily on a patient history revealing a recent febrile illness and typical clinical features. Other tests include the following:
• Lumbar puncture reveals increased protein levels in the CSF.
• EMG and nerve conduction studies are markedly abnormal; an abnormal wave pattern indicates Guillain-Barré syndrome.

Complications

The most serious complication of Guillain-Barré syndrome is respiratory failure, which occurs as paralysis progresses to the nerves that innervate the thoracic area. Most deaths are attributed to respiratory failure. Immobility from the paralysis can cause such problems as paralytic ileus, deep vein thrombosis, thrombophlebitis, pulmonary emboli, muscle atrophy, and orthostatic hypotension.

How it's treated

Treatment is primarily supportive with special attention to the respiratory, neurologic, and cardiovascular systems and with early recognition of deteriorating status. In addition:
• Plasmapheresis, a process that temporarily reduces the number of antibodies in the blood's circulation, is useful during the initial phase but offers no benefit if begun 2 weeks or more after onset.
• High-dose immunoglobulin can be given if plasmapheresis fails or is unavailable.
• The child's nutritional status—including body weight, serum albumin levels, and calorie counts—should be continuously evaluated.
• The child may require mechanical ventilation for respiratory difficulties, and continuous electrocardiogram monitoring for possible cardiac arrhythmias.

Be prepared when the child with Guillain-Barré syndrome can no longer speak. Age-appropriate tools can help the child communicate.

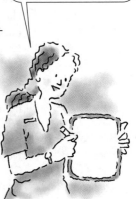

What to do

Because of the progressive nature of this disorder, it's extremely important to establish a communication system in anticipation of the time when the child can't communicate verbally:
• Perform frequent neurologic, cardiovascular, and respiratory assessments, and report changes to the doctor.
• Watch for ascending sensory loss, which precedes motor loss.

- Frequently assess respiratory status by monitoring pulse oximeter readings, pulmonary function tests, arterial blood gas values, and auscultating breath sounds.
- Perform chest physiotherapy to help prevent complications of immobility.
- To prevent aspiration, test the gag reflex and elevate the head of the bed before giving the child anything to eat.

Survey the signs

- Watch for signs of urine retention and constipation.
- Assess the need for nasogastric tube or gastrostomy feedings, which may become necessary.
- Perform passive ROM exercises to help maintain function and prevent contractures. (See *Care of the immobilized child*.)

Squash the stress

- Help relieve anxiety in the child and his parents, and facilitate the child's development with age-appropriate activities.
- Refer the parents to social workers, who can help with financial arrangements and school considerations, and to other health care professionals to help the family cope with the diagnosis.

Advice from the experts

Care of the immobilized child

An immobilized child requires meticulous care to prevent complications. Without constant care, a bedridden patient is more susceptible to skin breakdown caused by increased pressure on tissues over bony prominences. To care for an immobilized child, follow these steps:

- Change the child's position from side to side every 2 hours.
- Place the child on a sheepskin pad, a convoluted foam mattress, or an alternating–air current mattress.

- Keep the child's body in proper alignment with rolls made of towels or blankets, or with splints.
- Perform passive range-of-motion exercises at least three or four times per day, or as ordered by the doctor, to prevent contractures.
- Emphasize the importance of coughing and deep breathing. Teach the older child to use an incentive spirometer. Younger children can achieve the same effect by blowing bubbles or blowing up a medical glove like a balloon.
- Change soiled or wet diapers frequently to prevent excoriation of the perianal area.

Hydrocephalus

Hydrocephalus is an excessive accumulation of CSF within the ventricles of the brain, resulting from interference with normal circulation or absorption of the fluid.

CSF overload

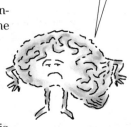

Too much CSF in my ventricles compresses me against the skull.

As excess CSF accumulates in the ventricular system, the ventricles become dilated and the brain is compressed against the skull. This results in enlargement of the skull if the sutures are open or in signs and symptoms of increased ICP if the sutures are fused.

What causes it

Hydrocephalus that results from an obstruction in CSF flow is called *noncommunicating hydrocephalus*. Causes include faulty fetal development, infection, a tumor, a cerebral aneurysm, or a blood clot after intracranial hemorrhage.

    Communicating hydrocephalus results from faulty absorption of CSF. Causes of communicating hydrocephalus include a surgical complication, adhesions, or meningeal hemorrhage. (See *Hydrocephalus and CSF circulation.*)

How it happens

In healthy children, CSF circulation is unimpeded:
• CSF is produced from blood in a capillary network (choroid plexus) in the brain's lateral ventricles.
• From the lateral ventricles, CSF flows through the interventricular foramen (foramen of Monro) to the third ventricle.
• From there, it flows through the aqueduct of Sylvius to the fourth ventricle, through the foramina of Luschka and Magendie, to the cisterna of the subarachnoid space.
• The fluid then passes under the base of the brain, upward over the brain's upper surfaces, and down around the spinal cord.
• Eventually, CSF reaches the arachnoid villi, where it's reabsorbed into venous blood at the venous sinuses.

What to look for

The signs and symptoms of hydrocephalus vary with the age of the child. In infants, the unmistakable sign of hydrocephalus is rapidly increasing head circumference that's clearly disproportionate to the infant's growth. Other characteristic changes include:
• widening and bulging of the fontanels
• distended scalp veins

Hydrocephalus and CSF circulation

In noncommunicating hydrocephalus, the obstruction of CSF circulation occurs most commonly between the third and fourth ventricles, at the aqueduct of Sylvius. However, it can also occur at the outlets of the fourth ventricle (foramina of Luschka and Magendie) or, rarely, at the foramen of Monro.

Absorption distortion

In communicating hydrocephalus, faulty absorption of CSF may result from surgery, adhesions between meninges at the base of the brain, or meningeal hemorrhage. Rarely, a tumor in the choroid plexus causes overproduction of CSF, resulting in hydrocephalus.

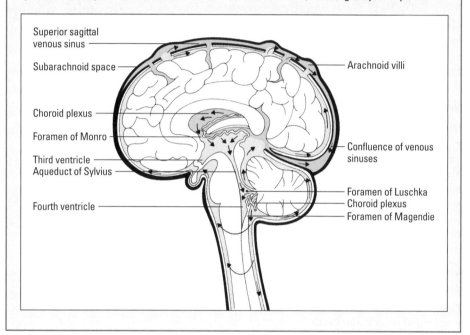

Superior sagittal venous sinus

Subarachnoid space

Choroid plexus

Foramen of Monro

Third ventricle

Aqueduct of Sylvius

Fourth ventricle

Arachnoid villi

Confluence of venous sinuses

Foramen of Luschka

Choroid plexus

Foramen of Magendie

- thin, shiny, fragile-looking scalp skin
- underdeveloped neck muscles. (See *Signs of hydrocephalus.*)

The setting sun

In severe hydrocephalus, the roof of the orbit is depressed, the eyes are displaced downward, and the sclerae are prominent. When the sclera is seen above the iris, it's called the *setting-sun sign*. Other common signs and symptoms include:
- high-pitched, shrill cry
- abnormal muscle tone of the legs
- irritability
- anorexia
- projectile vomiting.

Signs of hydrocephalus

In infants, characteristic changes in hydrocephalus include:
- marked enlargement of the head
- distended scalp veins
- thin, shiny, fragile-looking scalp skin
- weak muscles that can't support the head.

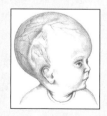

In older children, indicators of hydrocephalus include decreased LOC, ataxia, incontinence, and impaired intellect.

Arnold-Chiari malformation

Arnold-Chiari malformation commonly accompanies hydrocephalus, especially when a myelomeningocele is present. In this condition, an elongated or tonguelike downward projection of the cerebellum and medulla extends through the foramen magnum into the cervical portion of the spinal canal, impairing CSF drainage from the fourth ventricle.

Rigid, noisy, and irritable

Infants with this malformation also demonstrate nuchal rigidity, noisy respirations, irritability, vomiting, weak sucking reflex, and a preference for hyperextension of the neck.

What tests tell you

Diagnostic tests for hydrocephalus include:
• daily measurement of head circumference, because rapid head enlargement is the first indication of the problem
• skull X-rays, which show thinning of the skull with separation of sutures and widening of the fontanels
• a CT scan and an MRI, which are used to confirm the diagnosis, assess ventricular dilatation or enlargement, and demonstrate the Arnold-Chiari malformation.

Complications

Potential complications of hydrocephalus include:
• mental retardation
• impaired motor function
• vision loss.
    The most serious complication associated with shunt placement is infection. Shunt malfunction is the other major complication and is caused by such mechanical problems as kinking, plugging, migrating, and tubing separation.

How it's treated

Treatment involves removal of the obstruction (such as surgical removal of a tumor) or creation of a new CSF pathway to divert excess CSF. The goal of treatment is to bypass the obstruction and drain the fluid from the ventricles to an area where it can be reabsorbed.

It's tubular

This bypass is accomplished with insertion of a VP shunt or tube, which leads from the ventricles, out of the skull, and passes under the skin to the peritoneal cavity. (See *VP shunt.*)

Straight to the heart

An alternative to the VP shunt is the less commonly used ventro-atrial shunt, which drains the fluid from the ventricles to the right atrium of the heart.

What to do

Several preoperative and postoperative nursing interventions are indicated for the child with hydrocephalus.

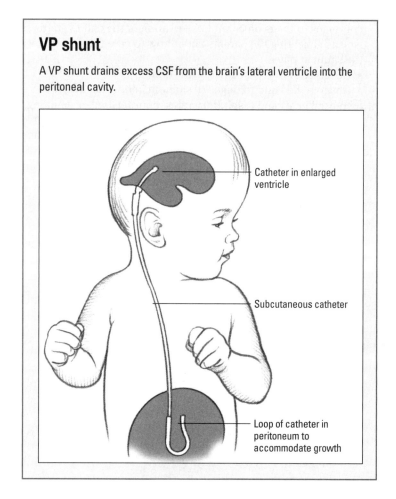

VP shunt

A VP shunt drains excess CSF from the brain's lateral ventricle into the peritoneal cavity.

Catheter in enlarged ventricle

Subcutaneous catheter

Loop of catheter in peritoneum to accommodate growth

Preoperative care

Preoperative care involves careful monitoring:
• Head circumference should be measured daily, watching for signs of increased ICP.
• Assess respiratory status every 4 hours or more often if necessary.
• Measure intake and output of all fluids.
• Monitor nutritional status and provide small feedings because the child is prone to vomiting. (During feedings, the child's head must be supported carefully and he must be burped frequently.)

Postoperative care

Postoperatively, the child is placed in a flat position on the non-operative side to prevent rapid CSF drainage and pressure on the valves. If CSF is drained too rapidly, the child is at risk for subdural hematoma caused by tears in the vessels secondary to the cerebral cortex pulling away from the dura. Nursing care continues to focus on careful observation of the child's status as well as educating the parents about how to care for the child with the shunt in place:
• Observe for decreased LOC and vomiting.
• Observe the child for signs of shunt infection, such as fever, increased heart and respiratory rates, poor feeding or vomiting, altered mental status, seizures, and redness along the shunt tract.
• Observe for abdominal distention or discomfort because shunt placement may cause a paralytic ileus or peritonitis.
• Measure head circumference daily; any increase of more than 0.5 cm is significant and should be reported to the doctor.

Shunt care 101

• Explain all procedures to the parents.
• Teach the parents signs and symptoms of shunt infection and malfunction and what to do if they suspect either.
• Teach the parents to foster normal growth and development in their child; the child shouldn't be overprotected but should avoid contact sports.

Neural tube defects

Neural tube defects (NTDs) are serious birth defects that involve the spine or the brain. They result from failure of the neural tube to close at approximately 28 days after conception. The most common forms of NTD are:
• spina bifida (50% of cases)
• anencephaly (40%)
• encephalocele (10%).

Spina bifida

Spina bifida occulta is a visible defect with an external saclike protrusion. It's characterized by incomplete closure of one or more vertebrae without protrusion of the spinal cord or meninges.

What's in the sac?

Spina bifida cystica is a visible defect with an external saclike protrusion. It has two classifications:
• *myelomeningocele*, in which the external sac contains meninges, CSF, and a portion of the spinal cord or nerve roots distal to the conus medullaris
• *meningocele*, in which the sac contains only meninges and CSF and may produce no neurologic symptoms. (See *Forms of spina bifida*, page 252.)

Anencephaly

Anencephaly occurs when both cerebral hemispheres are absent. The closure defect occurs at the cranial end of the neuroaxis and, as a result, part of the entire top of the skull is missing and the brain is severely damaged. It's the most severe NTD and is incompatible with life.

Gone too soon

Many infants with anencephaly are stillborn. If the infant does survive, there's no specific treatment. Because the infant has an intact brain stem, he can maintain vital functions, such as temperature regulation and respiratory and cardiac function. Most live for a few weeks and then die of respiratory failure.

Encephalocele

In encephalocele, a saclike portion of the meninges and brain protrudes through a defective opening in the skull.

What causes it

NTDs may be isolated birth defects, may result from exposure to a teratogen (factor that increases risk of congenital disorder in an embryo), or may be part of a multiple malformation syndrome. It's believed that isolated NTDs (those not due to a specific teratogen or associated with other malformations) are caused by a combination of genetic and environmental factors. Although most of the specific environmental triggers are unknown, research has identified a lack of folic acid in the mother's diet as one of the risk factors.

Forms of spina bifida

The most common forms of spina bifida are listed below, along with their major characteristics.

Spina bifida occulta
Spina bifida occulta is the least severe of the spinal cord defects. It's characterized by incomplete closure of one or more vertebrae without protrusion of the spinal cord or meninges.

Spina bifida cystica
Spina bifida cystica is a visible defect with an external saclike protrusion. It has two classifications: meningocele and myelomeningocele.

Meningocele
In meningocele, the sac contains only meninges and CSF.

Myelomeningocele
In myelomeningocele, the external sac contains meninges, CSF, and a portion of the spinal cord or nerve roots distal to the conus medullaris.

Spina bifida occulta

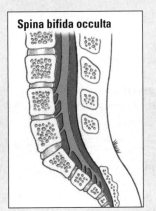

Meningocele

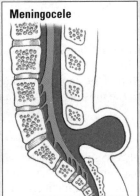

Myelomeningocele

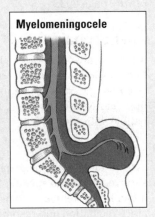

How it happens

During the fourth week of gestation, ventral induction of the neural tube fails to occur. The degree of impairment depends on the size and level of the defect and whether it involves the spinal cord and nerves. Associated malformations include hydrocephalus and Arnold-Chiari malformation.

What to look for

The signs and symptoms of NTDs vary widely according to the type of the defect.

Search the sacrum

In spina bifida occulta, a depression or dimple, a small tuft of hair, a hemangioma, or a port-wine nevi in the lower lumbar or sacral area usually accompanies the defect. Because there's no herniation of the spinal cord or meninges, spina bifida occulta usually doesn't cause neurologic dysfunction, but it's occasionally associated with foot weakness or bowel and bladder disturbances.

Sac on the back

In myelomeningocele and meningocele, a saclike structure protrudes over the spine. Meningocele seldom causes neurologic symptoms. Myelomeningocele is associated with permanent neurologic symptoms, such as flaccid or spastic paralysis; bowel and bladder incontinence; clubfoot; knee contractures; hydrocephalus and, possibly, mental retardation; Arnold-Chiari malformation; and curvature of the spine.

Poor prognosis

Clinical effects of encephalocele include paralysis, hydrocephalus, and severe mental retardation. Anencephaly is invariably fatal.

What tests tell you

Diagnostic tests include the following:
• Alpha-fetoprotein (AFP) screening to measure AFP levels in the blood at 16 to 18 weeks' gestation. AFP is a fetal-specific gamma-1 globulin in the amniotic fluid that indicates the presence of myelomeningocele. If the AFP screen is abnormal, amniocentesis and fetal ultrasound are performed.
• Amniocentesis may reveal the presence of AFP in the amniotic fluid.
• Ultrasound may be used to detect open NTDs or ventral wall defects.
• Transillumination of a protruding spinal sac can sometimes distinguish between myelomeningocele (in which the sac transilluminates) and meningocele (in which the sac doesn't transilluminate).
• Skull X-rays and CT scans identify the defects.

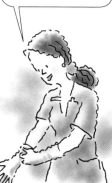

Latex-free is the way to be when caring for a child with spina bifida.

Complications

Complications of NTDs include decreased motor activity below the defect, paralysis, multiple musculoskeletal deficits, neurogenic bladder and bowel, CNS infections, hydrocephalus, and death.

Latex liability

Children with spina bifida are at high risk for developing latex allergies, possibly because of frequent exposure to latex during catheterizations and multiple surgical procedures. Allergic reactions can range from mild signs and symptoms to anaphylactic shock.

How it's treated

Immediate surgical closure (within 48 hours) is the most common choice of treatment, although spina bifida occulta usually requires no surgery. The rationale for early surgical closure is to decrease the risk of infection, morbidity, and mortality and to prevent further spinal cord and spinal nerve damage. Surgery doesn't reverse neurologic deficits.

Scheduled for surgery

A shunt may also be needed to relieve related hydrocephalus. Treatment of encephalocele includes surgery during infancy to place protruding tissues back in the skull, excise the sac, and correct associated craniofacial abnormalities.

What to do

Nursing interventions begin prenatally and, after the child is born, continue with preoperative and postoperative care.

Prenatal care

Prenatally, care focuses on educating and supporting the parents:
• Refer the prospective parents to a genetic counselor who can provide information and support the couple's decision on how to manage the pregnancy.
• Inform women of childbearing age to take a folic acid supplement until menopause or the end of childbearing potential. Research has indicated that the risk of an open NTD may be reduced 50% to 100% in pregnant women who take folic acid.
• Provide psychological support to help the parents accept the diagnosis and prognosis.

Preoperative care

Before surgery, many nursing interventions focus on preventing complications associated with the sac:
• Prevent the sac from drying by covering it with warmed saline-soaked sterile dressings.
• Check for leakage from the sac, monitor for redness and infection around the sac, and assess for signs and symptoms of CNS infection.
• Assess for sensory and motor activity below the sac, including bowel and bladder function.

No pressure, please

• Prevent trauma by keeping pressure off the sac; keep the child on his abdomen with hips flexed and legs abducted.

• Institute measures to keep the sac free from infection; avoid contamination from urine and stool. (A "mud flap" can be made using a strip of plastic with adhesive backing on the top portion; this is placed directly below the defect and will prevent contamination from stool.)
• Measure head circumference to establish baseline data.
• Be aware of the increased incidence of latex allergies in these children, and take appropriate precautions.

Teach and support

• Provide emotional support to the parents. Be aware that surgery is usually performed 24 to 48 hours after birth.
• Teach parents and other family members about measures to prevent contractures, pressure ulcers, urinary tract infections, and other complications.

Postoperative care

After surgery, provide routine postoperative care, including monitoring vital signs, positioning, and observation of the operative site. In addition, follow these steps:
• Provide thorough skin care if paralysis is present (to prevent complications such as pressure ulcers).
• Infant may be positioned on side (with order) or abdomen.
• Assess motor activity and bowel and bladder function to compare with the preoperative condition.
• Measure head circumference daily, and perform ROM exercises.
• Teach clean intermittent catheterization to parents.
• Maintain splints, braces, and casts; use wheelchairs, walkers, and other assistive devices as needed.

Reye's syndrome

Reye's syndrome is an acute childhood illness that causes fatty infiltration of the liver with concurrent hyperammonemia, encephalopathy, and increased ICP. Fatty infiltration of the kidneys, brain, and myocardium may occur.

Equal opportunity syndrome

Reye's syndrome affects children from infancy to adolescence and occurs equally in boys and girls.

What causes it

Reye's syndrome typically begins within 1 to 3 days of an acute viral infection, such as an upper respiratory tract infection, type B influenza, or varicella.

Nada to ASA

Use of aspirin in children younger than age 15 is not recommended because of its link to Reye's syndrome. Fortunately, Reye's syndrome has become rare because most parents now give their children acetaminophen instead of aspirin for flulike symptoms or fever.

> To prevent Reye's syndrome, never give aspirin to a child younger than age 15. Use acetaminophen or NSAIDs instead.

How it happens

In Reye's syndrome, damaged hepatic mitochondria disrupt the urea cycle, which normally changes ammonia to urea for its excretion from the body. This disruption results in hyperammonemia, hypoglycemia, and an increase in serum short-chain fatty acids, leading to encephalopathy. Fatty infiltration occurs simultaneously in renal tubular cells, neuronal tissue, and muscle tissue (including the heart).

What to look for

The severity of the child's signs and symptoms varies with the degree of encephalopathy and cerebral edema. In all cases, Reye's syndrome develops in five stages:

The first stage is the initial viral infection.

A brief recovery period follows, when the child doesn't seem seriously ill.

A few days later, he develops intractable vomiting, lethargy, rapidly changing mental status (mild to severe agitation, confusion, irritability, and delirium), rising blood pressure and respiratory and pulse rates, and hyperactive reflexes.

The syndrome commonly progresses to coma.

As coma deepens, seizures develop, followed by decreased tendon reflexes and, usually, respiratory failure.

What tests tell you

Diagnosis of Reye's syndrome is based on the abrupt change in the child's LOC and on findings from diagnostic tests. At the time of diagnosis, the child usually has already progressed to stage III—coma and decorticate posturing:
• Blood studies reveal liver enzyme levels (aspartate aminotransferase or alanine aminotransferase) elevated to twice their normal levels as well as elevated ammonia levels, below normal blood glucose levels, and prolonged prothrombin time.

• Liver biopsy, which is usually performed to confirm the diagnosis, reveals small fat deposits.

Complications

Developmental and neurologic deficits may occur and are more severe in children younger than age 2 years. Cerebral edema is the major factor contributing to morbidity and mortality. Other complications may include respiratory failure and death.

> Respiratory failure and cerebral edema can cause death in children with Reye's syndrome.

How it's treated

The goal of medical management is to provide supportive treatment to prevent the secondary effects of cerebral edema and metabolic injury; it includes assisted ventilation for the comatose child, monitoring for signs of increased ICP (caused by cerebral edema), and I.V. glucose for hypoglycemia. Close monitoring of electrolytes, blood chemistry, and blood pH is also done.

What to do

In stage I, follow these steps:
• Assess hydration status.
• Monitor skin turgor, mucous membranes, intake and output, and urine specific gravity.
• Maintain a patent I.V. line for hydration.

Respiratory inventory

In stages II through V, follow these steps:
• Assess respiratory status, noting changes in rate and pattern, presence of circumoral cyanosis, restlessness, or agitation.
• Assess circulatory status by taking vital signs frequently.
• Note skin color, temperature, and the presence of abnormal heart sounds or neck vein distention.

Know your neuro

In all stages, follow these steps:
• Assess neurologic status.
• Immediately report to the doctor signs of coma that require invasive, supportive therapy such as intubation.
• Monitor LOC, pupil response, motor coordination, extremity movement, orientation, posturing, and seizure activity.
• Support the child and his family. Explain treatments and procedures, incorporating family members in treatments as appropriate. Organize regular family and patient care conferences, and use support services as needed.
• Provide additional parental and community education to ensure early recognition and treatment.

Seizure disorders

A seizure is a sudden, episodic, involuntary alteration in consciousness, motor activity, behavior, sensation, or autonomic function caused by abnormal electrical discharges by the neurons in the brain. Seizures can accompany a variety of disorders, or they may occur spontaneously without apparent cause. Epilepsy is a condition in which a person has spontaneously recurring seizures.

What causes it

The most common causes of seizure during the first 6 months of life are:
- severe birth injury
- congenital defects involving the CNS
- infections
- inborn errors of metabolism.
    Other causes include birth trauma (inadequate oxygen supply to the brain, blood incompatibility, or hemorrhage), infectious diseases (meningitis, encephalopathy, or brain abscess), ingestion of toxins, head trauma, metabolic disorders (hypoglycemia, hypocalcemia, hyponatremia, hypernatremia, or hyperbilirubinemia), and high fever.

How it happens

In recurring seizures (epilepsy), a group of abnormal neurons seem to undergo spontaneous firing.

Consciously electric

Electrical discharges come from central areas in the brain that affect consciousness. The discharges may be localized in one area of the brain and cause responses specific to the anatomic focus controlled by that area. They may be initiated in a localized area of the brain and then spread to other areas, resulting in a generalized response.

Cellular excitement

Hyperexcitable cells, called the *epileptogenic focus*, spontaneously release the discharges. These discharges can be triggered by either environmental or physiologic stimuli, such as emotional stress, anxiety, fatigue, infection, or metabolic disturbances.

What to look for

Seizures can take various forms, depending on their origin and whether they're localized to one area of the brain (as in partial seizures) or occur in both hemispheres (as in generalized seizures). If a partial seizure generalizes, it's still classified as a partial seizure. (See *Classifying seizures*, page 260.)

What tests tell you

A complete history, physical, and neurologic examination—including birth and development history, significant illnesses and injuries, family history, history of febrile seizures, and a comprehensive neurologic assessment—should be performed. Laboratory and other tests include:
• CBC and blood chemistry to detect electrolyte imbalances
• blood glucose levels to detect hypoglycemic episodes
• lumbar puncture to rule out meningitis as a cause of the seizures
• EEG to help differentiate epileptic from nonepileptic seizures (each seizure has a characteristic EEG tracing).

CT, MRI—both can help identify

If the child is taking anticonvulsants, blood levels should be monitored. Lead levels, toxicology screening, and radiologic tests, such as CT scanning or MRI, may be performed to identify structural lesions.

Complications

Complications from seizures include physical injury during the seizure, brain damage, and respiratory insufficiency or arrest.

How it's treated

Most children are treated with anticonvulsants, preferably a single medication to minimize adverse effects. Children who continue to have seizures with the single medication are treated with multiple anticonvulsants. Medication dosage adjustments are usually needed as the child grows. Serum drug levels are monitored to achieve therapeutic levels or when toxicity is possible. Surgery may be necessary to remove a tumor, lesion, or portion of the brain that has been identified as causing the seizure. Older children and adolescents may be candidates for a vagal nerve stimulator.

Kudos for ketogenic

A ketogenic diet may occasionally be used for children younger than age 8 years with myoclonic or absence seizures. A ketogenic diet is a high-fat, low-carbohydrate, low-protein diet that causes ketosis as the body uses fat for metabolism. Ketosis is believed to slow the electrical impulses that cause seizures.

Classifying seizures

This chart lists and describes each type of seizure, along with signs and symptoms.

Type	Description	Signs and symptoms
Partial		
Simple partial	Seizure activity begins in one hemisphere or focal area. There's no change in LOC.	May have motor (change in posture), sensory (hallucinations), or autonomic (flushing, tachycardia) symptoms; no loss of consciousness
Complex partial	Seizure activity begins in one hemisphere or focal area. There's an alteration in consciousness.	Loss of consciousness, aura of visual disturbances; postictal seizures
Generalized		
Absence (petit mal)	Sudden onset; lasts 5 to 10 seconds; can have 100 daily; precipitated by stress, hyperventilation, hypoglycemia, fatigue; differentiated from daydreaming	Loss of responsiveness but continued ability to maintain posture control and not fall; twitching eyelids; lip smacking; no postictal symptoms
Myoclonic	Sudden, short contractures of a muscle or muscle group	No loss of consciousness; sudden, brief shocklike involuntary contraction of one muscle group
Clonic	Opposing muscles contract and relax alternately in rhythmic pattern; may occur in one limb more than others	Mucus production
Tonic	Muscles are maintained in continuous contracted state (rigid posture)	Variable loss of consciousness; pupils dilate; eyes roll up; glottis closes; possible incontinence; may foam at mouth
Tonic-clonic (grand mal, major motor)	Violent, total-body seizure	Aura first (20 to 40 seconds); clonic next; postictal symptoms
Atonic	Drop-and-fall attack; needs to wear protective helmet	Loss of posture tone
Akinetic	Sudden brief loss of muscle tone or posture	Temporary loss of consciousness
Miscellaneous		
Febrile	Seizure threshold lowered by elevated temperature; only one seizure per fever; common in 4% of population under age 5; occurs when temperature is rapidly rising	Lasts less than 5 minutes; generalized, transient, and nonprogressive; doesn't generally result in brain damage; EEG is normal after 2 weeks
Status epilepticus	Prolonged or frequent repetition of seizures without interruption; may result in anoxia and cardiac and respiratory arrest	Consciousness not regained between seizures; lasts more than 30 minutes

Keep it cool

Children with febrile seizures may be treated with an anticonvulsant throughout the presenting febrile illness; long-term anticonvulsants aren't generally used. Parents are taught to lower fever by administering antipyretics and to keep the child cool. Rectal diazepam may be given during the seizure episode.

What to do

The nurse caring for a child who has seizures should focus on maintaining airway patency, ensuring safety, administering medications, observing and treating the seizure, educating the child and his parents, and providing psychosocial intervention. In addition, she should:
• stay with the child during a seizure
• move the child to a flat surface, out of danger; if he's standing, gently assist him to the floor
• provide a patent airway and place the child on his side to allow saliva to drain out
• avoid trying to interrupt the seizure (Instead, she should gently support the child's head and keep his hands from inflicting self-harm but not restrain him.)
• pad the crib or bed rails to prevent physical injury.

Out with the noise, in with the calm

• reduce external stimuli and environmental noise
• administer anticonvulsants as ordered by a doctor
• record seizure activity, and assess neurologic status and vital signs after the seizure subsides
• monitor serum levels of anticonvulsants to ensure therapeutic levels and prevent toxicity.

Never try to interrupt a seizure. Instead, stay with the child and take appropriate measures to keep him safe.

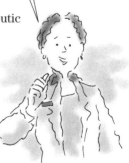

A helping hand

Having a seizure can be extremely frightening to a child; it can also be embarrassing, especially when a seizure occurs in the presence of peers. To the child's parents, and others who witness a seizure, the experience can be terrifying. The child and his parents need a great deal of education and emotional support:
• Instruct the parents (and the child, if old enough) in all aspects of seizure control measures such as how to control fever if the child has febrile seizures.
• Stress to the parents the need to treat the child as normally as possible.
• Encourage the parents and the child to express their fears and anxieties; answer their questions honestly.

It takes a village

• Instruct the parents to make sure that the child's teachers, day care providers, babysitters, coaches, and other caregivers know what to do in the event of a seizure.
• If the child has had a seizure at school, suggest that the parents arrange to have a doctor, nurse, or other health care professional go to the school and talk to the child's classmates.
• Refer the family to organizations that will provide them with more information and support such as the Epilepsy Foundation.
• Remind the parents that their child should wear some form of medical identification such as a medical identification bracelet.

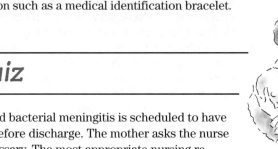

Always make sure that all of a child's potential caregivers know what to do—and what not to do—in the event of a seizure.

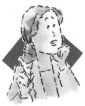

Quick quiz

1. A child who had bacterial meningitis is scheduled to have his hearing tested before discharge. The mother asks the nurse why the test is necessary. The most appropriate nursing response is:

    A.   "It's necessary to make sure your child is developing appropriately."
    B.   "The test will identify attention deficit problems related to your child's illness."
    C.   "It's necessary to make sure the steroid therapy your child had in the hospital didn't affect his ability to hear."
    D.   "Despite treatment, some children with bacterial meningitis suffer neurologic damage, especially to the nerve responsible for hearing."

Answer: D. The most common neurologic complications of meningitis are hearing loss, mental retardation, seizures, visual impairment, and behavioral problems.

2. A nurse is caring for a 2-year-old child with a VP shunt. Assessment indicates the child is afebrile but irritable and less responsive than he was previously. The most appropriate nursing action is to:

    A.   lower the head of the bed and position the child on his stomach.
    B.   increase the oxygen to 100%.
    C.   increase the fluids the child is receiving.
    D.   notify the doctor.

Answer: D. The nurse should notify the doctor of indications of increased ICP, including irritability and lethargy.

3. An 18-month-old is admitted to the emergency department with a diagnosis of seizure. Upon assessment, his vital signs are temperature of 104° F (40° C), respirations at 26 breaths/minute, pulse at 120 beats/minute, and blood pressure of 90/69 mm Hg. The nurse should:

    A.   give a tepid sponge bath.

    B.   administer phenytoin (Dilantin).

    C.   do an Accu-Check.

    D.   aggressively hydrate the child with I.V. fluids.

Answer: A. An elevated temperature could lead to a febrile seizure. The nurse should intervene to lower the core body temperature by offering oral fluids, giving the child a tepid sponge bath, and administering doctor-ordered antipyretics.

4. A 9-year-old is admitted with weakness in his legs and a history of the flu. He's diagnosed with Guillain-Barré syndrome. The nurse must notify the doctor immediately if what symptom is observed?

    A.   Tingling in the hands

    B.   Increasing hoarseness

    C.   Weak muscle tone in the arms

    D.   Weak muscle tone in the feet

Answer: B. The most serious complication of Guillain-Barré syndrome is respiratory failure, which occurs as paralysis progresses to the nerves that innervate the thoracic area. Increasing hoarseness may be a sign of impending respiratory distress.

Scoring

⭐⭐⭐ If you answered all four items correctly, fantastic! There's no deficit in your understanding of neurologic problems.

⭐⭐ If you answered three items correctly, great work! Your brain is in tip-top condition.

⭐ If you answered fewer than three items correctly, don't despair! Just scan the chapter again (no MRI needed).

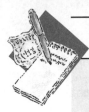

8

Cardiovascular problems

Just the facts

In this chapter, you'll learn:

♦ anatomy and physiology of the cardiovascular system

♦ diagnostic testing for cardiovascular problems

♦ treatments and procedures for cardiovascular problems

♦ cardiovascular system disorders that occur in children

♦ nursing care for the child with cardiovascular problems.

Anatomy and physiology

Understanding cardiovascular problems in children requires a sound, working knowledge of normal cardiac structure and function.

Structures of the heart

The *heart* is a muscular organ located behind the sternum in the chest and covered by a sac called the *pericardium*. Its main purpose is to pump blood throughout the body by continuous rhythmic contractions. The heart is composed of four chambers (two atria and two ventricles) and four valves.

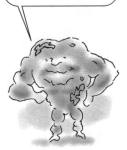

It isn't bragging to say I'm muscular. After all, it's my impressive physique that allows me to pump blood throughout the entire body.

Heart chambers

The four chambers of the heart are the right and left atria and the right and left ventricles.

Atria

The atria serve as reservoirs during ventricular contraction (systole) and as pumps during ventricular relaxation (diastole). The

A look inside the heart

Within the heart lie four chambers (two atria and two ventricles) and four valves (two atrioventricular and two semilunar valves). A system of blood vessels carries blood to and from the heart.

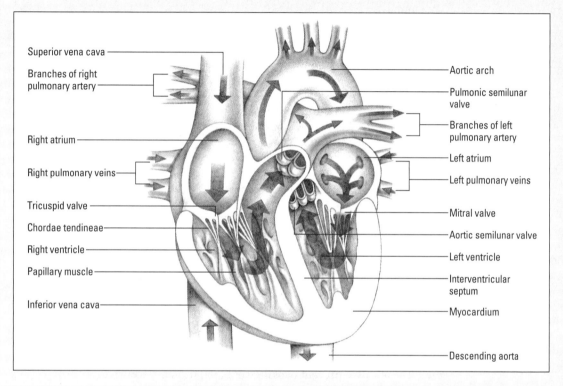

Superior vena cava

Branches of right pulmonary artery

Right atrium

Right pulmonary veins

Tricuspid valve

Chordae tendineae

Right ventricle

Papillary muscle

Inferior vena cava

Aortic arch

Pulmonic semilunar valve

Branches of left pulmonary artery

Left atrium

Left pulmonary veins

Mitral valve

Aortic semilunar valve

Left ventricle

Interventricular septum

Myocardium

Descending aorta

right atrium and left atrium are separated by an *atrial septum*.

Ventricles

The left ventricle propels blood through the aorta to the rest of the body. The right ventricle sends blood through the pulmonary artery to the lungs. The ventricles are separated by an *interventricular septum*.

Equal at birth

At birth, the ventricles are relatively equal in size because of low-resistance placental circulation. When the left ventricle begins functioning against systemic resistance that increases after birth, however, it becomes thicker than the right ventricle. (See *A look inside the heart*.)

Heart valves

The heart has four valves:

 tricuspid valve

 mitral valve

 aortic valve

 pulmonic valve.

Tricuspid and mitral valves

The tricuspid and mitral valves are known as the *atrioventricular (AV) valves*. They prevent blood backflow from the ventricles to the atria during ventricular contraction.

Location, leaflets, and muscles

The tricuspid valve is located between the right atrium and ventricle. It has three leaflets, or cusps, and three papillary muscles. The mitral valve is situated between the left atrium and ventricle. It has two leaflets and two papillary muscles.

Lovely leaflets

The leaflets of both the tricuspid and the mitral valve are attached to the papillary muscles of the ventricles by thin, fibrous bands called *chordae tendineae.*

Aortic and pulmonic valves

The aortic and pulmonic valves are known as the *semilunar valves*. These valves prevent backflow of blood from the aorta and pulmonary artery into the ventricles during ventricular relaxation. The aortic valve is located between the left ventricle and the aorta. The pulmonic valve is located between the right ventricle and the pulmonary artery.

Circulation

Blood is returned to the heart via the veins. *Veins* are small, thin-walled blood vessels that carry deoxygenated blood from the capillaries to the heart.

A long day's journey

Blood enters the right atrium from the inferior and superior vena cavae and then goes into the right ventricle. From there, it's pumped into the pulmonary artery to the lungs, where it gains oxygen and loses carbon dioxide.

Return to sender

The pulmonary veins bring the oxygenated blood from the lungs to the left atrium. The oxygenated blood then passes into the left ventricle, is pumped into the aorta, and is delivered to the rest of the body via the arteries. *Arteries* are large, thick-walled blood vessels that distribute oxygenated blood to the capillaries.

Pulmonary role reversal

The pulmonary artery is the only artery in the body that carries deoxygenated blood. The pulmonary veins are the only veins in the body that carry oxygenated blood.

Conduction system

The heart's conduction system is an electrical system that initiates myocardial contractions to move blood through the heart and maintain its rhythmic pumping action. This system is composed of several specialized cells:

- The *sinoatrial node* (also called *the pacemaker of the heart*) is located within the right atrial wall near the opening of the superior vena cava. It initiates electrical impulses and sends them throughout the atria.
- The *AV node* is located within the right atrium near the lower end of the septum. It transmits impulses from the atria to the ventricle.

I've got rhythm, I've got pumping. Blood moves through me. Who could ask for anything more?

Bundles and branches

- The *AV bundle* (bundle of His) extends from the AV node to each side of the interventricular septum and divides into right and left bundle branches. It facilitates rapid conduction of the impulses through the ventricles.
- The *Purkinje fibers* extend from the AV bundle into the walls of the ventricles and rapidly conduct impulses through the heart muscle.

Cardiac physiology

The heart's primary purpose is to pump the blood that delivers oxygen and nutrients to tissues throughout the body and to remove waste products such as carbon dioxide. To do this, the heart must maintain an adequate cardiac output.

Cardiac output is the amount of blood ejected by the heart in 1 minute. Cardiac output can be determined by multiplying the heart rate in 1 minute by the stroke volume. *Stroke volume* is the amount of blood ejected by the heart at each heartbeat (or contraction).

Stroke volume is affected by three factors:

☝ *Preload*, or the stretch of the myocardial fibers, is simply the circulating blood volume.

✌ *Afterload* is the resistance against which the ventricle must pump during its contraction, which can be affected by blood pressure. (Hypertension will increase afterload, as the heart must pump harder to force blood into circulation.)

🤟 *Contractility* is the force of left ventricular ejection.

Chillin' with homeostasis

To maintain homeostasis, the body will make many adjustments to the factors that contribute to cardiac output.

Cardiac adaptations at birth

During fetal circulation, blood is oxygenated and waste products are removed in the placenta. Blood is shunted away from those organs that aren't yet fully functional, such as the lungs and the liver.

> Right now I get all the oxygen I need from the placenta. But as soon as I get out of here, my lungs will take over.

Perfusion only—no exchange

In the fetus, the lungs are filled with fluid and aren't yet the site of gas exchange. The amount of blood that passes through the lungs is just enough to perfuse lung tissue.

Farewell placenta, hello lungs!

At birth, however, the neonate must transition from a reliance on the placenta to a reliance on his lungs for oxygenation. This transition is normally accomplished within the first few breaths after birth.

Many keys, one lock

Key structures that maintain fetal circulation include:
• *umbilical vein*, which carries oxygenated blood from the placenta to the fetus
• *umbilical arteries*, which carry deoxygenated blood from the fetus to the placenta
• *foramen ovale*, which serves as the septal opening between the atria of the fetal heart
• *ductus arteriosus*, which connects the pulmonary artery to the aorta, allowing blood to bypass the fetal lungs

• *ductus venosus*, which carries oxygenated blood from the umbilical vein to the inferior vena cava (IVC), bypassing the liver.

Out with fluid, in with air

Cardiac adaptations at birth occur gradually, resulting from structural and pressure changes in the lungs, heart, and major vessels. With the first few breaths after birth, the fluid in the neonate's lungs is absorbed and replaced with air. Inspired oxygen dilates the pulmonary vessels, resulting in decreased pulmonary vascular resistance and increased pulmonary blood flow as the lungs fill with air and expand. More blood will now travel to and from the lungs.

After only a few breaths, I'm breathing oxygen, dilating my pulmonary vessels, and sending more blood to my lungs. How about me!

The drama unfolds

The pressure in the right atrium, right ventricle, and pulmonary artery decreases. Simultaneously, a gradual increase in systemic vascular resistance occurs when the umbilical cord is clamped and the low-resistance placental circulation is removed. At that point, left atrial pressure increases more than right atrial pressure. The foramen ovale, which was a one-way door, closes as a result of this unequal pressure. The ductus arteriosus begins to close because of increased pulmonary blood flow and the dramatic reduction in pulmonary vascular resistance. Later, the ductus arteriosus (and ductus venosus) will become ligaments and will be closed structurally.

Out of a job

Function of the foramen ovale ceases immediately or soon after birth. Ductus arteriosus functioning ceases after the infant is about 4 days old. Anatomic closure, however, takes considerably longer. If the foramen ovale or ductus arteriosus fails to close, persistent shunting of fetal blood away from lungs will result. (See *From fetal to neonatal circulation*, page 270.)

Murmurs

Murmurs are produced by vibrations within the chambers of the heart or major arteries from the back-and-forth flowing of blood through these structures. In children, murmurs may be called:
• *innocent*, which means there's no anatomic or physiologic cause
• *functional* when there's a physiologic cause, such as anemia, but no anatomic abnormality
• *organic* when there's some anatomic defect in the heart, with or without the existence of a physiologic abnormality.

From fetal to neonatal circulation

These illustrations show the changes in circulation that occur at birth, allowing all neonatal blood to pass through the lungs.

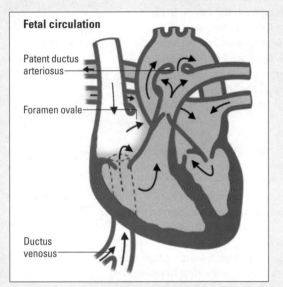

Fetal circulation

Patent ductus arteriosus

Foramen ovale

Ductus venosus

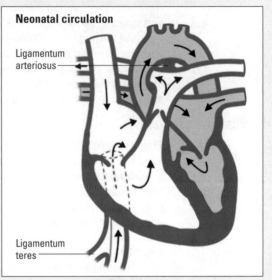

Neonatal circulation

Ligamentum arteriosus

Ligamentum teres

Sit, stand, recline

When auscultating for murmurs, position the child in the sitting and reclining positions. Also, auscultate the heart with the child standing, sitting and leaning forward, and in a left side-lying position. (See *Grading murmurs*.)

Diagnostic tests

Diagnostic tests of the cardiovascular system in children include:
- echocardiography
- electrocardiography (ECG)
- magnetic resonance imaging (MRI).

Echocardiography

Echocardiography is used to evaluate cardiac structures and functions using echoes from pulsed, high-frequency sound waves. An ultrasound transducer is placed on the chest, and the sound waves produce an image of the heart. The test is noninvasive and painless and is one of the most commonly used tests to detect cardiac problems in children.

Ultrasound-endoscopy combo

Transesophageal echocardiography (TEE) combines ultrasound with endoscopy. It's an alternative method for detecting cardiovascular problems in children and is used when the transthoracic approach isn't possible or would be difficult. During the procedure, the transducer is passed into the esophagus to an area behind the atria. The procedure is more complicated than the transthoracic approach and may require sedation and intubation to preserve the airway in young children.

Nursing considerations

Explain the procedure to the child and his parents; tell the child what he'll see, hear, and feel and be honest about any pain or discomfort he might experience. In addition, follow these steps:
• Stress the importance of holding still during the test and assist as necessary. (Tell the child that holding still is his "very important job.")
• Administer mild sedation if needed. Use distractions such as a videotape to help calm the child.
• For TEE, administer sedation as ordered and assist with endotracheal intubation as necessary. Explain that the child must have nothing to eat or drink before the procedure.

Electrocardiography

ECG provides a graphic representation of the heart's electrical activity. It's used to detect the presence of ischemia, injury, necrosis, bundle-branch block, fascicular blocks, conduction delay, chamber enlargement, and arrhythmias.

Nursing considerations

Explain the test to the child and his parents, stressing that there's no pain involved. In addition:
• Describe the equipment that will be used for the test; show the child a picture or, if possible, the actual equipment.
• Explain that the child may have to lie on his left side, inhale and exhale slowly, or hold his breath at intervals during the test.
• Encourage the child to be still during the test; he may sit on his parent's lap if necessary.

Grading murmurs

Use the system outlined here to describe the intensity of a murmur. When recording your findings, use Roman numerals as part of a fraction, always with "VI" as the denominator. For example, a grade III murmur would be recorded as "grade III/VI."

Grade I is a barely audible murmur.

Grade II is audible but quiet and soft.

Grade III is moderately loud, without a thrust or thrill.

Grade IV is loud, with a thrill.

Grade V is very loud, with a thrust or a thrill.

Grade VI is loud enough to be heard before the stethoscope comes into contact with the chest.

Magnetic resonance imaging

MRI uses magnetic fields and radio frequencies to show a cross-sectional view of the heart and its structures. It's useful in identifying some congenital heart defects. MRI is generally a noninvasive test; however, contrast media may be used.

Nursing considerations

When explaining the test to the child, show him a picture of the scanner or, whenever possible, let the child see the actual scanner. Tell the child that no pain is involved; prepare him if contrast media must be used. In addition:
• Tell the child that his parents may stay in the room with him during the scan.
• Prepare the child for the movements and the loud, clicking noises made by the scanner; reassure him that the machine won't touch him.
• Because no metal can go in the scanner, assist the child in removing hair clips, jewelry, and other metal items as necessary.
• If necessary, provide sedation to ensure that the child remains still during the test.
• Assess for a history of iodine or seafood allergies before the procedure if a contrast medium is to be used.

Exercise testing

Exercise testing may be done for some children, depending on their age and general condition. With it, the child's doctor can evaluate the extent of disease from any heart or lung disease that may be present. In addition, it can help to determine what kinds of activity ease or aggravate the child's condition, as well as his or her conditioning, both aerobic and musculoskeletal. Either a treadmill or a stationary bike may be used while the child's heart and respiratory rate are monitored. The blood pressure and pulse oximetry are also monitored during the exercise test.

Nursing considerations

Most children know what a bicycle looks like, but they may not be familiar with the concept of a stationary bike. They may not recognize a treadmill at all. So, good instructions and explanations may be necessary. Pictures or other visual aids may be helpful. Let the child know that there will be monitoring equipment, which may contain several wires that may be attached to him or her. Assure the child that there is no pain involved. In addition:
• The child's parents may remain in the room with the child, unless the child prefers to test alone (a possibility for an older school-age child or an adolescent).

• Be sure the child knows that the doctor needs to be notified right away if there is any discomfort, or if there is any difficulty keeping up with the exercise.

Treatments and procedures

Treatments and procedures used for cardiac problems in childhood include:
• valve replacement
• cardiac catheterization
• cardiac surgery
• cardiac transplantation.

Teach expectations

Many of the treatments and procedures done for children with cardiac problems involve surgery. When a child knows what to expect before a surgical procedure, he'll be less frightened, more cooperative, and more trusting of the nurses who provide his care. (See *Preparing children for surgery*, page 274.)

Valve replacement

Valve replacement with a prosthetic valve is indicated for heart valve narrowing (stenosis) and heart valve leaking (insufficiency). Valvular problems are commonly caused by rheumatic fever and congenital heart defects. They may also be caused by heart failure and infective endocarditis.

Nursing considerations

Nursing interventions focus on monitoring and educating the patient and his parents.
• After surgery, monitor for hypotension, arrhythmias, and thrombus formation.
• Monitor vital signs, arterial blood gas (ABG) values, intake, output, daily weight, blood chemistries, chest X-rays, and pulmonary artery catheter readings.

Heed the signs

• Because lifelong anticoagulant therapy will be necessary, teach the parents (and the child, if old enough) to recognize the signs and symptoms of bleeding, including black, tarry stools (from GI bleeding); oral bleeding (a small, soft bristle toothbrush should be used to prevent this); and excessive bleeding from minor cuts and scrapes.

Preparing children for surgery

Many of the interventions performed for cardiac problems involve major surgery. What a child imagines about surgery is likely much more frightening than the reality. A child who knows what to expect ahead of time will be less fearful and more cooperative and will learn to trust his caregivers. A child who's well prepared for medical procedures is much less likely to experience emotional trauma, which can have long-lasting effects.

Developmental concerns

Many of the concerns that children may have about hospitalization and surgery relate to their particular stage of development.

Infants, toddlers, and preschoolers

• Infants and toddlers are most concerned about separation from their parents. Stranger anxiety may make a necessary separation (during surgery) especially difficult.
• Because toddlers think concretely, showing is a necessary adjunct to telling when preparing a toddler for surgery.
• Preschoolers may view medical procedures, including surgeries, as punishments for some type of perceived bad behavior.
• Preschoolers are also likely to have many misconceptions about what will happen during surgery.

School-age children

• School-age children have concerns about fitting in with peers and may view surgery as something that sets them apart from their friends.
• A desire to appear "grown up" may make the school-age child reluctant to express his fears.

• Because this age is a time when children are especially curious and interested in learning, school-age children are very receptive to preoperative teaching and will likely ask many important questions (although they may need to be given the "permission" to do so).

Adolescents

• Adolescents struggle with the conflict between wanting to assert their independence and needing their parents (and other adults) to take care of them during illness and treatment.
• Adolescents may want to discuss their illness and treatment without a parent present.
• In addition, adolescents may have a hard time admitting that they're afraid or experiencing pain or discomfort.

Before surgery

Whenever the situation permits, arrange for the child to visit the hospital before he's admitted for surgery. Ideally, the formal preparation for surgery is done during the preadmission visit.

Explanations should be honest and age-appropriate and should involve the parents (unless the adolescent would rather be prepared alone). The explanation should focus on what the child will see, hear, and feel; where his parents will be waiting for him; and when they'll be reunited.

If a child will initially be cared for in an intensive care setting, allow him to visit the area ahead of time and to meet some of the nurses who will be caring for him. Prepare him for the equipment and the other patients he'll see.

Principles of preparation

Here are some principles to keep in mind when preparing a child for surgery:
• Begin by asking the child to tell you what he thinks is going to happen during his surgery.
• Ask the child about worries or fears. He may be worried about something that isn't going to happen at all.
• Provide a developmentally appropriate explanation of why the surgery is being performed; encourage the child to ask questions. Pictures or illustrations can be very helpful in assisting the child to understand the explanations.
• Reassure the child that he won't wake up during the surgery but that the doctor knows how and when to wake him up afterward.
• Show the child an induction mask (if it will be used) and allow him to "practice" by placing it on his face (or yours).
• Prepare the child for equipment (monitors, drains, and intravenous [I.V.] injections, for example) he'll wake up with.
• Tell the child about the sights and sounds of the operating room.
• Tell the child that his doctor and nurse will be in the operating room with him. Reassure him that they'll talk to him and tell him what's happening.
• If possible, show the child where he'll be waking up in the recovery room and where his parents will be waiting for him.
• Tell the child it's perfectly fine to be afraid and to cry.
• After the surgery, encourage the child to talk about the experience; he may also express his feelings through art or play.

• Stress to the child and parents the importance of antibiotic therapy before dental work and other invasive procedures to prevent infective endocarditis. Children who undergo valve replacement will always need this type of prophylactic antibiotic therapy.
• Teach the child and parents the importance of good oral hygiene to reduce the risk of oral infection, which may lead to bacteremia.
• Inform the child and parents that clicking of the mechanical heart valve may be heard outside of the chest. Reinforce that this sound is normal.

Cardiac catheterization

Cardiac catheterization is performed with a radiopaque catheter that's passed through the femoral artery directly into the heart and lungs. It may also be performed in conjunction with angiography, in which a radiopaque contrast medium is injected through the catheter into the circulation, allowing visualization of blood circulation through the heart chambers.

Measure for measure

Cardiac catheterization is used to evaluate ventricular function and measure heart chamber pressures and oxygen saturation in the blood. It also serves as a method for obtaining cardiac muscle biopsy specimens and for performing electrophysiologic studies.

Complications

Complications of cardiac catheterization include acute hemorrhage, transient arrhythmias, temporary diminished circulation to the catheterized extremity because of clot or hematoma formation, allergic reaction to the contrast medium, nausea and vomiting, and the possibility of infection.

Nursing considerations

Nursing interventions for cardiac catheterization begin when the procedure is scheduled and continue throughout the recovery period.

Before the procedure

Before catheterization, nursing interventions focus on preparing the child for the procedure, both physically and emotionally.
• Describe to the child and parents the procedure room as well as the equipment that will be used during the procedure. Show the child where on his body the catheter will be inserted, using doll play to prepare him, as necessary.

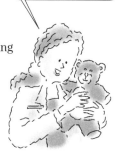

"Performing" a procedure on a "friend" gives the child a sense of control and helps him learn what to expect—in a non-threatening way.

• Tell the child that the lights in the room will be dimmed after the catheter is placed. Reassure him that you'll be right there with him and will talk to him throughout the procedure.
• Tell the child that he may feel warm after the contrast medium is injected.
• Weigh the child and take his vital signs.
• Assess the child's color, temperature of his extremities, and pedal pulses. Mark the dorsalis pedis and posterior tibial pulses with indelible ink before the procedure, allowing for easy assessment after the procedure.

After the procedure
After catheterization, nursing care focuses on preventing complications, monitoring the catheterized extremity, and ensuring adequate fluid intake.
• Keep the affected extremity immobile to prevent hemorrhage, usually for 4 to 6 hours after the procedure.
• Keep the catheter site clean and dry; monitor for bleeding and hematoma formation.
• Compare postcatheterization assessment data to precatheterization baseline data, paying special attention to pulses and neurovascular status in the catheterized extremity.
• Ensure adequate fluid intake (I.V. and oral) to compensate for blood loss during the procedure and the diuretic action of some contrast media used. Doing so will also aid in flushing the contrast medium from the circulation.
• Because cardiac catheterization is commonly done on an outpatient basis, provide thorough postprocedure teaching for the parents. (See *Instructions after cardiac catheterization*.)

Cardiac surgery

Treatment of almost all congenital heart defects is achieved through cardiac surgery. The specific procedure performed will depend on the defect. Even so, certain methods are used no matter which procedure is performed.

Heart-lung vacation

Cardiopulmonary bypass machines are typically used to oxygenate body tissues because surgery may necessitate stopping the heart. During the procedure, the patient is placed in a hypothermic state to minimize blood loss (which enhances patient recovery) and to reduce the body's need for oxygen. An incision into the chest (thoracotomy) is commonly performed, and chest tubes are placed.

It's all relative

Instructions after cardiac catheterization

Cardiac catheterizations are commonly performed on an outpatient basis. Provide parents with these clear instructions about caring for their child at home:
- Remove the pressure dressing the day after the procedure.
- Keep the site covered with an adhesive bandage for several days after the procedure.
- Keep the insertion site clean and dry; give only sponge baths until the site is healed.
- Observe the site for redness, swelling, drainage, and bleeding.
- Monitor the child's temperature, and report fever promptly.
- Have the child avoid strenuous exercise.
- Provide a regular diet for the child.
- Administer acetaminophen or ibuprofen as needed for discomfort or pain.
- Keep follow-up appointments.

Complications

Complications of cardiac surgery may include arrhythmias, acid-base and electrolyte imbalances, hypoxia, and trauma to the conduction pathways of the heart.

Nursing considerations

Prepare the child (and his parents) for what he'll see, hear, and feel after surgery. When a child and his parents know ahead of time that certain events are "normal," those events will be less stressful and frightening when they occur.
- Monitor the patient's heart rate closely. (It will normally increase after surgery.) Changes in regularity and rhythm should be reported to the doctor immediately.
- Auscultate the lungs every hour, assessing for diminished or absent breath sounds, which may require further medical evaluation and intervention.

Keep the heat

- Keep the child warm to prevent heat loss. (Infants may be placed under radiant heat warmers.)
- Monitor body temperature closely. It may rise to about 100° F (37.8° C) in the first 48 hours after surgery due to the inflammatory process initiated by tissue trauma. (Further temperature elevation may indicate an infection, requiring immediate action to determine the cause.)

Advice from the experts

Chest tube removal

Follow these guidelines to prepare the child for chest tube removal and to reduce complications:
• Tell the child he'll experience momentary sharp pain as the chest tube is removed.
• Administer anesthetics or analgesics as ordered.
• Instruct the child to take a deep breath. (The tube should be removed at the end of inspiration.)

• Cover the wound with sterile petroleum gauze, topped with a clear, occlusive film dressing, such as Tegaderm, making sure all sides are securely attached to the skin for an airtight seal.
• Monitor the site for drainage, bleeding, and infection. Change the dressing according to your facility's policy.

• Maintain mechanical ventilation of the child in the immediate postoperative period. Extubation may occur in the operating room or in the early postoperative period.
• After extubation, an oxygen mask, hood, or tent or nasal cannula is used to deliver humidified oxygen. If the patient is in an oxygen tent, change his linens and clothes frequently to keep them dry, preventing excessive chilling that would increase metabolic needs and, consequently, increase cardiac and oxygen demand.

Turn and breathe

• Implement turning and deep breathing hourly, using adjunct analgesics and splinting of the incision to minimize discomfort and pain. Firm stuffed animals can be used effectively for incisional support during deep-breathing and spirometry exercises.
• Prepare the child for chest tube removal (typically between the first and third postoperative day), which can be a painful and frightening procedure for a child. Topical anesthetics or analgesics are commonly administered before removal. (See *Chest tube removal*.)

Rx: TLC

• Provide emotional support and comfort because surgery can be frightening as well as painful to the child. (Encourage parental involvement in the child's care to foster feelings of comfort and security.)

• Provide detailed discharge teaching. (See *Teaching about cardiac surgery*.)

Cardiac transplantation

For infants and children with worsening heart failure and limited life expectancy, heart transplantation has become an option. Indications for transplantation in children include cardiomyopathy and end-stage congenital heart disease.

One of two

There are two surgical options for cardiac transplantation:
• *orthotopic procedure*, in which the diseased heart is removed in its entirety and a new, healthy heart from a donor (who has been declared brain dead) is implanted
• *heterotopic procedure* (rarely performed in children), in which the patient's own heart is kept in place and a "piggyback" heart is implanted to serve as an additional pumping organ to assist the diseased heart.

Who knows UNOS?

The process begins by placing the child on the United Network for Organ Sharing (UNOS) list to match a donor with the recipient. Due to limited donor supply, 30% of infants on the UNOS list die before a new heart can be found for them. Approximately 300 to 400 transplants are performed per year on pediatric patients.

Crucial 6 months

Complications are most common during the first 6 months to 1 year after transplantation. During this period, the family must adjust to a totally new lifestyle that will require lifelong management. The leading cause of demise after heart transplantation is organ rejection. Because lifelong immunosuppressive therapy is required, infection is always a risk.

Nursing considerations

The child and his parents must be prepared thoroughly for this major procedure. Preparation should include a brief visit to the coronary intensive care unit (CICU) and, if possible, the child should be introduced to the nurses who will be providing his care. Parents should be made aware of the visiting policies in the CICU and should be assisted in making arrangements (in the hospital and at home) to spend as much time with their child as possible.

It's all relative

Teaching about cardiac surgery

Be sure to include these points in your teaching plan for the parents of a child who has undergone cardiac surgery:
• dietary restrictions, if any
• fluid requirements and restrictions
• activity and exercise restrictions
• operative site care and inspection
• medication regimen
• follow-up tests and doctor visits
• home care needs
• importance of encouraging the child to talk and express his feelings about the surgery and hospitalization.

The hard part is over

Postoperative care involves:
• monitoring the patient closely for signs of rejection, infection, and adverse reactions from immunosuppressive therapy
• restricting fluids as ordered to prevent hypervolemia and heart strain
• providing adequate rest periods with gradual activity increases to further decrease the workload of the heart
• encouraging compliance with the complex drug regimen required, especially in adolescents
• providing emotional support to the child and family and offering resources for additional support
• helping the parents (and the child, if age appropriate) come to terms with the reality that someone had to die for a heart to become available. (This concept is too confusing and upsetting for most young children; parents should be encouraged to provide age-appropriate explanations when the child begins to ask where his new heart came from.)

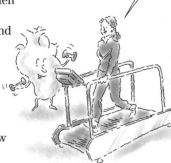

Activity is important after heart transplantation. Teach patients to go slowly, and intersperse gradual activity increases with lots of rest.

Congenital heart defects that increase pulmonary blood flow

Congenital heart defects that increase pulmonary blood flow include atrial septal defect (ASD), patent ductus arteriosus (PDA), and ventricular septal defect (VSD).

Atrial septal defect

In a child with ASD, an opening between the left and right atria allows blood to flow from the left side of the heart to the right side, resulting in ineffective pumping of the heart, thus increasing the risk of heart failure. (See *Looking at ASD*.)

ASDs come in threes

The three types of ASDs are:

ostium secundum defect, the most common type, which occurs in the region of the fossa ovalis at the center of the atrial septum and, occasionally, extends inferiorly, close to the vena cava

sinus venosus defect, which occurs in the superior-posterior portion of the atrial septum, sometimes extends into the vena cava, and is almost always associated with abnormal drainage of pulmonary veins into the right atrium

ostium primum defect, which occurs in the inferior portion of the septum primum and is usually associated with AV valve abnormalities (cleft mitral valve) and conduction defects.

Benign when small

ASD accounts for about 10% of congenital heart defects and is almost twice as common in females as in males, with a strong familial tendency. Although an ASD is usually a benign defect during infancy and childhood, delayed development of symptoms and complications makes it one of the most common congenital heart defects diagnosed in adults.

The prognosis is excellent for asymptomatic patients and for those with uncomplicated surgical repair. The prognosis is poor, however, in patients with cyanosis caused by large, untreated defects.

What causes it

The cause of ASD is unknown. Ostium primum defects commonly occur in patients with Down syndrome.

How it happens

In ASD, blood shunts from the left atrium to the right atrium because the left atrial pressure is normally slightly higher than the right atrial pressure. The difference in pressure forces large amounts of blood through the defect. This shunt results in right heart volume overload, affecting the right atrium, right ventricle, and pulmonary arteries.

Enlarge and dilate

Eventually, the right atrium enlarges, and the right ventricle dilates to accommodate the increased blood volume. If pulmonary artery hypertension develops, increased pulmonary vascular resistance and right ventricular hypertrophy follow.

What to look for

Signs and symptoms of ASD include:
• fatigue after exertion
• early to midsystolic murmur at the second or third left intercostal space
• low-pitched diastolic murmur at the lower left sternal border (more pronounced on inspiration)

Looking at ASD

An ASD is an opening between the left and right atria that allows blood to flow from the left side of the heart to the right side, as shown here.

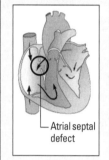

Atrial septal defect

- fixed, widely split S_2 due to delayed closure of the pulmonic valve
- systolic click or late systolic murmur at the apex
- clubbing and cyanosis if a right-to-left shunt develops. (See *Cyanosis and crying.*)

What tests tell you

A history of increasing fatigue and characteristic physical features suggest ASD. These tests confirm the diagnosis:
- Chest X-ray shows an enlarged right atrium and right ventricle, a prominent pulmonary artery, and increased pulmonary vascular markings.
- ECG results may be normal but commonly show right-axis deviation, prolonged PR interval, varying degrees of right bundle-branch block, right ventricular hypertrophy, atrial fibrillation and, in ostium primum defect, left-axis deviation.
- Echocardiography measures right ventricular enlargement, may locate the defect, and shows volume overload in the right side of the heart. (It may also reveal right ventricular and pulmonary artery dilation.)
- Two-dimensional echocardiography with color Doppler flow and contrast echocardiography have supplanted cardiac catheterization as the confirming tests for ASD. (Cardiac catheterization is used if inconsistencies exist in the clinical data or if significant pulmonary hypertension is suspected.)

Complications

Complications of ASD may include physical underdevelopment, respiratory infections, heart failure, atrial arrhythmias, and mitral valve prolapse.

How it's treated

Operative repair is advised for uncomplicated ASD with evidence of significant left-to-right shunting. Ideally, this is performed when the patient is between ages 2 and 4. An operative repair shouldn't be performed on a patient with a small defect and trivial left-to-right shunt.

Procrastination preferred

Because ASD seldom produces complications in an infant or toddler, surgery can be delayed until preschool or early school age. A large defect may need immediate surgical closure with sutures or a patch graft. Alternatively, placement of an atrial occluder during cardiac catheterization is becoming a more common intervention than open-heart surgery.

Cyanosis and crying

An infant may be cyanotic because he has a cardiac or pulmonary disorder. Cyanosis that worsens with crying is most likely associated with cardiac causes because crying increases pulmonary resistance to blood flow, resulting in an increased right-to-left shunt. Cyanosis that improves with crying is most likely due to pulmonary causes because deep breathing improves tidal volume.

What to do

Before cardiac catheterization, explain pretest and posttest procedures to the child and his parents. Whenever possible, use drawings or other visual aids to enhance the explanation.
• As needed, teach the parents (and child) about antibiotic prophylaxis to prevent infective endocarditis.
• If surgery is scheduled, prepare the child and his parents for what they'll experience in the intensive care unit and introduce them to the staff. Show the parents where they can wait during the operation, and explain postoperative procedures, tubes, dressings, and monitoring equipment.
• After surgery, closely monitor the patient's vital signs, central venous and intra-arterial pressures, and intake and output. (Watch for atrial arrhythmias, which may remain uncorrected.)

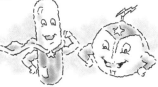

It's a bird, it's a plane, it's ... antibiotics! For the child with ASD, we're the first line of defense against the evil endocarditis!

Patent ductus arteriosus

The ductus arteriosus is a fetal blood vessel that connects the pulmonary artery to the descending aorta, just distal to the left subclavian artery. Normally, the ductus closes within days after birth. In PDA, the lumen of the ductus remains open after birth. This defect creates a left-to-right shunt of blood from the aorta to the pulmonary artery and results in recirculation of blood through the lungs.

Postdated PDA

Initially, PDA may not produce clinical effects. Over time, however, it can precipitate pulmonary vascular disease, causing symptoms to appear by age 40. PDA affects twice as many females as males. (See *Looking at PDA*, page 284.)

Smaller is better

In PDA, prognosis is good if the shunt is small or surgical repair is effective. Otherwise, PDA may advance to intractable heart failure, which may be fatal.

What causes it

PDA is associated with:
• premature birth, probably as a result of abnormalities in oxygenation or the relaxant action of prostaglandin E, which prevents ductal spasm and contracture necessary for closure
• rubella syndrome
• coarctation of the aorta
• VSD
• pulmonic and aortic stenosis
• living at high altitudes.

How it happens

The ductus arteriosus normally closes as prostaglandin levels from the placenta fall and oxygen levels rise. This process should begin as soon as the neonate takes his first breath but may take as long as 3 months in some children.

Back to the aorta

In PDA, relative resistance in pulmonary and systemic vasculature and the size of the ductus determine the quantity of blood that's shunted from left to right. Because of increased aortic pressure, oxygenated blood is shunted from the aorta through the ductus arteriosus to the pulmonary artery and the lungs. The blood returns to the left side of the heart and is pumped out to the aorta once more.

The left atrium and left ventricle must accommodate the increased pulmonary venous return by increasing filling pressure and workload on the left side of the heart. This compensation causes left-sided hypertrophy and, possibly, heart failure.

Reverse to cyanosis

In the final stages of untreated PDA, the left-to-right shunt leads to chronic pulmonary artery hypertension that becomes fixed and unreactive. This condition causes the shunt to reverse so that unoxygenated blood enters systemic circulation, causing cyanosis.

What to look for

Signs and symptoms of PDA may include:
• respiratory distress with signs of heart failure in infants, especially those who are premature
• classic machinery murmur (Gibson murmur), a continuous murmur heard throughout systole and diastole
• thrill palpated at the left sternal border
• prominent left ventricular impulse
• bounding peripheral pulses
• widened pulse pressure
• slow motor development
• failure to thrive
• fatigue and dyspnea on exertion, which may develop in adults with undetected PDA.

What tests tell you

These tests help diagnose PDA:
• Chest X-rays may show increased pulmonary vascular markings, prominent pulmonary arteries, and enlargement of the left ventricle and aorta.

Looking at PDA

In PDA, the lumen of the ductus arteriosus stays open after birth, causing a left-to-right shunt of blood from the aorta to the pulmonary artery, resulting in recirculation of arterial blood through the lungs. This shunt reversal (from fetal circulation) occurs because of the lower pressure in the lungs and pulmonary artery after birth.

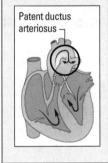

Patent ductus arteriosus

• ECG may be normal or may indicate left atrial or ventricular hypertrophy and, in pulmonary vascular disease, biventricular hypertrophy.
• Echocardiography detects and estimates the size of a PDA. It also reveals an enlarged left atrium and left ventricle or right ventricular hypertrophy from pulmonary vascular disease.

Complications

Possible complications of PDA may include infective endocarditis, heart failure, and recurrent pneumonia.

How it's treated

Correction of PDA may involve:
• indomethacin (Indocin), a prostaglandin inhibitor, to induce ductus spasm and closure in premature infants
    • As an alternative to indomethacin (Indocin), some facilities are using ibuprofen, with findings of equally good closure of the PDA but fewer renal side effects and complications.
• left thoracotomy to ligate the ductus if medical management can't control heart failure (asymptomatic infants with PDA don't require immediate treatment; if symptoms are mild, surgical ligation of the PDA is usually delayed until the child is 1 year old)
• visual assisted thoracoscopic surgery (VATS) to ligate the ductus as an alternative to surgery with a thoracotomy (VATS may be done at the bedside or in a procedure room and involves three small incisions in the left chest through which a clip is placed on the ductus)
    • Alternatively, procedures can be done through a cardiac catheterization to block the flow of blood through the ductus by inserting umbrella or coil-type devices into the ends of the ductus, thus blocking the shunt.
• prophylactic antibiotics to protect against infective endocarditis
• treatment of heart failure with fluid restriction, diuretics, and digoxin

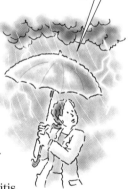

Plug up the ductus! In a child with a PDA, shunting can sometimes be stopped by inserting an "umbrella," or plug.

What to do

PDA necessitates careful monitoring, patient and family teaching, and emotional support.
• Watch carefully for signs of PDA in all premature neonates.
• Be alert for respiratory distress symptoms resulting from heart failure, which may develop rapidly in a premature neonate. Frequently assess vital signs, ECG, electrolyte levels, and intake and output and document the child's response to diuretics and other therapy.

• If the infant receives indomethacin for ductus closure, watch for possible adverse effects, such as diarrhea, jaundice, bleeding, and renal dysfunction. Obtain blood tests before each dose of indomethacin as ordered.

Explain, prepare, meet, and greet

• Before surgery, carefully explain all treatments and tests to the parents and child, if age-appropriate.
• Arrange for the family to meet the intensive care unit staff. Discuss the expected I.V. lines, monitoring equipment, and postoperative procedures.
• Immediately after surgery, the child may have a central venous pressure catheter and an arterial line in place. Carefully assess vital signs, intake and output, and arterial and venous pressures. Provide pain relief as needed.

Tell one, tell all

• Stress the need for regular medical follow-up examinations and advise the parents to inform any doctor who treats their child about his history of surgery for PDA—even if the child is being treated for an unrelated medical problem.
• Before discharge, review instructions with the parents about activity restrictions based on the child's tolerance and energy levels. (Advise the parents to avoid becoming overprotective as their child's tolerance for physical activity increases.)

Ventricular septal defect

In the child with VSD, an opening in the septum between the ventricles allows blood to shunt between the left and right ventricles. This opening results in ineffective pumping of the heart and increases the risk of heart failure. (See *Looking at VSD*.)

VSDs account for up to 30% of all congenital heart defects. The prognosis is good for defects that close spontaneously or are correctable surgically. Prognosis is poor, however, for untreated defects, which are sometimes fatal in children by age 1 year, usually from secondary complications.

What causes it

VSD may be associated with:
• fetal alcohol syndrome
• Down syndrome and other autosomal trisomies
• renal anomalies
• PDA and coarctation of the aorta
• prematurity.

Looking at VSD

In a VSD, an opening in the interventricular septum allows blood to shunt between the left and right ventricles.

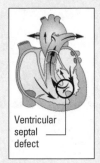

Ventricular septal defect

How it happens

In infants with VSD, the ventricular septum fails to close completely by gestation week 8. VSDs are located in the membranous or muscular portion of the ventricular septum and vary in size. Some defects close spontaneously; in other defects, the septum is entirely absent, creating a single ventricle. Small VSDs are likely to close spontaneously. Large VSDs should be surgically repaired before pulmonary vascular disease occurs or while it's still reversible.

Undercover VSD

VSD isn't readily apparent at birth because right and left pressures are approximately equal and pulmonary artery resistance is elevated. Alveoli aren't yet completely opened, so blood doesn't shunt through the defect. As the pulmonary vasculature gradually relaxes between 4 and 8 weeks after birth, right ventricular pressure decreases, allowing blood to shunt from the left to the right ventricle.

Because it isn't readily apparent at birth, VSD can sometimes go undiagnosed until an infant is 8 weeks old.

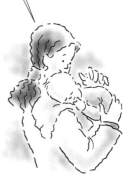

Leading with the left

Initially, large VSD shunts cause left atrial and left ventricular hypertrophy. Later, an uncorrected VSD causes right ventricular hypertrophy due to increasing pulmonary resistance. Eventually, right- and left-sided heart failure and cyanosis (from reversal of the shunt direction) occur. Fixed pulmonary hypertension may occur much later in life with right-to-left shunting, causing cyanosis and clubbing of the nail beds.

What to look for

Signs and symptoms of VSD may include:
• thin, small infant who gains weight slowly (when a large VSD is present)
• loud, harsh, widely transmitted systolic murmur heard best along the left sternal border at the third or fourth intercostal space
• palpable thrill
• loud, widely split pulmonic component of S_2
• point of maximal impulse displacement to the left
• prominent anterior chest
• liver, heart, and spleen enlargement
• feeding difficulties
• diaphoresis, tachycardia, and rapid, grunting respirations
• cyanosis and clubbing if right-to-left shunting occurs later in life.

What tests tell you

These tests help diagnose VSD:
• Chest X-rays appear normal in children with small defects. In children with large defects, X-rays may show cardiomegaly, left atrial and left ventricular enlargement, and prominent vascular markings.
• ECG may be normal with small VSDs, whereas in large VSDs, it may show left and right ventricular hypertrophy, suggesting pulmonary hypertension.
• Echocardiography can detect a VSD in the septum, estimate the size of the left-to-right shunt, suggest pulmonary hypertension, and identify associated lesions and complications.
• Cardiac catheterization determines the size and exact location of the VSD and the extent of pulmonary hypertension, detects associated defects, and calculates the degree of shunting by comparing the blood oxygen saturation in each ventricle. (The oxygen saturation of the right ventricle is greater than normal because oxygenated blood is shunted from the left to the right ventricle.)

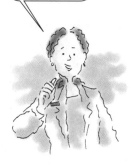

Small VSDs might not be detected by chest X-rays or ECG.

Complications

Complications of VSD may include pulmonary hypertension, infective endocarditis, pneumonia, and heart failure.

How it's treated

Many VSDs (20% to 60%) may close spontaneously during the first year of life, especially small VSDs. Correction of VSD may involve:
• early surgical correction for a large VSD, usually performed using a patch graft, before heart failure and irreversible pulmonary vascular disease develop
• placement of a permanent pacemaker, which may be necessary after VSD repair if complete heart block develops from interference with the bundle of His during surgery
• surgical closure of small defects using sutures (such defects may not be surgically repaired if the patient has normal pulmonary artery pressure and a small shunt)
• pulmonary artery banding to normalize pressures and flow distal to the band and to prevent pulmonary vascular disease if the child has other defects and will benefit from delaying surgery
• digoxin, sodium restriction, and diuretics before surgery to prevent heart failure
• prophylactic antibiotics before and after surgery to prevent infective endocarditis.

What to do

Although the parents of an infant with VSD commonly suspect something is wrong with their child before diagnosis, they may need psychological support to help them accept the reality of a serious cardiac disorder. Also, because surgery may take place months after diagnosis, parent teaching is vital to prevent complications until the child is scheduled for surgery or the defect closes. Thorough explanations of all tests are also essential. In addition, follow these steps:

• Instruct the parents to watch for signs of heart failure, such as poor feeding, sweating, and heavy breathing.
• If the child is receiving digoxin or other medications, tell the parents how to give it and how to recognize adverse effects. (Caution them to keep medications out of the reach of all children.)
• Teach the parents how to recognize and report early signs of infection and to avoid exposing the child to people with obvious infections.
• Encourage the parents to let the child engage in normal activities.
• Stress the importance of prophylactic antibiotics before and after surgical procedures.

Congenital obstructive defects

Defects that obstruct the flow of blood out of the heart include coarctation of the aorta, aortic stenosis, and pulmonic stenosis.

Coarctation of the aorta

Coarctation is a narrowing of the aorta, usually just below the left subclavian artery, near the site where the ligamentum arteriosum (the remnant of the ductus arteriosus) joins the pulmonary artery to the aorta.

Coarctation may occur with aortic valve stenosis (usually of a bicuspid aortic valve) and with severe cases of hypoplasia of the aortic arch, PDA, and VSD. The obstruction to blood flow results in ineffective pumping of the heart and increases the risk of heart failure. (See *Looking at coarctation of the aorta.*)

What causes it

Although the cause of this defect is unknown, it may be associated with Turner's syndrome. Turner's syndrome is a chromosome abnormality affecting only females, caused by the complete or partial deletion of the X chromosome.

Looking at coarctation of the aorta

In coarctation of the aorta, a narrowing of the aorta occurs, usually near the site of insertion of the ductus arteriosus.

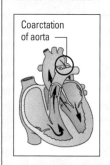

Coarctation of aorta

How it happens

Coarctation of the aorta may develop as a result of spasm and constriction of the smooth muscle in the ductus arteriosus as it closes. This contractile tissue may extend into the aortic wall, causing narrowing. The obstructive process causes hypertension in the aortic branches above the constriction (arteries that supply the arms, neck, and head) and diminished pressure in the vessel below the constriction (that supplies the trunk and lower extremities).

Under pressure

Restricted blood flow through the narrowed aorta increases the pressure load on the left ventricle and causes dilation of the proximal aorta and ventricular hypertrophy.

A leggy problem

As oxygenated blood leaves the left ventricle, a portion travels through the arteries that branch off the aorta proximal to the coarctation. If PDA is present, the rest of the blood travels through the coarctation, mixes with deoxygenated blood from the PDA, and travels to the legs. If the PDA is closed, the legs and lower portion of the body must rely solely on the blood that gets through the coarctation.

Untreated, this condition may lead to left-sided heart failure. If coarctation remains asymptomatic in infancy, it usually remains so throughout adolescence as collateral circulation develops to bypass the narrowed segment.

> Walking can be difficult and painful for a child with coarctation of the aorta.

What to look for

Signs and symptoms of coarctation of the aorta may include:
• tachypnea, dyspnea, pulmonary edema, pallor, tachycardia, failure to thrive, cardiomegaly, and hepatomegaly during an infant's first year of life
• claudication (cramping pain in arms and/or legs)
• hypertension in the upper body
• headache, vertigo, and epistaxis
• pink upper extremities and cyanotic lower extremities
• bounding pulses in the arms and absent or diminished femoral pulses
• in most cases, normal heart sounds unless a coexisting cardiac defect is present
• more developed chest and arms than legs
• upper extremity blood pressure greater than lower extremity blood pressure.

What tests tell you

Physical examination reveals the cardinal signs of coarctation of the aorta, including resting systolic hypertension in the upper body, absent or diminished femoral pulses, and a wide pulse pressure. In addition, these tests may indicate the condition:
• Chest X-rays may demonstrate left ventricular hypertrophy, heart failure, a wide ascending and descending aorta, and notching of the undersurfaces of the ribs due to erosion by collateral circulation.
• ECG may reveal left ventricular hypertrophy.
• Echocardiography may show increased left ventricular muscle thickness, coexisting aortic valve abnormalities, and the coarctation site.

Complications

Possible complications may include heart failure, severe hypertension, cerebral aneurysms and hemorrhage, rupture of the aorta, aortic aneurysm, and infective endocarditis.

How it's treated

Correction of coarctation of the aorta may involve:
• digoxin, diuretics, oxygen, and sedatives in infants with heart failure
• prostaglandin infusion to keep the ductus open
• antibiotic prophylaxis against infective endocarditis before and after surgery
• antihypertensive therapy for children with previous undetected coarctation until surgery is performed.

Resect, patch, ligate

Surgery may be performed early for infants with heart failure or hypertension, or it may be delayed until the preschool years. Options include:
• end-to-end anastomosis, in which the area of coarctation is resected and the distal and proximal aorta are anastomosed end-to-end
• patch aortoplasty, in which the area of coarctation is incised and an elliptical Dacron patch is sutured in place to widen the diameter
• subclavian flap aortoplasty, in which the distal subclavian artery is divided and the flap of the proximal portion of this vessel is used to expand the coarcted area.

The ductus arteriosus is always ligated with each of these surgical techniques. Balloon angioplasty may be performed if recoarctation occurs.

What to do

When providing care to an infant:
• If coarctation requires rapid digitalization, monitor vital signs closely and watch for digoxin toxicity (poor feeding and vomiting).
• Monitor intake and output carefully, especially if the infant is receiving diuretics with fluid restriction.
• Weigh the child daily.

Bigger and bigger

For an older child:
• Assess blood pressure in his extremities regularly, explain exercise restrictions, stress the need to take medications properly and to watch for adverse effects, and teach him about tests and other procedures.

Postop checklist

After corrective surgery, follow these steps:
• Monitor blood pressure closely using an intra-arterial line. Take blood pressure in all extremities.
• Monitor intake and output.
• If the patient develops hypertension and requires antihypertensives, administer the medication as ordered. Watch for severe hypotension and regulate the dosage carefully.
• Provide pain relief as needed and encourage a gradual increase in activity.
• Stress the importance of continued endocarditis prophylaxis if prescribed.

Stenosis, aortic

In aortic stenosis, narrowing or fusion of the aortic valve interferes with left ventricular outflow to the aorta. This defect, which is most common in males, causes left ventricular hypertrophy, causing pulmonary venous and arterial hypertension. (See *Looking at aortic stenosis*.)

What causes it

Aortic stenosis may result from congenital aortic bicuspid valves, congenital stenosis of valve cusps, or rheumatic fever.

Looking at aortic stenosis

In aortic stenosis, narrowing or fusion of the aortic valve causes left ventricular hypertrophy and interferes with ventricular outflow to the aorta.

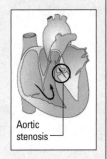

Aortic stenosis

How it happens

Increased left ventricular pressure attempts to overcome the resistance of the narrowed valvular opening. The added workload increases the demand for oxygen, and diminished cardiac output causes poor coronary artery perfusion, ischemia of the left ventricle, and left-sided heart failure. If left-sided heart failure develops, increased pressure in the left atrium with resulting increased pressure in the pulmonary veins can cause pulmonary edema.

What to look for

Signs and symptoms of aortic stenosis may include:
- rough, systolic murmur heard loudest at the second intercostal space
- diminished carotid pulses
- systolic thrill
- syncope
- hypotension
- poor feeding
- angina-like chest pain on activity and exercise intolerance.

What tests tell you

Tests used to diagnose aortic stenosis and determine its severity include:
- chest X-ray, which shows left ventricular hypertrophy and prominent pulmonary vasculature
- ECG, which shows left ventricular hypertrophy
- echocardiography, which shows a thickened aortic valve and left ventricular wall
- cardiac catheterization, which demonstrates the degree of stenosis.

Complications

Complications of aortic stenosis may include infective endocarditis, pulmonary edema, heart failure, and sudden death due to myocardial ischemia.

How it's treated

Digoxin and diuretics are given for signs of heart failure. Anticoagulant therapy is used to prevent thrombus formation around the stenotic or replaced valve. Prophylactic antibiotics are given to prevent infective endocarditis.

Surgery may involve aortic valvulotomy or prosthetic valve replacement. Balloon angioplasty, done through a cardiac catheterization, may be used to dilate the stenotic valve.

What to do

When caring for a child with aortic stenosis:
• Watch closely for signs of heart failure or pulmonary edema and for adverse effects of drug therapy.
• Teach the patient (and his parents) about the importance of his medications and consistent follow-up care.

Postsurgical steps

If the patient has had surgery:
• Watch for hypotension, arrhythmias, and thrombus formation.
• Monitor vital signs, ABG values, intake and output, daily weights, blood chemistries, chest X-rays, and pulmonary artery catheter readings.

Stenosis, pulmonic

In pulmonic stenosis, a narrowing or fusing of pulmonic valve leaflets at the entrance of the pulmonary artery interferes with right ventricular outflow to the lungs, decreasing blood flow to the lungs. (See *Looking at pulmonic stenosis.*)

What causes it

Pulmonic stenosis results from congenital stenosis of the valve cusp or rheumatic heart disease. It's also one of the four defects present that comprise tetralogy of Fallot.

How it happens

Obstructed right ventricular outflow causes right ventricular hypertrophy, eventually resulting in right-sided heart failure.

What to look for

Patients with pulmonic stenosis may be asymptomatic, or they may show:
• cyanosis
• signs of heart failure
• systolic murmur heard loudest at the upper left sternal border and a split S_2.

Looking at pulmonic stenosis

In pulmonic stenosis, a narrowing or fusing of the pulmonic valve interferes with right ventricular outflow to the lungs.

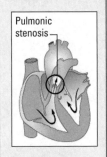

Pulmonic stenosis

What tests tell you

Evidence of right ventricular hypertrophy may be seen on chest X-ray, ECG, and echocardiography. Cardiac catheterization demonstrates the degree of the stenosis.

Complications

Complications of pulmonic stenosis may include infective endocarditis and heart failure.

How it's treated

Digoxin and diuretics are given for signs of heart failure, and anticoagulant therapy is used to prevent thrombus formation around the stenotic or replaced valve. Prophylactic antibiotics are given to prevent infective endocarditis. Balloon angioplasty during cardiac catheterization is widely used to relieve pulmonic stenosis, but in some cases, surgical valvulotomy may be necessary.

What to do

The child and his parents should be taught about the importance of medications and consistent follow-up care. The patient must be watched closely for signs of heart failure or pulmonary edema and for adverse effects of drug therapy.

If the patient has had surgery:
• Watch for hypotension, arrhythmias, and thrombus formation.
• Monitor vital signs, ABG values, intake and output, daily weight, blood chemistries, chest X-rays, and pulmonary artery catheter readings.

Mixed congenital heart defects

In defects that cause mixed blood flow, oxygenated and deoxygenated blood mix in the heart or great vessels. Such defects include hypoplastic left heart syndrome and transposition of the great arteries.

Hypoplastic left heart syndrome

Hypoplastic left heart syndrome refers to underdevelopment of the left side of the heart. The defects of this syndrome include:
• aortic valve atresia or stenosis
• mitral valve atresia or stenosis
• diminutive or absent left ventricle

Looking at hypoplastic left heart syndrome

Hypoplastic left heart syndrome consists of these defects:
- aortic valve atresia or stenosis
- mitral valve atresia or stenosis
- diminutive or absent left ventricle
- severe hypoplasia of the ascending aorta and aortic arch.

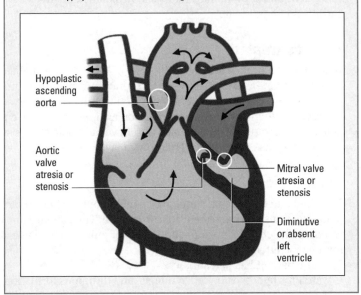

Hypoplastic ascending aorta

Aortic valve atresia or stenosis

Mitral valve atresia or stenosis

Diminutive or absent left ventricle

• severe hypoplasia of the ascending aorta and aortic arch. (See *Looking at hypoplastic left heart syndrome.*)

What causes it

The cause of hypoplastic left heart syndrome is unknown.

How it happens

Blood from the left atrium travels through a patent foramen ovale to the right ventricle and pulmonary artery, entering the systemic circulation via the ductus arteriosus. Patency of the ductus arteriosus, which allows blood flow to the systemic circulation, is necessary to sustain life.

What to look for

Signs and symptoms may include:
- cyanosis
- weak or absent pulses
- signs of heart failure, such as tachycardia, sweating, cardiomegaly, tachypnea, cyanosis, and peripheral edema.

Close call

If the ductus arteriosus closes, the infant will progressively deteriorate with worsening cyanosis, decreased cardiac output, and eventual cardiovascular collapse.

What tests tell you

Echocardiography provides visualization of the defect.

Complications

Complications of hypoplastic left heart syndrome can include heart failure and death.

How it's treated

Prostaglandin E is used to maintain patency of the ductus arteriosus. Digoxin and diuretics are administered to control heart failure.

Certain surgery

Without surgery, death will occur in early infancy. Surgical procedures include heart transplantation in the neonatal period (although not common because of the shortage of neonate organs, risk of rejection, and need for chronic immunosuppression) or the more commonly performed *staged reconstruction*, which is a series of surgeries to restructure the heart to be as efficient as possible without an adequately functioning left ventricle. Typically, three procedures are performed in stages:

• Norwood procedure (performed soon after birth)—Blood flow from the right ventricle is rerouted to provide systemic circulation (a task normally performed by the left ventricle). Because the right ventricle is now providing circulation to the rest of the body instead of to the lungs, an alternative source of pulmonary circulation must be provided. An aortopulmonary shunt is created to connect the aorta to the main pulmonary artery to provide pulmonary blood flow.

• bidirectional Glenn procedure (also called a hemi-Fontan) (performed at ages 4 to 6 months)—The pulmonary arteries are disconnected from their existing blood supply (e.g., a shunt created during a Norwood procedure). The superior vena cava (SVC), which carries blood returning from the upper body, is disconnected from the heart and instead redirected into the pulmonary arteries. The IVC, which carries blood returning from the lower body, continues to connect to the heart.

• modified Fontan procedure (the final stage performed at ages 2 to 3 years)—The blood from the IVC is redirected to the lungs. At this point, the oxygen-poor blood from upper and lower body flows through the lungs without being pumped (driven only by the pressure that builds up in the veins). This corrects the hypoxia associated with hypoplastic left heart and leaves the single ventricle responsible only for supplying blood to the body.

The ultimate goal of these surgeries is to make it possible for the right ventricle (fully functioning) to work as two normal ventricles would and to allow the separation of oxygenated and deoxygenated blood as the blood passes through the pulmonary and systemic circulations.

What to do

Explain the heart defect to the parents, prepare the child for surgery, and answer any questions. In addition, follow these steps:
• Monitor vital signs, pulse oximetry, and intake and output to assess renal function and detect changes.
• Assess cardiovascular and respiratory status to detect early signs of decompensation.
• Take the patient's apical pulse for 1 minute before giving digoxin and withhold the drug to prevent toxicity if the heart rate is below 90 to 110 beats/minute in infants and young children (below 70 beats/minute in older children).
• Monitor fluid status, enforcing fluid restrictions as appropriate to prevent fluid overload. Weigh the child daily.
• Organize nursing care activities around long periods of uninterrupted rest to decrease the child's oxygen demands.

Transposition of the great arteries

In transposition of the great arteries, the aorta rises from the right ventricle and the pulmonary artery rises from the left ventricle. This defect produces two noncommunicating circulatory systems. (See *Looking at transposition of the great arteries*.)

What causes it

The cause of transposition of the great arteries is unknown.

How it happens

The transposed pulmonary artery carries oxygenated blood back to the lungs rather than to the left side of the heart. The transposed aorta returns unoxygenated blood to the systemic circulation rather than to the lungs.

Communication between the pulmonary and systemic circulation is necessary for survival; the presence of other congenital defects, such as PDA, ASD, and VSD, allows for such communication. These defects cause holes in the heart that allow blood to flow from one side of the heart to the other so that oxygenated and deoxygenated blood can mix and flow to the lungs and the rest of the body, which is necessary to sustain life.

Looking at transposition of the great arteries

In transposition of the great arteries, the aorta rises from the right ventricle, and the pulmonary artery from the left ventricle, producing two noncommunicating circulatory systems.

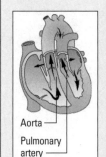

Aorta

Pulmonary artery

What to look for

Signs and symptoms of transposition of the great arteries include:
- cyanosis from birth and tachypnea (worsening with crying)
- gallop rhythm
- tachycardia
- dyspnea
- cardiomegaly
- hepatomegaly
- murmurs of ASD, VSD, or PDA, and loud S_2
- diminished exercise tolerance
- fatigue
- clubbing of the fingers and toes.

What tests tell you

Chest X-rays may show increased pulmonary vascular markings; right atrial and ventricular enlargements give the heart a characteristic oblong appearance. In addition:
- ECG may indicate right axis deviation and right ventricular hypertrophy.
- Echocardiography demonstrates the reversed position of the aorta and pulmonary artery and may detect other cardiac defects.
- Cardiac catheterization shows decreased oxygen saturation in left ventricular blood and aortic blood; increased right atrial, right ventricular, and pulmonary artery oxygen saturation; and right ventricular systolic pressure equal to systemic pressure. (Dye injection reveals transposed vessels and the presence of any other cardiac defects.)

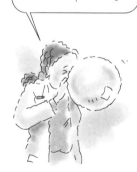

In a child with transposition of the great arteries, the patent foramen ovale is sometimes enlarged with atrial balloon septostomy.

Complications

Complications of transposition of the great arteries may include infective endocarditis and death.

How it's treated

Prostaglandin E is given to maintain patency of the ductus arteriosus. Prophylactic antibiotics will be needed to prevent infective endocarditis.

Up, up and away

Atrial balloon septostomy may be done during cardiac catheterization to enlarge the patent foramen ovale, which improves oxygenation by allowing greater mixing of the pulmonary and systemic circulations.

Go with the flow

Corrective surgery may be performed to redirect blood flow by switching the positions of the major blood vessels. This procedure is typically performed in the first few weeks of life.

What to do

Nursing care begins with patient education. Teach the parents about the defect and answer any questions they may have. The child should be prepared for surgery and other invasive procedures.
• Monitor vital signs, pulse oximetry, and intake and output to assess renal function and detect changes.
• Assess cardiovascular and respiratory status to detect early signs of decompensation.
• Monitor fluid status, enforcing fluid restrictions as appropriate to prevent fluid overload. Weigh the child daily.
• Offer the child high-calorie foods that are easy to ingest and digest.
• Encourage parents to help their child assume new activity levels and independence.

Congenital heart defects that decrease pulmonary blood flow

Defects that decrease pulmonary blood flow include tetralogy of Fallot and tricuspid atresia.

Tetralogy of Fallot

Tetralogy of Fallot is a combination of four cardiac defects:
• VSD
• right ventricular outflow obstruction (pulmonic stenosis)
• right ventricular hypertrophy
• overriding aorta (aorta positioned above the VSD).
    Blood shunts from right to left through the VSD, allowing unoxygenated blood to mix with oxygenated blood, which results in cyanosis. This heart defect accounts for about 10% of all congenital defects and occurs equally in males and females. (See *Looking at tetralogy of Fallot.*)

What causes it

The cause of tetralogy of Fallot is unknown, but it is thought to be due to environmental or genetic factors or a combination of both. It is associated with chromosome 22 deletions and DiGeorge syndrome.

How it happens

In tetralogy of Fallot, unoxygenated venous blood returning to the right side of the heart may pass through the VSD to the left ventricle, bypassing the lungs, or it may enter the pulmonary artery, depending on the extent of the pulmonic stenosis. Rather than originating from the left ventricle, the aorta overrides both ventricles.

Looking at tetralogy of Fallot

Tetralogy of Fallot is a combination of four defects:
• VSD
• right ventricular outflow obstruction (pulmonic stenosis)
• right ventricular hypertrophy
• overriding aorta (aorta positioned over the VSD).

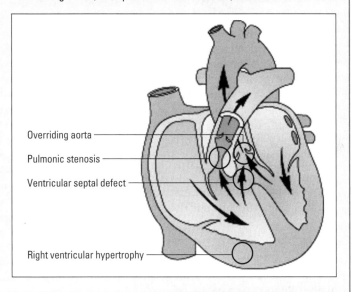

Overriding aorta

Pulmonic stenosis

Ventricular septal defect

Right ventricular hypertrophy

VSD usually lies in the outflow tract of the right ventricle. Severe obstruction of right ventricular outflow produces a right-to-left shunt, causing decreased systemic arterial oxygen saturation, cyanosis, reduced pulmonary blood flow, and hypoplasia of the entire pulmonary vasculature. Right ventricular hypertrophy develops in response to the extra force needed to push blood into the stenotic pulmonary artery.

What to look for

Cyanosis is the hallmark of tetralogy of Fallot. Children may have cyanotic or "blue" spells ("tet" spells), characterized by dyspnea; deep, sighing respirations; bradycardia; fainting; seizures; and loss of consciousness after exercise, crying, straining, infection, or fever. Not all children are cyanotic, and these children may be referred to as "pink tets."

Other signs and symptoms include:
• clubbing, diminished exercise tolerance, increasing dyspnea on exertion, growth retardation, and eating difficulties in older children
• squatting during episodes of shortness of breath

• loud systolic murmur best heard along the left sternal border, which may diminish or obscure the pulmonic component of S_2
• continuous murmur of the ductus in a patient with a large PDA
• thrill at the left sternal border
• obvious right ventricular impulse and prominent inferior sternum associated with right ventricular hypertrophy.

What tests tell you

Findings from chest X-rays, ECG, and echocardiography demonstrate the defects:
• Chest X-ray demonstrates a boot-shaped cardiac silhouette and decreased pulmonary vascular markings.
• ECG shows right ventricular hypertrophy, right axis deviation and, possibly, right atrial hypertrophy.
• Echocardiography and cardiac catheterization provide visualization of the defects.

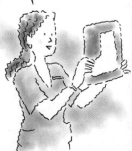

Tetralogy of Fallot gives the heart "the boot." Actually, the cardiac silhouette is boot-shaped on X-ray.

Complications

Complications of tetralogy of Fallot may include hypercyanotic tet spells, right ventricular dysfunction, infective endocarditis, polycythemia, and death.

How it's treated

Tetralogy of Fallot may be managed by:
• knee-chest position and administration of oxygen and morphine to improve oxygenation
• beta-blockers, such as propranolol, to prevent tet spells and prophylactic antibiotics to prevent infective endocarditis
• palliative surgery to reduce hypoxia during tet spells (involving the Blalock-Taussig procedure, which joins the subclavian artery to the pulmonary artery)
• complete surgical closure to relieve pulmonic stenosis and close the VSD, directing left ventricular outflow to the aorta (Brock procedure).

What to do

Educating the parents (and the child, if old enough) is a major part of nursing care:
• Explain tetralogy of Fallot to the parents; explain that their child will set his own exercise limits and will know when to rest.
• Teach the parents how to recognize tet spells, which can cause dramatically increased cyanosis; deep, sighing respirations; and syncope (tell them to place the child in the knee-chest position and to report such spells immediately; emergency treatment may be necessary). Older children may often squat during a tet spell.
• During hospitalization, alert the staff to the child's condition.

• Because of the right-to-left shunt through the VSD, treat I.V. lines like arterial lines, and remember that a clot dislodged from a catheter tip in a vein can cross the VSD and cause cerebral embolism (which can also happen if air enters the venous lines).
• If the child requires medical attention for an unrelated problem, advise the parents to inform the doctor immediately of the child's history of tetralogy of Fallot; any treatment must take this serious heart defect into consideration.

Tricuspid atresia

Tricuspid atresia is failure of the tricuspid valve to develop. This defect prevents blood from entering the right ventricle from the right atrium. (See *Looking at tricuspid atresia.*)

What causes it

The cause of tricuspid atresia is unknown, but it may be associated with pulmonic stenosis or transposition of the great arteries.

How it happens

Deoxygenated blood shunts from the right atrium through an ASD or a patent foramen ovale to the left atrium, where it mixes with oxygenated blood. This mixed blood then passes to the left ventricle and through a VSD to the right ventricle, pulmonary artery, and lungs, or mixed blood from the aorta refluxes back through the PDA to the lungs.

What to look for

Signs and symptoms may include cyanosis, tachycardia, dyspnea, and a heart murmur.

What tests tell you

In a patient with tricuspid atresia:
• Chest X-ray shows an enlarged right atrium and decreased pulmonary blood flow.
• ECG indicates left-axis deviation and absent right ventricular forces.
• Echocardiography provides visualization of the defect and shunting.

Complications

Complications of tricuspid atresia include infective endocarditis, brain abscess, and stroke.

Looking at tricuspid atresia

In tricuspid atresia, the tricuspid valve fails to develop, preventing blood from entering the right ventricle from the right atrium.

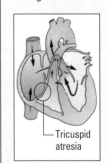

Tricuspid atresia

How it's treated

Prostaglandin E is administered to maintain ductal patency until surgery. Surgical repair may involve a subclavian-to-pulmonary artery shunt to improve blood flow to the lungs, or the modified Fontan procedure, which connects the right atrium directly to the pulmonary artery.

What to do

Explain the heart defect to the child and his parents, prepare the child for surgery, and answer any questions. In addition, follow these steps:
• Monitor vital signs, pulse oximetry, and intake and output to assess renal function and detect changes.
• Assess cardiovascular and respiratory status to detect early signs of decompensation.
• Monitor fluid status, enforcing fluid restrictions as appropriate to prevent fluid overload. Weigh the child daily.
• Organize nursing care around periods of uninterrupted rest to reduce the child's oxygen demands.

Other cardiovascular disorders

Other cardiovascular disorders that are common among children and adolescents include endocarditis, heart failure, Kawasaki disease, and rheumatic fever and rheumatic heart disease.

Endocarditis

Endocarditis (also known as *infective* or *bacterial endocarditis*) is an infection of the endocardium, heart valves, or cardiac prosthesis resulting from bacterial or fungal invasion.

Untreated endocarditis is usually fatal but, with proper treatment, 70% of patients recover. The prognosis is worst when endocarditis causes severe valvular damage, leading to insufficiency and heart failure, or when it involves a prosthetic valve.

What causes it

Most cases of endocarditis in children occur in patients with:
• abnormal heart valves
• prosthetic heart valves
• congenital heart defects (especially VSD, PDA, and tetralogy of Fallot)
• rheumatic heart disease.

Other predisposing conditions include Marfan syndrome, degenerative heart disease, I.V. drug use and, rarely, a syphilitic aortic valve.

The root of the problem

Some patients with endocarditis have no underlying heart disease. Infecting organisms differ among these groups. In patients with native valve endocarditis who aren't I.V. drug abusers, causative organisms usually include (in order of frequency) streptococci (especially *Streptococcus viridans*), staphylococci, and enterococci. Although other bacteria occasionally cause the disorder, fungal causes are rare in this group. The mitral valve is involved most commonly, followed by the aortic valve.

In patients who are I.V. drug abusers, *Staphylococcus aureus* is the most common infecting organism. Less commonly, streptococci, enterococci, gram-negative bacilli, or fungi cause the disorder. The tricuspid valve is involved most commonly, followed by the aortic valve, and then the mitral valve.

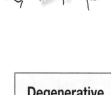

Bacteremia from something as simple as a dental extraction may be enough to cause endocarditis.

Postprosthesis predicament

In patients with prosthetic valve endocarditis, early cases (those that develop within 60 days of valve insertion) are usually due to staphylococcal infection. However, gram-negative aerobic organisms, fungi, streptococci, enterococci, or diphtheroids may also cause the disorder.

The course is usually fulminant and is associated with a high mortality rate. In late cases (occurring after 60 days), patients show signs and symptoms similar to those of native valve endocarditis.

How it happens

In endocarditis, bacteremia—even transient bacteremia following dental or urogenital procedures—introduces the pathogen into the bloodstream. This infection causes fibrin and platelets to aggregate on the valve tissue and engulf circulating bacteria or fungi that flourish and form friable wartlike vegetative growths on the heart valves, the endocardial lining of a heart chamber, or the epithelium of a blood vessel. (See *Degenerative changes in endocarditis*.)

It's a cover up

Such growths may cover the valve surfaces, causing ulceration and necrosis, or extend to the chordae tendineae, leading to rupture and subsequent valvular insufficiency. Ultimately, they may embolize to the spleen, kidneys, central nervous system, and lungs.

Degenerative changes in endocarditis

This illustration shows typical growths on the endocardium produced by fibrin and platelet deposits on infection sites.

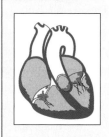

What to look for

Early clinical features of endocarditis are usually nonspecific and include malaise, weakness, fatigue, weight loss, anorexia, arthralgia, night sweats, chills, valvular insufficiency and, in 90% of patients, an intermittent fever that may recur for weeks. A more acute onset is associated with organisms of high pathogenicity such as *S. aureus*.

Murmur by megaphone

Endocarditis commonly causes a loud, regurgitant murmur typical of the underlying heart lesion. A sudden change in the murmur or the discovery of a new murmur in the presence of fever is a classic physical sign of endocarditis.

In about 30% of patients, embolization from growing lesions or diseased valvular tissue may produce:
• splenic infarction—pain in the left upper quadrant, radiating to the left shoulder, and abdominal rigidity
• renal infarction—hematuria, pyuria, flank pain, and decreased urine output
• pulmonary infarction—cough, pleuritic pain, pleural friction rub, dyspnea, and hemoptysis (most common in right-sided endocarditis, which commonly occurs among I.V. drug abusers and after cardiac surgery)
• cerebral infarction—hemiparesis, aphasia, or other neurologic deficits
• peripheral vascular occlusion—numbness and tingling in an arm, leg, finger, or toe or signs of impending peripheral gangrene.

Pinpoint spots

Other signs of endocarditis may include splenomegaly; petechiae of the skin (especially common on the upper anterior trunk) or buccal, pharyngeal, or conjunctival mucosa; and splinter hemorrhages under the nails.

Osler, Roth, and Janeway

Rarely, endocarditis produces Osler's nodes (tender, raised, subcutaneous lesions on the fingers or toes), Roth's spots (hemorrhagic areas with white centers on the retina), and Janeway lesions (purplish macules on the palms or soles).

What tests tell you

Three or more blood cultures in a 24- to 48-hour period (each from a separate venipuncture) identify the causative organism in up to 90% of patients. Blood cultures should be drawn from three different sites, with 1 hour between each venipuncture.

The remaining 10% of patients may have negative blood cultures, possibly suggesting fungal infection or infections that are difficult to diagnose such as *Haemophilus parainfluenzae*.

Other abnormal but nonspecific laboratory test results may include:
- normal or elevated white blood cell (WBC) count
- abnormal histiocytes (macrophages)
- elevated erythrocyte sedimentation rate (ESR)
- normocytic, normochromic anemia (in 70% to 90% of patients)
- proteinuria and microscopic hematuria (in about 50% of patients)
- positive serum rheumatoid factor (in about 50% of all patients after endocarditis is present for 3 to 6 weeks)
- valvular damage, identified by echocardiography
- atrial fibrillation and other arrhythmias that accompany valvular disease, identified by ECG.

Complications

Complications of endocarditis may include heart failure, aortic root abscesses, myocardial abscesses, pericarditis, cardiac arrhythmia, meningitis, cerebral emboli, brain abscesses, septic pulmonary infarcts, arthritis, glomerulonephritis, acute renal failure, and death.

How it's treated

The goal of treatment is to eradicate the infecting organism. First-line therapy is usually a combination of penicillin and an aminoglycoside, usually gentamicin (Garamycin). I.V. antimicrobial therapy should start promptly and continue over 4 to 6 weeks.

The right fit

Selection of an antibiotic is based on identification of the infecting organism and on sensitivity studies. While awaiting results, or if blood cultures are negative, empiric antimicrobial therapy is based on the likely infecting organism.

Supportive treatment includes bed rest, acetaminophen for fever and aches, and sufficient fluid intake. Severe valvular damage, especially aortic or mitral insufficiency, may require corrective surgery if refractory heart failure develops or in cases requiring that an infected prosthetic valve be replaced.

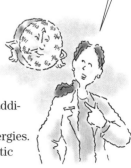

Watch the clock! Giving antibiotics at their prescribed times will keep blood levels consistent in a child with endocarditis.

What to do

Provide reassurance by teaching the patient and his family about this disease and the need for prolonged treatment. In addition, follow these steps:
- Before giving antibiotics, obtain the patient's history of allergies. Administer antibiotics on time to maintain consistent antibiotic blood levels.

Monitoring marathon

• Observe for signs of infiltration or inflammation at the venipuncture site—possible complications of long-term I.V. drug administration. To reduce the risk of these complications, rotate venous access sites at least every 3 days (72 hours).
• Watch for signs of embolization (hematuria, pleuritic chest pain, left upper quadrant pain, or paresis), a common occurrence during the first 3 months of treatment. Tell the parents—and the child, if old enough—to watch for and report these signs, which may indicate impending peripheral vascular occlusion or splenic, renal, cerebral, or pulmonary infarction.
• Monitor the patient's renal status (blood urea nitrogen [BUN] levels, creatinine clearance, and urine output) to check for signs of renal emboli or evidence of drug toxicity.
• Observe for signs of heart failure, such as dyspnea, tachypnea, tachycardia, crackles, jugular vein distention, edema, and weight gain.
• Teach the patient about antibiotic prophylaxis against endocarditis.

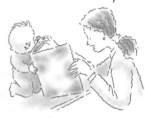

A book, song, or board game is a good choice for a child who needs some diversion but can't handle physical exertion, depending on the child's age.

The education edge

• Instruct the parents to watch closely for fever, anorexia, and other signs of relapse after treatment stops. Suggest quiet diversionary activities to prevent excessive physical exertion.
• Make sure that the patient who is susceptible to endocarditis (or his parents) understands the need for prophylactic antibiotics before, during, and after dental work, and genitourinary, gynecologic, or gastrointestinal (GI) procedures.
• Teach the patient how to recognize symptoms of endocarditis and to notify the doctor immediately if such symptoms occur.
• Teach the child and parents the importance of meticulous oral care when the child is susceptible to endocarditis.

Heart failure

Heart failure occurs when the heart can't pump enough blood to meet the body's metabolic needs. It results in intravascular and interstitial volume overload and poor tissue perfusion.

What causes it

Heart failure most commonly occurs in children secondary to structural defects (such as congenital heart defects), resulting in increased blood volume and pressure within the heart itself. Other causes include:

- ventricular impairment from myocardial infarction (MI)
- cardiomyopathy
- arrhythmias
- lung disease
- severe electrolyte imbalances
- sepsis or severe anemia, which can place excessive demands on the normal heart muscle.

How it happens

Right-sided heart failure results from ineffective right ventricular contractile function; blood isn't pumped effectively through the right ventricle to the lungs, causing it to back up into the right atrium and the peripheral circulation. The patient gains weight and develops peripheral edema and engorgement of the liver, kidneys, and other organs.

Left-sided heart failure occurs as a result of ineffective left ventricular contractile function. As the pumping ability of the left ventricle fails, cardiac output falls. Blood is no longer effectively pumped out into the body; it backs up into the left atrium and then into the lungs, causing pulmonary congestion, dyspnea, and activity intolerance. If the condition persists, pulmonary edema and right-sided heart failure may result.

Increased ventricular muscle mass improves my output, but it also increases my oxygen needs.

Reverse, reverse!

The body will attempt to compensate for heart failure by increasing cardiac output through such mechanisms as increased sympathetic activity, ventricular dilation, and ventricular hypertrophy.

Increased sympathetic activity

Increased sympathetic activity—a response to decreased cardiac output and blood pressure—enhances peripheral vascular resistance, contractility, heart rate, and venous return. Signs such as cool extremities and clamminess may indicate impending heart failure.

Ventricular dilation

In ventricular dilation, an increase in end-diastolic ventricular volume (preload) causes increased stroke work and stroke volume during contraction, stretching cardiac muscle fibers so that the ventricle can accept the increased intravascular volume. Eventually, the muscle becomes stretched beyond optimum limits and contractility declines.

Ventricular hypertrophy

In ventricular hypertrophy, an increase in ventricular muscle mass allows the heart to pump against increased resistance to the outflow of blood, improving cardiac output. This increased muscle mass, however, also increases myocardial oxygen requirements. An increase in the ventricular diastolic pressure necessary to fill the enlarged ventricle may compromise diastolic coronary blood flow, limiting the oxygen supply to the ventricle, and causing ischemia and impaired muscle contractility.

What to look for

In children, total adequate heart functioning depends on both the right and left sides of the heart because they work together to pump blood. Because a failure of one chamber causes reciprocal change in the opposite chamber, children don't show separate right- or left-sided signs and symptoms, as observed in adults. Typically, a combination of symptoms is seen because right- and left-sided heart failure occur simultaneously in children.

Gallops, wheezes, and weight

Signs and symptoms of heart failure in children may include:
• tachycardia (one of the earliest signs)
• gallop heart rhythm
• diaphoresis
• poor feeding
• failure to thrive
• peripheral edema
• tachypnea, dyspnea, orthopnea
• retractions and flaring nares in the infant
• rales, rhonchi, and wheezes
• hepatomegaly
• ascites
• weight gain.

What tests tell you

A chest X-ray may reveal cardiomegaly with pulmonary vascular markings resulting from increased pulmonary blood flow. ECG may identify ventricular hypertrophy, and echocardiography may reveal the cause of heart failure such as a congenital heart defect.

Complications

Acute complications of heart failure include pulmonary edema, acute renal failure, and arrhythmias. Chronic complications include activity intolerance, renal impairment, metabolic impairment, and thromboembolism.

How it's treated

Because heart failure in children occurs mainly as a result of congenital heart defects, treatment guidelines are directed toward the specific defect involved. Other therapies for heart failure in children may include:
- digoxin to increase myocardial contractility, improve cardiac output, reduce the volume of the ventricle, and decrease ventricular stretch
- angiotensin-converting enzyme (ACE) inhibitors to reduce the production of angiotensin II, resulting in preload and afterload reduction
- diuretics to reduce fluid volume overload and venous return
- sodium-restricted diet to reduce accumulated sodium (less common in children)
- oxygen administration to improve tissue oxygenation, especially in those with pulmonary edema and increased pulmonary vascular resistance.

Give the heart a break!

To reduce the workload on the heart, minimize metabolic demands by:
- maintaining a normothermic state in a neutral thermal environment
- providing treatment for infection, if present
- decreasing respiratory effort (providing oxygen and keeping the patient in a semi-Fowler's position)
- providing sedation or analgesics as needed for pain or discomfort
- decreasing stimuli to promote a quiet, restful environment.

What to do

Children with heart failure tend to require close monitoring. Because congenital heart defects are the main cause of heart failure in children, be alert for signs and symptoms of heart failure when caring for a child with a congenital heart defect.
- Prepare the child for the intensive care environment and various equipment that may be in use. Also, make sure parents are aware of visiting policies.

Oxygen as ordered

- Place the child in semi-Fowler's position and provide supplemental oxygen as ordered to help him breathe more easily.
- Weigh the patient daily, and check for peripheral edema.
- Carefully monitor vital signs and I.V. intake and output. Auscultate the heart for murmur or gallop rhythm and the lungs for crackles or rhonchi. Report changes at once.

Shhhhhh . . . he's sleeping

- Group nursing care measures to allow for periods of uninterrupted sleep.
- Frequently monitor BUN, creatinine, serum potassium, sodium, chloride, and magnesium levels.
- Minimize fatigue by providing gavage feedings if necessary.

Feed the heart well

- Increase caloric intake to meet the body's increased metabolic needs as the heart is working harder.
- Monitor the patient's apical pulse for 1 full minute before administering a digoxin dose. Although the drug may be given to adults with apical rates above 60 beats/minute, digoxin should be withheld in infants and young children if the apical rate is below 90 to 110 beats/minute (below 70 beats/minute in older children).
- Stress the importance of taking digoxin exactly as prescribed, and tell parents to watch for and immediately report signs of toxicity, such as anorexia, nausea, vomiting, and bradycardia.

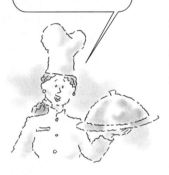

A child with heart failure has higher metabolic needs, so bring on the healthy high-calorie treats!

Kawasaki disease

Kawasaki disease (KD), also known as *mucocutaneous lymph node syndrome*, is an acute systemic vasculitis. It has become a leading cause of acquired heart disease in children in the United States. The majority of cases occur in children younger than age 5, with 1½ times the incidence in boys than in girls.

Although KD is a self-limiting disorder, cardiac sequelae may develop in about 20% of children who aren't treated. These sequelae may include damage to the coronary arteries and myocardium.

What causes it

The cause of KD is unknown. It has geographic or seasonal outbreaks in late winter or early spring, suggesting an infectious process. However, it isn't spread person to person.

How it happens

In KD, inflammation of the small to medium blood vessels occurs throughout the body. However, the coronary arteries and, subsequently, the myocardium are most vulnerable to damage. Later progression of the vasculitis may damage the walls of medium-sized vessels, possibly leading to coronary artery aneurysms. Systemic vasculitis usually begins to subside in 6 to 8 weeks.

What to look for

The three phases of KD are acute, subacute, and convalescent.

Acute phase

The acute phase of KD involves abrupt onset of high fever that doesn't respond to antipyretics and antibiotic therapy. Signs and symptoms during this phase include:
• fever
• irritability (possibly inconsolable)
• cervical lymphadenopathy
• congested conjunctivae and dry eyes
• erythema of the oral cavity, lips, and tongue, leading to the characteristic "strawberry tongue"
• desquamation of the palms of the hands and soles of the feet
• myocarditis
• intermittent signs of heart failure
• transient arthritis of the small joints. (See *Clinical criteria for KD*.)

Subacute phase

The subacute phase begins as fever subsides and continues until all clinical signs have resolved. Because the damaged coronary arteries will stretch to their maximum diameter during this phase, the child is at risk for coronary thrombosis and aneurysms. Signs and symptoms that may occur during this phase include:
• irritability
• periungual desquamation (peeling that occurs around the nails of the fingers and toes)
• arthritis of larger, weight-bearing joints.

Convalescent phase

By the convalescent phase, all of the clinical signs of KD have resolved. Laboratory results may, however, still be abnormal, and this phase will end when those results are normal. This phase usually occurs 6 to 8 weeks after the onset of fever, and the child usually seems to be "back to normal" by the end of the convalescent phase.

What tests tell you

Along with the clinical findings, diagnostic tests may show:
• elevated ESR
• tissue biopsy showing initial proliferation of the adventitia and intima of vessels and thickening of vessel walls

---

Clinical criteria for KD

To be diagnosed with KD, a child must have a fever that lasts for more than 5 days and show four of the following five signs and symptoms:

1) bilateral conjunctivitis without discharge

2) strawberry tongue and mucous membrane dryness with possible fissures

3) erythema of the palms or soles with peeling (usually at week 2 or 3) and peripheral edema

4) polymorphous rash

5) cervical lymph node swelling (one node greater than 1.5 cm).

• echocardiogram showing changes to the myocardium or coronary arteries.

Complications

Cardiac complications of KD include myocarditis, mitral regurgitation, dysrhythmias, and vasculitis—usually the coronary arteries that supply blood to the heart. Inflammation of the coronary arteries can lead to an aneurysm. Aneurysms increase the risk of blood clots forming and blocking the artery, which could lead to a heart attack or cause life-threatening internal bleeding.

How it's treated

High-dose I.V. immune globulin (IVIG) may reduce the duration of fever as well as coronary artery involvement (if given in the first 10 days of the disease course). Aspirin therapy is used to reduce fever and inflammation. Kawasaki treatment is a rare exception to the rule against aspirin use in children. For the occurrence of giant aneurysms, anticoagulation therapy may be instituted.

Most children recover completely following treatment, but cardiovascular involvement may lead to serious morbidity, usually due to coronary thrombosis.

What to do

Monitor cardiovascular status and intake and output carefully, including daily weights. Observe the child for fluid volume overload due to myocarditis, and assess him frequently for signs of heart failure. In addition, follow these steps:
• Administer IVIG as you would a blood product, obtaining vital signs during and immediately following the infusion and being alert for signs of allergic reaction (the single infusion is usually given over 10 to 12 hours).

The inconsolable crying of a child with Kawasaki disease is as hard on the parents as it is on the child.

Soft and soothing

• Decrease skin inflammation with cool compresses, unscented lotions, and the use of soft clothing.
• Provide gentle mouth care during the acute phase of the illness along with a diet of clear, nonirritating liquids and soft foods.
• Maintain a quiet environment to promote rest and reduce irritability. Teach parents that irritability is a hallmark symptom of KD (because parents are, at times, surprised by their child's uncharacteristic behavior).

Hush little baby, don't you cry

• Support the parents' efforts to console their crying child, and reassure them that irritability usually subsides during the convalescent phase.

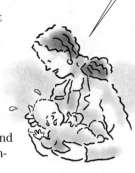

- Because antibody development may be suppressed, don't administer live immunizations, such as the measles-mumps-rubella or varicella vaccines, until at least 11 months after IVIG administration.

Come on in—the water's fine

- Because arthritis symptoms may persist for several weeks in weight-bearing joints, provide warm baths and passive range-of-motion exercises to maintain joint function and reduce stiffness.
- Teach the parents signs and symptoms of MI in children, such as abdominal pain, vomiting, restlessness, inconsolable crying, and pallor (possibly chest pain in older children). Instruct the parents in cardiopulmonary resuscitation of the child.

Rheumatic fever and rheumatic heart disease

A systemic inflammatory disease of childhood, *acute rheumatic fever* develops after infection of the upper respiratory tract with group A beta-hemolytic streptococci. It primarily involves the heart, joints, central nervous system, skin, and subcutaneous tissues, and it commonly recurs.

Rheumatic heart disease refers to the cardiac manifestations of rheumatic fever. It includes pancarditis (myocarditis, pericarditis, and endocarditis) during the early acute phase and, later in the course of the disease, chronic valvular disease. Cardiac involvement develops in up to 50% of patients with rheumatic fever.

Millions "served"

Worldwide, 15 to 20 million new cases of rheumatic fever are reported each year. The disease typically strikes during cool, damp weather in the winter and early spring. In the United States, it's most common in the north.

A family affair

Rheumatic fever tends to run in families, lending support to the existence of genetic predisposition. Environmental factors also seem to be significant in the development of the disorder. For example, in lower socioeconomic groups, the incidence is highest in children between ages 5 and 15 years, probably because of crowded living conditions.

Prognosis

Patients without carditis or with mild carditis have a good long-term prognosis. Severe pancarditis occasionally produces fatal heart failure during the acute phase. Of patients who survive this complication, about 20% die within 10 years.

Antibiotic therapy has greatly reduced the incidence of mortality from rheumatic heart disease.

What causes it

Rheumatic fever is caused by group A beta-hemolytic streptococcal pharyngitis.

How it happens

Rheumatic fever appears to be a hypersensitivity reaction to group A beta-hemolytic streptococcal infection. Because very few people (3%) with streptococcal infections go on to contract rheumatic fever, altered host resistance must be involved in its development or recurrence.

The antigens of group A streptococci bind to receptors in the heart, in muscle, and in the brain and synovial joints, causing an autoimmune response. Because of a similarity between the antigens of the streptococcus bacteria and the antigens of the body's own cells, antibodies may mistakenly attack healthy body cells.

When carditis gets complicated

- Carditis may affect the endocardium, myocardium, or pericardium during the early acute phase. Later, the heart valves may be damaged, causing chronic valvular disease.
- Pericarditis produces a serofibrinous effusion.
- Myocarditis produces characteristic lesions called *Aschoff bodies* (fibrin deposits surrounded by necrosis) in the interstitial tissue of the heart as well as cellular swelling and fragmentation of interstitial collagen. (These lesions lead to progressively fibrotic nodule and interstitial scar formation.)
- Endocarditis causes valve leaflet swelling; erosion along the lines of leaflet closure; and blood, platelet, and fibrin deposits, which form beadlike growths. Eventually, the valve leaflets become scarred, lose their elasticity, and begin to adhere to one another. (Endocarditis strikes the mitral valve most commonly in females and the aortic valve in males. In both genders, it occasionally affects the tricuspid valve and, rarely, the pulmonic valve.)

> Most children with rheumatic fever and rheumatic heart disease have joint pain—as if they don't have enough problems!

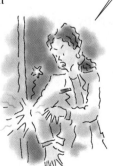

What to look for

The classic symptoms of rheumatic fever and rheumatic heart disease include:
- polyarthritis or migratory joint pain, caused by inflammation (in most patients)
- erythema marginatum, a nonpruritic, macular, transient rash on the trunk or inner aspects of the upper arms or thighs, that gives rise to red lesions with blanched centers

Under the skin

- subcutaneous nodules, which are firm, movable, and non-tender nodules, about 3 mm to 2 cm diameter, usually near tendons or bony prominences of joints, especially the elbows, knuckles, wrists, and knees (most commonly accompanying carditis and possibly lasting a few days to several weeks)
- chorea (rapid, jerky movements), possibly developing up to 6 months after the original streptococcal infection (hyperirritability, a deterioration in handwriting, or inability to concentrate in mild chorea and purposeless, nonrepetitive, involuntary muscle spasms; poor muscle coordination; and weakness in severe chorea).

But wait, there's more

Other signs and symptoms of rheumatic fever and rheumatic heart disease include:
- streptococcal infection a few days to 6 weeks earlier (in 95% of those with rheumatic fever)
- temperature of at least 100.4° F (38° C) due to infection and inflammation.

Aye, that's the rub

- pericardial friction rub caused by inflamed pericardial membranes rubbing against one another (if pericarditis exists)
- new mitral or aortic heart murmur or a worsening murmur in a person with a preexisting murmur
- chest pain, typically pleuritic, due to inflammation and irritation of the pericardial membranes (Pain may increase with deep inspiration and decrease when the patient sits up and leans forward, pulling the heart away from the diaphragmatic pleurae of the lungs.)
- dyspnea, tachypnea, nonproductive cough, bibasilar crackles, and edema due to heart failure in severe rheumatic carditis.

What tests tell you

Several tests are used to help diagnose rheumatic fever and rheumatic heart disease:
- Jones criteria (revealing two major criteria, or one major and two minor criteria, plus evidence of a previous group A streptococcal infection) are necessary for diagnosis. (See *Jones criteria for rheumatic fever.*)

Jones criteria for rheumatic fever

The Jones criteria are used to standardize the diagnosis of rheumatic fever. Diagnosis requires that the patient have either two major criteria, or one major criterion and two minor criteria, plus evidence of a previous streptococcal infection.

Major criteria
- Carditis
- Migratory polyarthritis
- Sydenham's chorea (involuntary muscular movements of the face and extremities)
- Subcutaneous nodules
- Erythema marginatum (the presence of pink rings on the trunk and inner surfaces of the arms and legs)

Minor criteria
- Fever
- Arthralgia
- Elevated acute phase reactants
- Prolonged PR interval

It's in the blood

- Laboratory testing may reveal an elevated WBC count and elevated ESR during the acute phase.
- Hemoglobin level and hematocrit may show slight anemia due to suppressed erythropoiesis during inflammation.
- C-reactive protein may be positive, especially during the acute phase.
- Cardiac enzyme levels may be increased in severe carditis.
- Antistreptolysin-O titer may be elevated in 95% of patients within 2 months of onset.
- Throat cultures may continue to show the presence of group A beta-hemolytic streptococci; however, they usually occur in small numbers.
- ECG may show changes that aren't diagnostic, but the PR interval is prolonged in 20% of patients.

Regular or extra-large

- Chest X-rays may show normal heart size or cardiomegaly, pericardial effusion, or heart failure.
- Echocardiography can detect valvular damage and pericardial effusion, measure chamber size, and provide information on ventricular function.
- Cardiac catheterization provides information on valvular damage and left ventricular function.

Complications

Possible complications of rheumatic fever and rheumatic heart disease include destruction of the mitral and aortic valves, pancarditis, and heart failure.

How it's treated

The goals of treatment for rheumatic heart disease are to destroy any remaining group A streptococcal bacteria, relieve symptoms, and control inflammation. Treatment typically involves:

- prompt treatment of all group A beta-hemolytic streptococcal pharyngitis with penicillin (or erythromycin for patients with penicillin hypersensitivity)
- anti-inflammatory treatment (with aspirin or naproxen) to relieve fever and pain and minimize joint swelling
- corticosteroids if the patient has carditis or if the anti-inflammatory agents fail to relieve pain and inflammation.

Lullaby and good night

Strict bed rest is advised for about 5 weeks for the patient with active carditis to reduce cardiac demands. Bed rest, sodium restriction, ACE inhibitors, digoxin, and diuretics are used to treat heart failure.

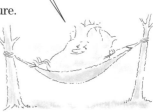

Give me a break and stay in bed! It makes my life easier when I'm dealing with the demands of rheumatic heart disease.

Surgery for severity

Corrective surgery is reserved for severe mitral or aortic valvular dysfunction that causes persistent heart failure. Procedures may include:
• commissurotomy—separation of adherent, thickened valve leaflets of the mitral valve
• valvuloplasty—inflation of a balloon within a valve
• valve replacement—replacement of the diseased valve.

On second thought

Secondary prevention of rheumatic fever begins after the acute phase subsides. The child will be prescribed long-term prophylactic antibiotics. Treatment usually continues for at least 5 years or until age 21, whichever duration is longer.

Pop a pill before the drill

Prophylactic antibiotics for dental work and other invasive or surgical procedures will be necessary to prevent infective endocarditis.

What to do

Because rheumatic fever and rheumatic heart disease require prolonged treatment, the care plan should include comprehensive patient (and parent) teaching to promote compliance with the prescribed therapy:
• Before giving penicillin, ask the parent if the child has ever had a hypersensitivity reaction to it, and warn that such a reaction is possible even if it hasn't occurred previously. (Instruct parents to stop giving the drug and call the doctor immediately if the child develops a rash, fever, chills, or other signs of allergy at any time during penicillin therapy.)

Be on alert

• Instruct the patient and his family to watch for and report early signs of heart failure, such as dyspnea and a hacking, nonproductive cough.

• Stress the need for bed rest during the acute phase and suggest appropriate, physically undemanding diversions.

Prescription for quality time

• After the acute phase, encourage family members and friends to spend as much time as possible with the patient to minimize boredom. Advise parents to secure tutorial services to help the child keep up with schoolwork during the long convalescence.
• Help parents overcome guilty feelings they may have about their child's illness. Tell them that failure to seek treatment for streptococcal infection is common because this illness typically seems no worse than a cold, and encourage them (and the child) to vent their frustrations during the long, tedious recovery.
• If the child has severe carditis, help the parents and child prepare for permanent changes in the child's lifestyle.
• Teach the patient and his family about the disease and its treatment, and stress the need to watch for and immediately report signs of recurrent streptococcal infection, including sudden sore throat; diffuse throat redness and oropharyngeal exudate; swollen, tender cervical lymph glands; pain on swallowing; temperature of 101° to 104° F (38.3° to 40° C); headache; and nausea. (Urge the parents to keep the child away from people with respiratory tract infections.)

Brush and floss at any cost

• Promote good dental hygiene to prevent infection. Stress the need to comply with prolonged antibiotic therapy and follow-up care and the need for additional antibiotics before dental surgery or other invasive procedures. Arrange for a home health nurse to oversee care, if necessary.
• Teach the patient (and his parents) to follow current recommendations of the American Heart Association for prevention of infective endocarditis; antibiotic regimens used to prevent recurrence of acute rheumatic fever are adequate for preventing infective endocarditis.

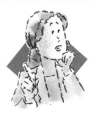

Quick quiz

1. Which sign best indicates the presence of coarctation of the aorta?

    A.   Clubbing of fingers and toes

    B.   Generalized cyanosis, especially with crying

    C.   Rapid and irregular apical heartbeat

    D.   Bounding brachial pulses with weak femoral pulses

Answer: D. The child with coarctation of the aorta has bounding pulses in the upper extremities and weak pulses in the lower extremities because the narrowed aorta causes higher blood pressure in the upper extremities.

2. Which nursing intervention is most important to perform before administering digoxin (Lanoxin) to a child?

    A.   Checking apical pulse for 1 full minute

    B.   Positioning the child with the head slightly elevated

    C.   Counting the child's respiratory rate for 1 full minute

    D.   Calculating the child's urine output

Answer: A. The child's apical heart rate should be counted for 1 full minute before digoxin administration. If the heart rate is below the rate specified in the order (typically, 90 to 110 beats/minute for infants and young children or below 70 beats/minute in older children), the dose should be withheld and the doctor notified.

3. An infant is diagnosed with PDA. Which drug may be administered to achieve pharmacologic closure of the defect?

    A.   digoxin (Lanoxin)

    B.   prednisone (Deltasone)

    C.   furosemide (Lasix)

    D.   indomethacin (Indocin)

Answer: D. Indomethacin is administered to an infant with PDA in an effort to close the defect.

4. Which cardiac defect is associated with VSD, right ventricular hypertrophy, right ventricular outflow obstruction, and an overriding aorta?
    A.   Tricuspid atresia
    B.   Hypoplastic left heart syndrome
    C.   PDA
    D.   Tetralogy of Fallot

Answer: D. Tetralogy of Fallot has four cardiac defects: VSD, right ventricular outflow obstruction, right ventricular hypertrophy, and an overriding aorta.

5. In a child with KD, the greatest concern is:
    A.   avoiding aspirin because of the risk of Reye's syndrome.
    B.   monitoring the child for any signs of heart failure.
    C.   meticulously bathing the child with soap and water.
    D.   ensuring that the child drinks plenty of orange juice daily.

Answer: B. With Kawasaki disease, the child has problems with the skin, mucous membranes, lymph nodes, joints, and heart and circulatory system. By far, the most serious, and therefore of greatest concern, is the cardiovascular system, with the risk of heart failure.

Scoring

★★★ If you answered all five items correctly, fabulous! You've gone straight to the heart of cardiac problems.

★★ If you answered three or four items correctly, good work! Your knowledge of cardiac problems is heartfelt.

★ If you answered fewer than three items correctly, don't take it to heart! A quick review will get your knowledge pumping.

Respiratory problems

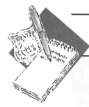

Just the facts

In this chapter, you'll learn:

♦ respiratory anatomy and physiology

♦ tests used to diagnose respiratory disorders in children

♦ treatments and procedures used for children with respiratory problems

♦ respiratory disorders that affect children and nursing interventions for each.

Anatomy and physiology

In with the oxygen, out with the carbon dioxide. Breathe easy—we're on the job!

The structures of the respiratory system are responsible for oxygen distribution and gas exchange. A child's respiratory tract is constantly growing and changing for the first 12 years of life. It differs anatomically from an adult's respiratory system in ways that predispose the child to respiratory difficulties, making respiratory problems common during childhood. (See *Structures of the respiratory system,* page 324.)

Chest and lungs

The *lungs* are the main component of the respiratory system. They inspire air, extract oxygen, and exhale the waste product carbon dioxide.

Totally lobular

The right lung has three lobes; the left has two. The mediastinum is the space between the two lungs. The lungs are surrounded by a framework of ribs, vertebrae (posteriorly), and the sternum (anteriorly), creating the *chest.*

Structures of the respiratory system

This illustration shows the structures of the respiratory system.

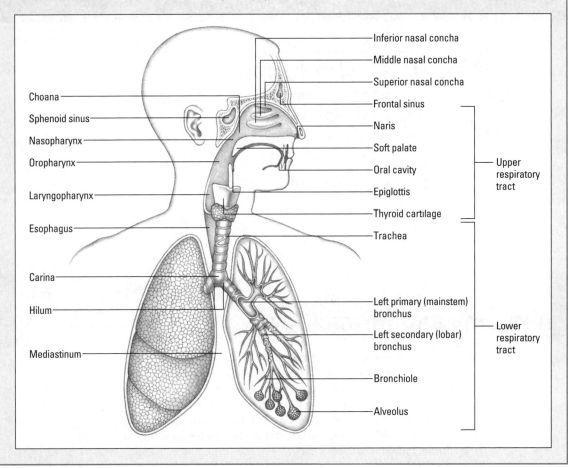

Choana

Sphenoid sinus

Nasopharynx

Oropharynx

Laryngopharynx

Esophagus

Carina

Hilum

Mediastinum

Inferior nasal concha

Middle nasal concha

Superior nasal concha

Frontal sinus

Naris

Soft palate

Oral cavity

Epiglottis

Thyroid cartilage

Trachea

Left primary (mainstem) bronchus

Left secondary (lobar) bronchus

Bronchiole

Alveolus

Upper respiratory tract

Lower respiratory tract

Roll out the barrel

At birth, the chest is relatively round-shaped. It will gradually develop into a flattened shape across the front and back as the child grows. However, certain respiratory diseases can alter the shape of the chest. For example, obstructive diseases like asthma and cystic fibrosis can produce a barrel-shaped chest when they become severe.

Upper respiratory tract

The upper respiratory tract consists of the:
- nose and nasal passages
- mouth and oropharynx
- pharynx
- larynx.

Nose and nasal passages

The nose and nasal passages serve as a conduit for air to and from the lungs. They're lined with ciliated mucous membranes that filter, warm, and moisten the air.

Nasal for 4 weeks

Infants and young children have smaller nares and narrow nasal passages, making them prone to airway occlusion. Because neonates prefer to breathe through their noses, nasal patency is essential for such life-sustaining activities as breathing and feeding. The neurologic pathways that will coordinate mouth breathing won't develop until age 4 weeks.

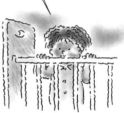

Hey, give me a break. I don't know that I'm supposed to open my mouth if my nose is blocked!

Mouth and oropharynx

After about age 4 weeks, air may also enter the respiratory system via the mouth and oropharynx. The child's small oral cavity and large tongue leave the child prone to airway occlusion.

Pharynx

The pharynx, or throat, serves as a conduit for the respiratory and digestive tracts. It's composed of smooth muscle and mucous membranes. The tonsils and adenoids, located in the pharynx, grow rapidly in early childhood and can leave the child prone to occlusion if they become inflamed. The tonsils and adenoids may decrease in size after age 12. (See *Locating the tonsils and adenoids*, page 326.)

Larynx

The larynx, or the upper end of the trachea, consists of a rigid framework of cartilage. It contains the epiglottis, a flaplike structure that overhangs the entrance to the trachea, and the glottis, the opening to the trachea.

Locating the tonsils and adenoids

These illustrations show the locations of the tonsils and adenoids. Because of their locations, inflammation of these structures can cause airway occlusion.

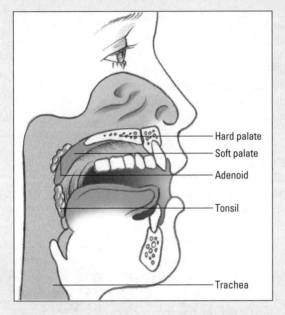

Hard palate
Soft palate
Adenoid
Tonsil
Trachea

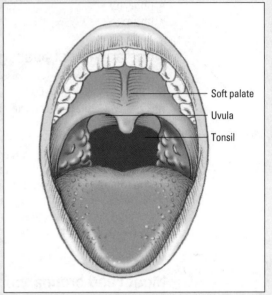

Soft palate
Uvula
Tonsil

No solids or fluids beyond this point

The epiglottis and glottis prevent solids and fluids from entering the air passages during swallowing. The glottis contains the vocal cords, which produce vocal sounds when they vibrate. The child's long, floppy epiglottis is vulnerable to swelling that may lead to obstruction.

Lower respiratory tract

The lower respiratory tract is composed of the:
- trachea
- bronchi
- alveoli.

Trachea

The trachea acts as a passageway for air into the lungs. It's made up of C-shaped rings of cartilage and is supported by smooth muscle. In infants, the cartilage is soft, making the airway more easily collapsible when the neck is flexed. A child's trachea is higher than an adult's and gives rise to two major bronchi: the right and the left. The right bronchus is shorter, wider, and situated more vertically than the left. Because of this, aspirated foreign bodies are more likely to become lodged in the right bronchus. (See *Estimating tracheal diameter.*)

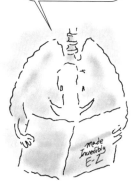

Says here that my larger air passages are called bronchi.

Bronchi

The bronchi, the larger air passages of the lungs, are composed of the same cartilaginous rings and smooth muscle as the trachea. The bronchi divide into progressively smaller passages called *bronchioles.*

As a child grows taller in stature, there's increased branching of the bronchioles, leading to greater lung surface area. The cartilaginous rings disappear as the bronchioles get smaller, leaving the smallest divisions with a lining of a single layer of cells. The bronchioles terminate in alveoli.

Alveoli

Alveoli are the small, saclike structures in which the exchange of oxygen for carbon dioxide takes place. Each alveolus is surrounded by many capillaries.

Throughout the first 12 years of life, the alveoli change in size and shape and increase in number, resulting in an increased area available for gas exchange as the child grows. A neonate's lung tissue contains about 25 million alveoli; this number increases to about 300 million by age 8.

No confusion—it's diffusion

The alveoli promote gas exchange by diffusion (the passage of gas molecules through the respiratory membranes). By diffusion, oxygen from the alveoli passes to the blood, and carbon dioxide, a by-product of cellular metabolism, passes out of the blood into the alveoli, where it's channeled away during exhalation.

Airway resistance

Airway resistance (the effort or force required to move air into the lungs) is greater in children than in adults because children's airways are narrower than those of adults. In infants, airway resistance is about 15 times that of an adult. When there's edema or swelling in the airway due to an irritant or infectious

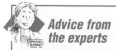

Advice from the experts

Estimating tracheal diameter

One way to estimate the size of a child's trachea is to remember the "rule of the finger." The diameter of a child's trachea is roughly equal to the diameter of his little (or pinky) finger. This rule may come in handy when selecting the appropriate size of endotracheal tube if intubation becomes necessary.

process, the airway is further narrowed, increasing the airway resistance even more.

Child labor

Increased airway resistance makes the child work harder to breathe. This is indicated by:
- increased respiratory rate
- retractions
- nasal flaring
- use of accessory muscles.

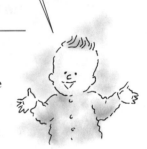

Being a kid isn't all fun and games. My airway is narrower than my mom's, so I have to work harder to breathe than she does.

Pulmonary circulation

In pulmonary circulation, blood passes through the lungs to obtain oxygen to distribute to the cells and tissues of the body in a four-step process:

Oxygen-depleted blood enters the lungs from the pulmonary artery that arises from the heart's right ventricle.

Blood then flows through the main pulmonary arteries into the smaller vessels of the main bronchi, through the arterioles and, eventually, into the capillary networks that surround the alveoli.

There, oxygen diffuses into the capillaries from the alveoli, and the oxygenated blood flows through progressively larger vessels, enters the main pulmonary vein, and flows into the left atrium.

From there, the oxygenated blood passes into the left ventricle and exits the heart through the aorta for distribution throughout the body.

Inspiration and expiration

An infant's ribs are primarily cartilage and are very flexible, making them inefficient in ventilating. Infants primarily engage in diaphragm breathing, also known as *abdominal breathing*. As the diaphragm moves downward during inspiration, a negative pressure is created, allowing the lungs to expand to draw air in.

Muscles to stabilize, muscles to breathe

The intercostal muscles of the chest are used for stabilization. However, after age 6, a child will begin to use the intercostal muscles for breathing. Then, contraction and relaxation of

Normal pediatric respiratory rates

This chart shows the normal respiratory rates from birth to age 18.

Age	Breaths per minute
Birth to 6 months	30 to 60
6 months to 2 years	20 to 30
3 to 10 years	20 to 28
10 to 18 years	12 to 20

these respiratory muscles moves air into and out of the lungs. Normally, expiration is passive. (See *Normal pediatric respiratory rates.*)

Retractions reveal distress

When an infant or child is having difficulty breathing, retractions of the respiratory muscles will occur. The depth and location of the retractions will indicate the severity of the respiratory distress:
• In mild distress, there are isolated intercostal retractions.
• In moderate distress, there are subcostal, suprasternal, and supraclavicular retractions.
• In severe distress, there are all of the retractions mentioned above along with accessory muscle use. (See *Looking for retractions.*)

Adventitious breath sounds

Adventitious breath sounds are sounds not normally heard on auscultation of the lungs. Due to the thinness of the chest wall, breath sounds seem louder and harsher in infants and young children, and adventitious breath sounds may transmit over larger areas.

Looking for retractions

This illustration shows you where to look for retractions. The types of retractions you see in a child can indicate the severity of his respiratory distress.

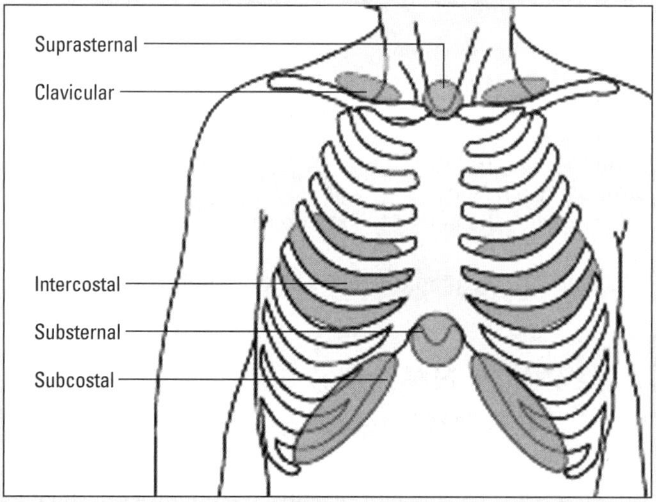

Suprasternal
Clavicular
Intercostal
Substernal
Subcostal

Types of adventitious breath sounds

This chart describes the types of adventitious breath sounds you might hear in a pediatric patient.

Breath sound	Characteristics	Causes
Wheezing	• Continuous, musical, high-pitched sounds heard in mid- to late expiration (may be audible without a stethoscope)	• Indicative of edema and obstruction in small airways
Crackles	• Intermittent, medium- to high-pitched popping sounds heard during inspiration (may clear with coughing)	• Caused by fluid in the alveoli, bronchioles, or bronchi
Rhonchi	• Continuous, snoring, low-pitched sounds heard throughout respiration (may clear with coughing)	• Due to edema and obstruction in large bronchi and the trachea
Stridor	• High-pitched crowing sound heard on inspiration	• Caused by upper airway obstruction at or above the vocal cords
Pleural friction rub	• Grating, rubbing, loud, high-pitched sound heard during inspiration and expiration	• Due to inflamed pleural surfaces

Ventriloquist lungs

Sounds may seem to originate in the lungs when they're actually referred from the upper airway, such as when there's mucus in the nose or throat. Auscultating in the axillae of infants and small children is a good way to hear adventitious breath sounds if they're present. (See *Types of adventitious breath sounds*.)

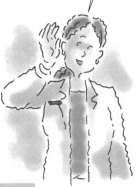

Hmmm. Sounds like adventitious breath sounds to me.

Blown away

When assessing breath sounds:
• Encourage small children to breathe deeply by asking them to pretend they're blowing out candles or have them blow away a tissue.
• Listen with the bell of the stethoscope for low-pitched sounds.
• Listen with the diaphragm for higher pitched sounds.

Diagnostic tests and monitoring techniques

Children with suspected or diagnosed respiratory problems may need to undergo invasive or noninvasive diagnostic tests as well as monitoring procedures.

Arterial blood gas

An arterial blood gas (ABG) analysis assesses gas exchange. It also assesses the ventilatory control system, determines the blood's acid-base balance, and monitors respiratory therapy. The respiratory and metabolic systems work together to keep the body's acid-base balance within normal limits. (See *Understanding acid-base disorders*.)

ABG analysis is done on a blood sample taken from a peripheral arterial puncture or an arterial catheter, such as an umbilical arterial catheter, arterial line, or central catheter. The normal pediatric values are similar to those for adults.

Understanding acid-base disorders

Acid-base disorders may have several causes and signs and symptoms, as outlined in the chart below along with arterial blood gas (ABG) analysis findings for each disorder.

Disorder and ABG findings	Possible causes	Signs and symptoms
Respiratory acidosis (excess carbon dioxide retention) pH <7.35 HCO_3^- >26 mEq/L (if compensating) $Paco_2$ >45 mm Hg	• Central nervous system depression from drugs, injury, or disease • Asphyxia • Hypoventilation from pulmonary, cardiac, musculoskeletal, or neuromuscular disease	Diaphoresis, headache, tachycardia, confusion, restlessness, apprehension, flushed face
Respiratory alkalosis (excess carbon dioxide excretion) pH >7.45 HCO_3^- <22 mEq/L (if compensating) $Paco_2$ <35 mm Hg	• Hyperventilation from anxiety, pain, or improper ventilator settings • Respiratory stimulation from drugs, disease, hypoxia, fever, or high room temperature • Gram-negative bacteremia	Rapid, deep respirations; paresthesia; light-headedness; twitching; anxiety; fear
Metabolic acidosis (bicarbonate loss, acid retention) pH <7.35 HCO_3^- <22 mEq/L $Paco_2$ <35 mm Hg (if compensating)	• Bicarbonate depletion from diarrhea • Excessive production of organic acids from hepatic disease, endocrine disorders, shock, or drug intoxication • Inadequate excretion of acids from renal disease	Rapid, deep breathing; fruity breath; fatigue; headache; lethargy; drowsiness; nausea; vomiting; coma (if severe); abdominal pain
Metabolic alkalosis (bicarbonate retention, acid loss) pH >7.45 HCO_3^- >26 mEq/L $Paco_2$ >45 mm Hg (if compensating)	• Loss of hydrochloric acid from prolonged vomiting or gastric suctioning • Loss of potassium from increased renal excretion (as in diuretic therapy) or steroids • Excessive alkali ingestion	Slow, shallow breathing; hypertonic muscles; restlessness; twitching; confusion; irritability; apathy; tetany; seizures; coma (if severe)

Nursing considerations

If the sample will be drawn from an arterial catheter, reassure the child that he won't feel any pain. If the sample will be taken via arterial puncture, keep in mind that this is typically more painful than a venous puncture. Help minimize the trauma from a peripheral arterial puncture:

• Be honest about the painful part of the procedure. (For example, say, "This is going to hurt for a few seconds. It's OK to be scared, but you're going to do a great job and it's going to be over very quickly.")

Blood borrowing

• Explain that only a small amount of blood will be taken, and that the child's body will quickly make new blood to replace it. (Young children think they have a finite amount of blood and may have many misconceptions about what happens to them when some of that blood is removed.)

• Allow the parent to comfort the child during the blood drawing. A parent's presence reassures the child that nothing terrible will happen to him.

See, now, that wasn't so bad, was it?

Count and squeeze

• Give the child coping mechanisms. (For example, say, "Count to 5 and the hurting part will be over," or, "Squeeze your mother's hand if it hurts.")

• Praise the child for doing a good job regardless of how he reacts.

• Comfort the child and apply a bandage as soon as the sample has been drawn; covering the site reassures the child that the hurting part is truly over.

Obtaining the sample

If a peripheral arterial puncture is performed, check arterial circulation to the area (for example, with the Allen test) before the puncture is made. After the puncture, apply firm pressure to the arterial site to stop the bleeding; then frequently assess the site for bleeding or hematoma formation.

To obtain the sample, follow these steps:

• Draw the blood sample into a heparinized syringe because unclotted blood is required.

• Remove air bubbles from the sample to avoid altering the gas concentration.

• Keep the blood sample on ice and transport it immediately to the laboratory.

Chest X-ray

A chest X-ray is used to visualize internal structures on film. On a chest X-ray, soft tissues, such as organs and muscles, appear as gray forms.

Dem bones, dem bones

Dense tissue such as bone appears white and clearly defined. The chest X-ray is used to rule out foreign body aspiration, determine infectious process, and gain information on cardiac size and contour, vessel and cardiac chamber size, and status of pulmonary blood flow.

Inspiration, expiration, front and back

Inspiratory and forced expiratory films are best to rule out foreign body aspiration. Anterior-posterior and lateral films are best to view internal structures for diagnosis of disease processes in the chest.

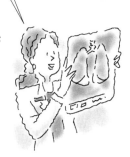

You'd be surprised what a child can aspirate! On a chest X-ray, an aspirated foreign body will appear white.

Nursing considerations

Explain the procedure to the child, assuring him that there are no "hurting parts" to the test. If possible, show the child an actual X-ray film to illustrate what the X-ray can and can't show. (Young children may think an X-ray machine will be able to tell what he's thinking and feeling.)
• Protect the child from radiation exposure by covering his gonads and thyroid gland with lead shields during the test.
• Make sure the child holds still during the test and tell him that doing so is his special job. (You may need to assist the child to do so.)

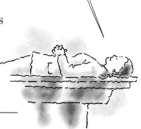

Some kids may think an X-ray can tell what they're thinking.

Pulmonary function tests

Pulmonary function tests (PFTs) are a series of measurements used to evaluate ventilatory function. They aid in the assessment of lung function in children with acute or chronic respiratory disorders. (See *Understanding PFT results*, page 334.)

Serial testing

Normal values can change dramatically with growth. For this reason, serial determination of pulmonary function is more informative than a single PFT, especially when evaluating a disorder for severity or progression, or when evaluating the effects of treatment.

Understanding PFT results

You may need to interpret pulmonary function test (PFT) results in your assessment of a patient's respiratory status. Use this chart as a guide to common PFTs.

Restrictive and obstructive

The chart mentions restrictive and obstructive defects.

• A restrictive defect is one in which a person can't inhale a normal amount of air; it may occur with chest wall deformities, neuromuscular diseases, or acute respiratory tract infections.

• An obstructive defect is one in which something obstructs the flow of air into or out of the lungs; it may occur with such disorders as asthma, chronic bronchitis, emphysema, and cystic fibrosis.

Test	Implications
Tidal volume (V$_T$): amount of air inhaled or exhaled during normal breathing	Decreased V$_T$ may indicate restrictive defect and indicates the need for further tests such as full chest X-rays.
Minute volume (MV): amount of air breathed per minute	Normal MV can occur in emphysema. Decreased MV may indicate other diseases such as pulmonary edema.
Inspiratory reserve volume (IRV): amount of air inhaled after normal inspiration	Abnormal IRV alone doesn't indicate respiratory dysfunction. IRV decreases during normal exercise.
Expiratory reserve volume (ERV): amount of air that can be exhaled after normal expiration	ERV varies, even in healthy people.
Vital capacity (VC): amount of air that can be exhaled after maximum inspiration	Normal or increased VC with decreased flow rates may indicate reduction in functional pulmonary tissue. Decreased VC with normal or increased flow rates may indicate respiratory effort, decreased thoracic expansion, or limited movement of the diaphragm.
Inspiratory capacity (IC): amount of air that can be inhaled after normal expiration	Decreased IC indicates restrictive defect.
Forced vital capacity (FVC): amount of air that can be exhaled after maximum inspiration	Decreased FVC indicates flow resistance in the respiratory system from obstructive disorders, such as chronic bronchitis, emphysema, and asthma.
Forced expiratory volume (FEV): volume of air exhaled in the first (FEV$_1$), second (FEV$_2$), or third (FEV$_3$) FVC maneuver	Decreased FEV$_1$ and increased FEV$_2$ and FEV$_3$ may indicate obstructive disease. Decreased or normal FEV$_1$ may indicate restrictive defect.

Breathing on cue

PFTs require the child to cooperate and understand instructions. Most children aren't able to perform the testing until about age 5, because it requires manipulating equipment, holding their breath, and exhaling on cue with directions.

Nursing considerations

Explain the test to the child and his parents, stressing that there's no pain involved. Tell the child that his job will be to follow instructions related to handling equipment, holding his breath, and inhaling on cue. Have him practice doing these things before the actual test. In addition:
• Note that results may not be accurate because the young child may have difficulty following the necessary directions.
• Instruct the child and his parents that he should have only a light meal before the test.
• Withhold bronchodilators and intermittent positive-pressure breathing therapy before the test.

Pulse oximetry

Pulse oximetry is a noninvasive monitoring technique used to estimate arterial oxygen saturation through a probe that measures saturation by the absorption of red and infrared light as it passes through tissue. It measures the amount of oxygen carried by hemoglobin by reading the amount of light that passes through a vascular bed and converting the amount of light absorbed by the oxygen-carrying hemoglobin, which gives a saturation value.

Sensing saturation

The sensor can be located on an extremity, a digit, a palm, or an earlobe or wrapped around the foot (in an infant) and works best when there's adequate peripheral perfusion. A reading of 95% or greater is ideal for most children.

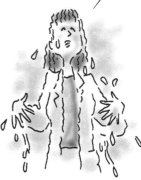

95% and above is a pretty good saturation rate.

Nursing considerations

Explain this type of monitoring to the child and his parents, and put the probe on a parent or nurse so the child can see that it's painless. Reassure him that even though it's used to measure oxygen in the blood, no needles are needed. In addition:
• Place the probe on a site with good perfusion, such as the finger, foot, or toe.
• Periodically rotate sites for probe placement to prevent skin breakdown under the probe.
• To ensure that the value is accurate, make sure the pulse reading on the pulse oximeter matches the child's heart rate.

Treatments and procedures

Respiratory treatments and procedures commonly used for the pediatric patient include aerosol therapy, assisted ventilation, chest physiotherapy (CPT), endotracheal (ET) intubation, oxygen administration, and tracheotomy.

Aerosol therapy

Metered-dose inhalers (MDIs) are used to administer medications such as bronchodilators and inhaled corticosteroids to children.

Spaced out

Children need to use a spacer with a valve if they can't coordinate inspiration with medication release or if they're younger than age 5. The spacer is a tube that captures the aerosol released, allowing the child to breathe it in over a couple of minutes.

Under-age aerosol

Nebulizer therapy is sometimes used for infants. A nebulizer aerosolizes the medication, releasing it into a small mask that's placed over the child's face. The child can then breathe in the medication through his mouth by taking deep, slow breaths.

Liquid to vapor

Vaporizers are used to create vapor from a liquid. They're most commonly used to vaporize cool water to increase the humidity in a room for the benefit of children with swollen, reactive airways. They can relieve many symptoms of upper airway irritation and congestion in young children.

Nursing considerations

Before beginning treatment, show the child the MDI with spacer or nebulizer mask. Let the child place the MDI/spacer to his mouth or the mask to his face before the medication has been added.
• To determine the effectiveness of aerosol therapy, assess the patient's breath sounds before and after treatment.
• Monitor the patient's tolerance of the procedure. An infant or young child may fight the MDI with spacer mask or the mask over his face during nebulizer therapy. (Calming techniques such as swaddling may be necessary.)
• After teaching the child and his parents how to use the device correctly (which is necessary for optimal effectiveness), observe

while they demonstrate their technique; provide support and correct technique as needed. (See *Using an MDI*.)

Assisted ventilation

Assisted ventilation can be administered to children via mechanical ventilation or nasal continuous positive airway pressure (CPAP).

Mechanical ventilation

Mechanical ventilation involves inflation of the lungs with compressed gas. It may be needed for children who are unable to maintain adequate gas exchange due to airway obstruction, neuromuscular disease, or other pulmonary pathology.

Compress and pressurize

The compressed gas is pushed into the lungs with pressure, and the exhalation is then passive. Oxygen may also be administered. Mechanical ventilation requires the child to be intubated or to have a tracheostomy, whereas positive-pressure ventilations may also be given by a bag and mask apparatus.

Inflate and expand

Inflation pressures are limited to what's necessary to provide sufficient lung expansion for adequate ventilation and prevention of atelectasis, while keeping a careful watch for damage to airways and lung parenchyma.
• Pressure-cycle ventilators, most commonly used in infants, deliver an indefinite volume of gas at a fixed inflation pressure.
• Volume-cycled ventilators, most commonly used in children and adolescents, deliver a fixed volume of gas at whatever inflation pressure is necessary, up to a preset maximum.
  With any ventilator, the nurse must assess the child carefully and frequently for breath sounds, chest wall excursion, and ABG measurements and pulse oximetry.

Continuous positive airway pressure

CPAP is used to infuse oxygen or air under a preset pressure through nasal prongs or a small mask. The pressure increases the alveolar volume by preventing the alveoli from collapsing on expiration, which leads to an increased functional residual capacity and improves the diffusion time of oxygen.

It's all relative

Using an MDI

To optimize treatment, make sure your patient (and his parents) know how to use a metered-dose inhaler (MDI) properly by providing them with the following instructions:

   Shake the canister while taking a deep breath in and out.

   Use a spacer with each use of the MDI.

   Depress the button on the canister at the beginning of the next inhalation.

   Breathe the mist in deeply and hold your breath for the count of 10, then exhale.

   Repeat as needed to complete the dosage. (Dosages are usually set in numbers of puffs or inhalations.)

Nasal fashion statement

Some CPAP systems come with small, triangular-shaped masks that fit only over the nose. These masks help prevent skin breakdown and irritation around and inside the nares that can occur with long-term use of nasal prongs and for preterm neonates whose nares are very small to begin with.

Nursing considerations

Before beginning assisted ventilation, explain the procedure to the parents and the child. If ventilation must be initiated in an emergent situation, tell the child (and his parents) what's happening as it's being done.
• Place the patient on a cardiorespiratory monitor and pulse oximeter during any form of assisted ventilation.
• Obtain blood gases to monitor gas exchange and oxygenation status as ordered. (Prepare the child if an arterial puncture must be performed.)

When there's no time to prepare a child before an emergency procedure, talk him through it—step-by-step—while it's being done.

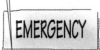

Suction secretions

• For infants who have an ET tube or tracheostomy, suction the airway as needed to prevent occlusion with secretions.
• Frequently assess breath sounds and watch for signs of ET tube or tracheostomy dislodgment. Make sure the ET or tracheostomy tube is appropriately secured to prevent dislodgment.

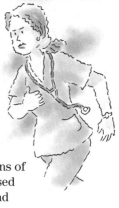

Assess for distress

• In patients who are mechanically ventilated, observe for signs of pneumothorax, such as respiratory distress, absent or decreased breath sounds on one side (the affected side), hypotension, and oxygen desaturation on pulse oximetry.
• For patients receiving CPAP via nasal prongs, cut and place a cushioning dressing (such as Duoderm) over the edges of the nares and the tip of the nose to protect the skin.

Chest physiotherapy

CPT includes breathing exercises and postural drainage. These therapies help to strengthen respiratory musculature and develop more efficient patterns of breathing.

Drain and clear

Postural drainage is usually done in combination with other techniques to enhance the clearance of mucus from the airway. It can be done with manual percussion, vibration, and squeezing of the chest followed by a cough or forceful expiration.

Percussion section

The most common technique involves manual percussion of the chest wall with the patient placed in a postural drainage position with the head down, while the provider strikes the chest wall with a cupped hand or a special device for percussing small areas. CPT is contraindicated in children who have pulmonary hemorrhage, pulmonary embolism, increased intracranial pressure, osteogenesis imperfecta, or minimal cardiac reserves. (See *Percussion devices.*)

Nursing considerations

Explain the purpose of physiotherapy to the child and his parents. In addition, follow these steps:
• Administer bronchodilators, if ordered, before CPT to enhance airway clearance.
• Perform percussion over the ribs only; don't percuss over the spine or the sternum.
• Encourage the child to cough (which may be easier while sitting up) and give him a soft pillow or stuffed toy to hug while coughing to provide support.
• Encourage the child to perform deep breathing exercises; use techniques to make this fun, such as having the child blow soap bubbles, blow through a straw, or blow cotton balls or tissues across a table.

Percussion devices

Percussion is done to clear secretions from the airway. It can be performed by striking areas over the patient's lungs using either the hand (positioned as in the top illustration) or a percussion device (such as the one in the bottom illustration) that's used for infants.

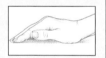

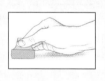

Endotracheal intubation

ET intubation is a short-term measure that may be needed in an emergency. It's used to stabilize the airway if a child is losing the ability to keep the airway open due to swelling or exhaustion that leads to a deteriorating level of consciousness. The ET tube can be inserted orally (orotracheal) or nasally (nasotracheal). The ET tube prevents vocal cord vibration; when the child is intubated, he's unable to cry or talk. If long-term intubation is required, a tracheostomy may be necessary.

Nursing considerations

If there's time, explain the procedure before intubation. If the tube is inserted as an emergency measure, explain each step as it's taken. In addition, follow these steps:
• Suction the ET tube as needed to maintain patency.

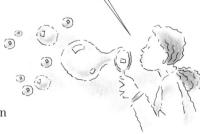

Soap bubbles and a bubble wand can do wonders for deep breathing—and for morale. (It's fun for the kids, too!)

• Securely retape the tube to the child's face as needed to prevent dislodgment.
• Monitor skin integrity around the tube, such as around the nares if nasotracheally intubated or on the lips and gums if orotracheally intubated.

Separate but equal

• Frequently monitor breath sounds to assess lungs and for positioning of the tube; breath sounds should be equal bilaterally.
• Observe for signs of tube dislodgment, such as audible crying or talking, oxygen desaturations on pulse oximetry, and decreased breath sounds.

Silent cry

• Monitor the child's facial expressions. Although you may not hear him cry, his face will still make the grimaces of crying. Provide support, calming and comforting techniques, and pain medication as necessary.
• Because the tube passes through the child's vocal cords, facilitate communication with the child by providing alternatives, such as using sign language, allowing the child to write information, or using a communication board.

Oxygen administration

Some children require more than the 21% oxygen that's present in room air to maintain an adequate oxygenation status. Oxygen is usually required for children who have a partial pressure of arterial oxygen (PaO_2) less than 60 mm Hg or an oxygen saturation range of 89% to 92% on pulse oximetry.

When oxygen therapy is used, the goal is usually to keep oxygen saturation above 92%. Because oxygen is a drug, it should be administered only in the prescribed dosage. It's usually administered in liters per minute (if via nasal cannula) or as a percentage (if via mechanical ventilation or an oxygen hood or tent). Oxygen can be drying, so it must be humidified before it's delivered to the patient.

Oxygen can be administered through an ET or tracheostomy tube during mechanical ventilation or via an anesthesia bag and mask. For children breathing on their own, oxygen can be delivered via nasal cannula, an oxygen hood or tent, or mask.

> Always remember that oxygen needs to be administered as prescribed—just like any other drug.

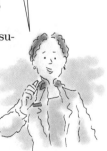

Nursing considerations

Explain to the parents (and the child, if he's old enough) why oxygen is being administered and how it will help the child's

condition. If an ET tube must be used, prepare the child for its insertion, explaining what he'll feel and reassuring him that he'll get used to the tube quickly. In addition:
• Monitor the effectiveness of oxygen therapy by assessing the child's color, pulse oximetry, and PaO_2 using ABG analysis.
• Make sure that the patient is receiving the appropriate concentration of oxygen; also make sure that the oxygen is being humidified before delivery to the patient.

Indoor camping

• For infants in an oxygen tent, keep the flaps of the tent closed snugly around the patient; openings in the tent will allow oxygen to rapidly escape, so the tent must be kept fully enclosed.
• Try to cluster care and procedures to avoid frequently opening the tent.
• Check the infant's clothes and bed linens frequently for moisture, and change as necessary to keep them dry.

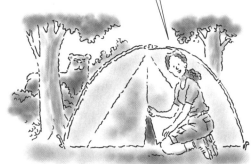

No matter what kind of tent you're in, it's always a good idea to keep the flaps closed tightly!

Tracheostomy

Tracheostomy is a surgically created opening in the anterior neck at the cricoid cartilage leading directly to the trachea. This may be done in the emergency department, in the field where immediate intervention is necessary, or in the more controlled setting of the operating room. A tracheostomy tube is inserted to keep the opening patent; the tube must be secured in place to prevent accidental extubation.

Tracheostomies are used for patients requiring long-term ventilation, or they can be created urgently for children with epiglottitis, croup, or foreign body aspiration. The tracheostomy is usually only needed short-term for these urgent indications. (See *Tracheostomy*, page 342.)

Nursing considerations

If time permits, prepare the child and his family before the procedure. Discuss how the tracheostomy will look and feel, and decide on a method of communication to be used after the procedure.
• After the procedure, monitor the child for complications such as hemorrhage, infection, edema, decannulation (dislodgment of the tracheostomy tube), and tube obstruction.
• Frequently assess the child's breath sounds and monitor respiratory status with blood gases.
• Suction the tracheostomy tube as needed to maintain patency.

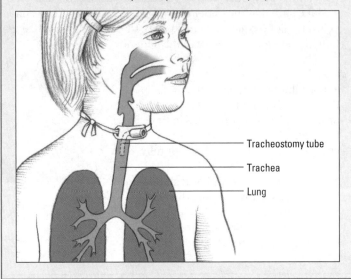

Tracheostomy

This illustration shows a tracheostomy tube in place in the trachea. Note how the tied cloth tapes keep the tube securely in place.

Tracheostomy tube

Trachea

Lung

- Provide stoma care per facility policy. The stoma can usually be gently cleaned with half-strength hydrogen peroxide to remove secretions. The skin around the stoma should be kept clean and dry. Monitor the skin for signs of breakdown.
- Keep the tracheostomy tube ties clean and dry, and change as needed.
- Keep the tracheostomy tube ties secured tightly, but with enough room to slip a fingertip between the ties and the neck to help prevent accidental decannulation.

Respiratory disorders

Disorders of the respiratory system that can occur during childhood include acute otitis media (AOM), asthma, bronchiolitis, croup, cystic fibrosis, epiglottitis, pneumonia, and tuberculosis (TB).

Acute otitis media

AOM is the most commonly diagnosed illness in childhood; it's an inflammation of the middle ear with a rapid onset of symptoms and clinical signs. AOM occurs most commonly in children between ages 6 months and 3 years and is uncommon after age 8. The incidence is higher during the winter months. Breast-fed infants have a lower incidence than formula-fed infants because breast milk provides an increased immunity that protects the eustachian tube and middle ear mucosa from pathogens.

What causes it

AOM is often caused by bacteria but can also be caused by viruses. The most common causative bacterial organisms are *Haemophilus influenzae*, *Moraxella catarrhalis*, and *Streptococcus pneumoniae*. The viruses that most commonly cause AOM are respiratory syncytial virus (RSV), rhinoviruses, influenza viruses, and adenoviruses.

How it happens

Infants and young children are more predisposed to AOM because they have:
• short, horizontally positioned eustachian tubes
• poorly developed cartilage lining, which makes eustachian tubes more likely to open prematurely
• enlarged lymphoid tissue, which obstructs the eustachian tube opening
• immature humoral defense mechanisms, which increase the risk of infection. (See *Characteristics of a child's ear*.)

Characteristics of a child's ear

You'll recognize three major differences between an infant's or a young child's ear and an adult's ear. These anatomic differences make the infant and young child more susceptible to ear infection:
• A child's tympanic membrane slants horizontally, rather than vertically.

• A child's external canal slants upward.
• A child's eustachian tube slants horizontally; this causes fluid to stagnate and act as a medium for bacteria.

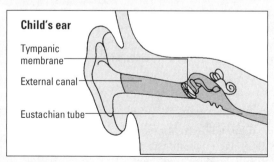

Child's ear

Tympanic membrane

External canal

Eustachian tube

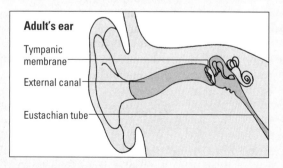

Adult's ear

Tympanic membrane

External canal

Eustachian tube

The great equalizer

The eustachian tube connects the middle ear to the nasopharynx and is normally closed and flat, thus preventing organisms in the pharyngeal cavity from entering the middle ear. The tube opens to allow drainage of secretions produced by the middle ear and equalizes air pressure between the middle ear and the environment.

No escape

When swelling or other predisposing factors cause eustachian tube dysfunction, secretions are retained in the middle ear. Air is also unable to escape through the obstructed tubes and causes negative pressure within the middle ear. If the tube opens, the difference in pressure causes bacteria to be drawn into the middle ear chamber where they proliferate and invade the mucosa, causing infection.

Supine? Not this time

Bottle-feeding an infant in the supine position increases the risk of infection because this position promotes pooling of milk in the pharyngeal cavity, creating an excellent medium for the spread of infection.

> Hear ye, hear ye! Infants and young toddlers communicate ear pain by tugging at their ears.

What to look for

Common acute symptoms of AOM include:
• ear pain that may present as pulling at the ears in younger children or difficulty eating or lying down due to ear pressure and pain
• fever
• irritability
• loss of appetite
• purulent drainage in the external ear canal
• nasal congestion and cough
• vomiting and diarrhea.

The trouble with tympany

Otoscopy reveals:
• tympanic membrane injection (sometimes bright red)
• bulging tympanic membrane, which is dull, with no visible landmarks or light reflex
• diminished mobility of the tympanic membrane with air insufflation (pneumatic otoscopy).

What tests tell you

These tests are used for diagnosis and to guide treatment:
• A culture and sensitivity of any drainage may indicate what the organism is and which antibiotic is indicated for treatment.

- Tympanometry is used to measure the change in air pressure in the external auditory canal (from movement of the eardrum).
- Audiometric testing establishes a baseline or detects any hearing loss secondary to recurring infection. (Hearing evaluation is recommended for any child who has recurrent ear infections or chronic otitis media with effusion that lasts 3 months or longer.)

Complications

Complications of AOM include effusion (which may persist beyond 3 months), hearing impairment, spontaneous rupture of the tympanic membrane, and mastoiditis.

How it's treated

In March 2013, the American Academy of Pediatrics and the American Academy of Family Physicians issued new guidelines for treating AOM to help inhibit the development of antibiotic-resistant organisms and contain the escalating costs of AOM, both direct (treatment) and indirect (lost time from school and work). These guidelines are intended for otherwise healthy children without underlying medical conditions that may complicate AOM (such as cleft palate, Down syndrome, and other genetic or immune system disorders) and include:

Never fear, the antibiotics are here! We'll have the patient feeling better in only 2 or 3 days.

- using analgesics, such as ibuprofen (Motrin) and acetaminophen (Tylenol), to relieve pain, especially in the first 24 hours of infection (Parents should be aware that analgesics—not antibiotics—will relieve the ear pain of AOM.)
- on the basis of joint clinical management in children aged 6 to 23 months with nonsevere unilateral otitis media, giving parents the option of allowing their child's immune system to fight the infection for 48 to 72 hours, then only starting antibiotics if the child's condition doesn't improve after that time
- encouraging the prevention of AOM by breast-feeding for the first 6 months of life, avoiding "bottle-propping," and eliminating the child's exposure to tobacco smoke.

But wait, there's more!

The guidelines also recommend that antibiotics should be used without a waiting period for infants younger than 6 months of age, children ages 6 months to 2 years with a confirmed diagnosis of AOM (bulging tympanic membrane, ear pain, fever greater than 39° C), and children ages 2 and older with severe symptoms.

Most children should receive amoxicillin (Amoxil) as a first-line agent. With severe illness or if additional antibacterial coverage is necessary, amoxicillin-clavulanate (Augmentin) may be initiated. In cases of allergic reaction to amoxicillin or penicillin, alternative therapies may include cephalosporins, azithromycin (Zithromax), clarithromycin (Biaxin), the combination drug erythromycin and sulfisoxazole (Pediazole), or co-trimoxazole (Bactrim). With antibiotic therapy, the child should experience symptom resolution within 48 to 72 hours.

If drugs don't do it

After antibiotic therapy is completed, the child should be reevaluated to make sure that treatment was effective and there are no complications. Other treatments for repeated or complicated infections may include:
• myringotomy, which is an incision in the posterior inferior aspect of the tympanic membrane and may be necessary to promote drainage of exudate and release pressure
• tympanoplasty ventilating tubes, or *pressure-equalizing tubes*, which may be surgically inserted into the middle ear to create an artificial auditory canal that equalizes pressure on both sides of the tympanic membrane. (See *Ventilating tubes in the ear.*)
• prophylactic antibiotics are not recommended for recurrent ear infections.

Ventilating tubes in the ear

This illustration shows where tubes are placed in the ear to equalize pressure on both sides of the tympanic membrane.

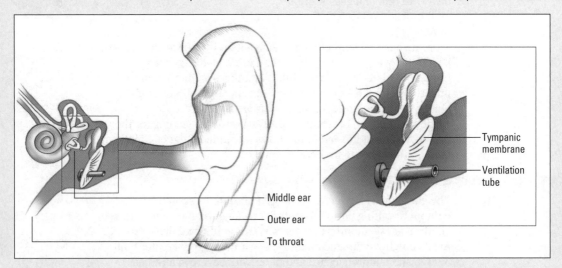

Tympanic membrane

Ventilation tube

Middle ear

Outer ear

To throat

What to do

To care for a child with AOM, follow these steps:
• Relieve pain by administering analgesics, offering liquid or soft foods to limit the need for chewing, and applying local heat or a cool compress over the affected ear.
• Reduce fever by administering antipyretics and removing extra clothing.
• Facilitate drainage by having the child lie with the affected ear in a dependent position.
• Help prevent skin breakdown by keeping the external ear clean and dry; apply zinc oxide or petroleum jelly to protect the skin if needed.

Testing, 1, 2

• Assess for hearing loss and refer for audiology testing if necessary.
• Administer prescribed medication as ordered.

Teach your children well

• Provide appropriate preoperative and postoperative teaching if the child requires surgical intervention.
• Educate parents about the indications for and use of earplugs postoperatively for bathing and swimming.

Asthma

Asthma is a chronic, inflammatory airway disorder that causes episodic airway obstruction and hyperresponsiveness of the airway to multiple stimuli. It results from bronchospasms, increased mucus secretion, and mucosal edema. It's characterized by:
• recurrent cough
• wheezing
• shortness of breath
• reduced expiratory flow
• exercise intolerance
• respiratory distress.

What causes it

Asthma exacerbations or attacks are caused by inflammation of the lungs, including the protective mechanisms of mucus formation, swelling, and airway muscle contraction.

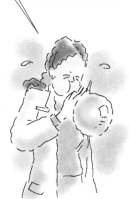

Asthma can take your breath away! That causes stress, which worsens asthma, which causes more stress, which . . . well, you get the idea.

Over-reacting

The lungs react excessively in response to a stimulus (trigger), increasing anxiety and physical responses, in addition to releasing histamine and intracellular chemical mediators that result in bronchospasm. The result is a vicious cycle of anxiety and physiologic response to anxiety.

Gentleman, choose your triggers

Common asthma triggers include:
• exercise
• viral or bacterial agents
• allergens, such as mold, dust, and pollen
• pollutants
• changes in weather
• food additives
• animal dander.
    Many people with asthma, especially children, have intrinsic and extrinsic asthma.

Outside and sensitive

Extrinsic, or *atopic*, asthma begins in childhood. Patients are typically sensitive to specific external (extrinsic) allergens and have a family history of asthma or other allergies. Extrinsic allergens that can trigger an asthma attack include such elements as pollen, animal dander, house dust or mold, kapok or feather pillows, food additives containing sulfites, and other sensitizing substances. Extrinsic asthma in childhood is commonly accompanied by other hereditary allergies, such as eczema and allergic rhinitis.

A look within

Patients with *intrinsic*, or *nonatopic*, asthma react to internal, nonallergenic factors. Intrinsic factors that can trigger an asthma attack include irritants, emotional stress, fatigue, endocrine changes, temperature variations, humidity variations, exposure to noxious fumes, anxiety, coughing or laughing, and genetic factors. Most episodes occur after a severe respiratory tract infection, especially in adults.
    Exercise-induced asthma is a narrowing of the airways that makes it difficult to move air out of the lungs. Symptoms include coughing; wheezing; chest tightness; and prolonged, unexpected shortness of breath after 5 to 20 minutes of exercise. These symptoms are commonly worse in cold, dry air.

Genetic messes

Asthma is associated with two genetic influences:
• ability to develop asthma because of an abnormal gene (atopy)
• tendency to develop hyperresponsive airways (without atopy).

A potent mix

Environmental factors interact with inherited factors to cause asthmatic reactions with associated bronchospasms.

How it happens

Asthma attacks follow a predictable course of bronchospasm, inflammation, and airway narrowing. Here's how asthma develops:

The tracheal and bronchial linings overreact to various stimuli, causing episodic smooth-muscle spasms that severely constrict the airways.

Mucosal edema and thickened secretions also block the airways.

Immunoglobulin (Ig) E antibodies, attached to histamine-containing mast cells and receptors on cell membranes, initiate intrinsic asthma attacks.

When exposed to an antigen such as pollen, the IgE antibody combines with the antigen.

On subsequent exposure to the antigen, mast cells de-granulate and release mediators. These mediators cause the bronchoconstriction and edema of an asthma attack.

Ready, set, spasm!

As a result, expiratory airflow decreases, trapping gas in the airways and causing alveolar hyperinflation.

Atelectasis may develop in some lung regions. The increased airway resistance initiates labored breathing.

Repeat and damage

With repeated episodes of bronchospasm, swelling airways, and mucus plugging, cells that line the airways suffer damage, leaving a chronically irritated and scarred lining that results in air trapping or hyperinflation.

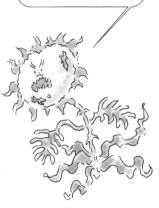

You can't always trust a pretty face. Exposure to my pollen makes mast cells in the lung release histamine. Sorry about that!

What to look for

An acute asthma attack may begin dramatically, with simultaneous onset of multiple, severe symptoms, or insidiously, with gradually increasing respiratory distress. Look for these signs and symptoms:
• sudden onset of breathing difficulty
• frequent coughing or frequent respiratory infections such as pneumonia or bronchitis (which may be an indication that the child's airway is overly sensitive to stimuli)

Working overtime

- rapid and labored respirations and a tired appearance due to the ongoing exertion of breathing
- nasal flaring and intercostal retractions
- productive cough and expiratory wheezing

Four levels of asthma severity

There are four major classifications of asthma severity based on the frequency of symptoms and exacerbations, effects on activity level, and lung function study results. The four levels are mild intermittent, mild persistent, moderate persistent, and severe persistent.

Level of severity	Clinical findings
Intermittent	• Symptoms occur less than two times per week. • The patient is asymptomatic with normal peak expiratory flow (PEF) between exacerbations. • No interference with normal activity. • Nighttime symptoms occur less than two times per month. • Short-acting β-agonist less than 2 days/week • Lung function studies show forced expiratory volume in 1 second (FEV_1) or PEF greater than 80% of normal values; PEF may vary by less than 20%.
Mild persistent	• Symptoms occur more than two times per week, but less than once per day; exacerbations may affect activity. • Nighttime symptoms occur more one to four times per month. • Short-acting β-agonist greater than 2 days/week but not daily. • Minor limitations in normal activity. • Lung function studies show FEV_1 or PEF greater than 80% of normal values; PEF may vary by 20% to 30%.
Moderate persistent	• Symptoms occur daily. • Exacerbations occur more than two times per week and may last for days; exacerbations affect activity. • Bronchodilator therapy is used daily. • Nighttime symptoms occur three to four times per month or more than once weekly but not nightly. • Daily use of short-acting β-agonist. • Some limitation in normal activity. • Lung function studies show FEV_1 or PEF 60% to 80% of normal values; PEF may vary by greater than 30%.
Severe persistent	• Symptoms occur throughout the day. • Exacerbations occur frequently and limit physical activity. • Nighttime symptoms occur more than once per week. • Use short-acting β-agonist several times a day. • Extremely limited normal activity. • Lung function studies show FEV_1 less than 60%.

• use of accessory muscles, decreased air movement, and respiratory fatigue
• barrel chest and use of accessory muscles after repeated acute exacerbations. (See *Four levels of asthma severity.*)

What tests tell you

Several tests are used to diagnose asthma, assess its severity, and identify allergens:
• Pao_2 and partial pressure of arterial carbon dioxide ($Paco_2$) are usually decreased, except in severe asthma, when $Paco_2$ may be normal or increased, indicating severe bronchial obstruction.

Function or obstruction?

• PFTs reveal signs of airway obstructive disease, low-normal or decreased vital capacity, and increased total lung and residual capacities. (Pulmonary function may be normal between attacks.)
• Serum IgE levels may increase from an allergic reaction.
• Sputum analysis may indicate the presence of Curschmann's spirals (casts of airways), Charcot-Leyden crystals, and eosinophils.
• Chest X-rays can be used to diagnose or monitor the progress of asthma and may show hyperinflation with areas of atelectasis.
• ABG analysis detects hypoxemia (decreased Pao_2; decreased, normal, or increasing $Paco_2$) and guides treatment.
• Skin testing may identify specific allergens.

Up to the challenge?

• Bronchial challenge testing evaluates the clinical significance of allergens identified by skin testing.
• Electrocardiogram shows sinus tachycardia during an attack; during a severe attack, this test may show signs of cor pulmonale (right axis deviation, peaked P wave) that resolve after the attack.

Complications

Status asthmaticus, in which there's unrelenting, severe respiratory distress and bronchospasm, may occur despite pharmacologic and supportive interventions. Mechanical ventilation may be needed due to respiratory failure. Death may occur if a child in acute exacerbation isn't treated in a timely manner and proceeds to respiratory failure without intubation.

How it's treated

The best treatment for asthma is prevention of exacerbations. Management includes medications, environmental management of asthma triggers, and education and support of the child and parents. Choice of medications to promote optimal respiratory function is typically based on the asthma's level of control and severity.

Anti-inflammatory agents

Anti-inflammatory medications to reduce mucosal edema in airways include inhaled corticosteroids, such as fluticasone (Flovent) and budesonide (Pulmicort). These drugs are preventive medications, usually taken on a daily basis to stop the release of chemicals such as histamine during the inflammatory process.

Anti-inflammatories must be taken consistently to be effective. These medications aren't effective after wheezing starts but may help gain control and speed the resolution of an asthma attack.

Cortico-reactions

Adverse reactions of corticosteroids include glucose metabolism abnormalities, increased appetite, fluid retention, weight gain, moon face, mood alteration, growth suppression, and hypertension, all of which may be severe if used daily for long-term therapy.

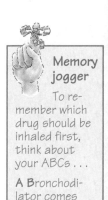

> Leukotriene modifiers can help control seasonal allergies.

Bronchodilators

Bronchodilators are used to relax smooth muscle in the airway for moderate to severe symptoms resulting in rapid bronchodilation within 5 to 10 minutes. Short-acting β-agonists (SABAs) are the first line of treatment for quick relief of acute symptoms and for prevention of exercise-induced bronchospasm. These medications include albuterol (Proventil), metaproterenol (Alupent), levalbuterol (Xopenex), and pirbuterol (Maxair).

Open wide

Bronchodilators relax the muscle bundles that constrict airways for airway dilation and relaxation and are used for acute or daily therapy, nocturnal symptoms, and exercise-induced bronchospasm. When used for long-term control, they work best when a specific amount is maintained in the bloodstream, so serum level checks and dosage adjustments may be required. Adverse effects include tachycardia, nervousness, nausea and vomiting, and headaches.

Leukotriene modifiers

Leukotriene modifiers such as montelukast (Singulair) may be used as a steroid-sparing adjunct for the prevention of bronchospasm. They improve pulmonary function and enhance the effect of corticosteroids, allowing for lower dosages of corticosteroids.

Memory jogger

To remember which drug should be inhaled first, think about your ABCs . . .

A Bronchodilator comes before a Corticosteroid.

Adverse reactions include diarrhea, laryngitis, pharyngitis, nausea, otitis media, sinusitis, or headache. Administering leukotriene modifiers daily, at bedtime, may promote compliance.

Allergy shots and oxygen

The use of allergy shots for hyposensitization—to reduce sensitivity to environmental allergens that may be unavoidable, such as mold or pollen—is controversial because their actual effect is questionable.

Oxygen is administered by nasal cannula or face mask for the child exhibiting difficulty breathing. The oxygen must be humidified to decrease drying and thickening of mucus secretions.

What to do

Nursing interventions are focused on maintaining airway patency and fluid status, promoting rest, and decreasing stress for the child and his parents.

• Upon arrival at the clinic or hospital setting, evaluate the child's current respiratory status, remembering the *ABCs* (airway, breathing, and circulation); move on to other activities only after establishing that the child doesn't need immediate intervention to promote oxygenation.

• If the child isn't moving air or is unable to talk, take emergency action.

• Continue to assess the quality of the child's breathing, obtain oxygen saturation via pulse oximeter, and peak expiratory flow rate in an older child (the frequency of assessment is based on the severity of symptoms).

Top to bottom, looking for problems

• Assess skin and intake and output, and perform a head-to-toe assessment to identify associated problems contributing to the asthma exacerbation.

• Assess the child's psychosocial status, looking for indications of anxiety or fear, and promote comfort for the child and his family. (Encouraging the parents' presence can be reassuring for the child and can decrease his anxiety and fear.)

• Place the child in a sitting (semi-Fowler's) position to facilitate respiratory effort.

• Administer fluids, which are important for restoring and maintaining fluid balance as adequate hydration helps break up trapped mucus plugs in a narrowed airway. (Intravenous [I.V.] fluids may be necessary if adequate fluid intake isn't

> Always think about your ABCs when evaluating a child's respiratory status.

A is for AIRWAY
B is for BREATHING
C is for CIRCULATION

> Good hydration is essential for a child with asthma.

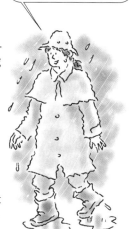

possible due to compromised respiratory status and risk of aspiration with tachypnea.)

Please do not disturb

- Promote rest and stress reduction by grouping nursing tasks and avoiding repeated disturbances.
- Support the family by encouraging them to rest and giving them the opportunity to assist with the child's treatments as they wish; give them frequent updates on the child's condition.
- Provide discharge planning and home care teaching that gives the parents a thorough understanding of the disease and how to prevent attacks and maintain the child's health to avoid illness that leads to hospitalization. (Include education on medication therapy and stress the need for follow-up care.)

> Smoking and asthma don't mix! Teach parents that being around cigarette smoke is particularly dangerous for a child with asthma.

Smoke provokes

- Teach parents about the dangers of smoking around a child with asthma. Encourage them to quit or, at the very least, never smoke indoors, even if the child isn't in the home at the time. Even if parents smoke outside, they should be encouraged to wear a smoking jacket so that the child does not inhale smoke residue from the parent's clothing.
- Teach the older child signs of early respiratory distress so he can seek treatment before the signs get more serious. (A plan should be communicated to the child's school to ensure that medications are given as needed and school officials can recognize respiratory distress.)

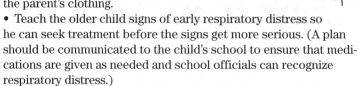

Bronchiolitis

Bronchiolitis is an illness that usually occurs after an upper respiratory infection causes inflammation and obstruction of the small airways (bronchioles)—either early in life as a single episode or with multiple occurrences in the first year of life. It most commonly affects toddlers and preschoolers, but can become severe in infants younger than 6 months old, causing life-threatening respiratory distress that requires hospitalization.

What causes it

RSV is the leading cause of bronchiolitis. Other causes exist, however, including viruses, bacteria, and mycoplasmal organisms. Premature infants and those with bronchopulmonary dysplasia, immunodeficiency, or congenital heart disease are at especially high risk.

How it happens

Bronchiolitis occurs when viruses or other infectious agents invade the mucosal cells lining the bronchi and bronchioles, causing the cells to die. Cell death results in cell debris that clogs and obstructs the bronchioles and irritates the airway. The airway lining responds by swelling and producing excessive mucus resulting in partial airway obstruction and bronchospasm. The process continues as both lungs are invaded and the obstructed airways allow air in, but the swollen airways and mucus buildup don't allow for expulsion of the air, creating wheezing and crackles in the airways.

Diminishing returns

Air trapped below the obstructed airways interferes with gas exchange, leading to decreased oxygen and increased carbon dioxide levels. Airflow continues to decrease and breath sounds diminish.

What to look for

The diagnosis of bronchiolitis is based on clinical findings, the child's age, and the season. Clinical findings may include:
• recent history of upper respiratory symptoms, including nasal stuffiness or serous nasal discharge accompanied by mild fever and a cough in older toddlers and preschoolers
• wheezing, deep and frequent cough, and labored breathing
• rapid, shallow respirations accompanied by nasal flaring and retractions
• tachypnea, paroxysmal cough, and increasing irritability with increasing respiratory distress

The child commonly appears ill, is less playful, and has little interest in eating or has a history of spitting up food with thick, clear mucus.

What tests tell you

Bronchiolitis is diagnosed primarily by history and physical examination.
• Chest X-rays usually show nonspecific findings of inflammation, but may show areas of consolidation that are difficult to differentiate from bacterial pneumonia.
• Viral cultures or antigen testing by nasal swab or a direct aspiration of nasal secretions or nasopharyngeal washings may indicate RSV.

• If the bronchiolitis is severe and advanced, there may be a rise in Pa_{CO_2}, leading to respiratory acidosis and hypoxemia.

Complications

Some children with more severe cases require intubation and assisted ventilation if they become too fatigued to breathe effectively, and they progress to respiratory failure. Death may result due to severe RSV bronchiolitis in children with preexisting cardiopulmonary disease. Bronchiolitis in infancy may increase the chances of childhood wheezing and asthma.

How it's treated

Usually, supportive management with high humidity, adequate fluid intake, and rest is all that's needed when the bronchiolitis is mild to moderate in severity. The child with more severe bronchiolitis will need:
• monitoring with pulse oximetry
• postural drainage and CPT to loosen trapped mucus

Hydrate and humidify

• humidified oxygen therapy via nasal cannula or an oxygen hood or tent to alleviate dyspnea and hypoxia
• I.V. hydration if the child is tachypneic and unable to maintain hydration status (due to decreased intake with respiratory distress or insensible fluid loss due to fever and increased respiratory rate).

Drugs to the rescue

Pharmacologic therapy includes:
• aerosol medications, such as bronchodilators, steroids, and beta-adrenergic agonists to act directly on inflamed and obstructed airways
• antipyretics to reduce fever
• antibiotics (only if a secondary bacterial infection such as otitis media is present)
• ribavirin (Virazole), an antiviral drug delivered via hood, tent, or mask, to treat RSV. (Ribavirin's effectiveness is controversial, and is usually reserved for life-threatening cases.)

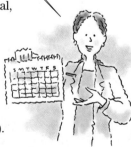

Palivizumab is given from November to April—RSV season.

'Tis the season

Preventative therapy may be indicated for RSV bronchiolitis in high-risk infants or children with congenital heart disease, bronchopulmonary dysplasia, chronic lung problems, cystic fibrosis, or prematurity. Palivizumab (Synagis) is given for 5 consecutive months during RSV season (November to April).

What to do

Nursing care focuses on careful attention to respiratory function:
• Assess airway and respiratory function carefully and frequently because it's important to intervene in a timely manner for worsening respiratory symptoms to prevent respiratory distress.
• Maintain respiratory function by administering oxygen and pulmonary care therapies.

Head's up

• Elevate the head of the bed to ease the work of breathing and assist mucus to drain from upper airways.
• Use oxygen saturation level as an indicator of the severity of the disease and to spot early signs of deterioration.
• Maintain isolation in a separate room or cohort room for RSV infection and use meticulous hand washing and contact precautions such as gowns and gloves to prevent spreading infection. (RSV is highly contagious and has the potential to spread during close contact.)

Assess and de-stress

• Perform psychosocial assessment by observing the child and his parents for signs of fear and anxiety, which can worsen respiratory distress.
• Help to reduce anxiety by providing thorough explanations and updates and encouraging parents to participate in the child's care as able (to promote emotional security).
• Cluster nursing activities to promote rest and decrease stress as rest is required to improve the child's breathing and healing.
• Administer antipyretics to control temperature and promote comfort as needed.
• Assist in hydrating the child by encouraging oral fluid intake if possible or maintaining I.V. infusion.
• Assist in discharge planning and home care teaching when the child is able to go home; supportive therapies may be needed at home until resolution of all symptoms, which may take weeks.

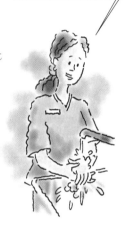

Never skimp on hand washing when caring for a child with RSV. The virus is one thing you definitely don't want to share.

Croup

Croup, also known as *acute laryngotracheobronchitis*, is a self-limiting upper airway obstructive disease that affects young children (usually younger than age 5). It involves severe inflammation and obstruction of the upper airway and is most common from the late fall to early spring, although it may occur throughout the year.

What causes it

Croup usually results from viral infection with common causative organisms, typically parainfluenza, RSV, *H. influenzae*, or *Mycoplasma pneumoniae*. It also may be of bacterial origin (diphtheria or pertussis). It affects more boys than girls and is typically seen in children between ages 6 months and 3 years.

How it happens

Croup is usually preceded by an upper respiratory infection that proceeds to laryngitis and then descends into the trachea (and sometimes the bronchi), causing inflammation of the mucosal lining and subsequent narrowing of the airway. Profound airway edema may lead to obstruction and seriously compromised ventilation. (See *How croup affects the upper airway*.)

If it barks like a seal . . .

The flexible larynx of a young child is particularly susceptible to spasm, which may cause complete airway obstruction. When the child's airway is significantly narrowed, he struggles to inhale air past the obstruction and into the lungs, producing the

How croup affects the upper airway

In croup, inflammatory swelling and spasms constrict the larynx, reducing airflow. This cross-sectional drawing (from chin to chest) shows the upper airway changes caused by croup. Inflammatory changes obstruct the larynx (which includes the epiglottis) almost completely and significantly narrow the trachea.

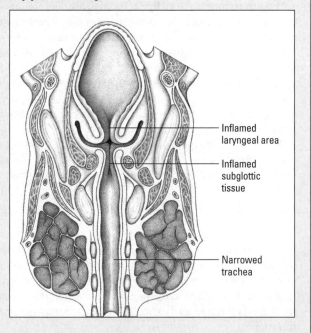

Inflamed laryngeal area

Inflamed subglottic tissue

Narrowed trachea

characteristic inspiratory stridor and suprasternal retractions, and the classic barking or seal-like cough.

It's always darkest before the dawn

Croup is characterized by gradual onset of a low-grade fever. Worsening of symptoms at night and a cough are common. The airway obstruction increases, leading to retractions, restlessness, anxiety, tachycardia, and tachypnea. Severe obstruction leads to respiratory exhaustion, hypoxemia, carbon dioxide accumulation, and respiratory acidosis.

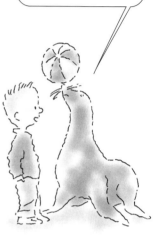

This child with croup has my bark down pat! I guess imitation really is the sincerest form of flattery.

What to look for

History and physical examination typically reveal:
• history of upper respiratory infection
• inspiratory stridor and substernal and suprasternal retractions
• barking cough and hoarseness
• pallor or cyanosis
• restlessness and irritability
• low-grade fever
• crackles, rhonchi, expiratory wheezing, and localized areas of diminished or absent breath sounds
• retractions, wheezing, and cyanosis (in severe cases).

What tests tell you

The diagnosis of croup is based primarily on history and clinical findings. Croup is differentiated from epiglottitis by a lateral neck radiograph that shows a normal epiglottis. X-rays show symmetrical narrowing of the subglottic space ("steeple sign").

Complications

If the child experiences obstruction that's severe enough to prevent adequate exhalation of carbon dioxide, respiratory acidosis results and the child eventually experiences respiratory failure.

How it's treated

The majority of children with croup don't require hospitalization. The mainstays of at-home treatment are vaporizers, oral fluids, and antipyretics. The major objectives of treatment are to maintain an airway and provide for adequate respiratory exchange. High humidity with cool mist provides relief for most children and can be accomplished using a cool air vaporizer or a steamy bathroom at home. In the hospital, hoods for infants or mist tents for toddlers are sometimes used to increase humidity and provide supplemental oxygen if needed.

Reading the signs

Parents must learn the signs of respiratory distress so they can seek medial attention if symptoms progress. Indications for hospitalization include:
- dusky or cyanotic skin color
- severe stridor
- significant retractions
- agitation, restlessness, or obtundation (mental dullness).

Epi for edema

These medications are used to treat croup:
- Nebulized racemic epinephrine (Isuprel) is used for its alpha-adrenergic properties, which decrease subglottic inflammation and edema by causing mucosal vasoconstriction. This drug acts quickly—within 10 to 15 minutes—last about 2 hours, and can be administered as a nebulization every 20 to 30 minutes for severe croup and every 4 to 6 hours for moderate croup.
- Corticosteroids reduce subglottic edema and inflammation. Dexamethasone (Decadron) given one time early in the course of croup results in a shorter hospital stay and reduces cough and dyspnea and, commonly, the need for intubation.
- Acetaminophen reduces fever and oxygen consumption in the febrile child with croup.

What to do

The most important nursing intervention for the child with croup is continuous observation and accurate assessment of respiratory status, including careful monitoring of color, respiratory effort, evidence of fatigue, and vital signs to assess for worsening of symptoms that would require further management.

Continually assess for possible respiratory failure, and have intubation equipment readily accessible at the bedside.
- Assess for airway obstruction by evaluating respiratory status.
- Administer prescribed medications as ordered, which may include racemic epinephrine via nebulizer, antibiotics if croup is bacterial in origin, and corticosteroids to reduce inflammation.

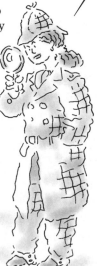

Careful monitoring is key. Hmmm . . . what do we have here?

I get misty

- Provide humidified air via a cool mist vaporizer or mist tent and oxygen as necessary. The parents may need to stay with the child in the mist tent to decrease crying or apprehension that would contribute to more respiratory distress and hypoxia.

• Because oral hydration is essential to help loosen secretions, encourage the child to drink unless his respiratory rate is greater than 60 breaths/minute, putting him at risk for aspiration. If aspiration risk exists, fluids may need to be administered I.V.

• Help the child find the most comfortable position for the best oxygenation. Most infants and small children prefer sitting upright and many want to be held.

A friend from home

• Help reduce the child's anxiety by maintaining a quiet environment, promoting rest and relaxation, and minimizing intrusive procedures. Encourage the parents to bring a favorite toy for the child.

• Support the parents, who may be frightened by the rapid progression of croup and the alarming sound of the cough and stridor, by answering questions and explaining treatments and procedures. Encourage them to be present and participate in their child's care as appropriate.

• Educate the parents about caring for the child at home. (See *Croup class.*)

It's all relative

Croup class

Teach parents how to care for their child with croup at home by telling them:

• medication dosages, administration techniques, and possible adverse reactions

• symptoms of croup to watch for and report

• how to manage home vaporizer or mist treatments

• how to alleviate symptoms (such as awakening with a barking cough) by putting the child in the bathroom and running hot water to produce steam (always with adult supervision).

Cystic fibrosis

Cystic fibrosis is a chronic, autosomal-recessive, inherited disorder of the exocrine glands that affects multiple organ systems. It's characterized by chronic airway infection that leads to bronchiectasis, bronchiolectasis, exocrine pancreatic insufficiency, intestinal dysfunction, abnormal sweat gland function, and reproductive dysfunction. The disease is the most common fatal genetic disease in white children. Cystic fibrosis is accompanied by many complications. Life expectancy for the person with the disease is currently 37 years—but, because of advances in treatment and technology, some people live much longer.

What causes it

The gene responsible for cystic fibrosis is located on chromosome 7q. It encodes a membrane-associated protein called the *cystic fibrosis transmembrane regulator (CFTR)*. The exact function of CFTR remains unknown, but it appears to help regulate chloride and sodium transport across epithelial membranes. Causes of cystic fibrosis include abnormal coding found on as many as 350 CFTR alleles and autosomal-recessive inheritance.

How it happens

Abnormally thick secretions affect the normal function of multiple organ systems, including the:
• bronchi, resulting in chronic bronchial pneumonia and obstructive emphysema
• small intestine, causing intestinal obstruction and failure of the neonate to pass meconium (meconium ileus)
• pancreatic ducts, leading to malabsorption syndromes
• bile ducts, leading to biliary cirrhosis and portal hypertension
• salivary and sweat glands, leading to increased sodium and chloride excretion
• autonomic nervous system, which may lead to hyperactivity.

Parents of a child with cystic fibrosis may travel a difficult road; they need ongoing education, support, and encouragement.

What to look for

Clinical manifestations may appear at birth or may take years to develop and can vary in severity. Respiratory assessment findings may include:
• dyspnea
• dry, nonproductive cough
• wheezing
• atelectasis and generalized obstructive emphysema due to mucoid obstruction as the disease progresses with the characteristic features of barrel-shaped chest, cyanosis, and clubbing of fingers and toes
• chronic sinusitis
• bronchitis
• bronchopneumonia.

Eye on the GI

Gastrointestinal (GI) assessment findings include:
• meconium ileus in a neonate
• weight loss despite increased appetite
• malnourishment and vitamin deficiency
• obstruction of pancreatic ducts and absence of pancreatic enzymes, leading to malabsorption syndrome with chronic diarrhea and large, frothy, foul-smelling stools
• abdominal cramping and distention; foul-smelling flatus
• cirrhosis leading to possible portal hypertension with resultant splenomegaly and esophageal varices.

The legacy stops here

Reproductive system assessment findings include:
• decreased fertility due to increased viscosity of cervical mucus, blocking the entry of sperm in females

• sterility in males due to blockage of the vas deferens with abnormal secretions, preventing sperm formation.

To the heart of it all

Cardiovascular system assessment findings include:
• right-sided heart enlargement (cor pulmonale) and heart failure resulting from obstruction of pulmonary blood flow
• hyponatremia, which may lead to circulatory collapse if sodium isn't replaced.

What tests tell you

Elevated sodium and chloride levels detected on a sweat test are used to establish a diagnosis. Stool analysis reveals steatorrhea (fat in the stool). Chest X-rays show evidence of generalized obstructive emphysema.

Complications

One complication of cystic fibrosis is pneumothorax, which is most commonly caused by rupture of subpleural blebs through the visceral pleura. This condition occurs most commonly in children with more advanced disease. Other complications include bronchiectasis, intestinal obstruction, rectal prolapse, cor pulmonale, diabetes mellitus, and nasal polyps.

How it's treated

Pulmonary treatment of cystic fibrosis is aimed at prevention and treatment of pulmonary infection by improving aeration, removing mucopurulent secretions, and administering antimicrobial agents.

Twice per day keeps infection away

Prevention of infection is maintained with good pulmonary hygiene with a daily routine of CPT, which is usually performed twice daily and more often if needed during pulmonary infections. Some children can use a flutter mucus clearance device, a handheld device that facilitates removal of mucus by increasing sputum expectoration. The child blows into the plastic pipe that contains a stainless steel ball on the inside.

Dilate and stimulate

Bronchodilators delivered in an aerosol help open the bronchi for easier expectoration and are administered before CPT if the child has reactive airway disease or wheezing. Recombinant human deoxyribonuclease, known generically as *dornase alpha* (Pulmozyme), is used to decrease the viscosity of mucus. Physical exercise is also an important adjunct to daily CPT as it stimulates mucus secretion and provides a sense of well-being. Oxygen is administered to children with acute episodes, as needed, but is used cautiously as many of these children have chronic carbon dioxide retention.

What to do

Nursing care will vary depending on where a child is in the disease process and whether he's being treated for an acute exacerbation of pulmonary infection or is simply undergoing routine care.

Oil change not included

When PFTs are low or when children have difficulty breathing or experience a flare-up of infection, they may need to be hospitalized for a "pulmonary tune-up." This type of treatment may include:
• I.V. antibiotic therapy for *Pseudomonas* infection when it interferes with daily functioning
• rigorous CPT
• inhalation therapy.

The deluxe treatment

Nursing care also involves:
• encouraging pulmonary hygiene (such as CPT, postural drainage, aerosol treatments with bronchodilators, and breathing exercises) to aid in sputum expectoration
• monitoring respiratory status by evaluating breathing patterns and vital signs

> Make sure the patient with cystic fibrosis has a high-calorie, high-protein diet.

No dieting here

• promoting adequate nutrition by providing a diet high in calories and protein, with fats as tolerated and increased salt intake during hot weather or febrile periods
• maintaining calorie counts, monitoring intake and output, and recording daily weights
• administering medications as ordered, including aminoglycosides to prevent or treat infection, bronchodilators, and pancreatic enzymes
• administering vitamin supplements and iron and medium-chain triglycerides as dietary supplements

Infection-free zone

• monitoring for signs of infection and limiting exposure to persons with respiratory infections
• promoting adequate rest by clustering nursing interventions and scheduling regular rest periods

• providing and encouraging activities according to the child's developmental level and physical capabilities, and arranging for a school tutor or help with schoolwork if a school-age child is hospitalized
• providing family support through education and referrals for counseling, support groups, and other resources, such as a dietitian, social worker, physical therapist, tutor, or pastor.

Epiglottitis

Epiglottitis is an acute inflammation of the epiglottis that occurs most commonly in children between ages 2 and 5. Epiglottitis obstructs the airway and needs immediate attention.

What causes it

Epiglottitis commonly results from infection with *H. influenzae* type B (Hib) but other possible causative organisms include *S. pneumoniae* and streptococci A, B, and C.

How it happens

Epiglottitis is commonly preceded by a minor upper respiratory infection and sore throat of several days duration that rapidly progresses to severe respiratory distress. The child usually goes to bed with no symptoms and then awakens later complaining of a sore throat and difficulty swallowing. If untreated, it may rapidly progress to increasing upper airway obstruction that results in hypoxia, hypercapnia, and acidosis, closely followed by decreased muscle tone, altered level of consciousness and, if obstruction becomes complete, sudden death.

What to look for

Health history and physical assessment typically reveal one or more of these signs and symptoms:
• sudden onset of symptoms, commonly preceded by upper respiratory infection
• sore throat, pain on swallowing, and refusal to eat or drink due to dysphagia

There's a frog in my throat

• muffled, thick voice; wheezy inspiratory stridor; and snoring expiratory sound with a froglike croaking sound on inspiration (not hoarseness as with croup)
• characteristic positioning of sitting upright, leaning forward, with chin thrust out, mouth open, and tongue protruding (tripod position)
• drooling because of difficulty or pain with swallowing

Hot and toxic

- high fever, toxic appearance
- irritability; restlessness; and an anxious, apprehensive, frightened expression
- suprasternal and substernal retractions
- tachycardia and thready pulse.

Hypoxia

Late signs of hypoxia include listlessness, cyanosis, bradycardia, and decreased respiratory rate with decreased aeration. On inspection, the child's throat appears red and inflamed with a large, cherry-red, edematous epiglottis.

A job for the experts

When symptoms of epiglottitis occur, throat inspection should be done only by an otolaryngologist or other properly trained personnel. In addition, equipment should be readily available for performing emergency ET intubation or tracheotomy because examination may precipitate complete airway obstruction.

> Give me a call if you suspect epiglottitis. Unless it's done by an expert, a throat inspection can make matters worse.

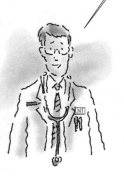

What tests tell you

- A lateral neck film showing epiglottal enlargement confirms the diagnosis of epiglottitis.
- Elevated white blood cell (WBC) count and increased bands and neutrophils on differential count may also indicate the diagnosis.
- Identification of causative bacteria through blood cultures will assist with antibiotic selection.

Complications

Complications of epiglottitis include rapid progression of the illness to the point at which the airway is swollen shut. The child can't be intubated and suffers from respiratory distress. If respiratory distress isn't reversed in a timely manner, the child can die or suffer from the long-term disabling results of brain anoxia.

How it's treated

The child is immediately transported to a facility that's set up to manage this type of emergency. When a diagnosis is confirmed, the child is usually intubated or a tracheotomy is performed to maintain an airway so the child can be ventilated if necessary.

The best treatment for epiglottitis is prevention, and it's recommended that all children receive the Hib conjugate vaccine beginning at age 2 months.

First by vein, then by mouth

Children with epiglottitis are treated with antibiotics, first I.V. and then orally, to complete a 7- to 10-day course. Sometimes, corticosteroids are used to reduce edema during initial treatment. Most intubated children will be treated with corticosteroids for 24 hours before extubation.

The child continues to require intensive observation for the first 24 hours of antibiotic therapy, after which the epiglottal swelling usually decreases. By the third day the epiglottis is near normal and most children can be extubated at that time.

What to do

Nursing care focuses primarily on maintaining airway patency and observing for any signs of respiratory distress or infection:
• Closely monitor respiratory status to ensure airway patency; if the child presents with symptoms of epiglottitis, ensure that a throat examination is performed only by a trained professional with emergency equipment on hand.
• After the child is intubated, monitor closely and maintain a patent airway. Suction as needed, and provide oxygen therapy as ordered.
• Observe closely for signs of respiratory distress after extubation.
• Monitor for signs and symptoms of infection.
• Ensure adequate hydration by monitoring I.V. fluid administration and keeping strict intake and output records.
• Help relieve anxiety by maintaining a calm, relaxing atmosphere; limiting intrusive procedures; encouraging the parents to bring in security objects from home; providing age-appropriate play activities; assisting the child to the most comfortable position for breathing before intubation; and administering sedative agents, as ordered, after the child is intubated.
• Support the family by answering their questions and providing information about diagnosis and treatment. Allow the parents to be present to participate in their child's care, as appropriate.
• Administer prescribed medications, which may include antibiotics, sedation if the child is being intubated, and corticosteroids to reduce edema.

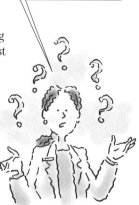

Making sure a parent's questions are answered is the best prescription for stress reduction.

Pneumonia

Pneumonia is an acute inflammation or infection of the respiratory bronchioles, alveolar ducts and sacs, and alveoli (the parenchyma) of the lungs that impairs gas exchange. It occurs in about 4% of children younger than age 4; the incidence decreases with advancing age.

What causes it

Infection can result from viruses, bacteria, mycoplasma, or aspiration of foreign substances. Viral pneumonia is the most common type, with RSV the most common causative organism. Other viral causes include influenza and parainfluenza viruses, rhinovirus, and adenovirus.

Major causative organisms in bacterial pneumonia include pneumococci, streptococci, and staphylococci. Children with bacterial pneumonia appear more ill than those with viral pneumonia and have more localized physical findings.

How it happens

Bacterial and viral pneumonia begin as upper respiratory infections:
• Bacterial pneumonia typically begins as a mild upper respiratory infection in which bacteria circulate through the bloodstream to the lungs, leading to cell damage throughout one or more lobes of a single lung.
• Viral, or mycoplasma, pneumonia begins as an upper respiratory tract infection. The virus infiltrates the alveoli near the bronchi of one or both lungs, where they replicate and burst out to kill cells and send out cell debris.

Invasion of the cell snatchers

Invasion of the virus, bacteria, or mycoplasma results in exudate from cell death. This exudate fills the alveolar spaces, with pooling and clumping in dependent areas of the lung to create areas of consolidation. Bacterial pneumonia most commonly causes lobular involvement and sometimes consolidation. Viral pneumonia most commonly results in inflammation of interstitial tissue. (See *Types of pneumonia*.)

What to look for

Regardless of the causative agent, symptoms of pneumonia may include:
• elevated temperature
• rhonchi
• crackles

Types of pneumonia

Pneumonia is classified according to location and extent of involvement:
• *Lobar pneumonia* involves a large segment of one or more lung lobes; if it involves both lungs it's known as *bilateral* or *double pneumonia*.
• *Bronchopneumonia* begins in the terminal bronchioles and involves nearby lobules, which become clogged to form consolidated patches.
• *Interstitial pneumonia* is confined to the alveolar walls and peribronchial and interlobular tissues.
• *Aspiration pneumonia* is caused by aspiration of fluid or food substance in a child who has difficulty swallowing; who's unable to swallow due to paralysis, weakness, congenital anomalies; or who has an absent cough reflex. It can also occur if the child is fed while crying or breathing rapidly.

- wheezes
- dyspnea
- tachypnea
- restlessness
- decreased breath sounds if consolidation exists.

Fretful and feverish

Infants may also demonstrate vomiting, seizures, poor feeding, fretfulness, fever, stiff neck, bulging anterior fontanel, circumoral cyanosis, respiratory distress, diminished breath sounds and crackles, and pleural friction rub.

Headache and hacking

Older children usually experience headache, abdominal or chest pain, high fever with chills, intermittent drowsiness and restlessness, tachycardia, tachypnea, hacking nonproductive cough, expiratory grunting, circumoral cyanosis, diminished breath sounds and disappearance of crackles (indicating consolidation), and moist crackles and cough that produce copious, blood-tinged mucus (as the disease resolves).

What tests tell you

Diagnosis of pneumonia is made by chest X-ray, which shows abnormal density of tissue such as lobar consolidation. Other tests include:
- sputum specimen, Gram stain and culture, and sensitivity tests help differentiate the type of infection and the drugs that are effective against it
- blood cultures reflect bacteremia and are used to determine the causative organism
- WBC count reveals leukocytosis in bacterial pneumonia; the WBC count is normal or low in viral or mycoplasmal pneumonia
- ABG levels vary, depending on the severity of pneumonia and the underlying lung state
- bronchoscopy or transtracheal aspiration enables collection of material for culture
- pulse oximetry may show a reduced oxygen saturation level.

Complications

Hospitalization is reserved for seriously ill children. Complications of pneumonia include pleural effusion, empyema, and tension pneumothorax. Some effusions require surgical drainage.

How it's treated

Treatment for all types of pneumonia consists mainly of symptomatic therapy, such as pain and fever control, supportive care of the airway and hydration status, and rest promotion.

• Bacterial pneumonias are treated with organism-sensitive antibiotics; mycoplasma pneumonias may also be treated with antibiotics to prevent secondary bacterial infection.

• Some children may also be treated with anti-inflammatory medications.

• To help prevent pneumonia, immunization with pneumococcal conjugate vaccine (PCV-13) is recommended for all children in the United States beginning at 2 months of age. Additionally, pneumococcal polysaccharide vaccine (PPSV or PPV-23) is recommended for children older than age 2 who are immunosuppressed or have chronic diseases, such as asthma and sickle cell disease.

What to do

The goal of nursing care is to restore optimal respiratory function:

• Ease respiratory effort by administering oxygen therapy as ordered.

• Perform ongoing respiratory assessment, watching for respiratory distress by monitoring vital signs and respiratory status.

• Use a humidifier or mist tent to create a high-humidity atmosphere.

• Perform CPT, postural drainage, and suctioning as needed to remove mucus from airways.

• Reposition the child frequently and elevate the head of the bed to prevent pooling of secretions and ease respirations.

• Provide relief from pain when coughing and deep breathing with such medications as acetaminophen and ibuprofen; antitussives may sometimes be used before periods of rest and before eating.

• Administer prescribed medications as ordered, including antibiotics and antipyretics.

Thanks for elevating the head of the bed. It makes my work a lot easier when I'm dealing with pneumonia.

What goes in must come out

• Monitor intake and output, and weigh the child daily.

• Encourage adequate oral intake or administer I.V. fluids to prevent dehydration.

• Promote rest by clustering nursing care to minimize disturbances, and maintain bed rest as necessary to conserve energy.

• Provide a diet of high-calorie foods in small amounts in a relaxed atmosphere.

Keeping parents in the loop

• Provide support to the child and his family by answering questions, providing updates, and encouraging the parents to participate in the child's care.

• Begin discharge planning early, providing teaching on medications, especially antibiotics that must be taken at prescribed intervals for the full course.

Tuberculosis

TB, one of the major chronic diseases today, is increasing in incidence. This increase is due to the rise in homelessness, the increase in foreign-born immigrants in the United States, and the human immunodeficiency virus (HIV) epidemic.

Individuals at highest risk include the homeless, those with weakened immune systems (such as those with HIV infection or leukemia or those on corticosteroid therapy), young infants and children with immature immune systems, and those in correctional facilities. Cases of TB are most common in urban and low-income areas.

Lying in wait

TB is considered *latent* when the patient is asymptomatic and can't spread the disease to others, but has a positive purified protein derivative (PPD) test result. In these individuals, the body has been able to prevent the infection from growing; however, the infection retains the ability to become active disease in the future, especially if the individual becomes immunocompromised. *Active TB* occurs when the body can't prevent the bacteria from multiplying and the individual becomes symptomatic.

What causes it

TB is caused by *Mycobacterium tuberculosis*. The main source of infection in children is an infected adult or adolescent in the household.

How it happens

The lung is the usual portal of infection for human beings. Transmission occurs as the child inhales the microorganisms into the respiratory tract after an infected individual coughs or sneezes. Epithelial cells proliferate around multiplying bacilli of *M. tuberculosis* in an attempt to wall off the invading organisms. This forms the typical tubercle. There's progressive tissue destruction as the primary lesion extends and spreads within the lung, which can produce pneumonia and erode blood vessels.

> One kid sneezed and another inhaled. It's into the respiratory tract we go to spread, destroy, and erode.

What to look for

Contact with an infected individual is the most important finding of the history. A child may be asymptomatic, but if signs and symptoms do occur, they may include:

- chronic cough
- anorexia
- weight loss or failure to gain weight
- fever.

What tests tell you

The tuberculin test is used to determine if the child has been exposed to the tubercle bacillus. The Mantoux test, which uses PPD injected intradermally, is the recommended procedure. A positive reaction (defined as 10 mm or more induration in 48 to 72 hours) indicates that the child has been exposed and his body has developed sensitivity to the protein of the tubercle bacillus; it doesn't, however, confirm the presence of active disease.

Once positive, always positive

After a child has a positive reaction, he'll continue to have positive reactions. Some children born in other countries may have been vaccinated against TB using the Bacillus Calmette–Guérin (BCG) vaccine. Children vaccinated with BCG may have a positive PPD skin test. A previously negative reaction that converts to a positive indicates that the child has been exposed since the last skin test.

Chest X-rays may be helpful in diagnosis as they may demonstrate hilar lymphadenopathy in active disease or calcification if the disease is in the healing phase.

Complications

Very young children (younger than age 2), adolescents, and children who are HIV-positive are more affected by the disease and have a higher incidence of disseminated disease. Death seldom occurs in treated children but may be an outcome in those who contract TB meningitis.

How it's treated

Treatment for TB lesions in children consists of drug therapy, general supportive care, and prevention of unnecessary exposure to other infections that may further compromise the body's defenses. Hospitalization isn't usually necessary except for needed diagnostic tests or, when indicated, surgery.

Teaming up to treat TB

The use of two or more drugs simultaneously has been found to be optimal, with isoniazid and rifapentine given in a 3-month regimen. Isoniazid may also be used alone in a 9-month treatment regimen. Treatment must be modified if the patient is a contact of an individual with drug-resistant TB. Consultation with a TB expert is advised if the known source of TB infection has drug-resistant TB. The guidelines for drug therapy are based on chest X-ray findings after a positive skin test has been verified.

> Two or more are better than one when it comes to treating TB—and we're the team for the job!

Removing the source

Surgery may be required to remove the source of infection in tissues that aren't affected by drug therapy or tissue that has been destroyed by the disease. Bronchoscopy for removal of a tuberculous granulomatous polyp or resection of a portion of a diseased lung may also be performed.

What to do

The majority of nursing care for children with TB is provided in the ambulatory care setting, in schools, and through public health agencies:

• Assist with radiographic examinations, perform skin tests, and obtain specimens for laboratory examination.
• Encourage the child to attend school and continue life activities as usual. However, older children should be restricted from vigorous activities, such as competitive games and contact sports, during the active stage of TB.
• Encourage compliance with the drug regimen to optimize treatment success. (Parents must be instructed to give the medication at the correct times and for the length of time it's ordered.)

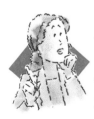

Quick quiz

1. In which anatomic structure does gas exchange take place?
    A. Nasopharynx
    B. Trachea
    C. Bronchioles
    D. Alveoli

Answer: D. The exchange of oxygen for carbon dioxide occurs in the alveoli.

2. A child with difficulty breathing and a "barking cough" is displaying signs associated with which condition?
- A. Cystic fibrosis
- B. Asthma
- C. Epiglottitis
- D. Croup

Answer: D. A "barking cough" and difficulty breathing indicate croup. These signs arise as the child attempts to inhale air around a laryngospasm that obstructs the airway.

3. The nurse is assessing the lung sounds of a child with asthma. Which sound is the nurse most likely to hear?
- A. Murmur
- B. Wheezing
- C. Crackles
- D. Pleural friction rub

Answer: B. When listening to the lung sounds of a child with asthma, the most commonly heard adventitious sound is wheezing, which sounds like a musical note.

4. Which condition can rapidly obstruct the airway, requiring immediate attention?
- A. Tonsillitis
- B. Bronchiolitis
- C. Epiglottitis
- D. Tuberculosis

Answer: C. Epiglottitis is an acute inflammation of the epiglottis that can rapidly progress to upper airway obstruction. It requires immediate attention because, if the obstruction becomes complete, death can result unless emergency treatment such as tracheotomy is initiated.

5. Which sign or symptom suggests cystic fibrosis?
- A. Steatorrhea (fat in the stool)
- B. Decreased appetite
- C. Decreased respiratory rate
- D. Early passage of meconium in the neonatal period

Answer: A. Cystic fibrosis causes thick secretions that block the pancreatic ducts and prevent essential pancreatic enzymes from reaching the duodenum. This condition causes stools that are greasy, foul-smelling, and frothy from undigested fats.

Scoring

☆☆☆ If you answered all five items correctly, excellent work! You can breathe easy about your knowledge of respiratory problems.

☆☆ If you answered four items correctly, good job! Your knowledge of respiratory problems in children is unobstructed.

☆ If you answered fewer than four items correctly, don't hyperventilate! Take a deep breath, review the chapter, and move on.

Urinary problems

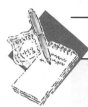

Just the facts

In this chapter, you'll learn:

♦ anatomy and physiology of the urinary tract

♦ assessment of the child with a urinary problem

♦ diagnostic tests and treatments used for urinary problems

♦ specific acquired and congenital urinary disorders.

Anatomy and physiology

The key structures of the urinary system are the kidneys and urinary tract.

> I filter waste from the blood and form urine. It's a dirty job, but someone's gotta do it.

Kidneys

The kidneys are bean-shaped organs located near the middle of the back. Their primary functions are to filter waste products from the blood and form urine and send it to the bladder through the ureters. Other functions of the kidneys include regulation of volume, electrolyte concentration, acid-base balance of body fluids, and blood pressure and support of red blood cell (RBC) production (erythropoiesis).

The kidney is divided into two distinct areas:

renal cortex—the outside, superficial area of the kidney

renal medulla—the internal portion of the kidney in which the nephrons are located.

A closer look at a nephron

The nephron is the kidney's basic functional unit and the site of urine formation:

The renal artery, a large branch of the abdominal aorta, carries blood to each kidney.

Blood flows through the interlobular artery (running between the lobes of the kidneys) to the afferent arteriole, which conveys blood to the glomerulus.

Blood passes through the glomerulus into the efferent arteriole and into the peritubular capillaries, venules, and the interlobular vein.

The peritubular capillary network of vessels then supplies blood to the tubules of the nephron.

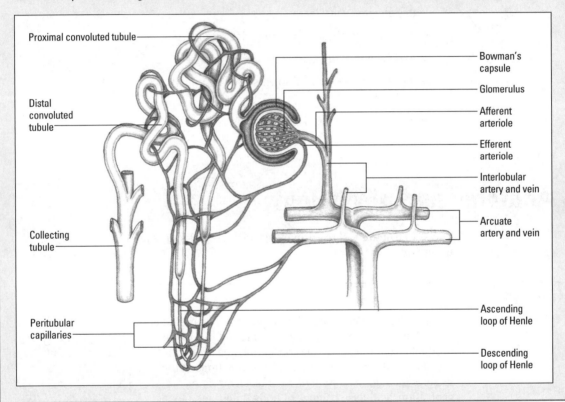

Proximal convoluted tubule

Distal convoluted tubule

Collecting tubule

Peritubular capillaries

Bowman's capsule

Glomerulus

Afferent arteriole

Efferent arteriole

Interlobular artery and vein

Arcuate artery and vein

Ascending loop of Henle

Descending loop of Henle

Nephrons

Nephrons are the kidney's functional units. These microscopic structures form urine. (See *A closer look at a nephron.*)

A child acquires the adult number of nephrons shortly after birth, although these structures continue to mature throughout early childhood. The renal corpuscle within the nephron filters blood plasma. The renal tubules within the nephron allow the filtered fluid to pass through on its way to the bladder.

Multitasking kidneys

To produce urine, the various parts of the kidney perform three basic functions:

glomerular filtration (the process of filtering blood as it flows through the kidneys)

tubular resorption

tubular secretion.

While waste products and excess fluids are filtered out of the blood for elimination, necessary fluids, electrolytes, proteins, and blood cells are retained (resorbed) into the bloodstream.

Urinary tract

The urinary tract consists of the bladder, urethra, and ureters. The bladder is a balloon-shaped pouch of a thin, flexible muscle, in which urine is temporarily stored before being eliminated from the body through the urethra. Urine is produced by the kidneys and passed into the bladder through two ureters, one from each kidney.

A friendly nudge

Peristaltic contractions within the ureters push urine from the kidneys toward the urinary bladder. A valve mechanism prevents urine from backing up into the kidneys as the bladder fills. When the bladder is full:
• The micturition reflex is triggered, and nervous innervation causes relaxation of the internal sphincter muscle.
• Relaxation of the internal sphincter muscle sends a message to the person's conscious mind to indicate the need to void.
• The person then releases the external sphincter, and urine passes through the urethra and out of the body.

Any volunteers?

Voluntary control of these urethral sphincters usually occurs in a child between ages 18 and 24 months. However, the psychological readiness to initiate toilet training may develop much later.

Urine

Urine is a liquid waste product that's filtered out of the blood by the kidneys, stored in the bladder, and expelled from the body through the urethra during urination. About 96% of urine is water, and the other 4% is waste product.

A child's bladder can hold 1 to 1.5 oz of urine for every year of age. Average urine output will vary according to age. (See *Urine output in children.*)

Diagnostic tests

Diagnostic tests commonly used to assess urinary system problems in the pediatric population include:
• urinalysis and urine culture
• blood urea nitrogen (BUN) and creatinine levels
• X-ray of the kidneys, ureters, and bladder (KUB)
• excretory urography
• voiding cystourethrogram (VCUG)
• renal ultrasound
• renal biopsy.

Urinalysis and urine culture

Urinalysis determines urine characteristics, such as specific gravity, pH, and physical properties (color, clarity, odor), and detects the presence of RBCs, white blood cells (WBCs), casts, and bacteria.

Culture on a plate

In a urine culture, the urine specimen is placed on a medium and bacteria that may be present are allowed to grow and are then counted. As soon as bacteria are identified, sensitivity testing can determine which antibiotics would be most effective for treating the infection.

Catch 'em while you can

Specimens for urinalysis and urine culture are typically obtained as clean-catch specimens but may also be obtained from an infant's diaper (urinalysis only), a urine collection bag for infants and young children, bladder catheterization, or a suprapubic bladder tap.

Nursing considerations

Nursing considerations differ according to the child's age and gender. For boys, the head of the penis and the urinary meatus must be cleaned. For girls, the urinary meatus must be cleaned, carefully washing between the labia.

Urine output in children

This chart shows the average volume of urine output per 24 hours for children according to age.

Age-group	Urine output
Neonate	50 to 300 ml/day
Infant	300 to 550 ml/day
Preschool	500 to 800 ml/day
School-age	600 to 1,400 ml/day
Adolescent	1,000 to 1,500 ml/day

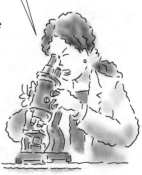

After bacteria are identified with a urine culture, sensitivity testing can be done to choose the best antibiotic.

Lather up, rinse away

For both boys and girls, soapy water, which is then rinsed away, is usually used for cleaning. If an antiseptic towelette is provided, it may be used without rinsing afterward. In addition, follow these steps:
• Instruct the child or parents on how to clean the penis or meatus.
• Instruct the child or parents on how to collect the urine specimen by starting to urinate into the toilet bowl to clear the urethra of contaminates and then catching 3 to 6 oz of urine in a sterile container.
• For neonates and infants, apply a urine bag to obtain a clean specimen; the bag fits over the perineum in females and the penis (and perhaps the scrotum) in males to catch urine as the infant voids (instruct the parents to inform you as soon as the child voids, so the container can be removed and fecal contamination can be avoided).
• When obtaining a urine specimen from a catheterized child, don't take the specimen from the collection bag; aspirate a specimen through the collection port in the catheter with a sterile needle and syringe.

Keep it clean

A clean-catch specimen may be needed to diagnose a urinary tract infection (UTI). In addition to the procedures used for routine urinalyses, it's useful to:
• Instruct the child or parents to use an antiseptic solution to clean the urethral meatus (with a prepared towelette or a cotton ball soaked in the solution); the urethral meatus should be cleaned at least three times, using a new towelette or cotton ball each time.
• Stress to the child and parents the importance of not touching the inside of the sterile container to maintain its sterility.

Blood urea nitrogen and creatinine

Serum BUN and creatinine levels are obtained from blood samples drawn from venipuncture.
• BUN levels can provide a great deal of information about kidney function; they measure the blood nitrogen that's part of the urea resulting from catabolism of amino acids (proteins). When the glomerular filtration rate (GFR) reduces suddenly and severely, the BUN level rises suddenly.
• Plasma creatinine levels become elevated when there's catabolism of creatinine phosphate in skeletal muscles. An elevation in these levels indicates poor renal function.
• The ratio between BUN and creatinine may also be examined. The ratio is usually between 10:1 and 20:1. Results vary with muscle damage, as in the case of a crushing injury or degenerative muscle disease.

Nursing considerations

Nursing considerations are aimed at making venipuncture less stressful for the child.

• Use lidocaine and prilocaine (eutectic mixture of local anesthetics [EMLA]) cream or some other form of topical anesthetic to make it easier and less traumatic to draw blood from a child; remember to apply it at least 1 hour before drawing blood.

• Allow the parent to be present, and allow the child to hold a comfort object, such as a stuffed animal or blanket, during the venipuncture.

• Follow dietary orders as necessary; sometimes, when BUN levels are elevated, protein intake may need to be limited.

KUB radiography

KUB assesses the size, shape, position, and possible areas of calcification of the kidneys, ureters, and bladder. A KUB may be required as a first step if a problem with these structures is suspected.

Nursing considerations

The nurse should help the child remain quiet and lie still during the X-ray. Tell the child that this is his "job" and that there's no "hurting part" involved.

Depending on facility policy, parents may be able to remain in the radiology room with the child. Instruct them that they must be shielded from radiation by wearing a lead apron.

> For a child, the hardest part of a KUB is holding still. It's a painless first step toward sorting out a problem in the urinary system.

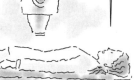

Excretory urography

Excretory urography is a form of X-ray of the lower urinary tract, during which a dye is injected intravenously (I.V.). A series of X-rays is taken as the dye passes through the bloodstream, is filtered through the kidneys, passed on through the ureters into the bladder, and then through the urethra to be eliminated from the body.

Nursing considerations

Begin by explaining the reason for the test to the child and parents and telling them what to expect.

• Prepare the child for insertion of the I.V. line and reassure him that it's the only needle stick he'll experience.

• Assess for a history of allergies to dyes, iodine, shellfish, or eggs because of the use of an iodine-based contrast medium.

- Administer a bowel preparation as ordered; the colon must be emptied because a full bowel won't allow proper visualization of the urinary tract.
- Insert an I.V. line to allow for the injection of the dye.
- Explain to the child that he may feel warm or a bit woozy when the dye is injected; reassure him that this is normal and that the feeling will pass quickly.
- On the day of the test, allow only clear liquids to be consumed until after the test is completed.

Voiding cystourethrogram

VCUG is an X-ray of the bladder and the lower urinary tract. A catheter is inserted through the urethra into the bladder, and a water-soluble contrast medium is injected through the catheter. The catheter is then withdrawn, and X-ray images are taken as the bladder is emptied.

This test is performed to determine if there are abnormalities of the lower urinary tract, particularly vesicoureteral reflux, a condition that increases the risk of or prolongs a UTI. Sedation is rarely required, nor is it desirable, because the child must urinate during the test.

Before a VCUG, reassure the child that the X-ray technician won't be watching him while he's voiding; he'll be looking at the X-ray instead.

Nursing considerations

VCUG can be a difficult test for children. Insertion of a catheter can be uncomfortable and embarrassing. The child will be asked to void during the test, and to do so without going into the bathroom, which can be confusing to a child who has recently been toilet trained. What's more, the thought of voiding in the X-ray room in full view of the technician can be embarrassing. Reassure the child that the hospital staff realizes he knows how to use the bathroom and that he'll be urinating during the test only because he's being asked to do so (explain why this is necessary).

In addition, follow these steps:
- Explain the reason for the test and prepare the child for insertion of the catheter.
- Before the test, make sure the child is dressed in comfortable clothing and is wearing no metal objects.
- Assess for a history of allergies to dyes, iodine, shellfish, or eggs because of the use of an iodine-based contrast medium.
- Tell the parents of infants and young children that the child may be wrapped tightly in a blanket to help him lie still during the procedure.
- Assure the parents that the amount of radiation received by the child is minimal.

• Inform the parents that a VCUG can't be performed while the child has an active UTI.

Behind closed doors

• Insert a urinary catheter just before the test; provide as much privacy as possible by closing the door or drawing curtains, and allow a parent to remain in the room if the child desires (depending on the child's age, a nurse of the same sex may be the best person to insert the catheter).
• After the procedure, remove the urinary catheter and encourage the child to drink fluids to reduce burning on urination and to flush out residual dye; pouring a glass of very cold water over the genital area during the first few voids after catheter removal helps to minimize burning.

> A little cold water can put out the "fire" during a postcatheter void.

Renal biopsy

Although renal biopsy isn't performed routinely in children, it may be used to evaluate decreased kidney function, persistent blood in the urine, or protein in the urine. It may also be performed to evaluate the functioning of a newly transplanted kidney.

In renal biopsy, a needle is inserted through the child's flank under ultrasound guidance. A small specimen of kidney tissue is withdrawn and sent for microscopic study.

Nursing considerations

Prepare the child and parents for the procedure, which can be frightening. Use a doll to show the child how it will be done. In addition, follow these steps:
• Reassure the parents that ultrasound will allow the doctor to see exactly where he'll be inserting the needle and will prevent damage to other organs.
• Provide analgesics as ordered.
• Assist with positioning and holding the child throughout the procedure.

Treatments and procedures

Common treatments and procedures used in the care of a child with a urinary disorder include bladder catheterization, hemodialysis, kidney transplantation, and peritoneal dialysis.

Always prepare children for treatments and procedures with an age-appropriate explanation of what to expect. When treatments and procedures involve surgery, preparation should include an explanation of the anesthesia and what to expect postoperatively.

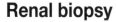

Bladder catheterization

Bladder catheterization may be performed for diagnostic or treatment purposes. In this procedure, the urethral meatus is thoroughly cleaned and an appropriate-sized catheter is inserted through the urethra into the bladder.

Insert and drain

In intermittent catheterization, a straight catheter is inserted and a urine specimen may be taken; the catheter is removed after the bladder is drained.

Insert and inflate

If the catheter is to remain in place, an indwelling catheter, also called a *Foley catheter*, may be used and attached to a drainage bag for urine collection. An indwelling catheter has an inflatable balloon near its tip to hold the catheter in place in the bladder.

Nursing considerations

Remember that catheterization can be uncomfortable and embarrassing for a child. The older child may feel more comfortable when a same-sex nurse inserts the catheter. The younger child may be confused and fearful if he has been told it's wrong for anyone to touch his "private parts." Have the parents explain to the child that this situation is different.

To minimize trauma, follow these steps:

- Educate the child and parents about the purpose of the catheterization; if it's being done to obtain a sterile specimen, explain why this is preferable to a clean-catch specimen.
- Prepare the child to facilitate the procedure and ease the child's fears; use a doll to show him what will happen.
- Be sure to choose the appropriate-sized catheter. (For a premature neonate, a size 5 French feeding tube may be used; for a larger infant or a small toddler, use a size 8 French feeding tube; for children ages 4 and older, use a size 8 French to 14 French catheter.)
- Provide as much privacy as possible; close the door, draw the room divider curtain, and allow the child to keep on as much clothing as possible.
- Allow the parent to be present if the child desires.
- Give the child coping mechanisms to deal with discomfort (such as "Squeeze your mother's hand if it hurts," or, "Count to 10 and the hurting part will be over").
- Use distraction techniques to help keep the child's mind off of what is happening. This can be accomplished with toys with which the child likes to play or with bubbles. Just be sure to keep everything clear of the sterile field that has been set up.

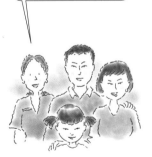

A young child may need her parents' okay for a doctor or nurse to touch parts of her body that are otherwise off-limits to adults.

Generous and gentle

When inserting the catheter:
• Clean the urethral meatus three times with an antiseptic swab, using a different swab each time.
• Generously lubricate the tip of the catheter and gently insert it through the urethra into the bladder until urine returns and is collected in the sterile specimen container.
• If the catheter doesn't easily enter the meatus, use a smaller catheter; never force it into the urethral meatus.
• If performing an intermittent catheterization, gently remove the catheter after the bladder is drained; clean off the antiseptic and lubricant with water.
• If inserting an indwelling urinary catheter, insert the inflatable balloon with sterile water and gently pull on the catheter to make sure it inflated; next, connect the catheter to the closed drainage system.

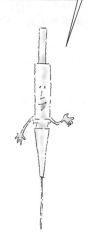

When it comes to kids and catheters, one size doesn't fit all.

Hemodialysis

Hemodialysis involves the use of a machine to clean waste products from the bloodstream if the kidneys are severely damaged or have failed. The blood travels through tubes to an artificial kidney in the machine, and waste products and excess fluid are removed from the body. The purified blood then flows back to the body through another set of tubes. Ideally, this would be done in a pediatric dialysis center.

To stick or not to stick

The child on hemodialysis may have a double-lumen central catheter in place in his chest to serve as a site for blood removal. Children needing long-term dialysis may have a subcutaneous graft, anastomosing a vein and an artery. This graft reduces the risk of infection but means the child will need two venipunctures each time dialysis is performed. EMLA cream should be used to reduce discomfort.

Nursing considerations

Provide diversional activities to prevent boredom, such as games, music, drawing or coloring materials, and videos; encourage a family member to stay with the child. In addition, follow these steps:
• Weigh the child before beginning hemodialysis.
• If the patient has a subcutaneous graft, check the blood access site every 2 hours for patency and signs of clotting; don't

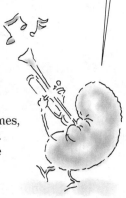

A set of headphones and a CD player can be a great antidote to boredom during hemodialysis.

use the arm with this site for taking blood pressure or drawing blood.
• During dialysis, monitor vital signs, clotting times, blood flow, the function of the vascular access site, and arterial and venous pressures.

Look out for losses

• Watch for complications, such as septicemia, embolism, hepatitis, and rapid fluid and electrolyte loss.
• After dialysis, monitor vital signs and the vascular access site; weigh the patient and watch for signs of fluid and electrolyte imbalances.
• Use standard precautions when handling blood and body fluids.

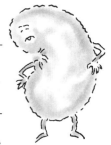

When I can't do my job, the professionals send in a replacement— a healthy kidney from a living person or a cadaver.

Kidney transplantation

Kidney transplantation involves replacing a patient's diseased kidney with a healthy kidney from another person. The donor kidney may come from a living donor or a cadaver donor. Although hemodialysis and peritoneal dialysis are life-preserving procedures and may even be carried out in the home, kidney transplantation is the preferred method of renal replacement therapy in the pediatric population because it offers the opportunity for a normal life.

Nursing considerations

By the time a child undergoes kidney transplantation, he most likely has a long history of procedures and hospitalizations. The child should be given as many choices as possible; a choice as simple as which arm to use for a blood draw can help to give the child a sense of control.

In addition, follow these steps:
• Provide emotional support and guidance to the child and parents; prepare them for the procedure, including what will occur preoperatively, during the procedure, and postoperatively.
• Arrange for the child and his parents to tour the intensive care unit and meet the nursing staff before the transplantation.
• Administer immunosuppressive medications as ordered; a child who will have or has had a kidney transplant will be taking immunosuppressive medications to decrease the risk of organ rejection.
• Monitor for signs and symptoms of infection; while immunosuppressed, the child is at increased risk for infection.

It isn't worth the risk. Even the common cold can pose a major threat to an immunosuppressed child.

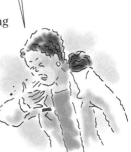

You sneeze, you leave

• Make sure that no one with obvious infection takes care of the child.

• Prepare the child (and parents) for the possibility of continuing to need hemodialysis temporarily after the transplant because the transplanted kidney might not work effectively right away.

Peritoneal dialysis

In peritoneal dialysis, the blood is cleaned of waste products and excess fluids using the lining of the abdomen as a filter. Peritoneal dialysis is especially useful for children who are poor risks for vascular access and for those who live far from a medical center. This procedure includes these steps:

• A peritoneal dialysis catheter is inserted through a small abdominal incision or a puncture hole into the peritoneal cavity. The catheter is then connected to fluid bags and tubing.
• A cleaning solution is drained from a bag into the abdomen.
• Fluids and waste products flow through the lining and are "caught" by the dialysis fluid.
• This fluid is then drained from the abdomen, taking the extra fluids and waste products with it.

Nursing considerations

Prepare the child and parents for the insertion of the catheter into the abdominal cavity. Make sure a valid informed consent form has been signed and included in the patient's chart. In addition, follow these steps:

• Monitor the child's reaction to the sedation, anesthesia, and pain management regimen.
• Make sure strict sterile technique is used at all times during catheter placement and peritoneal dialysis.
• Monitor the child's response to the therapy.
• Make the child as comfortable as possible and provide sufficient rest periods.
• Assess for bleeding from the catheter insertion site.
• Maintain patency of the peritoneal dialysis catheter; keep it in place, without kinks or pulling, and with the fluid bags at the correct level.
• Monitor for signs of infection at the insertion site.

Urinary disorders

Urinary disorders that may affect children include acute post-streptococcal glomerulonephritis, chronic glomerulonephritis, congenital urologic anomalies, hemolytic uremic syndrome (HUS), nephrotic syndrome, renal failure (acute and chronic), and Wilms' tumor.

Acute poststreptococcal glomerulonephritis

Glomerulonephritis is an inflammation of the tubules of the kidneys (glomeruli), which filter waste products from the blood. When this inflammation follows an infection with streptococcal bacteria (most commonly via strep throat), it's called *acute poststreptococcal glomerulonephritis*. It's most commonly seen in boys between ages 3 and 7 but can occur at any age. Up to 95% of children recover fully; the rest may progress to chronic renal failure.

An interesting point: The relationship between acute glomerulonephritis and scarlet fever was first recognized as early as the 18th century. Its relationship with hemolytic streptococcus was identified later in the 1950s.

What causes it

Acute poststreptococcal glomerulonephritis typically follows a group A beta-hemolytic streptococcal infection of the respiratory tract. Less commonly, it may follow a skin infection such as impetigo.

How it happens

The disease usually begins about 1 to 6 weeks after a streptococcal infection, although 2 weeks is the most common time of onset.

Clumping with the enemy

In this immunologic disorder, antigens from streptococci clump together with the antibodies that killed them and become trapped in the tubules of the kidneys. The tubules become inflamed, and edema of the capillary walls decreases the amount of glomerular perfusion. The kidneys then become incapable of filtering and eliminating body wastes.

What to look for

Edema may initially appear in the face, especially around the eyes. Later, edema may occur in the legs. Changes in urination may include low urine output (oliguria), blood in the urine (hematuria), protein in the urine (proteinuria), and cola-colored (smoky) urine. Other signs and symptoms may include:
- high blood pressure
- mild anemia, pallor
- joint pain and stiffness
- malaise, lethargy
- anorexia
- fever
- headache.

What tests tell you

Urinalysis reveals the presence of protein, RBCs, and WBCs in the urine. Blood studies show elevated levels of urea and creatinine.
• Antistreptolysin-O test confirms that the patient has had a streptococcal infection.
• Throat culture, if performed during an acute infection, confirms the presence of group A beta-hemolytic streptococci.
• Renal ultrasound shows slightly enlarged kidneys bilaterally.
• Renal biopsy may be performed to assess the renal tissue or confirm the diagnosis.

Complications

No complications are typically associated with acute poststreptococcal glomerulonephritis. Generally, a full recovery can be expected within a matter of weeks to months. If complications occur, they may include:
• hypertensive encephalopathy
• chronic or progressive problems of kidney function
• renal failure (in rare instances)
• pulmonary edema and heart failure (occasionally).

How it's treated

Treatment may involve antibiotics for 7 to 10 days to treat infections contributing to the ongoing antigen-antibody response. Other medications may include:
• antihypertensives to control high blood pressure
• diuretics to reduce fluid retention and edema
• corticosteroids to decrease antibody synthesis and suppress the inflammatory response.

Lay low

The patient may be placed on bed rest to reduce his metabolic demands. In the acute phase, a low-sodium, low-protein diet may be ordered to prevent fluid retention, and fluid restrictions may be ordered to decrease edema. In rare instances, dialysis may be necessary.

A child with acute poststreptococcal glomerulonephritis might have to wait a while for potato chips and pepperoni pizza.

What to do

Nursing care of the patient with acute poststreptococcal glomerulonephritis focuses on monitoring and education.
• Check vital signs and electrolyte values; monitor intake and output and measure the child's weight daily.
• Assess renal function daily through serum creatinine, BUN, and urine creatinine clearance levels; watch for and immediately report signs of acute renal failure (oliguria, azotemia, and acidosis) and monitor for ascites and edema.

Battle the boredom

- Provide quiet, age-appropriate activities that the child can enjoy while on bed rest; allow him to gradually resume normal activities as symptoms subside.
- Monitor for signs of complications, such as sudden major changes in vital signs, a change in the amount or appearance of urine output, significant weight gain, changes in vision, changes in motor abilities, seizure activity, severe pain, or behavioral changes.

Medication education

- Teach the child and parents about medications the child will be taking; tell them that the child should continue taking the prescribed medications even if he's feeling better and to report adverse effects.
- Teach the child and parents about necessary dietary restrictions. Most commonly, this would include limited water and sodium intake.

Strep alert

- Advise the child and parents to immediately report signs of a streptococcal throat infection, such as sore throat and fever.
- Teach the parents to monitor the child's weight and blood pressure on a regular basis; instruct them to report changes in the child's condition, such as increased edema, changes in appetite, signs of infection, abdominal pain, headaches, lethargy, or changes in urine output.

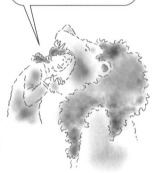

After a child has had acute poststreptococcal glomerulonephritis, a sore throat can take on gigantic significance!

Chronic glomerulonephritis

Chronic glomerulonephritis results from slow, progressive destruction of the glomeruli of the kidney with progressive loss of kidney function. It may eventually result in renal failure.

What causes it

Most cases of chronic glomerulonephritis are thought to be caused by an abnormality of the immune system. Other causes may include:
- systemic lupus erythematosus (SLE)
- bacteremia associated with a ventriculoperitoneal shunt
- infection with streptococcus or staphylococcus bacteria
- exposure to organic solvents, mercury, or certain nonsteroidal anti-inflammatory agents
- human immunodeficiency virus infection
- infection with hepatitis B virus.

How it happens

Because chronic glomerulonephritis may go undetected for years until renal function declines markedly, it's more commonly diagnosed during adolescence than in early childhood.

Damage, changes, impairment

Damage to the glomeruli of the kidneys is caused by abnormal immune responses—possibly a direct attack on the kidney itself or accumulated immune complexes in the glomerular filter. Chronic changes to the structure of the glomeruli result. These changes impair renal function—specifically, inefficient filtering of the blood. Blood and protein then spill into the urine.

What to look for

In chronic glomerulonephritis, symptoms of declining renal function may be present along with hematuria, proteinuria, and hypertension that don't respond to routine treatment. Nephrotic syndrome may develop.

What tests tell you

- Urinalysis shows a high specific gravity and the presence of blood, casts, and protein.
- Blood chemistry shows hyperkalemia, anemia, and azotemia.
- Ultrasound, computed tomography (CT) scan, or excretory urography may show small kidneys.
- Renal biopsy may show one of the forms of chronic glomerulonephritis or nonspecific scarring of the glomeruli.

Complications

Complications of chronic glomerulonephritis may include nephrotic syndrome, chronic renal failure, end-stage renal disease, chronic hypertension, malignant hypertension, heart failure, pulmonary edema, chronic or recurrent UTI, and increased susceptibility to other infections.

How it's treated

Treatment of chronic glomerulonephritis is largely symptomatic and may include:
- antihypertensive medications to control blood pressure
- corticosteroids or immunosuppressive medications to suppress inflammatory and immune responses
- restricted dietary intake of sodium, potassium, fluids, and proteins to help in the control of hypertension
- dialysis or kidney transplantation if renal failure develops.

What to do

Care of the child with chronic glomerulonephritis includes careful monitoring and long-term follow-up. Provide emotional support and reassurance to the child and his parents and be sure to include clear explanations of procedures. In addition, follow these steps:
• Weigh the patient daily. Carefully measure and record intake and output.
• Monitor vital signs and watch for and report signs of inadequate renal perfusion (hypotension) and acidosis.

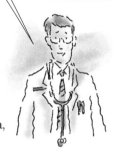

A good relationship with the health care provider is essential to help the child and his family deal with chronic glomerulonephritis.

Strike a balance

Maintain proper electrolyte balance by:
• strictly monitoring potassium levels
• watching for symptoms of hyperkalemia (malaise, anorexia, paresthesia, or muscle weakness)
• monitoring for and immediately reporting electrocardiogram (ECG) changes (tall, peaked T waves; widening QRS segment; and disappearing P waves)
• avoiding medications containing potassium. (See *Managing the child with hyperkalemia.*)

Follow through on the follow-up

In addition, the importance of long-term follow-up, including frequent visits to the child's health care provider should be stressed to the parents. They should also be informed that follow-up renal biopsies will be needed every 2 to 5 years. If renal failure occurs,

---

Advice from the experts

Managing the child with hyperkalemia

Emergency treatment is needed for the child with acute hyperkalemia (a serum potassium level higher than 7 mEq/L or ECG changes). Hypertonic glucose, insulin, and calcium gluconate may be administered because they provide a rapid, although temporary, reduction in potassium. However, these infusions won't remove potassium from the body. They may be used until a slower acting agent, such as sodium polystyrene sulfonate (Kayexalate), can be administered. Kayexalate can be administered orally or rectally to bind potassium and remove it from the body.

During emergency treatment to lower potassium levels, assess the patient frequently.
• If the child receives hypertonic glucose and insulin infusions, monitor potassium and glucose levels.
• If the child receives calcium gluconate, monitor calcium and potassium levels.
• If Kayexalate is given rectally, make sure the child doesn't retain it and become constipated (to prevent bowel perforation).

the child and parents should be prepared for the possibility of an eventual kidney transplant.

Congenital anomalies of the ureter, bladder, and urethra

Congenital anomalies of the ureter, bladder, and urethra are among the most common birth defects, occurring in about 5% of births. Some of these abnormalities are obvious at birth; others are recognized only after they produce symptoms.

What causes it

Causes of these congenital anomalies are unknown.

How it happens

The most common malformations include duplicated ureter, retrocaval ureter, ectopic orifice of the ureter, stricture or stenosis of the ureter, ureterocele, bladder exstrophy, congenital bladder diverticulum, hypospadias, and epispadias. Their pathophysiology, signs and symptoms, diagnosis, and treatments vary. (See *Congenital urologic anomalies.*)

What to look for

Signs and symptoms will vary. (See *Congenital urologic anomalies.*)

What tests tell you

With the exception of bladder exstrophy, hypospadias, and epispadias (which can be diagnosed on clinical examination), diagnostic tests are used to visualize the defect.

Complications

Complications will vary according to the specific anomaly but may include UTI, vesicoureteral reflux, voiding dysfunction, and hydronephrosis.

How it's treated

Surgical repair is needed. The specific procedure will depend on the anomaly. (See *Congenital urologic anomalies.*)

Congenital urologic anomalies

Three congenital urologic anomalies are described here, along with their pathophysiology, clinical features, and diagnosis and treatment.

Duplicated ureter	**Retrocaval ureter (preureteral vena cava)**	**Ectopic orifice of ureter**

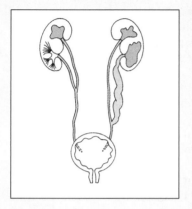 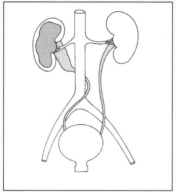 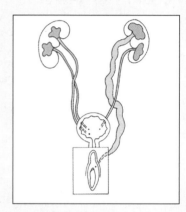

Pathophysiology
- Most common ureteral anomaly
- Complete—double-collecting system with two separate pelves, each with its own ureter and orifice
- Incomplete—two separate ureters that join before entering the bladder

Clinical features
- Persistent or recurrent infection
- Frequency, urgency, or burning on urination
- Diminished urine output
- Flank pain, fever, and chills

Diagnosis and treatment
- Excretory urography
- Voiding cystoscopy
- Cystoureterography
- Retrograde pyelography
- Surgery for obstruction, reflux, or severe renal damage

Pathophysiology
- Right ureter that passes behind the inferior vena cava before entering the bladder (with compression of the ureter between the vena cava and the spine that causes dilation and elongation of the pelvis, hydroureter, hydronephrosis, and fibrosis and stenosis of the ureter in the compressed area)
- Relatively uncommon; higher incidence in males

Clinical features
- Right flank pain
- Recurrent UTI
- Renal calculi
- Hematuria

Diagnosis and treatment
- Excretory urography demonstrating superior ureteral enlargement with spiral appearance
- Surgical resection and anastomosis of the ureter with the renal pelvis or reimplantation into the bladder

Pathophysiology
- Ureters single or duplicated in females (ureteral orifice usually inserting in urethra or vaginal vestibule, beyond external urethral sphincter)
- In males, in prostatic urethra, seminal vesicles, or vas deferens

Clinical features
- Symptoms rare if ureteral orifice opening between trigone and bladder neck
- Obstruction, reflux, and incontinence (dribbling) in 50% of females
- In males, flank pain, frequency, urgency

Diagnosis and treatment
- Excretory urography
- Urethroscopy, vaginoscopy
- Voiding cystourethrography
- Resection and ureteral reimplantation into the bladder for incontinence

What to do

Because these anomalies aren't always obvious at birth, carefully evaluate the neonate's urogenital function. Document the amount and color of urine, voiding pattern, strength of stream, and indications of infection, such as fever and urine odor.

Neighborhood watch

Tell parents to watch for these signs at home. In all children, watch for signs of obstruction, such as dribbling, oliguria or anuria, abdominal mass, hypertension, fever, bacteriuria, or pyuria.

When caring for the hospitalized child, follow these steps:
• Monitor renal function daily; record intake and output accurately; weigh diapers if necessary.
• Follow strict sterile technique in handling cystostomy tubes or indwelling urinary catheters.
• Make sure that ureteral, suprapubic, or urethral catheters remain in place and don't become contaminated; document type, color, and amount of drainage.
• Apply sterile saline pads to protect the exposed mucosa of the neonate with bladder exstrophy; don't use heavy clamps on the umbilical cord and avoid dressing or diapering the infant.

Moistening mist

• Place the infant with exstrophy in an Isolette, and direct a stream of saline mist onto the bladder to keep it moist; use warm water and mild soap to keep the surrounding skin clean, rinse well, and keep the area as dry as possible to prevent excoriation.
• Provide reassurance and emotional support to the parents and, when possible, allow them to participate in their child's care to promote normal bonding.
• As appropriate, suggest or arrange for genetic counseling.

Hemolytic uremic syndrome

HUS is a complex of symptoms that includes acute renal failure, hemolytic anemia, and thrombocytopenia. It's an acute renal disease that occurs mostly in infants and children from age 6 months to 3 years. It's one of the main causes of acute renal failure in the young child, with severity of symptoms ranging anywhere from subclinical to life-threatening.

What causes it

In pediatrics, the most common cause of HUS is an infection with a specific strain of *Escherichia coli*, usually the strain known as O157:H7. Such *E. coli* may be found in contaminated meat or produce and in swimming pools or lakes contaminated with feces.

The usual suspects

HUS usually follows an attack of infectious bacterial diarrhea caused by *E. coli*, *Shigella*, *Salmonella*, *Yersinia*, or *Campylobacter*. Viral infections, such as varicella, echovirus, and coxsackie A and B, may also cause it. Occasionally, HUS can appear, with no associated diarrhea. HUS may follow an upper respiratory infection and may be associated with such long-term illnesses as acquired immunodeficiency syndrome (AIDS) and cancer.

We cannot tell a lie. One of us is usually the culprit in a case of hemolytic uremic syndrome.

How it happens

The bacterial infection causes endothelial cell injury in the lining of the small glomerular arterioles. The endothelial cell damage triggers microvascular lesions with platelet-fibrin microthrombi that occlude the arterioles and capillaries. This platelet aggregation results in thrombocytopenia, and the kidneys become swollen and pale.

Although damage occurs mainly in the endothelial lining of the glomerular arterioles, other organs may be involved. Cardiac involvement may include heart failure and arrhythmias. Pancreatitis or type 1 diabetes mellitus may occur from pancreatic involvement. Ocular involvement may include retinal or vitreous hemorrhage.

What to look for

The patient's history typically shows a recent episode of diarrhea. Less commonly, there may be a history of upper respiratory tract infection or viral infection. Signs and symptoms may include:
- irritability, weakness, lethargy
- pallor
- fatigue
- dehydration
- edema
- ecchymosis and petechiae, purpura
- decreased or absent urine output (oliguria or anuria)
- hypertension
- gastrointestinal (GI) bleeding with blood in stool
- seizures
- heart failure.

What tests tell you

A urinalysis shows the presence of protein and RBCs, hemosiderin, WBCs, and casts.

In the blood

Blood studies show:
• microangiopathic hemolytic anemia (severe) and mild to moderate thrombocytopenia
• prothrombin time, activated partial thromboplastin time, and fibrinogen levels within normal ranges
• elevated lactate dehydrogenase and indirect bilirubin levels
• markedly elevated BUN and creatinine levels
• increased reticulocyte count
• negative Coombs' test
• moderately elevated WBC count
• plasma containing free hemoglobin, the concentration of which coincides with the degree of the anemia.

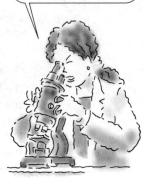

Blood work is the mainstay of diagnostic testing in a child with suspected hemolytic uremic syndrome.

I got cultcha

Other studies may include a stool culture, which may be positive for a specific type of *E. coli*. Bone marrow biopsy shows hyperplasia. Renal biopsy would clinically establish the diagnosis but is rarely required.

Complications

Complications of HUS may include:
• hypertension
• acute renal failure
• chronic renal failure
• need for hemodialysis
• neurologic deficits with seizures and coma
• stroke
• bleeding complications such as disseminated intravascular coagulation (DIC).

How it's treated

Antibiotics aren't effective in treating HUS, except when caused by *Shigella dysenteriae*. Treatment of HUS may include:
• daily plasma exchange until remission is achieved (in severe cases)
• maintenance of adequate fluid and electrolyte balance and correction of acidosis to prevent seizures and azotemia. In the early stages, the child should be given fluids *without* potassium.
• corticosteroids and aspirin
• early dialysis if fluid overload, hyperkalemia, hyponatremia, or other signs of acute renal failure occur

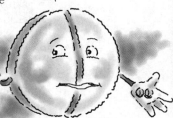

Sorry. Antibiotics aren't effective for hemolytic uremic syndrome unless *Shigella dysenteriae* is to blame.

- management of hypertension with antihypertensive medications and, if needed, fluid and salt restriction
- eculizumab (Soliris) for atypical HUS cases
- maintenance of optimal nutritional status.

What to do

Monitoring and maintaining fluid and electrolyte balance is important. Intake and output should be accurately recorded, and the child's weight should be recorded once or twice daily during the acute phase.

- Monitor blood pressure and pulse pressure at least every 4 hours.
- Assess hydration status at least every 4 to 6 hours.
- Monitor the child's nutritional status.
- Observe and report signs and symptoms of complications, such as seizures, shock, infection, and DIC.
- Prepare the child and his family for the possibility of hemodialysis or peritoneal dialysis.
- Teach the parents and child to avoid eating raw or partially cooked meat or drinking untreated water to decrease the risk of infection with *E. coli*.

Nephrotic syndrome

Nephrotic syndrome is a condition in which the kidneys lose a significant amount of protein in the urine, resulting in low blood levels of protein. The syndrome is characterized by proteinuria, hypoalbuminemia, hyperlipidemia, and edema. The prognosis is highly variable depending on the underlying cause.

Preschool predominance

Primary nephrotic syndrome occurs predominantly in preschool children; the incidence peaks between ages 2 and 3, and the syndrome is rare after age 8. It's more common in boys than in girls. Some forms of nephrotic syndrome may eventually progress to end-stage renal disease.

What causes it

Causes of nephrotic syndrome include:
- lipid nephrosis
- glomerulonephritis
- metabolic diseases such as diabetes mellitus
- collagen-vascular disorders such as SLE
- circulatory diseases, such as heart failure, sickle cell anemia, and renal vein thrombosis
- nephrotoxins, such as mercury, gold, and bismuth
- allergic reactions.

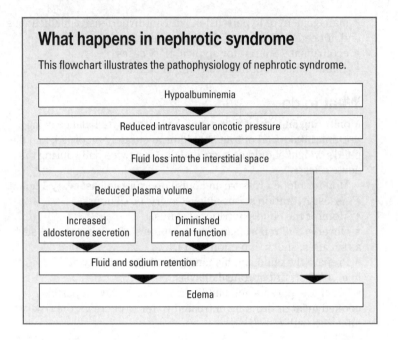

What happens in nephrotic syndrome

This flowchart illustrates the pathophysiology of nephrotic syndrome.

Hypoalbuminemia

Reduced intravascular oncotic pressure

Fluid loss into the interstitial space

Reduced plasma volume

Increased aldosterone secretion

Diminished renal function

Fluid and sodium retention

Edema

How it happens

In nephrotic syndrome, the injured glomerular filtration membrane allows the loss of plasma proteins, especially albumin and immunoglobulin, resulting in decreased levels of serum albumin (hypoalbuminemia). Hypoalbuminemia results in decreased colloidal osmotic pressure and fluid accumulation in the interstitial spaces. Edema subsequently results from sodium and water retention. (See *What happens in nephrotic syndrome.*)

What to look for

Signs and symptoms of nephrotic syndrome include:
• oliguria with dark, concentrated urine
• edema starting around the eyes (periorbital) and then becoming more generalized
• weight gain
• abdominal distention, which may be so severe that it causes respiratory difficulty, abdominal pain, anorexia, and diarrhea
• irritability
• lethargy, easy fatigability, and activity intolerance
• pallor
• hypertension (in later stages).

What tests tell you

Urinalysis shows severe proteinuria, hematuria, and casts; it also shows an elevated specific gravity because of the proteinuria. When performed, renal biopsy identifies the type of nephrotic syndrome the child has and can be used to monitor response to medical management.

Highs and lows

Blood studies show:
• high levels of lipids, especially cholesterol (hypercholesterolemia)
• low levels of protein, especially albumin
• normal to high hematocrit and hemoglobin level
• high platelet levels.

Complications

Complications of nephrotic syndrome may include:
• hypovolemic shock
• venous thrombosis
• respiratory difficulties
• impaired skin integrity from severe edema
• infection
• loss of proteins required to fight infections, resulting in increased risk of infections
• loss of proteins that prevent blood from clotting, resulting in clot formation within the blood vessels
• adverse effects of steroid therapy.

How it's treated

Prednisone commonly produces a rapid improvement in symptoms (remission). I.V. administration of albumin may be used, followed by I.V. furosemide (Lasix), to induce diuresis. If marked hypertension exists, antihypertensive medications may be used. Other medications may include:
• pain medication to lessen discomfort
• prophylactic antibiotics to control and prevent infection
• immunosuppressive medications for children who don't respond to steroids.

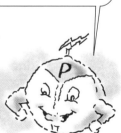

Prednisone is my name—nephrotic syndrome remission is my game!

Hold the salt

Dietary changes may include some restriction of salt intake. Bed rest may be required during the acute phase, especially when the child is hypertensive.

What to do

The child with nephrotic syndrome is likely to require multiple hospitalizations. Because these hospitalizations interrupt the child's normal routine, it's important to provide him with activities that support his continued development, and simply allow him to have fun.

A delicate balance

Other interventions focus on monitoring and assessment:
• Maintain fluid balance and monitor for signs of fluid volume excess, such as edema, ascites, weight gain, decreased and concentrated urine, and pulmonary congestion.
• Assess for signs of electrolyte imbalance—cardiovascular, neurologic, GI, and skin changes—and work with the health care providers to correct imbalances that may exist.
• Assess general nutritional status and work to improve it by providing a diet the child will eat (with sufficient protein and other nutrients and without excess sodium). Parents can help with this, too, by bringing in food from home that the child likes, as long as it fits within the child's dietary restrictions.
• Assess for adverse effects of medications, and report them to the health care provider as soon as possible.

Protection from infection

• Assess for signs of infection and work to prevent it; if infection occurs, report it as soon as possible.
• Monitor for pain and provide appropriate pain relief measures.
• Provide emotional support and education to the child and parents.

Renal failure, acute

Renal failure is a general term used to describe what happens when the kidneys aren't functioning at an optimum level. In *acute* renal failure, the kidneys suddenly stop filtering waste products from the blood.

What causes it

Most commonly, acute renal failure in children is a temporary condition resulting from dehydration or other condition that causes poor renal perfusion (which can be resolved by increasing the child's fluid volume). The causes of acute renal failure may be classified as prerenal, intrarenal, or postrenal. (See *Causes of acute renal failure.*)

Causes of acute renal failure

The causes of acute renal failure may be classified as prerenal, intrarenal, or postrenal.

Prerenal

Prerenal causes, which are most common in children, may include:
- arrhythmias that cause reduced cardiac output
- heart failure
- burns
- dehydration
- diuretic overuse, hemorrhage, hypovolemic shock
- disseminated intravascular coagulation
- sepsis.

Intrarenal

Intrarenal causes of acute renal failure include:
- poorly treated prerenal failure
- nephrotoxins
- transfusion reaction
- acute glomerulonephritis, acute interstitial nephritis, or acute pyelonephritis
- sickle cell anemia
- SLE.

Postrenal

Postrenal causes of renal failure are uncommon in children older than age 1 year. They may include:
- bladder obstruction
- ureteral obstruction
- urethral obstruction.

How it happens

The pathophysiology of acute renal failure varies depending on whether the cause is prerenal, intrarenal, or postrenal.

Prerenal failure

Prerenal failure ensues when a condition that diminishes blood flow to the kidneys leads to hypoperfusion.

It's rude to interrupt

When renal blood flow is interrupted, so is oxygen delivery. The ensuing hypoxemia and ischemia can rapidly and irreversibly damage the kidney. The renal tubules are most susceptible to hypoxemia's effects.

Azotemia (excess nitrogenous waste products in the blood) develops in 40% to 80% of patients with acute renal failure and is also a consequence of renal hypoperfusion. The impaired blood flow results in a decreased GFR and increased tubular resorption of sodium and water. Usually, restoring renal blood flow and glomerular filtration reverses azotemia.

Intrarenal failure

Intrarenal failure, also called *intrinsic* or *parenchymal renal failure*, results from damage to the filtering structures of the kidneys. Causes of intrarenal failure are classified as *nephrotoxic*, *inflammatory*, or *ischemic*.

Damage in the basement

When the damage is caused by nephrotoxicity or inflammation, the delicate layer under the epithelium (the basement membrane) becomes irreparably damaged, typically leading to chronic renal failure.

Severe or prolonged lack of blood flow caused by ischemia may lead to renal damage (ischemic parenchymal injury) and excess nitrogen in the blood (intrinsic renal azotemia).

Totally radical

Acute tubular necrosis is the precursor of intrarenal failure; it can result from ischemic damage to renal parenchyma during unrecognized or poorly treated prerenal failure. The ischemic tissue generates toxic, oxygen-free radicals, which cause swelling, injury, and necrosis.

Postrenal failure

Bilateral obstruction of urine outflow leads to postrenal failure. The obstruction may be in the bladder, ureters, or urethra.

What to look for

Acute renal failure is a critical illness in children. Its early signs are oliguria, azotemia, and, rarely, anuria.

System alert

Electrolyte imbalance, metabolic acidosis, and other severe effects follow as the patient becomes increasingly uremic and renal dysfunction disrupts other body systems:
• *GI*—anorexia, nausea, vomiting, diarrhea or constipation, stomatitis, bleeding, hematemesis, dry mucous membranes, uremic breath
• *central nervous system*—headache, drowsiness, irritability, confusion, peripheral neuropathy, seizures, coma
• *cutaneous*—dryness, pruritus, pallor, purpura, and, rarely, uremic frost
• *cardiovascular*—hypotension (early in the course of the disease), hypertension (later in the course of the disease), arrhythmias, fluid overload, heart failure, systemic edema, anemia, altered clotting mechanisms
• *respiratory*—pulmonary edema, Kussmaul's respirations.

What tests tell you

• Blood studies show elevated BUN, serum creatinine, and potassium levels; decreased sodium, calcium, bicarbonate, and hemoglobin levels; decreased hematocrit; and low blood pH.

• Urine studies show casts, cellular debris, and decreased specific gravity; in glomerular diseases, proteinuria and increased urine osmolality.
• ECG shows changes associated with electrolyte imbalance and heart failure.
• Ultrasound of the kidney shows the size of the kidneys and may reveal the presence of a tumor, cyst, or urinary tract obstruction.
• Excretory urography demonstrates the appearance of the kidney structure and, possibly, the presence of obstruction.

Complications

Renal failure affects many body processes. Complications may include fluid volume overload, arrhythmias or seizures from electrolyte imbalance, heart failure, hypertension or hypotension, tachypnea, pulmonary edema, infection, skin breakdown, malnutrition, or development of chronic renal failure.

How it's treated

The key to managing acute renal failure is prevention. For children with dehydration or any type of fluid loss, fluid volume should be restored as soon as possible to prevent disruption of perfusion to the kidneys. Caution should be exercised whenever nephrotoxic drugs are used in the pediatric population. Treatment of acute renal failure may include:
• diet high in carbohydrates and fats and low in protein, sodium, and potassium to meet metabolic needs
• fluid restriction
• careful monitoring of electrolytes and fluid status; I.V. therapy to maintain and correct fluid and electrolyte balance
• diuretic therapy with Lasix or mannitol (Osmitrol) to treat oliguria
• Kayexalate by mouth or enema to reverse hyperkalemia with mild symptoms (malaise, loss of appetite, muscle weakness); hypertonic glucose, insulin, and sodium bicarbonate I.V. for more severe hyperkalemic symptoms (numbness and tingling and ECG changes)
• antihypertensives to control elevated blood pressure
• blood products as needed to control anemia or reverse effects of bleeding
• hemodialysis or peritoneal dialysis (occasionally required).

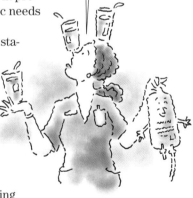

Fluid and electrolyte balance is essential for the child with renal failure.

What to do

Care of the child with acute renal failure includes careful monitoring and dietary education. The child and parents will need emotional support and reassurance, with clear explanations of all procedures.

No fluid shall go unmeasured

Measure and record intake and output, including body fluids, such as wound drainage, nasogastric output, and diarrhea; weigh the child daily. Monitor vital signs; watch for and report signs of inadequate renal perfusion (hypotension) and acidosis.

Maintain proper electrolyte balance by:
• strictly monitoring potassium levels
• watching for symptoms of hyperkalemia (malaise, anorexia, paresthesia, or muscle weakness)
• monitoring for and immediately reporting ECG changes (tall, peaked T waves; widening QRS segment; and disappearing P waves)
• avoid administering medications containing potassium.

Monitor and maintain

Other interventions focus on monitoring and maintaining nutritional status and preventing infection:
• Maintain nutritional status; provide a high-calorie, low-protein, low-sodium, and low-potassium diet with vitamin supplements. (Give the anorexic child small, frequent meals.)
• Use sterile technique because the child with acute renal failure is highly susceptible to infection; don't allow personnel with upper respiratory tract infections to care for the child and limit visitors who have symptoms of infection.
• Use guaiac tests to monitor stools for blood, a sign of GI bleeding.

Renal failure, chronic

Chronic renal failure is usually the end result of gradual tissue destruction and loss of renal function. It can also result from a rapidly progressing disease of sudden onset that destroys the nephrons and causes irreversible kidney damage.

Few symptoms develop until less than 25% of glomerular filtration remains. The normal parenchyma then deteriorates rapidly and symptoms worsen as renal function decreases. End-stage renal disease is the final stage of chronic renal failure. This disorder is fatal without treatment, but maintenance on dialysis (either hemodialysis or peritoneal dialysis) or kidney transplantation can sustain life.

What causes it

Chronic renal failure may be caused by:
• chronic glomerular disease (glomerulonephritis)
• chronic infection (such as chronic pyelonephritis)
• congenital anomalies (renal hypoplasia and dysplasia, obstructive uropathy)
• vascular disease (hypertension, nephrosclerosis)
• collagen disease (SLE)
• nephrotoxic agents (long-term aminoglycoside therapy).

How it happens

Chronic renal failure commonly progresses through four stages:

When renal reserve is reduced, GFR is 35% to 50% of normal function.

With renal insufficiency, GFR is 20% to 35% of normal function.

In renal failure, GFR is 20% to 25% of normal function.

In end-stage renal disease, GFR is less than 20% of normal function.

The point of no return

Nephron damage is progressive; damaged nephrons can't function and don't recover. The kidneys maintain relatively normal function until about 75% of the nephrons are nonfunctional. Surviving nephrons hypertrophy and increase their rate of filtration, reabsorption, and secretion. Compensatory excretion continues as GFR diminishes.

Toxin takeover

Eventually, the healthy nephrons and glomeruli are so overburdened that they become sclerotic, stiff, and necrotic. Toxins accumulate and potentially fatal changes ensue in all major organ systems. (See *Effects of chronic renal failure*, page 406.)

What to look for

In the early stages, the child may be asymptomatic (until normal kidney function has declined to 20% or less). The first signs are usually lethargy and fatigue. Progressing signs and symptoms may include:
• hypertension
• growth retardation evidenced by the child falling behind on growth charts
• edema

Effects of chronic renal failure

In addition to the retention of waste products, chronic renal failure may produce other physiologic changes; the presence and severity of these manifestations depend on the duration of renal failure and its response to treatment.

Hyperkalemia and acidosis

In early renal insufficiency, acid excretion and phosphate reabsorption increase to maintain normal pH. When the GFR decreases by 30% to 40%, progressive metabolic acidosis ensues (characteristic of chronic renal failure) and tubular secretion of potassium increases. Total-body potassium levels may increase to life-threatening levels, requiring dialysis.

Bone demineralization

Demineralization of the bone (renal osteodystrophy or renal rickets) manifested by bone pain and pathologic fractures is due to several factors:
• Decreased renal activation of vitamin D decreases absorption of dietary calcium.
• Retention of phosphate increases loss of calcium in urine (which decreases serum calcium levels).
• Decreased urinary excretion causes an increase in parathyroid hormone circulation.

Anemia

Anemia and platelet disorders with prolonged bleeding time ensue as diminished erythropoietin secretion leads to reduced RBC production in the bone marrow. Uremic toxins associated with chronic renal failure shorten RBC survival time. The patient may experience lethargy and dizziness.

Growth and hormonal alterations

Growth retardation induced by renal failure is one of the most profound effects on children. Its cause isn't clearly understood.

All hormone levels are impaired in excretion and activation, which may delay sexual maturation or prevent it from occurring. This impairment may also cause anovulation or amenorrhea in females and impaired spermatogenesis in males.

Skin changes

The skin of a child with chronic renal failure acquires a grayish-yellow tint as urine pigments (urochromes) accumulate. Inflammatory mediators released by retained toxins in the skin cause pruritus. Uric acid and other substances in the sweat crystallize and accumulate on the skin as uremic frost. High plasma calcium levels are also associated with pruritus.

Infection

Chronic renal failure increases the risk of death from infection. Children with chronic renal failure are at high risk for infection related to suppression of cell-mediated immunity and a reduction in the number and function of lymphocytes and phagocytes.

• signs of fluid overload, evidenced by abnormal heart and breath sounds and shortness of breath
• "uremic" odor on the breath
• anorexia, nausea, and vomiting
• general malaise
• headache
• generalized pruritus
• increased or decreased urine output, nocturia, enuresis
• easy bruising or bleeding
• decreased level of alertness, poor school performance
• muscle cramps and twitching
• seizures
• decreased sensation, especially in the hands or feet.

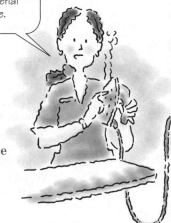

Decreased sensation in the hands may be a sign of chronic renal failure.

What tests tell you

Blood tests reveal:
- anemia that doesn't respond to oral iron therapy
- reduced levels of platelets
- elevated serum creatinine and BUN levels
- elevated potassium, sodium, calcium, and phosphorus levels
- metabolic acidosis.

What's in urine

Urine tests reveal:
- RBCs or casts in the urine
- alterations in urine electrolyte levels and specific gravity.

The also-rans

Other studies may include:
- ECG, which shows changes associated with electrolyte imbalances
- KUB, excretory urography, nephrotomography, renal scan, or renal arteriography (all of which show reduced kidney size)
- renal biopsy to identify underlying disease
- electroencephalogram (EEG) to identify metabolic encephalopathy.

Complications

Possible complications of chronic renal failure include:
- fluid and electrolyte imbalances
- arrhythmias
- heart failure, pulmonary edema
- respiratory failure
- seizures
- altered level of consciousness
- malnutrition, failure to thrive
- altered growth and sexual maturation
- bone pain and fractures
- skin breakdown
- progressive renal insufficiency.

How it's treated

Treatment of chronic renal failure involves:
- sodium and potassium limitations
- protein restricted only to the recommended daily allowance for children (because further protein restrictions may impede growth and neurodevelopment)
- fluid restrictions and diuretics to maintain fluid balance
- antihypertensives to control blood pressure and edema

• calcium carbonate (Caltrate) or calcium acetate (PhosLo) to treat renal osteodystrophy by binding to phosphate and supplementing calcium
• antiemetics to relieve nausea and vomiting
• iron and folate supplements and an iron- and folic acid–rich diet for anemia and, possibly, transfusion of RBCs if needed
• synthetic erythropoietin (Epogen) to stimulate the bone marrow to produce RBCs
• antipruritics such as diphenhydramine (Benadryl) to relieve itching
• supplementary vitamins, particularly B and D, and essential amino acids
• dialysis for hyperkalemia and fluid imbalances
• oral or rectal administration of cation exchange resins, such as Kayexalate, and I.V. administration of calcium gluconate, sodium bicarbonate, 50% dextrose, or regular insulin to reverse hyperkalemia
• peritoneal dialysis or hemodialysis to help control end-stage renal disease
• kidney transplantation (usually the treatment of choice if a donor is available).

What to do

Provide emotional support to the child and family and help them deal with the diagnosis and prognosis. They should be encouraged to express their feelings and to ask questions.

Because chronic renal failure has such widespread clinical effects, it requires meticulous and carefully coordinated supportive care.

In with the moisture, out with the itch

Good skin care is important. Bathe the child daily using superfatted soaps and oatmeal baths, and use skin lotion without alcohol to ease pruritus. Glycerin-containing soaps shouldn't be used because they cause skin drying.

Good oral hygiene is also important. Brush the child's teeth often with a soft brush or sponge tip to reduce breath odor. Sugarless hard candy and mouthwash minimize the metallic taste in the mouth and alleviate thirst.

The child should be given small, palatable meals that are also nutritious; try to provide favorite foods within dietary restrictions.

It's not just for breakfast anymore! A little oatmeal in the bath water keeps skin moist and eases the itch.

Other interventions focus on careful monitoring.
• Watch for hyperkalemia; observe for diarrhea and cramping of the legs and abdomen.
• As potassium levels rise, watch for muscle irritability and a weak pulse.
• Monitor for ECG changes.
• Assess hydration status carefully; measure daily intake and output carefully, including drainage, emesis, diarrhea, and blood loss. (Record daily weight, presence or absence of thirst, dryness of tongue, hypertension, and peripheral edema.)
• Monitor for bone or joint complications.
• Maintain strict sterile technique and watch for signs of infection (high fever, leukocytosis).
• Observe for signs of bleeding. Monitor hemoglobin levels and hematocrit and check stools, urine, and vomitus for blood.

Wilms' tumor

Wilms' tumor, also called *nephroblastoma*, is the most common form of kidney cancer in children as well as the most common intra-abdominal tumor in children. The average age at diagnosis is 2 to 4 years. The tumor favors the left kidney and is usually unilateral. It can remain encapsulated for a long time, and prognosis is excellent if metastasis hasn't occurred.

What causes it

Studies have shown an increased risk in children with specific chromosomal abnormalities. Wilms' tumor has also been associated with several congenital anomalies including hypospadias and cryptorchidism.

How it happens

Wilms' tumor is an embryonal cancer of the kidney originating during fetal life. In the early stages, the tumor is well encapsulated, but it may later spread into the lymph nodes, renal vein, or vena cava; metastasis to the lungs or other sites may occur.

Life is but a stage

The tumor is staged to determine the best treatment:
• *Stage I*—The tumor is limited to one kidney.
• *Stage II*—The tumor extends beyond the kidney but can be completely excised.
• *Stage III*—The tumor has spread but is confined to the abdomen and lymph nodes.

- *Stage IV*—The tumor has metastasized to the lung, liver, bone, and brain.
- *Stage V*—The tumor involves both kidneys.

What to look for

The child usually has a nontender abdominal mass, commonly first identified by the parents during bathing or dressing or by a pediatrician during a routine physical examination. The mass can be palpated in the region of the lower abdomen and is usually confined to one side. Other signs and symptoms may include an enlarged abdomen, hypertension, vomiting, hematuria, anemia, and constipation.

What tests tell you

- Ultrasound will determine if the mass originated within the kidney and if the mass is a solid tumor.
- CT scan or magnetic resonance imaging will determine the extent of the tumor and whether it has spread to other organs.
- Excretory urography assesses function of the unaffected kidney.
- Chest X-ray and CT scan of the chest will determine if the tumor has metastasized to the lungs.

Complications

Recurrence of Wilms' tumor may occur in several sites, such as the lungs, liver, and the surgical area. Other complications may include:

- musculoskeletal defects from radiation therapy
- possible development of other (metastatic) cancers in the bones, breast, and thyroid
- decreased fertility, especially after radiation therapy
- renal failure.

> Phhhew! That was close. After surgery for bilateral Wilms' tumor, my partner and I were spared!

How it's treated

Most commonly, treatment involves surgical removal of the entire affected kidney (radical nephrectomy). Exploratory surgery of the lymph nodes and the liver may be performed at the same time to determine if the tumor has spread outside the kidney.

Keep the kidney

If the tumor is bilateral, neither kidney is removed during the initial surgery. Rather, a biopsy of the tumor is taken to help determine the tumor type. Chemotherapy will reduce the size of bilateral tumors. Later, with bilateral tumors, the child has further surgery, removing just the tumors and a portion of the kidneys, saving most of both kidneys to maintain kidney function.

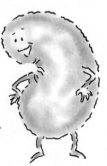

Chemotherapy is typically administered after nephrectomy. In addition, radiation therapy may be used, as it has been found to improve survival rates.

What to do

A great deal of emotional support is needed for the child and parents dealing with this diagnosis. The child should be thoroughly prepared for treatments and procedures, including surgeries, chemotherapy, and radiation and their adverse effects. The nurse should serve as an advocate for the child and his parents, making certain that questions are answered and concerns are addressed in a timely fashion.

In addition, follow these steps:

• Keep in mind that a Wilms' tumor is very soft, and the capsule can easily rupture before or during surgery; if this happens, there can be rapid metastasis to other organs.

• Make sure that after the diagnosis is suspected or confirmed, there's absolutely no further palpation of the abdomen because this can cause rupture of the capsule.

• Tell the parents and the child that he may need frequent imaging of the remaining kidney to detect recurrence of the tumor.

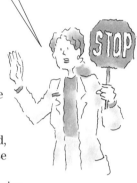

Stop—don't palpate! Abdominal palpation can rupture the surrounding capsule of Wilms' tumor, causing distant metastasis.

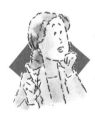

Quick quiz

1. The main functioning unit of the kidney is the:
   A.   renal cortex.
   B.   renal medulla.
   C.   nephron.
   D.   ureter.

Answer: C. The nephron, located within the renal medulla, is the main functional unit of the kidney; it filters out waste products and excess water, forming urine.

2. An X-ray done with I.V. contrast media to show the structure of the urinary system is called:
   A.   KUB.
   B.   excretory urography.
   C.   VCUG.
   D.   renal biopsy.

Answer: B. In excretory urography, I.V. contrast medium is injected, and then X-rays are taken to visualize the structures of the entire urinary elimination system.

3. A child has decreased output of pink-tinged urine, facial edema, and a history of a sore throat "a little while ago." The nurse anticipates the doctor will be evaluating the child for:

    A. cryptorchidism.

    B. adverse effects of hemodialysis.

    C. HUS.

    D. acute poststreptococcal glomerulonephritis.

Answer: D. Pink-tinged urine, facial edema, and a history of a sore throat are the typical signs and symptoms of acute poststreptococcal glomerulonephritis.

4. A child is admitted to the pediatric unit with a new diagnosis of nephrotic syndrome. Which set of symptoms would the nurse expect to see?

    A. Periorbital edema, polyuria, proteinuria, and hyperproteinemia

    B. Hypercholesterolemia, hypoproteinemia, proteinuria, and periorbital edema

    C. Pedal edema, hypolipidemia, hematuria, and oliguria

    D. Hyperlipidemia, glycosuria, hyperproteinemia, and generalized edema

Answer: B. The four classic signs and symptoms of early stages of nephrotic syndrome are hypercholesterolemia, hypoproteinemia, proteinuria, and periorbital edema.

5. A child on the pediatric unit has a Wilms' tumor. One of the most important nursing functions for this child is to:

    A. prepare the parents for the possible loss of the child.

    B. maintain the child's fluid volume.

    C. ensure the child's nutritional status.

    D. make sure that no abdominal palpation is performed.

Answer: D. Remember that a Wilms' tumor is very soft and the capsule surrounding it can rupture easily, causing distant and potentially devastating metastasis to other organs.

Scoring

✰✰✰ If you answered all five items correctly, bravo! Your knowledge of urinary problems flows unobstructed.

✰✰ If you answered three or four items correctly, good for you! Take a potty break and read on.

✰ If you answered fewer than three items correctly, go with the flow! You'll breeze through the rest of your work.

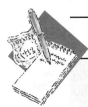

Musculoskeletal problems

Just the facts

In this chapter, you'll learn:

♦ basic anatomy and physiology of the musculoskeletal system

♦ common diagnostic tests for musculoskeletal problems

♦ orthopedic treatments and procedures

♦ selected musculoskeletal disorders in the pediatric population.

Anatomy and physiology

The musculoskeletal system is one of the most complex systems within the body. The muscles and bones allow the body to move and function. If a problem occurs in the musculoskeletal system, mobility and general activities of daily living may be impaired.

Bones

The body's form and function are supported by the skeletal system. The mature human skeleton is made up of 206 bones that are shaped according to their function. Newborn infants have over 300 bones, a number of which fuse together by the time a child is around 9 years old. The skeletal system:
• enables movement of the body by supporting soft tissues
• provides support and allows a person to stand erect
• protects underlying organs
• serves as a reservoir for storing such minerals as calcium and phosphorus
• serves as a site for red blood cell formation.

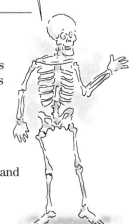

I support the body's form and function—no bones about it! (Actually, 206 bones, to be exact.)

The long and short of it

Long bones are found in the upper and lower extremities. They're responsible for carrying the body's weight and helping make ambulation possible. Short bones are found in the hands and feet and are shaped to provide strength in a compact area. Some bones, such as the ribs and sternum, are flat and thin; they provide structure. Other bones are large and irregularly shaped (for example, the pelvic bone).

Universal coverage

The composition of bone differs depending on the type of bone, but all are covered by a double layer of connective tissue, called the *periosteum*, which helps provide nourishment to the bone. In children, the periosteum is thick and vascular, so a child's bone tends to heal faster than that of an adult with the same injury.

Bone growth and formation

The epiphysis is the growth end of the long bones. The epiphyseal plate, or *growth plate*, is located in the epiphysis.

A plate of cartilage

The epiphyseal plate is composed of cartilage cells that grow and develop, thereby causing the bone to lengthen. The growth plate is gradually replaced by bone until only the epiphyseal line remains. When the plate is completely replaced by bone, the bones can no longer lengthen; they can only increase in breadth. Injury to the growth plate may seriously impede bone growth. Children are particularly susceptible to growth plate injuries.

Cartilage serves as a smooth surface for articulating bones. Because young children have a more cartilaginous skeleton, they may be less prone to severe fractures than adults.

Salty framework

Ossification is the process of developing new bones from tissue. Osteoblasts form bone cells that lay down a framework for the new bone. Calcium and phosphorus combine to form salts, which are then deposited into the framework. The thyroid and parathyroid glands regulate this deposition. (See *Bone growth and remodeling*.)

Bone bank deposit

To maintain equilibrium, bone is deposited where it's needed within the skeletal system. If increased stress is placed on a certain bone, more bone is deposited. If there's no stress on the bone, part of the bone mass is reabsorbed.

Bone growth and remodeling

The ossification of cartilage into bone, or *osteogenesis*, begins at about week 9 of fetal development. The diaphyses (shaft) of long bones are formed by birth, and the epiphyses (growth end) begin to ossify around that time. The stages of growth and remodeling of the epiphyses of a long bone are shown in these illustrations.

Creation of an ossification center

At about the ninth month of fetal development, an ossification center develops in the epiphysis. Some cartilage cells enlarge and stimulate ossification of surrounding cells. The enlarged cells die, leaving small cavities. New cartilage continues to develop.

Osteoblasts form bone

Osteoblasts (bone-forming cells) begin to form bone on the remaining cartilage, creating the scaffolding or trabeculae network of cancellous (spongy) bone. Cartilage continues to form on the outer surfaces of the epiphysis and along the upper surface of the epiphyseal plate.

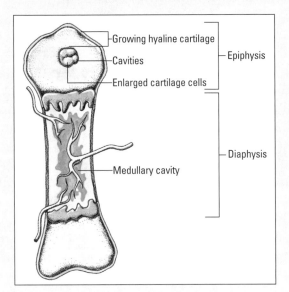

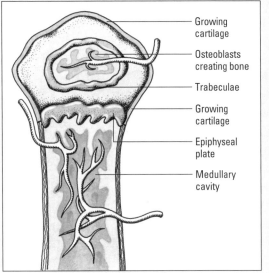

(continued)

Resorption is the process by which old bone is dissolved. The bone cells known as *osteocytes* and *osteoclasts* are responsible for the resorption of bone in this framework. This process can release calcium into the circulation.

Muscles

Muscles are the major organs that enable movement. They're fibrous bundles covered with thin connective tissue. They also serve as repositories for some metabolites. Muscles are

Bone growth and remodeling (continued)

Bone growth

Cartilage is replaced by compact bone near the outer surfaces of the epiphysis. Only cartilage cells on the upper surface of the diaphyseal plate continue to multiply rapidly, pushing the epiphysis away from the diaphysis. This new cartilage ossifies, creating trabeculae on the inner or medullary side of the epiphyseal plate.

Remodeling

Osteoclasts (cells associated with bone resorption) produce enzymes and acids that reduce trabeculae created by the epiphyseal plate, thus enlarging the medullary (bone marrow) cavity. In the epiphysis, osteoclasts reduce bone, making its calcium available for new osteoblasts that give the epiphysis its adult shape and proportion. In young adults, the epiphyseal plate completely ossifies (closes) and becomes the epiphyseal line; longitudinal growth of bone then ceases.

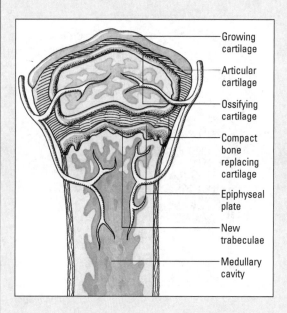

- Growing cartilage
- Articular cartilage
- Ossifying cartilage
- Compact bone replacing cartilage
- Epiphyseal plate
- New trabeculae
- Medullary cavity

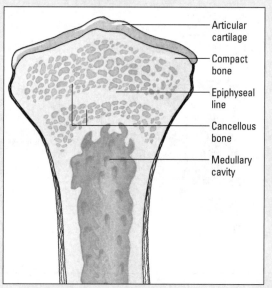

- Articular cartilage
- Compact bone
- Epiphyseal line
- Cancellous bone
- Medullary cavity

attached at each end directly to the bone or to a tendon, ligament, or fascia:

- *Tendons* hold muscles to bones and are formed by strong, non-elastic collagen cords.
- *Ligaments* hold bones to other bones; they encircle the joints and add strength and stability.
- The *fascia* is a fibrous membrane of supporting, connective tissue.

Muscles in opposition

The movement enabled by muscles occurs through the contracting and lengthening of opposing muscle groups. As a muscle shortens on contraction, it pulls the bones to which it's attached, bringing the bones closer together. Most muscles are attached to two bones that *articulate* (join or work together as a single unit) at an intervening joint.

Taking turns

For the most part, movement happens when one bone moves while the other is held stable. The body of the muscle that produces movement of the extremity usually lies proximal (closest) to the bone that's moved.

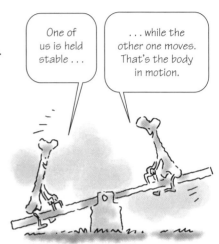

One of us is held stable . . .

. . . while the other one moves. That's the body in motion.

Six hundred volunteers

There are more than 600 *voluntary muscles* (muscles we control) in the body. These muscles are called *striated* or *skeletal muscles*. Other types of muscles include visceral muscles (also called *smooth* or *involuntary muscles*) and the cardiac muscle.

Joints

Joints are formed when two surfaces of bones come together and articulate.

Joints on the move

There are three types of joints, classified by the degree of movement:
- *Synarthrodial* (immovable) joints separate bone by a thin layer of cartilage—for example, the skull and various bones of the cranium.
- *Amphidiarthrodial* (semimovable) joints separate bone with cartilage or a fibrocartilaginous disk—for example, the joints between the vertebral bodies.
- *Diarthrodial* (freely movable) joints are commonly called *synovial joints*. Most joints in the body are synovial joints. They're lined with a membrane that secretes and lubricates the joint with synovial fluid—for example, the knees, shoulders, and hips. They're encased by the joint capsule, which is strengthened by ligaments that surround the capsule.

Flex or extend

Muscles are categorized according to the type of joint movement produced when the muscle is contracted. They're designated as flexor or extensor muscles depending on whether the joint is flexed or extended. Range of motion (ROM) is determined by the degree of movement in a joint. (See *Types of joint movement*, page 418.)

Diagnostic tests

Tests used to assess the musculoskeletal system and guide treatment include arthroscopy, bone scans, electromyography (EMG), muscle and bone marrow biopsy, and X-rays.

Arthroscopy

Arthroscopy is a surgical procedure used to visualize, diagnose, and treat problems inside a joint. It involves placing a fiber-optic instrument into the joint and then visualizing the area. Corrective surgery can be done at the same time, which helps eliminate the need for more extensive surgery.

The knee is the most common joint evaluated and treated with arthroscopy. It's most commonly done under a general anesthetic with younger children but can also be performed with a local or spinal anesthetic depending on the joint and the suspected problem.

Lean on me

There may be some swelling and pain after arthroscopy. With knee arthroscopy, the child may need to use crutches for 2 to 4 weeks after a surgical repair. It's important for the crutches to be the right size for the child and for the child to be instructed in their use. This instruction is best given by someone from the physical therapy (PT) department. The child can usually return to school within a few days.

Nursing considerations

Prepare the child for the procedure by explaining the general anesthesia or the anesthetic, what the child will experience in the operating room (if he'll be awake), and how he'll feel after the procedure. In addition, follow these steps:
• Note any allergies because of the anesthesia use.
• Tell the child he may feel a thumping sensation as the cannula is inserted into the joint capsule (if he'll be awake during the procedure).
• Cover the site with a small dressing after the procedure.

Bone scans

Bone scans are used to diagnose osteomyelitis and metastatic bone disease. They can also be used to aid diagnosis of joint infections and certain fractures. Special radiographic techniques

---

Types of joint movement

There are seven types of joint movement:
• *Flexion* is a bending forward of the joint; this decreases the angle between the bones that are connected.
• *Extension* is an increase of the joint angle that occurs with straightening of the limb.
• *Abduction* is the movement of the limb away from the midline, or *central axis*, of the body
• *Adduction* is the movement of the limb toward or beyond the midline, or *central axis*, of the body.
• *Internal rotation* is the turning of the body part inward, toward the midline, or *central axis*, of the body.
• *External rotation* is the turning of the body part away from the midline, or *central axis*, of the body.
• *Circumduction* is the movement of the body part in a circular motion.

can help diagnose a musculoskeletal problem. These techniques include computed tomography (CT) scans and magnetic resonance imaging (MRI).

Nursing considerations

The tubelike structures that house the imaging equipment can be frightening to a child. Whenever possible, show the child a picture of the scanning equipment, or the equipment itself, before the procedure. Reassure the child that the parent will be allowed to remain in the room.
• Explain the procedure to the parents and child. Tell the child that he'll be placed in a tube so that pictures may be taken.
• Instruct the child to remain still during the procedure; sedation may be necessary. Distraction techniques may help calm the child.
• Remove metallic objects.

Electromyography

EMG measures muscle response to nervous stimulation (the electrical activity within the muscle fibers). Needle electrodes are inserted into the muscle to be tested, and electrical activity is recorded when the muscle is at rest and during contraction.

A sign of weakness

EMG is used when there are symptoms of muscle weakness and decreased muscle strength. It can differentiate primary muscle conditions from weakness caused by neurologic disorders or a lack of use of the particular muscle. Conditions that may be diagnosed by EMG include muscular dystrophy, nerve dysfunction, and Guillain-Barré syndrome.

Nursing considerations

EMG can be frightening and uncomfortable for a child. When explaining the procedure to the child and parents, prepare the child for insertion of the needle and the feeling in the muscle when the electrical impulses are sent through (like a hard hit to the "funny bone"). Let them know that residual bruising may occur.
In addition, follow these steps:
• Explain that the child may be asked to voluntarily contract the muscle; help him practice the different positions or movements.
• Use deep breathing exercises and play preparation to help lessen the fear and anxiety the child may experience. Involving a child life specialist may be helpful.
• Reassure the child that his parent may stay with him during the procedure.

Muscle and bone marrow biopsy

Biopsy of the muscles and bones involves the removal of a small specimen of muscle or bone marrow for analysis. It's usually performed at the bedside and takes about 20 minutes. Local anesthetics or systemic analgesics are used to help alleviate the pain. The puncture site may remain tender for a few weeks. For bone marrow biopsy, the proximal tibia is the most commonly used site in young children. In older children, the vertebral bodies T10 through L4 are preferred.

Nursing considerations

Biopsy can be an extremely frightening procedure for a child (and his parents). Thoroughly prepare the child and his parents. Allowing the child to "perform" the procedure on a doll (using correct positioning, a syringe, and a bandage) will enhance his understanding of the procedure and may help to ease his fears.

In addition, follow these steps:
• Clarify the meaning of *biopsy* in context; many parents (and older children) automatically think of cancer when they hear the word *biopsy*.
• Provide analgesics as ordered.
• Assist the child into the desired position depending on the site to be used. If necessary, assist in holding the child still during the procedure. (Allow a parent to be present in a comforting capacity only, leaving the positioning and restraint of the child to the health care professionals.)
• When the specimen is obtained, apply direct pressure to the site for 5 to 10 minutes.
• Cover the site and make sure the child remains still for approximately 30 minutes after the procedure.

> A child who cries more when a parent is present probably does so because he feels safe. Feeling safe is the best antidote to emotional trauma.

X-rays

Radiography is the most widely used diagnostic test in the assessment of children with bone abnormalities or other conditions affecting the bones. X-rays can show pathology, such as a fracture, and can show bone density and irregularities. X-rays are used not only for initial evaluation but also for monitoring and evaluating the effectiveness of treatment.

Invisible bone

Normally, the calcium deposits in bones will make skeletal structures appear radiopaque, or white, on X-rays. However, in the infant and young child (whose skeleton is composed mostly of growth cartilage), structures are radiolucent and may not appear on X-ray. Thus, X-rays are less reliable in this population. High-resolution ultrasound may provide a more accurate picture.

Nursing considerations

Always explain to the child the reason for obtaining an X-ray. Explain that an X-ray simply takes pictures (of whatever part of the body is being X-rayed). Reassure the child that the X-ray itself doesn't hurt, but keep in mind that a child with an injury may experience discomfort during positioning for the X-ray.

It's common to allow the parents to remain with the child during the procedure as long as appropriate precautions are taken. In addition, follow these steps:
• Tell the child that it's his job to remain still during the procedure.
• Obtain previous X-rays if possible, which may be useful for comparison.
• If an adolescent female is sexually active, assess for possible pregnancy, a contraindication for radiography.
• Remove metallic objects, such as jewelry or snaps on gowns, before the X-ray because metallic objects may be mistaken for pathology.

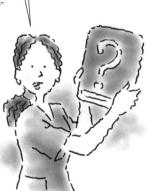

Where did they go? The skeletal structures of an infant or young child are radiolucent, meaning they may not be visible on X-ray.

Treatments and procedures

Children may experience dysfunction in any part of the musculoskeletal system. Treatment depends on a thorough assessment and appropriate interventions based on findings. These interventions are typically designed to promote healing and lessen the impact of the condition on mobility. Principles of body mechanics are used to maintain the integrity of the musculoskeletal system.

Prevent and restore

Nursing care of orthopedic conditions involves the correction of alterations in the musculoskeletal system. These preventive and restorative measures include:
• casting or splinting and traction, which are used to help correct, maintain, and support the body part in a functional position
• surgical repairs such as tendon release
• limb amputations, which may be necessary in some circumstances.

Casting or Splints

Casts or splints may be required when a child has a fractured bone, weakness, paralysis, or spasticity. They're also used following corrective orthopedic surgery.

The cast may be made of plaster or, more commonly, of synthetic material such as fiberglass or plastic. Polyester and cotton impregnated with water-activated polyurethane resin may also be used. (See *Types of casts for children*.)

Depending on the type of material that's used, drying time for the cast may be as little as 7 minutes or as much as 48 hours. Weight bearing on the affected part of the body is typically avoided until the cast has dried.

Types of casts for children

These illustrations show the types of casts commonly used for children.

Full spica cast

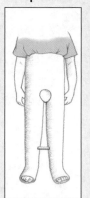

1½ spica cast

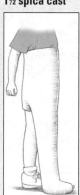

Single spica cast

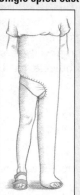

Long leg cast

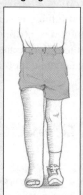

Cylinder cast

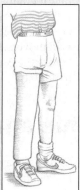

Short leg cast

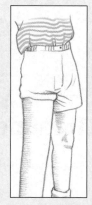

Bootie cast

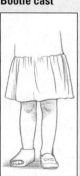

Bilateral long leg cast

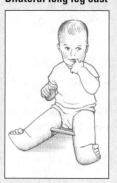

Shoulder spica cast

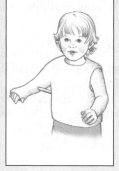

Long arm cast

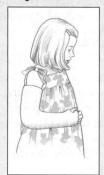

Short arm cast

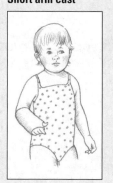

Splints

Splints are "half-casts" and offer a bit more flexibility than a standard cast. They also do not offer quite as much support as a cast. Splints may be custom-formed to the child or may be ready-to-wear. Most splints have Velcro straps to adjust to the child's body. Instruct the parent and the child to keep the splint on as much as possible and to avoid excess activities that would further compromise the injury.

A wash and a blow-dry

Some synthetic casts may be waterproof. Double check that the inner lining of the cast is waterproof as well before allowing the child to get the cast wet. If appropriate, instruct the patient and family to dry the cast after bathing or immersion by using a blow-dryer on a cool setting.

Nursing considerations

Explain each step of the procedure to the child before the procedure and again as the cast is being applied. If plaster will be used, explain that the child will experience a sensation of warmth when it's first applied. As it dries, the cast—and the child—will feel cold.

In addition, follow these steps:
• If a closed reduction is necessary, explain to the child that there will be some pain. Allow the parents to remain close to the child and hold his hand to help lessen anxiety.
• Assess the casted area every 30 minutes for the first few hours, then every hour for 24 hours, then every 4 hours for an additional 48 hours. Drainage from a wound under the cast should be noted.
• If there are signs and symptoms of compromise in the affected area, notify the doctor immediately. Also notify the doctor if cracks are noted in the cast.
• Assess for signs of skin breakdown, a common occurrence. The area around the cast edges will typically become pink and warm and swelling may also occur. (Provide skin care to prevent further breakdown.)

Cast scratch fever

• Because cool air can relieve the itchiness that accompanies casting, instruct the parents to blow cool air down into the cast using a blow-dryer on a cool setting. Also advise against putting an object down the cast in an attempt to scratch.

May I have your autograph?

• Ask the child if he would like his nurses and doctors to sign his cast to help him cheer up, feel important to the medical staff, and view the staff as friends.

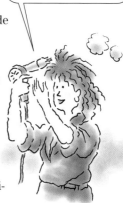

In addition to drying your hair, blow-dryers can be set on cool and aimed at the edges of the child's cast. It's a great itch reliever!

• Explain to the child and parents that the cast must be worn as recommended. It shouldn't be removed and overly rigorous activities should be discouraged (to prevent dislodgment or malalignment of a fracture).

The cut stops here—promise!

• When the fracture is healed, prepare the child for cast removal with the cast cutter. Let him hear the noise and feel the vibrations, and show him (on your body) how the cutter stops when it touches skin and won't, therefore, cut anything except the cast.

• Inform the child that his skin will look different after cast removal, especially if it has been in the cast for weeks. Reassure him that this is temporary, and apply baby oil, then gently wash the area to remove the dead skin. (See *Cast care.*)

• Instruct the child and parents in an exercise regimen to help regain muscle strength and function following the injury.

Traction

Although it is not as widely used now, traction is still used in some circumstances. Traction can be continuous or intermittent. It's used to:

• stabilize or immobilize a certain body part
• reduce muscle spasms
• relieve pressure on spinal nerves
• realign fractures or joint dislocations.

Just hanging out

Traction uses weights and pulleys to exert a pulling force and maintain the body part in correct alignment. Weights must hang freely and the ropes shouldn't have knots that could interfere with free movement.

Serial X-rays are taken while the child is in traction in order to monitor progress and determine the need for changes in the direction and amount of traction pull.

Central location

The child should be kept in the center of the bed to maintain countertraction and prevent complications. Traction can cause muscle spasms that may require analgesics or muscle relaxants. The child is in bed for extended periods; therefore, circulatory and skin assessment is vital.

Traction in twos

There are two basic types of traction:

 skin

 skeletal.

It's all relative

Cast care

Be sure to include these points in your teaching plan for the child with a cast and his parents:

• mechanism of bone healing and necessity for casting
• cast care, including air exposure, elevation, and movement
• measures to protect the cast
• measures for skin care
• methods to relieve itching
• measures to keep the cast dry
• ways to test for sensation, movement, and circulation
• measures for coping with swelling
• ways to relieve skin irritation
• monitoring for wound drainage
• exercises for the casted extremity.

Types of skin traction

This chart describes the various types of skin traction.

Traction	Purpose	Patient positioning
Buck's extension	Used for a fractured hip to prevent muscle spasms and dislocation	• Child lies flat in bed. • Head of the bed is elevated only for activities of daily living.
Cervical traction	Used for neck strain and arthritic or degenerative conditions of the cervical vertebrae	• Child lies flat in bed or with the head of the bed elevated 15 to 20 degrees.
Dunlop's traction	Used for a fractured humerus	• Child lies flat in bed. • Arm is suspended horizontally.
Pelvic girdle	Used for muscle spasms, lower back pain, or a herniated disc	• Child lies with head and knees raised to keep the hips flexed at a 45-degree angle.
Russell traction	Used for adolescents with a femur fracture or certain knee injuries	• Child lies with the head of the bed elevated 30 to 45 degrees.
Bryant's traction	Used for children with a fractured femur who are younger than age 2 years and weigh less than 31 lb (14 kg)	• Hips are flexed at a 90-degree angle. • Buttocks are raised 1" (2.5 cm) above the mattress.

Skin traction

Skin traction is a noninvasive traction that's especially useful for a child who may not require continuous traction. It's applied by placing foam rubber straps against the affected part and then securing the straps with elastic bandages.

Sometimes, the straps have an adhesive backing. If this type of strap is used, the nurse should protect the skin by first applying compound benzoin tincture or other skin protectant. Traction should be removed by two people. (See *Types of skin traction.*)

Skeletal traction

Skeletal traction exerts a greater force than skin traction by using wires or pins inserted into the bone. They're usually placed under anesthesia. Skeletal traction is continuous. (See *Types of skeletal traction*, page 426.)

Nursing considerations

The sight and idea of a body part in skeletal traction can be frightening to a child (and his parents). Explain what the child will see and feel before the traction is applied. Use dolls and toy traction

Types of skeletal traction

This chart describes the different types of skeletal traction.

Traction	Purpose	Special considerations
Thomas leg splint with Pearson attachment	Used for bone alignment and as a more effective line of pull	• Child is placed in the supine position with the knee flexed.
External fixation devices (Ilizarov)	Used to manage open fractures that have soft tissue damage or to provide stability for severe comminuted fractures	• Child is on bed rest (however, early mobility and active exercise of other joints are necessary).
Halo	Used to provide immobilization of the cervical spine and to support the neck following injury	• Early ambulation is recommended. • The anterior metal bars maintain traction. • The posterior bars can be used to position the patient.
Skeletal tongs (Crutchfield, Vinke, Gardner-Wells)	Used to maintain alignment of the cervical spine, for immobilization, and for reduction of cervical roll fractures	• Child is on bed rest. • Special frames may be used for turning.

devices to show the child what's about to happen and help familiarize him with the equipment and reduce fear.

In addition, follow these steps:

• Involve the family as much as possible to reduce anxiety, alleviate boredom, encourage cooperation with the recommended treatment, and minimize disruption of the family structure.

• Maintain the traction system and frequently check the ropes, pulleys, and weights for proper function.

• Maintain correct alignment of the affected body part.

Don't fall behind

• Provide age-appropriate activities to help maintain the child's developmental level, prevent developmental delay, and alleviate boredom.

• Frequently assess for signs of skin breakdown. Place sheepskin under the affected extremity to help alleviate pressure.

• Provide footplates for the affected side to prevent footdrop.

Pin and skin

• For the child in skeletal traction, assess the pin insertion sites for signs of infection or *tenting* (new skin that has attached to the insertion site, creating a tentlike configuration); tenting may cause the skin to tear, which can promote infection.

• Clean the area around the pin insertion sites frequently, and cover the tips of the pins to prevent injury to the skin or other parts of the child's body. Notify the doctor immediately if the pins become loose, and keep the child immobilized until skeletal traction is assessed.

Surgical repairs

At times, surgical repairs may be necessary to promote normal growth and development. Examples of these types of repairs include tendon release and leg-length corrections. Surgery to release a tendon involves cutting a part of the tendon in order to decrease the tension in the muscle that the tendon controls. Tendon release surgery is often used in correcting severe congenital clubfoot in young children. It can also be used on shoulder, hips, knees, or even thumbs.

Leg lengthening or shortening is often used to treat children who have an abnormally short or long leg causing a discrepancy between the two legs. Lengthening requires several surgeries over an extended length of time and is used if there is a significant difference (>5 cm or 2″) between the leg lengths. Plates and screws (some may be external) are used to hold the cut bone in place and slowly pull apart the bone, allowing new bone to fill in the gap, thereby lengthening the bone. Bone growth restriction or shortening is used if there is less than a 5 cm (2″) difference. Surgery is done to stop the epiphysis (growth plate) from promoting further growth. The metal plates and screws used may be removed after several months once complete healing has occurred.

Nursing considerations

As with any surgery, the child and family need to be prepared. Allow the child and the parents to express their fears and answer any questions they may have about the procedure itself. In addition, follow these steps:
• Following surgery, check the site for circulation, signs of infection, or complications.
• Notify the health care provider if there are any abnormal signs.
• Teach the parents how to care for the pin insertion site and signs and symptoms of any complications.

Amputation

Unfortunately, amputations occur in children as well as adults. An amputation may be needed because of a trauma; a disease process, such as osteosarcoma; or it may have occurred prenatally due to teratogens, metabolic diseases in the mother, or small pieces of the amnion that cut off circulation to a certain body part (known as an *amniotic band*). Only rarely is a congenital amputation genetically determined. Occasionally, a hair or a loose piece of thread can cause a tourniquet on an infant's toes and feet or fingers and hands. This strand of hair or thread can wrap itself so tightly around a wiggling infant that it can cause significant damage to the extremity and may even lead to amputation if not caught in enough time (known as a *hair tourniquet*). In rare circumstances, it may be caused by child abuse. Teach the parents to daily take off mittens or booties and inspect for any loose threads or hair.

A loss that lasts

Limb amputation that isn't congenital can be traumatic to a child or adolescent and his family. It may be particularly damaging to the child's self-image. Everyone deals with feelings of loss in his own way and in his own time; there's no right or wrong way to grieve. Families need extra time and support to deal with the grief and loss they feel when they're given the news that amputation is required.

Something in common

It may be helpful to introduce the child and family to another family who has gone through an amputation and has learned to cope successfully with day-to-day activities and enjoy life. Support groups such as the Amputee Coalition have pediatric support groups in many areas around the country.

Many amputations are treated with a prosthesis. Sometimes, stump shrink bandages are used to apply pressure, reduce swelling, and help mold the stump for fitting a prosthesis, which usually can be done within 4 to 6 weeks after the amputation.

> The best prescription for feelings of fear, loss, and grief is a nurse who simply listens and validates those feelings.

Quick studies

Children quickly learn how to function with a prosthesis and can lead very active, normal lives. They should be reassured that amputation doesn't have to mean permanent disability. Many children participate in sports and other strenuous activities while using a prosthesis. The nurse can play an essential role in helping the child and his family cope with this traumatic situation.

Nursing considerations

After the surgery, the nurse should provide basic postoperative care while keeping in mind some special considerations:
• Provide care to prevent contractures and perform ROM exercises to keep the stump from becoming permanently flexed or

abducted. (These exercises also increase muscle strength and improve mobility of the stump.)

Let's get physical

- Depending on the site and extent of the amputation, the child should begin to move and start PT as quickly as possible.
- Teach the child and parents about proper care of the stump and application and maintenance of the prosthesis.
- If the amputation is on a lower extremity, teach the child how to walk with crutches, then how to ambulate using a prosthetic device. Refer the child for PT as he may need extensive training.
- Assess for phantom limb pain, which is real pain and should be treated with analgesics as appropriate. (Tell the child and parents that this pain should gradually fade.)

Musculoskeletal disorders

Musculoskeletal disorders that may occur in children include congenital clubfoot, developmental dysplasia of the hip (DDH), Ewing's sarcoma, fractures, juvenile idiopathic arthritis (JIA) (formerly juvenile rheumatoid arthritis), Legg-Calvé-Perthes disease, slipped capital femoral epiphysis (SCFE), Osgood-Schlatter disease, and scoliosis.

Congenital clubfoot

Congenital clubfoot is a deformity that occurs in utero in approximately 1 of every 1,000 births.

Boys are twice as likely to be affected as girls. If a family has one child with a clubfoot, the chances of having another affected child increase markedly.

Although talipes equinovarus is the most commonly occurring type of clubfoot, other variations may be present and are identified according to the orientation of the deformity. (See *Recognizing clubfoot*, page 430.)

What causes it

Clubfoot may be caused by a mechanical force (the position in utero), through prenatal exposure to drugs or infections, or by an inherited factor. It can be a singular birth defect or associated with certain syndromes. An infant with a clubfoot should be carefully examined for additional anomalies.

How it happens

Regardless of the cause of the clubfoot, the result is a nonfunctional position of the foot and ankle due to abnormal muscles

Recognizing clubfoot

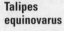 Clubfoot (talipes) may have various names, depending on the orientation of the deformity, as shown in these illustrations.

Talipes equinus

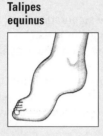

Talipes calcaneus

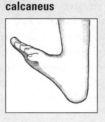

Talipes cavus

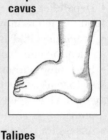

Talipes varus

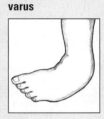

Talipes equinovarus

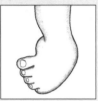

Talipes calcaneovarus

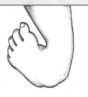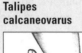

Talipes valgus

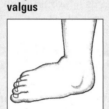

Talipes calcaneovalgus

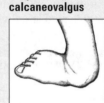

Talipes equinovalgus

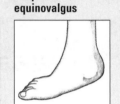

and joints and contracture of soft tissue. The position of the foot determines the classification of the clubfoot.

The classic definition of talipes equinovarus requires these three components:

- plantar flexion of the foot at the ankle joint
- inversion deformity of the heel
- turning in of the forefoot.

What to look for

The deformity is usually obvious at birth. The foot is usually inverted (turned in), also known as a *varus position*. An everted (turned outward) foot is known as a *valgus position*. A single foot or both feet may be affected. The deformity may be mild with some flexibility noted, or severe with the foot completely rigid. In the most severe form, the foot has a clublike appearance.

What tests tell you

Early diagnosis of clubfoot is usually relatively simple because the deformity is obvious. However, X-rays may show superimposition of the talus and calcaneus bones and a ladderlike appearance of the metatarsals.

Complications

If identification and treatment of clubfoot isn't instituted early on, chronic impairment may result. The prognosis is good, however, for infants who receive treatment.

How it's treated

Treatment of clubfoot consists of manipulation of the foot to stretch the contracted tissues. Splinting is then applied to maintain that correction. If treatment is begun shortly after birth, the correction is fairly rapid. If treatment is delayed for any reason, the foot quickly becomes more rigid, which can occur in a matter of days. Treatment is typically begun in the neonatal nursery. Straps and splints are applied and are quite effective until formal casting can be done.

Casting call

Casts are applied sequentially by first correcting the forefoot adduction, then the heel inversion, and then the flexion of the ankle. Casts are usually changed at 1- to 2-week intervals to allow the infant's foot to grow and to manipulate the foot gradually. Treatment lasts for several months depending on the severity of the deformation. To maintain the long-term correction, exercises and a night brace are commonly prescribed.

Please release me

In approximately one-half of patients with clubfoot, corrective surgery is required to release the tightened structures around the foot. The outcome of this surgery is usually good; the foot appears normal and is adequate for normal footwear and sports. For infants, surgery is usually limited to soft tissue to prevent interference with bone growth.

Successful surgery for congenital clubfoot is usually followed by successful shoe shopping!

From designer wedges . . .

For the older child or the child with severe clubfoot, the bones of the foot may need to be realigned by using bone wedges. Casts are worn for months following surgery. A specialized splint called the *Denis Browne boots* or *splint* may sometimes be used.

. . . to designer shoes

This splint consists of specially made shoes attached to an adjustable bar that provides the eversion, rotation, and dorsiflexion needed to achieve a slight overcorrection. It's worn for several weeks and then worn only at night to help maintain this position. Compliance in using this orthosis can be an issue. Make sure you teach the parents on the importance of using it regularly.

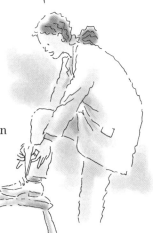

What to do

The primary concern related to clubfoot is the need for early recognition, preferably during the neonatal period. Look for exaggerated appearances in the infant's feet. Apparent clubfoot (resulting from positioning in utero) can be differentiated from true clubfoot because an apparent clubfoot will easily move back to normal position.

When caring for a child with clubfoot, follow these steps:

• Don't use excessive force when assessing a clubfoot.

• Stress to the parents the importance of prompt treatment; clubfoot demands immediate therapy and orthopedic supervision until growth is completed.

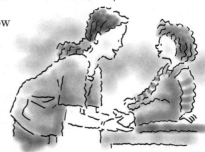

It takes a gentle touch to examine a child with clubfoot.

Put up your feet and relax

• After casting, elevate the child's feet with pillows; check the toes every 1 to 2 hours for temperature, color, sensation, motion, and capillary refill time and watch for edema.

• Before discharge, teach parents to recognize signs of circulatory impairment, such as numbness or tingling of the toes, coldness in the toes, or lack of capillary refill.

• Emphasize the need for long-term orthopedic care to maintain the correction.

The agony of de feet

• Help the parents (and child) deal with grief or other emotional issues that arise from this problem.

• Teach parents the prescribed exercises that the child should do at home.

• Urge parents to make sure the child wears his corrective shoes and splints during naps and at night. Make sure they understand that treatment for clubfoot continues throughout the entire growth period.

Developmental dysplasia of the hip

The hip joint develops early in utero. By the end of the first trimester, the shape of the joint is recognizable and the cartilage, ligaments, capsule, and vascular pattern are formed.

Relationship problems

DDH is a spectrum of conditions in which there's an abnormal relationship between the proximal femur and the acetabulum. It occurs in approximately 3 to 5 of every 1,000 live births. Females are six times more likely to be affected as males. A positive family history of DDH increases the risk fivefold.

Frankly breech

Another important risk factor for DDH is a breech presentation at birth. Children who present in a frank breech position have a risk of DDH almost 20 times higher than children who have a cephalic presentation. The way infants are carried in some cultures may also contribute to the development of DDH. (See *Carried away with DDH.*)

Other associated abnormalities include oligohydramnios (decreased amniotic fluid in utero), torticollis, and metatarsus adductus (a form of clubfoot).

What causes it

Dislocation of the hip is usually a developmental problem in an otherwise normal child. It isn't always clear when it occurs. A child who develops a deformity in utero is usually more severely affected than the child who has a hip that dislocates after birth.

What's in a name?

Although *congenital dislocation of the hip* is a common term for DDH, it implies that the dislocation occurs at birth. However, the problem may occur over several months after birth. Therefore, *developmental dysplasia of the hip* is a more accurate description of the hip pathology that exists in this disorder.

How it happens

There are three typical forms of DDH:
• *Dysplasia* is a result of the femoral head failing to exert appropriate pressure against the acetabulum. As a result, the femoral head becomes small and flattened and the acetabulum becomes shallow and eventually flat. A dysplastic hip may progress to a subluxated or dislocated hip. The abductor muscles of the hip will also shorten and contract.
• The hip is considered *subluxated* when the femoral head (the ball) is in contact with the acetabulum (the socket) but not deeply centered within it.
• *Dislocation* occurs when the femoral head (the ball) is no longer in contact with the acetabulum (the socket). (See *Forms of DDH*, page 434.)

What to look for

A dislocation diagnosed in the first few weeks of life can be treated conservatively. If the diagnosis is delayed until walking age, reconstructive surgery is usually required for correction, which greatly increases the likelihood of complications.

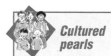

Cultured pearls

Carried away with DDH

Some experts suggest that the infant carrying practices of certain cultures may influence the development of DDH. For instance, the rate of DDH increases by 25 to 50 times among Native Americans, who traditionally carry their infants tightly swaddled, sometimes strapped to a cradleboard, which keeps the legs in an extended position. On the other hand, DDH is rarely seen in certain African populations in which the infant is carried with his front side bound to his mother's back. This position keeps the infant's legs flexed and abducted, which may prevent the development of DDH.

Forms of DDH

These illustrations show a normal hip and the three presentations of DDH.

Normal hip	Dysplasia	Subluxation	Dislocation
	The acetabulum is more flattened than cup-shaped.	The femoral head is in contact with the acetabulum but isn't deeply centered within it.	The femoral head is no longer in contact with the acetabulum.

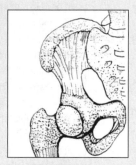 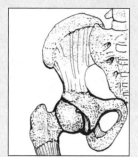 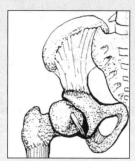 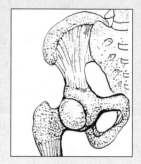

It's important for the nurse to be aware of risk factors for DDH and to assess the infant and child carefully for signs of a hip problem. Physical signs of DDH include asymmetrical skin folds, Galeazzi sign, limited hip abduction, and hip instability.

Asymmetrical skin folds

When the infant is lying on his back with his hips and knees flexed at a 90-degree angle, the same number of skin folds should appear in the medial (inner) aspect of both thighs. If a hip is dislocated, the soft tissues of the thigh may fold down on each other like an accordion, producing a larger number of skin folds on the affected side.

Galeazzi sign

If there's a dislocation, the femoral head may be placed superior to the acetabulum when the hips and knees are flexed at 90 degrees. This malpositioning will cause the knee on the affected side to be significantly lower than the other knee, a sign known as *Galeazzi sign*.

Limited hip abduction

The normal range of hip abduction in an infant is from 0 degrees (with thighs perpendicular to the table) to almost 90 degrees (with thighs resting on the table). In DDH, a shortening of the adductor muscle on the medial aspect of the thigh while the femoral head

Memory jogger

Here's an easy way to keep adduction and abduction straight.

Adduction is moving a limb toward the body's midline; think of it as adding two things together.

Abduction is moving a limb away from the body's midline; think of it as taking something away like abducting, or kidnapping.

is displaced superiorly causes the thigh to be limited in its range. This sign may not be apparent in the neonate because, at this age, there hasn't been enough time for muscle spasms and contractures to develop.

Hip instability

Testing hip stability is important in the diagnosis of DDH. In neonates, this test is usually the only clue to a problem.

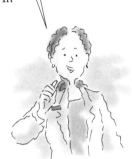

In neonates, a "clunk" during thigh adduction and abduction may be diagnostic of DDH.

A clunky diagnosis

Barlow test and Ortolani's test are used to evaluate hip stability.
• A positive Barlow test is noted when a clunk is heard as the examiner adducts the thigh toward the midline while trying to displace or dislocate the femoral head posteriorly.
• A positive Ortolani's test occurs when a clunk is felt as the examiner abducts the thigh to the table from the midline while lifting up the greater trochanter with the finger.

What tests tell you

A *Trendelenburg test* can be used to assess for hip dislocation in children who are old enough to stand and bear weight. When the child stands on the affected leg, the opposite hip slants downward instead of remaining level.

A limp or a waddle

As the child walks, there's a characteristic limp known as the *Trendelenburg gait*. This limp is due to a weakness of the hip abductor muscles. If both hips are dislocated, the child will have lordosis and a waddling gait.

X-rays will show the location of the femoral head and a shallow acetabulum. X-rays are also used to monitor treatment or deterioration.

Complications

For children who don't receive treatment before age 7, treatment is very unsatisfactory. Delayed treatment may have lifelong implications for walking, development of back problems, and self-esteem. DDH may cause:
• degenerative hip changes
• abnormal acetabular development
• lordosis (abnormally increased concave curvature of the lumbar and cervical spine)
• joint malformation
• sciatic nerve injury (paralysis)

- avascular necrosis of the femoral head
- soft tissue damage
- permanent disability.

How it's treated

Treatment of DDH depends on the severity of the dysplasia, how quickly the diagnosis is made, and the child's age and includes a Pavlik harness, spica cast, and surgical correction.

Pavlik harness

If treatment is instituted early, the success of treatment with a Pavlik harness is greater than 90%. As the child ages and treatment is delayed, the prognosis worsens. (See *Two views of the Pavlik harness.*) In some cases, a Pavlik harness cannot be used. If the family cannot consistently and correctly use the harness, another form of treatment should be used.

Whoa, Nellie!

In the child younger than age 6 months, careful positioning to maintain the hip in abduction with the head of the femur in the acetabulum is achieved with a Pavlik harness. This harness is worn at all times except for bathing until the hips are stable on examination. When the hips are stable, usually in 1 to 3 weeks, the harness is then used during sleep for 6 additional weeks.

Harness hip hooray!

If DDH is diagnosed during the neonatal period, the harness may be needed for only 2 to 3 months. The older infant may need to wear it for 4 or 5 months.

Don't double up

Parents should be taught how to apply the harness correctly and to avoid double and triple diapering (which can cause extreme abduction, leading to avascular necrosis). The harness doesn't interfere with the child's ability to receive immunizations as the thighs remain exposed.

Spica cast

For the child older than age 6 months, a Pavlik harness can't reliably treat the dysplasia. These children require a spica cast to hold the hips in a flexed and abducted position. Traction is commonly used before the application of the cast to gently stretch out the soft tissues around the hip that have contracted. Traction is usually used for 2 to 3 weeks before placement of the cast. Sometimes the traction can be done at home.

Two views of the Pavlik harness

These illustrations show an infant in a Pavlik harness. The Pavlik harness maintains the hip in abduction, with the femoral head in the acetabulum.

Front view

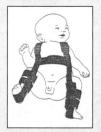

Back view

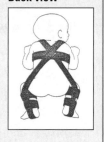

A temporary setback

When the cast has been applied, it usually remains on for several months and is removed and reapplied to accommodate growth. It may delay walking for a few months, but the child usually learns quickly how to walk when the cast is removed.

Hold and turn

Care for a child in a spica cast is essentially the same as that for a child in a Pavlik harness. Parents should be encouraged to hold the child as much as possible. The infant should be turned frequently to prevent skin breakdown.

Surgical correction

For the child older than age 18 months, surgical correction is usually required. Surgery enables the removal of tissues that block reduction and positioning of the femoral head into the acetabulum under direct visualization. Occasionally, a bone graft is required.

What to do

Listen sympathetically to the parents' expressions of anxiety and fear. Explain possible causes of DDH, and reassure them that early, prompt treatment will probably result in complete correction.

You'd be cranky too

During the child's first few days in a cast or harness, she may be prone to irritability due to the unaccustomed restriction of movement. Encourage her parents to stay with her as much as possible and to calm and reassure her. Assure parents that the child will adjust to this restriction and return to normal sleeping, eating, and playing behavior in a few days.

If treatment requires a spica cast, follow these steps:
• Position the child on a Bradford frame (a rectangular frame of pipe with attached sheeting used for immobile patients) elevated on blocks with a bedpan under the frame or on pillows to support the child's legs. Be sure to keep the cast dry and change the child's diapers often.
• Turn the child every 2 hours during the day and every 4 hours at night. Check color, sensation, and motion of the infant's legs and feet. (Be sure to examine her toes, and notify the doctor of dusky, cool, or numb toes.)

Investigate the itch

• If the child complains of itching, she may benefit from diphenhydramine (Benadryl) or another over-the-counter antihistamine, or you may aim a blow-dryer set on cool at the cast edges to

relieve itching. (Don't scratch or probe under the cast; investigate persistent itching.)
• Provide adequate stimuli to promote growth and development. If the child's hips are abducted in a frog-like position, tell parents that she may be able to fit on a tricycle that the parent can push (if the child can't pedal) or an electric child's car.

> Kids with DDH still need to be kids— and a tricycle is the perfect fit for hips that are abducted in a froglike position.

A change of scenery

• Encourage parents to let the child sit at a table (by sitting her on pillows on a chair), sit on the floor for short periods of play, and play with other children her age.
• Tell parents to watch for signs that the child is needing an adjustment of the cast and to notify the provider if any of the following are seen: skin breakdown, cyanosis, cool extremities, pain, or an ill-fitting or broken cast.

Ewing's sarcoma

Ewing's sarcoma is the second most common bone tumor in children and adolescents. It's fairly rare, with only approximately 150 new cases reported in the United States each year. It affects primarily young, white males younger than age 20. The tumor usually develops in the midshaft of the long bones of the arms and legs, although it's occasionally found in the pelvis, ribs, spine and, rarely, in the soft tissues or other bones.

What causes it

A consistent, chromosomal abnormality has been identified in the cells responsible for Ewing's sarcoma. The cause of this chromosomal problem hasn't yet been identified. It doesn't appear to be inherited, and it isn't thought to be due to exposure to chemicals or radiation or to an environmental factor.

How it happens

Although Ewing's sarcoma is considered a form of bone cancer, it arises from a type of primitive nerve cell, which explains why the tumor can be found in the soft tissues.

Off to a bad start

Ewing's sarcoma is a cancer that spreads quickly. The tumor is aggressively malignant and approximately 25% of patients diagnosed with the disease have experienced metastasis, with some experts feeling that the majority of those affected will have a subclinical form of metastatic disease. The most common sites of metastasis include the lungs, other bones, and the bone marrow.

What to look for

Signs and symptoms of Ewing's sarcoma include pain and swelling over the affected site (even causing awakening at night), possible tenderness over the affected area, and weight loss. Occasionally a soft, tissue mass may be felt. Fever occurs in 25% of patients. If the tumor is over the leg bone, a limp may be present. If it's on one of the ribs, shortness of breath may be evident. In physically active children, the disease may be initially diagnosed as a sports injury. In some cases, a fracture may occur with only a seemingly minor injury. This is known as a pathologic fracture.

> In athletes like me, the signs and symptoms of Ewing's sarcoma might initially be diagnosed as a sports injury.

Pelvic prognosis

The outcome for a child with Ewing's sarcoma is largely dependent on whether or not there has been metastasis. Prognosis is good in patients with a small, localized primary tumor. For patients with significant pelvic involvement or metastatic disease, survival rates are poor. New treatment options for these high-risk patients include autologous bone marrow transplants.

What tests tell you

• Serology reveals the cells of Ewing's sarcoma (the cells stain a characteristic blue color), which are described as small and round; they're tightly packed and arranged into compartments by bands of fibrous tissue.
• Blood tests include a complete blood count (CBC), serum chemistries, and a test for lactase dehydrogenase (LDH). Higher levels of LDH are associated with poorer prognoses.
• X-rays reveal the tumor and, commonly, an area of bone destruction around the tumor.
• CT scanning and MRI should be performed to determine as precisely as possible the extent of local disease.
• A chest X-ray, bone scan, and bone marrow biopsy may be performed to determine the extent of metastasis, if any.

Complications

As with any cancer, some complications arise due to treatment. Metastasis may result from the cancer itself. Children receiving prolonged, intensive treatments are forced to endure frequent venipuncture. Access devices are helpful to lessen the need for repeated needle sticks.

When chemo gets complicated

Complications of chemotherapy include nausea and vomiting, anorexia, weight loss, and bone marrow suppression. Hair loss is a noticeable adverse effect of chemotherapy. The child and family should be reassured that the hair will grow back after therapy, although the texture and color may be different. With prompt treatment, the prognosis is generally good.

How it's treated

Treatment includes chemotherapy, radiation, and surgery. Chemotherapy is given in cycles over the course of 1 year. When surgery is performed, the tumor is usually removed without needing to amputate the limb. The site of tumor excision is then filled in with a graft or prosthesis to allow for normal limb function. For all children with cancer, pain control is a must.

What to do

Caring for a child with cancer can be a difficult, yet rewarding part of nursing. By offering support, assisting with necessary treatments, and helping the family adjust to the diagnosis, the nurse can have a significant impact on the lives of a child and his family during this time.
• Because of the severity of the disease, be available to help the family and child cope with the diagnosis.

Nurse in shining armor

• Assure the child and parents that you're there to be their advocate; make sure their questions are answered promptly and facilitate communication between the family members and the health care team.
• Prepare the child and parents for treatments and procedures.
• Allow the child to make as many choices as possible during his day-to-day care; this helps give him a sense of control in a situation that's likely to make him feel helpless.
• Clarify the prognosis and help the child and family deal with their fears; to many people, a diagnosis of cancer is viewed as a death sentence.

Growing up too fast

• Help the child be a child while dealing with a very "adult" diagnosis; provide play activities and encourage interaction with peers.
• Refer the child and family (including siblings) to support groups and other professionals with expertise in helping families cope with a cancer diagnosis.

Cultured pearls

Different cultures and religions have very different practices when it comes to dealing with children with severe illness or are facing death. The child and family should determine the best care path for them.

Fractures

Bones are designed to withstand stress; however, when increased stress and traumatic force are exerted on the bone, a fracture will occur. Fractures can occur in almost any bone, but the long bones are the most commonly fractured. Other common sites of fracture include the wrists, fingers, toes, and skull.

What causes it

Fractures commonly occur during athletic activities and accidents. They may also result from child abuse (suspected in the case of infants without a known cause for a weakened bone, multiple or repeated episodes of fractures), bone tumors, or metabolic disease.

How it happens

Fractures occur when traumatic forces are exerted on the bone. Because children are more flexible than adults, they may not be as prone to fractures.

Sticks and stones may bend my bones

Rather than fracturing completely, children's bones tend to simply bend, buckle, or sustain an incomplete fracture.

A stressful situation

Stress fractures are associated with unusually strong physical stress and are commonly seen in children who suddenly begin a vigorous training program. (See *Common fractures in children*, page 442.)

The remodeling team

After a fracture occurs, the body quickly begins a repairing process. A blood clot is formed at the site of the fracture. Osteoblasts and fibroblasts then converge on the site and begin to lay down an organic matrix. This forms a callus into which calcium salts are deposited, evolving into bone tissue that connects the pieces of the original bone. After that happens, the callus is remodeled into a strong, permanent bone.

What to look for

Bone fractures are classified according to:
- type of injury to the bone or surrounding tissue
- whether they're *open* (in which the skin has been broken due to penetration of bone fragment or external trauma) or *closed* (in which the fracture is contained under the skin's surface)
- whether there's involvement of the epiphyseal (growth) plate.

Sudden and sharp

Fractures usually cause sudden, sharp pain at the fracture site. Pain increases with movement and limits motion in the affected

Common fractures in children

Bends, buckle fractures, greenstick fractures, and complete fractures commonly occur during childhood. Each of these fractures is described and illustrated below.

Bends	**Buckle fractures**	**Greenstick fractures**	**Complete fractures**
Bends are common in childhood because of the flexibility of children's bones. Children's bones can be bent up to 45 degrees, or possibly more, before breaking.	Buckle fractures occur due to compression of the porous bone, causing a raised area or bulge at the fracture site.	Greenstick fractures occur when the bone is bent beyond its limits, causing an incomplete fracture.	Complete fractures occur when the bone is broken into separate pieces.

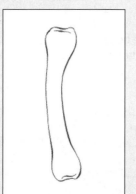 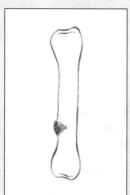 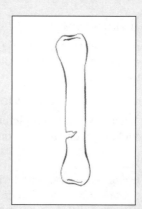 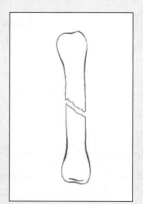

part. Swelling, bruising, or discoloration around the site may occur. There may be obvious deformity or abnormal positioning of the affected part.

What tests tell you

X-rays provide the definitive diagnosis for a fracture. Occasionally, an incomplete fracture isn't seen initially on the X-ray and appears only after the film has dried after several hours. Serial X-rays are taken to monitor healing and check the alignment of the bone.

Complications

Complications of fractures include infection, particularly in open fracture. A fracture that affects the growth plate can interrupt and alter growth. The impact of this alteration depends on the area of the epiphyseal plate that's affected.

The *Salter-Harris classification system* is used to determine the severity of the injury on the epiphyseal plate. Type I injuries typically

Salter-Harris classification system

The Salter-Harris classification system divides growth plate fractures into five categories. These categories are based on the type of damage to the growth plate.

Type I	Type II	Type III	Type IV	Type V
The epiphysis is completely separated from the metaphysis or end of bone. Although a type I fracture generally requires casting, it rarely requires manipulation. Growth disturbance isn't common unless the blood supply has been injured.	Type II is the most common type of fracture. The epiphysis and the growth plate are separated from the cracked metaphysis. This type of fracture must be manipulated and casted for normal growth to continue. Minimal shortening of the bone may occur but usually doesn't result in functional limitations.	Type III is a rare fracture that usually involves the lower tibia, or a long bone of the lower leg. It occurs when the fracture runs completely through the epiphysis and separates part of the epiphysis and the growth plate from the metaphysis. Surgery may be necessary. Growth usually isn't affected as long as the blood supply to the bone is intact.	A type IV fracture runs through the epiphysis, across the growth plate, and into the metaphysis. It occurs most commonly in the humerus near the elbow. Perfect alignment must be achieved for normal growth to occur.	A crush or compression injury, a type V fracture most likely occurs in the knee or ankle. It is an uncommon injury. Stunting of growth is possible and prognosis is poor. Surgery is required as well as future reconstructive or corrective surgery.

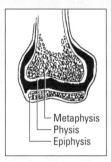

Metaphysis
Physis
Epiphysis

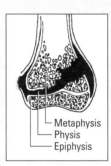

Metaphysis
Physis
Epiphysis

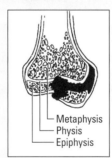

Metaphysis
Physis
Epiphysis

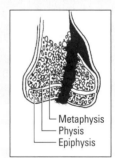

Metaphysis
Physis
Epiphysis

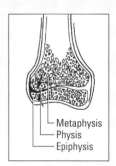

Metaphysis
Physis
Epiphysis

don't affect growth. Injuries identified as type III and above require intervention to prevent future dysfunction in the bone and affected body part. (See *Salter-Harris classification system.*)

From bone to lung

Fat embolism is a major, life-threatening complication of a fracture. Fat globules are released into the circulation and can become lodged in the capillaries of the lung, thereby decreasing the exchange of oxygen and carbon dioxide. Signs of an embolism are increasing blood pressure, dyspnea, and other signs of respiratory compromise.

How it's treated

Reducing or realigning the bone into proper placement and allowing it to heal is the treatment required for a fracture. The reduction may be closed (through external manipulation of the body part) or open (done through surgery).

Closed reductions are usually treated with casting. Surgical repair of a fracture involves the use of either internal or external fixation devices.

> A cast is usually applied after a closed reduction. It's a little easier on the eyes when there's clothing involved—not to mention skin.

Permanent hardware

Internal devices (rods, pins, or wires) are permanent; they remain in the child unless a problem develops. External devices are pins or wires that are inserted through the bone and then attached to an external frame. When the bone heals, the devices are removed. Follow-up evaluation is essential to prevent and quickly treat complications that may arise.

What to do

Fractures are usually treated in an emergency setting. Formal preparation for treatments and procedures may not be possible.

Prepare on the go

Tell the child (and parents) everything that's being done as it's happening and provide as much support as possible to help ease the child's fears and enhance cooperation.
• Provide emergency care to the child with a fracture; steps should be taken to quickly assess the injury, prevent further damage, and promote comfort.
• Frequently check for neurologic and circulatory compromise to the affected area.

Cast caution

• After the cast or splint has been applied, continue to assess the area around the cast.
• When a fracture requires long-term immobilization with traction, reposition the patient often to increase comfort and prevent pressure ulcers, assist with active ROM exercises to prevent muscle atrophy, and encourage deep breathing and coughing to prevent pneumonia.

> Telling the child his classmates will think his crutches are "cool"—priceless!

Are you shocked?

• Watch for signs of shock in the child with a severe open fracture of a large bone such as the femur.
• Assist the child to regain normal function as quickly as possible; encourage him to start moving around as soon as he can, help him walk, and demonstrate how to use crutches properly.

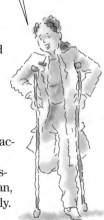

- Help the family deal with the fracture and help the child understand what's happening.

Postscript

- Encourage the child to talk about the experience and express his feelings after the emergency is over; use this time to answer questions and clear up misconceptions (as would usually be done before treatment).

> When things happen quickly, encourage the child to express concerns and ask questions after the emergency is over.

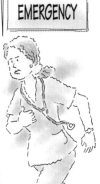

Juvenile idiopathic arthritis

JIA (formerly known as juvenile rheumatoid arthritis) is a chronic, autoimmune disease of the connective tissue. It's a group of conditions characterized by the presence of chronic synovial inflammation. Immunogenetic traits in children with JIA are different from those in adults with adult rheumatoid arthritis. These traits may be significant because of their effect on the formation of cellular antibodies, the immune system, and consequent chronic inflammation.

What causes it

The exact cause of JIA is unknown. Some experts believe that a two-step process takes place. First, the child is genetically more likely to develop JIA. Second, an environmental trigger in a joint causes normal immunoglobulins within the joint to release harmful chemicals which in turn damage the tissue. This tissue injury may be a result of infection, possibly viral. Researchers haven't pinpointed a specific infectious gene marker or even identified the mechanism that provokes the systemic and local immune responses in children with JIA.

How it happens

Autoantibodies develop in response to injured joint tissue. These autoantibodies are known as *rheumatoid factors*. These factors then lodge in the joint's synovial fluid and cause inflammation. As the inflammatory process continues, the synovial membrane thickens, production of synovial fluid increases, and cellular composition is altered. This process results in pain, swelling, and limited mobility.

What to look for

There are three major presentations of JIA. Most children with JIA exhibit some joint swelling, warmth, and morning stiffness. (See *Types of JIA*, page 446.)

Types of JIA

There are three major types of JIA, each with its own presentation.

Oligoarthritis (formerly known as pauciarticular disease)

Persistent oligoarthritis is characterized by chronic arthritis in four or fewer joints for the first 6 months of the disease. The large joints (knees, ankles, elbows) are most commonly affected. This presentation accounts for 50% of all JIA cases. The symptoms are typically mild with possibly little or no pain. Systemic features are uncommon but the eyes can be severely inflamed. If the disease progresses to affect more than four joints, it is known as extended oligoarthritis.

Polyarticular pattern

The polyarticular pattern of JIA most closely resembles the adult disease. Chronic pain and swelling occur in five or more joints, usually the knees, wrists, ankles, neck, and elbows. Systemic features are usually less prominent, although a low-grade fever, fatigue, and anemia may be present. This process may wax and wane over the course of years. It accounts for approximately 30% of all cases and affects girls more commonly than boys. Polyarticular arthritis can have either a positive or negative rheumatoid factor.

Systemic JIA

In systemic JIA, an acute presentation of the disorder, a salmon-pink rash appears on the trunk and extremities, often disappearing and reappearing quickly or moving to other areas. A high fever spikes intermittently over a couple of weeks, and anorexia and weight loss are common. Swelling of the lymph glands or the liver or spleen arises. Joint involvement occurs later in the disease process. Other areas of the body may be affected, including the heart, lungs, and blood. This type of presentation accounts for less than 10% of all JIA cases and may be episodic. Remission of the systemic features may occur within 1 year.

Psoriatic arthritis

Children with psoriatic arthritis also have the skin affliction known as psoriasis or have a close relative with the disease. They often have swelling and inflammation of a finger or toe and the nails will split or become discolored.

Enthesitis-related arthritis

The enthesis is the point where the tendon attaches to the bone. In this form of arthritis, the child has swelling and inflammation at the enthesis. The most commonly affected areas include the Achilles tendon and the knee. Other affected areas include the back (known as juvenile ankylosing spondylitis) or around the sacroiliac joint in relation to inflammatory bowel disease. In addition, the iris of the eye may become inflamed (iritis, uveitis, or iridocyclitis).

Undifferentiated arthritis is labeled for those types of arthritis that do not fit into the previously mentioned categories or fits into more than one category.

What tests tell you

There's no single diagnostic test for JIA. In early stages of the disease, only soft tissue swelling may be seen on X-ray. MRI of the involved joints may show joint damage.

Hematologic tests may help confirm the diagnosis if clinical manifestations are present:

- Rheumatoid factor is positive in only 15% of cases.
- Leukocytes may be elevated, suggesting an inflammatory process.
- Erythrocyte sedimentation rate may be normal or elevated.
- Antinuclear antibodies may be present.
- Anti-cyclic citrullinated peptide (anti-CCP) antibodies, which are commonly found in adult patients with arthritis, may or may not be present in children with JIA.

Complications

The prognosis for children with JIA is very good. It's a self-limiting disease, and 70% to 90% survive JIA without functional limitations. However, some complications do occur:
• In children with early-onset oligoarthritis disease involving only one knee, there may be a significant difference in leg length.

Thrown another curve

• The incidence of scoliosis may be up to 10 times higher in children with JIA than in the general population.
• Cervical spine involvement and other skeletal abnormalities may develop in up to 70% of children with arthritis.
• Anemia is a common feature of systemic and polyarticular arthritis.

The eyes have it

• Up to 30% of children with oligoarthritis develop an inflammation of the iris and ciliary bodies of the eye (uveitis), which produces no symptoms but may cause blindness if left untreated.
• Children with JIA are at increased risk for iridocyclitis (inflammation of the iris and ciliary body in the eye).

A child with JIA should be referred to an ophthalmologist who will follow her for signs of eye involvement.

CAUTION!

How it's treated

Treatment of JIA aims to reduce disease activity, relieve symptoms, and maintain function.

NSAIDs first unless pain is worse

Nonsteroidal anti-inflammatory drugs (NSAIDs) are prescribed to decrease inflammation and relieve pain; medications such as naproxen (Naprosyn/Aleve) or ibuprofen (Motrin/Advil) may be used. Aspirin should not be used in children due to the rare but serious risk of developing Reye's syndrome. If NSAIDs fail, alternative medications are used. These medications include methotrexate (Rheumatrex), which has replaced gold salts as the second-line medication. Occasionally, local corticosteroid injections or joint replacement is required. Systemic corticosteroids are not routinely used due to the high risk of side effects.

Up and active

ROM and muscle strengthening exercises are ordered and carried out by a physical therapist. Unless JIA is in the most acute stage, bed rest should be avoided. Involvement of the eye should be followed and treated by an ophthalmologist. A number of children find relief through complementary and alternative therapies. It is important to stress to the family that these therapies are used in addition to standard medical care and do not replace recommended medical treatments.

What to do

The child and his parents will need help adjusting to the realities of a chronic disease. Parents may tend to be over-protective and may need help to find the balance between allowing their child to live a normal life and protecting him from injury and complications.

In addition, follow these steps:
- Monitor the child for signs of joint limitation and pain.
- Teach the family about the disease process and how to monitor for complications.
- Help parents acquire the skills needed to parent a child with a chronic illness.

> It's a balancing act. There's a fine line between protecting and overprotecting a child with JIA.

Helpful or harmful?

- Help family members distinguish between harmless interventions and those that are potentially harmful; some studies show that most patients will try alternative treatments for JIA, including copper bracelets, acupuncture, herbs and other medicines, and diet.
- During inflammatory exacerbations, administer NSAIDs or prescribed medication on a regular schedule.

Legg-Calvé-Perthes disease

Legg-Calvé-Perthes disease is an avascular necrosis of the femoral head. It may involve the entire femoral head or only a portion of it. There may be a widening and flattening of the femoral head. The disorder can appear at any time between ages 2 and 12, although it's most commonly seen between ages 4 and 8. Boys are four times more likely to be affected than girls. The disorder is most prevalent in Whites and children of Chinese origin and rarely seen in African Americans. It usually affects only one hip. If both hips are symmetrically affected, an underlying systemic disorder should be considered.

What causes it

Necrosis (death) of the bone is caused by diminished blood supply to the femoral head. It isn't known what causes the blood supply to be interrupted.

Epidemiologic studies show an increased association of Legg-Calvé-Perthes disease with such factors as low birth weight, older parental age at conception, and lower socioeconomic status, to name a few. HIV and short stature as well as delayed bone maturation for age also seem to be risk factors.

Other theories have focused on conditions that could directly impede blood flow to the femoral head. Disorders of coagulation, such as thrombophilia, may predispose a child to Legg-Calvé-Perthes disease.

How it happens

Legg-Calvé-Perthes disease has three distinct stages:

The *avascular stage* is characterized by the interference of the blood supply to the head of the femur; without an appropriate blood supply, death of the bone cells (osteocytes) and bone marrow cells occurs. This stage can last several months to 1 year.

During the *revascularization stage*, vascular and connective tissue invade the dead bone in a process called *creeping substitution*; the necrotic tissue is replaced with living bone, although the bone isn't yet calcified.

In the final stage, also called the *healing stage*, ossification occurs; this process can take between 2 and 3 years to complete.

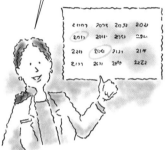

It's worth the wait. A few years of healing can result in completely normal bone in a child with Legg-Calvé-Perthes disease.

A job well done

The replacement of necrotic bone may be so complete and perfect that a completely normal bone results.

What to look for

Typically, children with Legg-Calvé-Perthes disease demonstrate a painless limp. Occasionally, pain is present and is made worse by activity. Pain is usually referred to the knee. Children may also complain of anterior thigh or groin pain. On examination, there is limited ROM in the hip joint.

What tests tell you

Symptoms may occasionally follow an injury, but studies usually show the disease was present before the injury.

X-rays correlate with the progression of the disease and the extent of the necrosis. There may be evidence of decreased bone mass and a smaller ossification center. A subchondral (below the cartilage—similar to the epiphyseal plate) fracture may be an early finding in the child with Legg-Calvé-Perthes disease. As the disease progresses, X-rays will show changes.

Complications

Osteochondritis dissecans occurs in less than 5% of patients with Legg-Calvé-Perthes disease. In this disorder, a wedge-shaped necrotic area of bone and cartilage develops adjacent to the joint.

It may break off and become lodged within the joint itself. The growth plate may be affected in severe disease.

Prognosis depends on the child's age, the extent of femoral head involvement, the disease's duration, and ROM. Some long-term studies have suggested that osteoarthritis leading to the need for total hip replacement will commonly develop later in life.

How it's treated

Legg-Calvé-Perthes disease is a self-limiting disease with no known treatments to speed the return of blood to the femoral head.

Keep it simple

Treatment consists simply of protecting the joint by keeping the femoral head within the acetabulum. If the joint is deeply seated within the acetabulum and normal joint motion is maintained, then a reasonably good result can be expected.

The goal of treatment is to reduce hip irritability, restore normal ROM, and prevent subluxation or dislocation. Surgical intervention is sometimes required. Children with Legg-Calvé-Perthes disease should be kept non–weight bearing.

Nonsurgical intervention includes PT, traction, and crutches. Casts and abduction bracing have been used in an attempt to hold the femoral head in place while the disease runs its course, but recent studies have shown no benefit from this type of treatment.

> When kids talk about hanging out, this isn't what they have in mind! Diversional activities keep boredom in check and will help keep development on track.

What to do

The child (and his parents) will need continuous emotional support. They should be encouraged to talk about their fears, anxiety, and frustration. Explaining all procedures as well as the need for no weight bearing will help reduce anxiety. In some cases, a period of bedrest is required.

In addition, follow these steps:
- Administer analgesics as ordered.
- Encourage parents to participate in their child's care.
- Stress the need for follow-up care to monitor rehabilitation.

Party at Tommy's bedside! RSVP

- Stress the need for home tutoring and socialization to promote normal mental and emotional growth and development.
- Offer tips for making home management of the bedridden child easier; tell parents what special supplies are needed, such as pajamas and trousers in a size larger than usually worn (with the side

seam opened and Velcro fasteners attached to close it), a bedpan, adhesive tape, moleskin and, possibly, a hospital bed.

It's hard to be a patient patient

• Remind the child and his parents that, although recovery may be a long and frustrating process, this is a self-limiting disease and the child will ultimately recover.

Slipped capital femoral epiphysis

As the name implies, a child with SCFE has a portion of the femoral head distal to the growth plate (physis) that slips out of the socket causing pain and a limp. In many cases, the pain is referred to the knee. The SCFE can occur in one or both of the hips. Depending on how severe the slip is and how long it has occurred, the treatment and prognosis can be short and sweet or long and complex.

What causes it

It is not fully understood what causes SCFE, but it is seen more commonly in younger teens who are obese. There may be a genetic predisposition. Kids with endocrine disorders such as diabetes, hypothyroidism, or growth hormone deficiencies are more prone to having an SCFE. This may be due to the abnormal cartilage growth and mineralization that occurs with these disorders.

How it happens

Any time the force placed on the femoral head exceeds that of the growth plate (the capital femoral physis), an SCFE is bound to happen. No one is quite sure what causes a weakening of the growth plate, but some factors include the normal thinning and widening of the growth plate during growth spurts or trauma. Other conditions that affect normal bone health such as cancer or certain medications may also predispose a child to SCFE.

What to look for

The biggest symptom of SCFE is pain in the knee, groin, thigh, or hip. The pain may be mild or severe depending on the severity of the slip. Some children with a mild slip may experience stiffness. A limp is often noticed. Increased activity frequently brings increased pain. SCFE is often classified according to the time of presentation.

Preslip—Children with preslip SCFE have pain but no overt signs of displacement. A widening of the proximal femoral physis may be seen on X-ray.

Acute—Children presenting with acute SCFE have pain that is recent (less than 2 to 3 weeks). It is commonly seen with traumatic injuries such as a fall and accounts for only 10% to 15% of cases. These children are in severe pain and may show a visible deformity. The child may refuse to bear weight. Children with an acute form of SCFE are at significant risk of further joint damage. They should be kept non–weight bearing until treatment is started.

Chronic—Chronic SCFE is the most common presentation of all types of SCFE. Pain can be vague and intermittent over a long period of time. The pain is commonly found in the knee, hip, groin, or thigh. On occasion, a diagnosis is missed or delayed because there is no actual hip pain. A limp is usually present with the foot of the affected side turning outward. ROM is decreased and painful in all directions. The upper thigh and gluteal muscles may begin to atrophy.

Acute on chronic—Children with chronic SCFE who suddenly have increased pain and symptoms are classified as acute on chronic presentation. Joint changes and effusion are typically seen. SCFE is also classified as stable or unstable or according to severity—mild, moderate, or severe.

What tests tell you

X-rays are the most common test used for the diagnosis of SCFE. A widening or irregularity of the physis is seen. If the slip is very mild, an MRI or bone scan may be used. Ultrasounds or CT scans have not been shown to be any more effective in the diagnosis of SCFE than regular X-rays. Other lab tests may be used to identify additional causes of SCFE (such as hypothyroidism).

Complications

Complications of SCFE can cause permanent joint damage or a discrepancy in leg length. Osteonecrosis or avascular necrosis is essentially the death of the bone. It can occur with severe slips, a delay in treatment, or due to a complication of the treatment itself. Chondrolysis is a narrowing of the joint itself and a loss of cartilage often due to untreated SCFE. It can also be seen in children whose severe SCFE requires a prolonged period of bedrest. Children with SCFE are at higher risk of developing osteoarthritis.

How it's treated

Surgery is the treatment for SCFE. The orthopedic surgeon places a screw through the growth plate and femoral head to stabilize the joint. In many cases, the surgeon will also stabilize the opposite hip due to the high risk of slippage bilaterally. Postoperative care includes teaching the child how to use crutches or a walker and the gradual return to normal activities.

What to do

SCFE can be a frightening diagnosis for a teen (or child) and his family. Reassure the family that with proper treatment, the outcomes are generally very good. Allow the child to express his fears and answer any questions he may have. Explain the importance of following the recommended treatment in order to prevent any long-term consequences.

Osgood-Schlatter disease

Osgood-Schlatter disease is not exactly a disease. It is an overuse injury of the knee in a growing adolescent. The patellar tendon becomes inflamed at the tibial junction, eventually leading to pain and swelling at the tibial tuberosity. It usually will go away as the child matures.

What causes it

Osgood-Schlatter disease happens when the repeated strain from activities exceeds the amount of give that the patellar tendon has. Athletic kids are more likely to develop Osgood-Schlatter disease than nonathletes. One-quarter to one-half of teens will have both knees affected.

How it happens

Active children often are involved in sports or other activities that require a lot of stress and contraction of the quadriceps. This contraction then exerts a pull on the developing patellar tendon. Repeated strain leads to inflammation of the tendon (apophysitis), thus causing a slight tear. As the body tries to repair the tear, a callus is formed. The result is pain and swelling at the tibial tuberosity—the bony protrusion on the tibia just below the kneecap.

What to look for

Knee pain is the hallmark symptom of Osgood-Schlatter disease. It starts out as a dull ache then increases with continued use. It is exacerbated by activities that require a lot of knee use (running, climbing stairs, kneeling, etc.). The pain goes away with rest. Other symptoms include tenderness and swelling at the tibial tuberosity and tight hamstrings and quads.

What tests tell you

The diagnosis of Osgood-Schlatter disease is made by clinical examination. Unless there are unusual signs and symptoms such as redness, warmth, nighttime pain, or an acute onset of severe pain, X-rays are not needed.

Complications

Complications of this process are rare. The most common complication is continued chronic pain. A persistent prominence of the
tibial tubercle may occur. Very rarely, Osgood-Schlatter disease
may cause a hyperextension of the knee known as *genu recurva-
tum* (backward-bending knee).

How it's treated

Because the biggest problem with Osgood-Schlatter disease is
pain due to overuse, treatment is geared toward controlling the
pain and resting the knee. NSAIDs such as ibuprofen (Motrin/
Advil) or naproxen (Naprosyn/Aleve) may be used for 4 to 7 days
to decrease the inflammation and provide pain control. Resting
the knee is paramount. Unfortunately, the kids who are most
likely to develop Osgood-Schlatter disease are also those most
likely not to rest the knee. Gradual return to sports after therapy
to stretch and strengthen the quadriceps is recommended. On
rare occasions, surgery is needed to resect the ossicle that has
developed or to remove the prominent tuberosity.

What to do

The name Osgood-Schlatter disease can frighten a child and the
family. Reassurance that this is not a disease and will usually
resolve after a short amount of rest and therapy is often all that
the child needs to be able to deal with this diagnosis. In addition,
follow these steps:
• Help the child and family understand the importance of resting
the knee as recommended and to not try to continue at the same
level the activities that caused this injury to begin with.
• Encourage the child, however, to be active as long as the pain is
tolerable and resolves within 24 hours.
• Educate the child and family on strengthening and stretching
exercises of the quadriceps and hamstrings.
• Encourage the use of a protective pad to prevent direct trauma
to the tibial tubercle.

Scoliosis

Scoliosis is a spinal deformity; it's defined as a lateral curvature
of the spine that's greater than 10 degrees and is always associated with some rotation of the involved vertebrae. Posterior
curvature of the spine is known as *kyphosis*, and anterior curvature is known as *lordosis*. Although some curvature is normal,
excessive curvature becomes pathologic. Scoliosis is classified as

either nonstructural (functional) or structural. (See *Looking at scoliosis*.)

Scoliosis can occur at any age, but idiopathic scoliosis is seen in greatest numbers in children after age 8. Girls are four to five times more likely to be affected than boys, and the incidence is higher if another family member is affected. The deformity progresses during growth periods and stabilizes when vertebral growth is complete.

What causes it

In nonstructural scoliosis, the spine is structurally normal and the disorder never progresses to structural scoliosis. Nonstructural scoliosis may be caused by poor posture, leg-length discrepancies, an irritated sciatic nerve, or an infectious process such as appendicitis. A very rare psychological scoliosis is known as *hysterical scoliosis*.

Not sure about structure

Structural scoliosis can be categorized by its major causes: neuromuscular, congenital, syndromic, or idiopathic. Neuromuscular disorders such as cerebral palsy, poliomyelitis, or muscular dystrophy can cause scoliosis. Birth defects, injuries, certain infections, tumors, and metabolic factors are also identified causes. Connective tissue disorders leading to Marfan syndrome, neurofibromatosis, osteogenesis imperfecta, or rheumatic disease may also cause structural abnormalities. The cause of *idiopathic scoliosis*, the most common type of structural scoliosis, is currently unknown. There may be a genetic component as some studies in identical twins show a higher incidence of idiopathic scoliosis than that of fraternal twins. Children also have a higher incidence of acquiring scoliosis if a parent had it.

How it happens

The spine is normally curved in order to maintain proper balance, with the muscles on either side of the spine supporting it. If a lateral curve has developed, a convex rotation of the spine and ribs will eventually cause the vertebrae to become rotated or wedge-shaped. Muscles become contracted and a compensatory curve develops so that the body can maintain balance and posture. The curve either stabilizes on its own or progress. The amount of progression depends on the child's sex, the initial severity of the curve, and the remaining growth potential. The curve will naturally worsen as the spine continues to grow.

Looking at scoliosis

The spinal deformity that occurs in scoliosis is shown in this illustration.

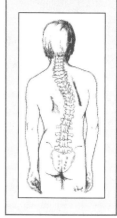

What to look for

Examination of the child usually begins with a general inspection of the back with the child in a standing position. Obvious asymmetries can be seen, including:
• one shoulder higher than the other
• prominent scapula
• uneven waistline
• rib hump.

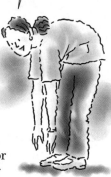

The signs of scoliosis are even more obvious when the child bends over.

Over for obvious

As the child bends over, these asymmetries become even more obvious. The shoulder and hip levels become uneven. The head should normally align directly over the sacrum but, in persons with a spinal deformity, there may be deviation from the midline. These differences disappear in nonstructural scoliosis.

Something suspicious

Scoliosis classically produces no symptoms. If the child has pain, the scoliosis is likely due to some other disorder such as a bone or spinal cord tumor. Neurologic symptoms, wasting of the hands or lower extremities, and an age of onset younger than 10 years suggests a different cause. These secondary causes must be ruled out. In cases of secondary scoliosis, the curvature often will resolve when the underlying cause is treated.

What tests tell you

X-rays are used to evaluate the entire spine in the standing position, looking at both the anteroposterior and lateral planes.
• Measurement of skeletal maturity and shoulder and hip levels determines the degree of scoliosis.
• An abnormal forward bending test, in which the patient bends forward 90 degrees with the hands joined at the midline, demonstrates asymmetry of the shoulders and height of the ribs.
• Two types of measurement devices—a level plane ruler, used for measurement while the patient is bending over, and a scoliometer, designed to assess the angle of trunk rotation—can be used to help determine the severity of the curve and guide management decisions. It can also be used to help reassure the child and her family.

Complications

Generally, scoliosis is mild and there are few problems. Some children with scoliosis will continue with back pain throughout adulthood. Complications can sometimes lead to serious, debilitating, or even life-threatening sequelae. The curve can cause the thoracic area to become smaller, thus crowding the heart and lungs. This can lead to pulmonary and cardiac compromise.

Negotiating the curves

The severity of complications increases with the severity of the curvature:

• Severe curves can affect vital lung capacity, causing tachypnea or even hypoxia; severe restrictive lung disease and even death from cor pulmonale may occur if scoliosis is left untreated.

• Large thoracic curves greater than 60 degrees are associated with a shortened life span.

• Large lumbar curvatures may lead to subluxation of the vertebrae and arthritic changes in the spine; disabling pain in adulthood may result because of these changes.

• Neurologic sequelae and paralysis may be a complication if the vertebral column is manipulated during surgery.

• Infection is always a risk after surgery.

How it's treated

Treatment of scoliosis depends on the magnitude of the curve, skeletal maturity, and the risk of progression. No treatment is necessary in children with functional scoliosis or in whom the curve is less than 20 degrees. Structural scoliosis is treated as early as possible in order to lessen or prevent progression. Stretching and strengthening the back muscles improve posture and maintain flexibility.

Brace yourself

Bracing is used in skeletally immature children with curves between 20 and 40 degrees. A silastic, thoracolumbosacral brace is molded to the child and exerts gentle pressure on the spine. This brace is worn 23 hours per day until growth is complete, usually for several years. It's removed only for hygiene and skin care. This brace, also known as an underarm brace, can be fairly well concealed under clothing. A more cumbersome under-chin brace is sometimes needed with more complex curvatures. This brace is less likely to be concealed under clothes and may not be tolerated by the child. Bracing usually does not cure scoliosis but does prevent it from progressing further and may even decrease the amount of curvature noted at the end of treatment.

No confusion, it's spinal fusion

Spinal fusion surgery, rod placement, and bone grafting may be required to correct curves greater than 45 degrees. Activities are restricted for several months until the fusion is solid.

What to do

It's essential to assess continually for compliance, as noncompliance with recommended treatment measures may be detrimental. In addition, follow these steps:
• Teach the prescribed treatment routines to the child and her parents, and explain the consequences of not following these recommendations (to help ensure the best possible outcome).
• Emphasize activity restrictions; provide alternative exercises and activities that are beneficial.

Stealth brace

• Help the child find clothing that minimizes the appearance of the brace to enhance her self-image; teach her to wear a light T-shirt or jersey underneath the brace and to place a smooth cloth over the chin pad (to minimize skin breakdown and promote skin integrity).

A strange new world

• For children requiring surgical correction, preoperative teaching is essential. Prepare the child for the presence of various catheters, a special bed (Stryker frame), and the use of certain body mechanics in order to restrict bending at the fusion site. Peer support groups may also be helpful when the child can return home.

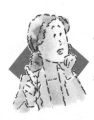

Quick quiz

1.   The growth plate of the bone is known as:
     A.   the epiphyseal plate.
     B.   the metaphyseal plate.
     C.   the diaphyseal plate.
     D.   the medullary plate.

Answer: A. The epiphyseal plate. The diaphysis is the shaft of the long bone. The metaphysis is the wider portion of the long bone next to the epiphysis. The medullary cavity is where the bone marrow is found.

2. When teaching parents about treatment for their baby's clubfoot, the nurse should educate the parents that the casts will be:

    A.   placed on the affected foot for 2 weeks only.

    B.   placed on both feet for 6 weeks.

    C.   placed on the affected foot initially then changed every 2 to 3 weeks as the baby's foot grows and is manipulated.

    D.   placed on both feet initially and then changed every 4 to 5 weeks as the baby's feet grow and are manipulated.

Answer: C. Serial casting is done on the affected foot (or both feet if affected) and changed every 2 to 3 weeks as the baby's foot grows and is manipulated. Treatment lasts for several months depending on the severity of the deformation.

3. Initial treatment of JIA includes:

    A.   gold salts.

    B.   methotrexate.

    C.   aspirin.

    D.   NSAIDs.

Answer: D. NSAIDs such as ibuprofen or naproxen are the first-line treatment for JIA. Methotrexate has replaced gold salts as a second-line treatment if NSAIDs are not sufficient. Aspirin should not be used in children due to the rare but severe risk of developing Reye's syndrome.

4. A nurse is caring for a child with an SCFE. What findings would she expect on exam?

    A.   Pain in the affected hip only and a noticeable limp

    B.   Pain in the knee, hip, groin, or thigh; possible complaints of stiffness; and perhaps a limp

    C.   Pain and swelling of the affected hip and a severe limp

    D.   Redness, swelling, and pain above the knee of the affected side

Answer: B. An SCFE often will refer pain to the knee, groin, or thigh. A mild slip may only cause stiffness. The severity of the limp depends on the severity of the slip. Redness and swelling would suggest a different cause.

5. Educating patients and families about Osgood-Schlatter disease should include teaching that:

    A.   the disease progresses to a point that the child can no longer participate in any activity.

    B.   the disease name is a misnomer and it is really an overuse injury.

    C.   the disease means the child must be on bedrest until the injury resolves.

    D.   the disease means the child can treat the pain with ice and medication and continue with all activities as before.

Answer: B. Osgood-Schlatter disease is not really a disease but an overuse injury to the patellar tendon. It will heal with rest and maturity of the muscles and tendons. Children should be encouraged to stay active but not at the same level as before to prevent further injury to the tendon. Icing and short-term use of NSAIDs may help the pain.

Scoring

☆☆☆ If you answered all five items correctly, hip-hooray! You've earned the right to flex your muscles.

  ☆☆ If you answered four items correctly, fine work! Now you're ready to bone up for the next quiz.

    ☆ If you answered fewer than four items correctly, don't let it rattle your bones! There are still four quizzes in your future—no bones about it.

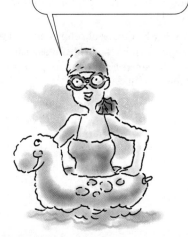

You did a swimmingly good job with musculoskeletal disorders! Next up: GI problems.

Gastrointestinal problems

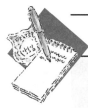

Just the facts

In this chapter, you'll learn:

♦ anatomy and physiology of the GI system

♦ diagnostic tests for children with GI disorders

♦ treatments and procedures used for children with GI disorders

♦ GI disorders that affect infants and children.

Anatomy and physiology

The functions of the gastrointestinal (GI) tract enable ingestion and propulsion of food, digestion and absorption of food and nutrients needed by the body, and elimination of waste products.

Structures of the GI system

The GI system consists of two major components:

  alimentary canal

  accessory organs of digestion.

It's alimentary, my dear Watson

The alimentary canal of the GI tract consists of a hollow, muscular tube that begins in the mouth and ends at the anus. It includes the:

- oral cavity
- pharynx
- esophagus
- stomach
- small intestine
- large intestine.

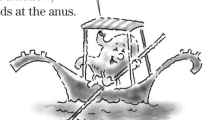

If neighbors make the neighborhood, the alimentary canal is the best! To my north is Mr. Esophagus, and to my south are the Intestines.

Accessories make the system

Accessory glands and organs that aid GI function include the:

- salivary glands
- liver
- biliary duct system (gallbladder and bile ducts)
- pancreas.

Digestion

Digestion starts in the oral cavity, where chewing (mastication), salivation (the beginning of starch digestion), and swallowing (deglutition) take place. (See *The growing GI system.*)

Growing pains

The growing GI system

Here are some highlights of the developing GI system during the first few years of life.

Salivary assistance

- Saliva production begins at age 4 months and aids in the process of digestion. Saliva contains mucus to protect oral mucosa and to coat food. Food breakdown begins in the mouth with the enzymes ptyalin and amylase.
- The sucking and extrusion reflex (a reflex that protects the infant from food substances his system is too immature to digest) persists until ages 3 to 4 months.

Stomach

- The stomach capacity of the neonate is 30 to 60 ml and gradually increases to 200 to 300 ml by age 12 months and to 1,500 ml in the adolescent.
- Up until ages 4 to 8 weeks, the neonatal abdomen is larger than the chest and the musculature is poorly developed.
- Spit-ups are frequent in the neonate because of the immature muscle tone of the lower esophageal sphincter and the low volume capacity of the stomach.
- Peristalsis occurs within 2½ to 3 hours in the neonate and extends to 3 to 6 hours in older infants and children.
- Digestive enzymes are deficient until at least ages 4 to 6 months; gas, diarrhea, sensitization for food allergies, and microscopic hemorrhages can develop if solid foods are introduced before this time.

Intestinal

- From ages 1 to 3 years, the composition of intestinal flora becomes more adultlike and stomach acidity increases, reducing the number of GI infections.
- Exposure to breast milk increases intestinal flora early on and provides some protection against viruses and pathologic flora.
- Increased myelination of nerves to the anal sphincter allows for physiologic control of bowel function, usually at about age 2; psychological readiness for toilet training may occur at a later age.

Liver

- The liver is immature at birth, resulting in inefficient detoxifying of substances and medications. Medication dosages may need to be adjusted.
- The liver's slow development of glycogen storage capacity makes the infant prone to hypoglycemia.
- Infants are more prone to dehydration and fluid and electrolyte imbalances due to greater body surface area, high rate of metabolism, and immature kidney function.

The rise and fall of hormones

Hunger is controlled by the lateral hypothalamus in the brain. A fall in blood nutrients, a rise or fall in hormones governing metabolism, hunger contractions from the stomach, and emotional input signal the hypothalamus to stimulate hunger. Fullness of the stomach, blood levels of nutrients and hormones, and emotions or habits stimulate the satiety center in the ventromedial area of the hypothalamus to decrease hunger.

The tasteful tongue

The tongue provides the sense of taste and is the strongest muscle in the body. Saliva secreted from the salivary glands moistens the mouth and lubricates the food bolus to ease swallowing.

Look out stomach, here it comes!

When a person swallows a food bolus:

The upper esophageal sphincter relaxes, allowing food to enter the esophagus.

The epiglottis closes with swallowing to prevent food from being aspirated into the trachea.

As food moves through the esophagus, glands in the esophageal mucosal layer secrete mucus, which lubricates the food and protects the esophageal mucosal layer from being damaged by poorly chewed foods. (See *Choking hazards.*)

Lower esophageal contractions (called *peristalsis*) gradually push the food down the esophagus and through the lower esophageal sphincter into the stomach.

Stomach

Until the child is approximately age 2 years, the stomach is round. It will gradually elongate and take the adult shape and position in the abdomen by age 7 years.

The stomach lies in the left upper quadrant of the abdomen and is made up of three parts:

The *fundus* is an enlarged portion above and to the left of the esophageal opening in the stomach; the *cardiac sphincter* is at the opening of the esophagus to the stomach.

The *body* is the middle portion of the stomach.

The *pylorus* is the lower portion of the stomach, lying near the junction of the stomach and the duodenum. The pyloric sphincter is at the opening of the stomach to the duodenum.

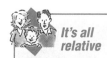

It's all relative

Choking hazards

Foods that are round and less than 1¼″ (3.2 cm) in diameter can obstruct the airway of a child when swallowed whole. Teach parents to cut foods into small pieces to prevent obstruction of the airway. Common foods that may cause choking include:

• hot dogs
• Vienna sausages
• nuts
• popcorn
• marshmallows
• grapes
• hard candy
• fruits with pits
• dried beans.

A gastric response

The secretory cells in the lining of the stomach are believed to be functional at birth. The lining of the stomach secretes gastrin in response to stomach wall distention. In turn, gastrin stimulates the release of highly acidic digestive secretions consisting mainly of pepsinogen, which is converted to pepsin, hydrochloric acid, intrinsic factor, and proteolytic enzymes. Limited amounts of water, alcohol, and some drugs are absorbed in the stomach. Intrinsic factor is necessary for vitamin B_{12} absorption.

> There's no such thing as a day off when you store the food, mix it with gastric juices, and send the chyme into the small intestine.

Triple overtime

The stomach's three functions are to store food, mix food with gastric juices via peristaltic contractions, and slowly distribute this food (now called *chyme*) into the small intestine through the pyloric opening for further digestion and absorption.

Small intestine

Nearly all digestion and absorption take place in the small intestine. The small intestine lies coiled in the abdomen and consists of three major sections:

 duodenum

 jejunum

 ileum.

Contractions and secretions

Peristaltic contractions and various digestive secretions break down carbohydrates, proteins, and fats, enabling the intestinal mucosa to absorb these nutrients, along with water and electrolytes. *Secretin* and *cholecystokinin* are the hormones that affect intestinal secretions and gastric motility.

Distribution center

The surface area of the small intestine is increased by millions of villi in the mucous membrane lining. Digested food is absorbed through the mucosal walls and into the blood for distribution throughout the body. Failure to feed, malnutrition, ischemia, and infections affect the small intestine's ability to absorb nutrients, resulting in growth delays.

Large intestine

The ileocecal valve is the sphincter between the ileum of the small intestine and the cecum of the large intestine. It prevents secretions from returning to the ileum. By the time chyme passes through the small intestine and enters the ascending colon of the large intestine, it has been reduced to mostly indigestible substances.

Downward spiral

From the ascending colon, chyme passes through the transverse colon and descending colon to the rectum, and finally into the anal canal, where it's expelled. The anal sphincter voluntarily controls defecation except in infants and patients with spinal cord injuries.

We aren't always the bad guys. As residents of the large intestine, we help synthesize vitamin K and break down cellulose. Newborn infants do not synthesize vitamin K for about the first week of life.

A large job description

The large intestine doesn't produce hormones or digestive enzymes; it is, however, the site of water and sodium and potassium absorption. The mucosa produces alkaline secretions that lubricate the intestinal wall as chyme pushes through and protect the mucosa from acidic bacterial actions. The large intestine also harbors bacteria, such as *Escherichia coli* and *Enterobacter aerogenes*, which help to break down cellulose into usable carbohydrates and synthesize vitamin K. Vitamin K is needed by humans for blood clotting. Older children and adults get most of their vitamin K from bacteria in the gut, and some from their diet. Babies have very little vitamin K in their bodies at birth. Vitamin K does not cross the placenta to the developing baby, and the gut does not have any bacteria to make vitamin K before birth. After birth, there is little vitamin K in breast milk and breast-fed babies can be low in vitamin K for several weeks until the normal gut bacteria start making it. Infant formula has added vitamin K, but even formula-fed babies have very low levels of vitamin K for several days. With low levels of vitamin K, some babies can have very severe bleeding—sometimes into the brain, causing significant brain damage. This bleeding is called *hemorrhagic disease of the newborn* (HDN). As a preventive measure, babies are routinely given vitamin K injections at birth.

Accessory glands and organs

Allied with the GI tract are the liver, biliary duct system, and pancreas, which contribute the hormones, enzymes, and bile that are vital to digestion.

Liver

The liver is located in the right upper quadrant (RUQ) of the abdomen and is the body's largest gland. It plays an important role in carbohydrate metabolism, detoxifies various endogenous and exogenous toxins in plasma, and synthesizes plasma proteins, nonessential amino acids, and vitamin A.

Essential storage

The liver also stores essential nutrients, such as iron and vitamins K, D, and B_{12}. It secretes bile and removes ammonia from body fluids, converting it to urea for excretion in urine.

Biliary duct system

Bile is a greenish fluid that aids the small intestine to emulsify and absorb fats and fat-soluble vitamins and also neutralizes stomach acids. Bile exits through bile ducts that merge into the right and left hepatic ducts to form the common hepatic duct. This common duct joins the cystic duct from the gallbladder to form the common bile duct to the duodenum.

> The stomach gets all the credit, but digestion would be a disaster without the accessory glands and organs!

Gallbladder

The gallbladder, located beneath the liver, stores and concentrates bile produced by the liver. Secretion of the hormone cholecystokinin causes the gallbladder to contract and relax the ampulla of Vater, releasing bile into the common bile duct for delivery to the duodenum.

Pancreas

The pancreas is a large gland located behind the stomach and attached to the duodenum. The pancreas performs exocrine and endocrine functions. Its exocrine function involves cells that secrete digestive enzymes, bicarbonate, and hormones into the small intestine to aid in digestion.

Alpha beta Langerhans

The endocrine function of the pancreas involves the islets of Langerhans, which house alpha and beta cells. Alpha cells secrete glucagon, which stimulates glycogenolysis in the liver. Beta cells secrete insulin to promote carbohydrate metabolism.

Diagnostic tests

Tests used to diagnose GI disorders include barium enema, barium swallow, endoscopic retrograde cholangiopancreatography (ERCP), endoscopy, and stool specimen testing.

Barium enema

A barium enema, also called a *lower GI series*, allows X-ray visualization of the colon. Barium is dripped into the rectum by gravity, and a series of X-rays is taken as the barium passes through the lower GI tract.

Nursing considerations

Explain the procedure to the child and his parents. Prepare the child for insertion of the barium, and explain that he may be slightly uncomfortable as he changes positions on the X-ray table. Also explain that the child will have to wait until the test is over to go to the bathroom and that his bowel movements may look whitish until the barium has passed through his system.
- Usually, the child will be on a liquid diet for 24 hours before the test.

An interesting way to start the day

- Bowel preparations are administered before the examination; an enema the night before the test, the morning of the test, or both may be used for children and infants. (Prepare the child for the enema and provide as much privacy as possible.)
- Tell the child that X-rays will be taken on a test table and that he must hold still (even though he'll feel like he has to go to the bathroom).
- Cover the genital area with a lead apron during the X-rays.

Exit the barium

- Hydrate the child well with electrolyte-containing fluids after the procedure to prevent dehydration and to help expel the barium to prevent barium impaction.

Barium swallow

A barium or diatrizoate meglumine (Gastrografin) swallow, also called an *upper GI series*, provides imaging of the upper GI tract. It's used primarily to examine the esophagus.

Follow the swallow

A series of X-rays is taken while the swallowed barium or Gastrografin moves into the esophagus, stomach, and duodenum to reveal abnormalities. The barium outlines the stomach walls and delineates ulcer craters and filling defects. Gastrografin and barium facilitate imaging through X-rays, but Gastrografin is less toxic if it escapes from the GI tract.

Seeking the ileocecal valve

A small bowel series is an extension of the upper GI series; additional imaging is done as the barium or Gastrografin flows farther down the GI tract through the small intestine to the ileocecal valve.

Nursing considerations

- Explain the procedure to the child and his parents. Tell the child that he'll need to take big swallows of a thick drink that looks like a milkshake (but doesn't taste as good). Explain

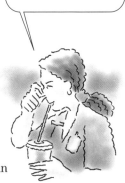

Barium preparations are disguised as milkshakes but they taste more like chalk! They're easier to swallow when they're ice cold.

that pictures will be taken while he's drinking and afterward, and that he'll need to hold still during the X-rays.
• Maintain the child on a nothing-by-mouth (NPO) status beginning at midnight before the test.
• After the test, monitor bowel movements for excretion of barium and monitor GI function.

Endoscopic retrograde cholangiopancreatography

In ERCP, a contrast medium is injected into the duodenal papilla to allow radiographic examination of the pancreatic ducts and hepatobiliary tree.

Nursing considerations

Obtain written, informed consent after explaining the procedure to the child and his parents. In addition:
• Check the child's history for allergies to cholinergics and iodine.
• Administer a sedative and monitor the child for the drug's effect.

It's all over

After the procedure:
• Monitor the child's gag reflex. (The child remains on NPO status until his gag reflex returns.)
• Protect the child from aspiration of mucus by positioning him on his side.
• Monitor the child for urine retention.

Endoscopy

Endoscopy allows visualization of the GI system (and, when needed, biopsy of tissue) with a fiber-optic scope.

The direct approach

Fiber-optic testing allows direct visualization of the GI tract. Different types of fiber-optic testing are used to examine different portions of the GI tract:
• *Esophagogastroduodenoscopy* allows visual inspection of the esophagus, stomach, and duodenum.
• *Colonoscopy* allows direct visualization of the descending, transverse, and ascending colon.
• *Proctosigmoidoscopy* allows inspection of the anus, rectum, and distal sigmoid colon.

Nursing considerations

• Explain the procedure to the child and his parents, and make sure that written, informed consent has been obtained.

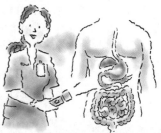

It's hard to hide from endoscopy! A fiber-optic scope can "shine a light" on the entire GI system.

• Oral and tongue piercings must be removed. They may accidently dislodge and enter airway as foreign bodies.
• Prepare the child for sedation by explaining that it will make him sleepy and will keep him from hurting during the procedure.
• A mild sedative may be administered before the examination; prepare the child for insertion of an intravenous (I.V.) line for sedation during this procedure.
• The child may be kept on NPO status beginning at midnight before the test for an upper GI series.
• The child may be placed on a liquid diet for 24 hours before the examination or require enemas and laxatives until the bowel is clear for a lower GI series.
• After the procedure, assess vital signs for dyspnea and fever with a decrease in blood pressure and an increase in pulse, indicating the possibility of bleeding from perforation.

Stool specimen

Stool specimens are obtained to examine the stool for suspected GI bleeding, infection, or malabsorption. Tests include the guaiac test for occult blood and microscopic tests for ova, parasites, and fat.

Nursing considerations

Nursing interventions focus on proper collection and handling of the specimen.
• Obtain the specimen in the correct container (the container may need to be sterile or contain a preservative).
• Be aware that the specimen may need to be transported to the laboratory immediately or placed in the refrigerator.
• For infants, stool specimens may be obtained from the diaper. However, apply a urine bag to prevent urine from contaminating the stool.

Treatments and procedures

Treatments and procedures for children with GI disorders include alternative feeding methods, total parenteral nutrition (TPN), GI intubation, and ostomy creation.

Alternative feeding methods

Children who are unable to take nutrients by mouth (for example, premature neonates with a poor sucking reflex, children who can't take in enough calories, or children with disorders of the mouth and esophagus, such as atresia and fistulas) are fed by alternative feeding methods. These methods include nasogastric (NG) gavage, orogastric (OG) gavage, duodenum and jejunum gavage, gastrostomy feedings, and jejunostomy feedings. These feedings may be administered intermittently or continuously.

Nursing considerations

Explain to the child and his parents why the alternative feeding method is needed, and prepare the child for insertion of the feeding tube.

Nasogastric and orogastric feedings

In NG and OG feedings, a tube is inserted into the stomach by way of one of the nares (NG) or the mouth (OG). Follow these steps:

• To determine the correct length of the feeding tube, measure from the tip of the child's nose to his ear and add to that amount the length from his ear to his xiphoid process.

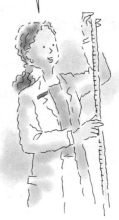

How long should it be? Do the math! The tip of the child's nose to the ear + the ear to the xiphoid process = the tube length.

Cold coil in a cup

• Lubricate the tube with sterile water or a water-soluble lubricant before administration.
• Facilitate insertion of the NG tube by having the child take large swallows of water as the tube is being inserted; allow the child to practice first.
• When the feeding tube is secured, check placement immediately, at the start of intermittent feedings, and at least every 4 hours thereafter.
• Inject 1 cc of air for infants and 5 cc of air for children into the feeding tube, and auscultate for gurgling sounds in the stomach when the air is injected. Alternate methods of checking placement are to aspirate a small amount of stomach contents and apply pH paper to check acidity level. Measure the tube from the nose or mouth to the end and record in the nurse's notes every shift. If the tube is to be left in place, an X-ray may be ordered to check placement.

Recycle the residual

• Check the residual amount of formula by aspirating stomach contents into a syringe. Record the amount of residual formula and the color, odor, and consistency of the gastric contents before refeeding the contents.
• Administer feeding by gravity or feeding pump.

Clear the clogs

• Irrigate the feeding tube with 10 ml of sterile water after each feeding to prevent stagnant formula from clogging the tube.

• Record the total amount of formula administered and describe how well it was tolerated. Observe for signs of aspiration and intolerance, including low oxygen saturation, difficulty breathing, increased crying or discomfort, and vomiting.

Pinch and position

• If the feeding tube will be removed after feeding, pinch the tube while withdrawing it to prevent aspirating fluid left in the tube.
• Position the child with his head elevated during the feeding and for 1 hour afterward to prevent aspiration.

Sucking for satiation

• When feeding infants by NG or OG tube, nonnutritive sucking is essential for oral stimulation. It helps the infant to relate a full stomach with oral sucking and fulfills the developmental need to suck.

> An infant who's receiving tube feedings still needs to suck. It provides stimulation and comfort.

Duodenum and jejunum gavage feedings

Duodenum and jejunum gavage feedings are administered with indwelling feeding tubes in the duodenum or jejunum.

Feedings are administered as they are with NG and OG feedings; however, the residual gastric contents and tube placement don't need to be checked. Duodenum and jejunum feeding tubes aren't removed after each feeding.

Gastrostomy and jejunostomy feedings

Gastrostomy and jejunostomy feedings are administered with a surgically placed feeding tube. The tube has one exit site on the abdomen but is composed of two separate chambers, each with a unique entry port. One side of the tube ends in the stomach and is typically used for medication administration. The other side of the tube ends in the jejunum and is typically used for formula administration.

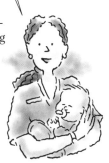

It wouldn't work in outer space

In gastrostomy and jejunostomy feedings:
• Boluses of formula or water are administered by gravity or by feeding pump.
• The feeding tube must be flushed with sterile water after each feeding to prevent clogs.
• The child should be positioned with his head elevated at a 30-degree angle after feeding to prevent aspiration and encourage gastric emptying.
• Long-term gastrostomy tubes have a button closure that allows for the removal of the gastrostomy tube between feedings.
• As with NG or OG tubes, infants fed by gastrostomy tube should engage in nonnutritive sucking for oral stimulation. It helps the infant to relate a full stomach with oral sucking and fulfills the developmental need to suck.

Total parenteral nutrition

TPN provides nutrients intravenously for infants and children who aren't able to take GI feedings, if GI feedings can't provide enough nutrition, or if feedings are needed long-term.

Concentrate on TPN

TPN is a highly concentrated solution of protein, glucose, vitamins, and minerals. It's infused through I.V. tubing with a special filter to remove particulate matter and microorganisms. Low-glucose solutions may be administered through a peripheral I.V. line. High-glucose solutions are administered through central I.V. lines. Some medications, such as heparin and ranitidine (Zantac), may be added to the TPN solution and, therefore, shouldn't be administered separately.

TPN is typically administered with an intralipid infusion that provides necessary lipids and calories.

Nursing considerations

Prepare the child for insertion of the peripheral or central line. It can be frightening to a child (or his parents) if a line is inserted in the neck or shoulder area. Using a doll to demonstrate may help the child understand what will happen.

In addition, follow these steps:
• Monitor the infusion rate via the I.V. pump. Cycling TPN, if ordered, involves tapering the drip rate at the start and end of the infusion, which commonly requires hourly rate changes.

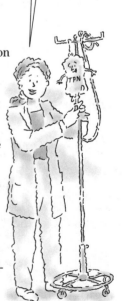

Parents may need reassurance that all the nutrition their child needs is in the TPN solution.

Infection inspection

• Assess the insertion site for signs of infection and infiltration because TPN can cause significant tissue damage.
• Bags of TPN should be changed every 24 hours; tubing should be changed according to your facility policy. The doctor will order changes to the contents of the TPN solution based on the child's daily laboratory values. Inspect the bag of TPN; don't hang it if the solution appears cloudy or if there are precipitates visible (if so, return it to the pharmacy).

Not too much, not too little

• Monitor electrolytes for excesses and deficits, particularly hyperkalemia and hypophosphatemia.
• Monitor the child's blood glucose for hyperglycemia and administer insulin as ordered.
• Reassure the parents that the TPN will provide all the nutrition the child needs.

GI intubation

GI intubation is the insertion of an NG tube for diagnostic and therapeutic purposes. It's used to:
• empty the stomach and intestine
• aid in diagnosis and treatment of stomach and upper GI tract disorders
• decompress obstructed areas
• detect and treat GI bleeding
• administer medications or feedings.

Nursing considerations

Prepare the child for insertion of the NG tube with a simple, age-appropriate explanation. Because many children panic at the sight of the tube, it's important to maintain a calm and reassuring manner and provide emotional support.

In addition, follow these steps:
• When inserting the tube, instruct the child to take swallows of water to ease insertion, which also gives the child a job to do and provides a degree of distraction.

A glass of water makes an NG tube easier to swallow.

What goes in must come out

• Maintain accurate intake and output records.
• Record the amount, color, odor, and consistency of gastric drainage every 4 hours.
• When irrigating the tube, note the amount of normal saline solution instilled and aspirated.
• Check for fluid and electrolyte imbalances.
• Provide good oral and nasal care. Make sure the tube is secure and doesn't put pressure on the nostrils.

Anchors away

• To support the tube's weight and prevent its accidental removal, anchor the tube to the child's clothing.
• After removing the tube from a child with GI bleeding, watch for signs and symptoms of recurrent bleeding.

Ostomy

An ostomy is an opening in the intestines with the intestinal wall drawn to the abdomen. A stoma is created to allow passage of intestinal contents. An ostomy can be permanent or temporary, depending on the reason for the ostomy and how much of the intestine has been removed.

Correct the defect

An ostomy is created to correct an anatomical defect, relieve an obstruction, or permit treatment of an infection or injury to the intestinal tract. The most common reasons for an ostomy in infants and children are imperforate anus, necrotizing enterocolitis, Hirschsprung's disease, and inflammatory bowel diseases.

Location, location, location

An *ileostomy* is placed in the ileum portion of the small intestine. A *colostomy* is placed in the large intestine and may be ascending, transverse, or descending, depending on where it's placed.

Nursing considerations

Explain the procedure in simple, age-appropriate terms, preparing the child and his parents for all aspects of the surgery. Prepare the child and his parents for the post-operative period, specifically, what the child will see on his body and feel.

Bad timing

For older children and adolescents who are already concerned with appearance and acceptance by their peers, concerns about body image and, for the adolescent, sexuality are likely. Encourage the child to express these concerns and ask questions. (A same-gender nurse may be easier for the child to talk with.)

I want to be just like my friends, and having an ostomy makes me feel different. It helps to talk about it and to have my questions answered.

Been there, done that

If possible, introduce the child to a peer who has had the procedure and is handling it well. Refer the child to other health care professionals who can help him deal with his body image issue. Also note the following:

• Mucus secretions begin within 48 hours after surgery.
• Fecal drainage begins within 72 hours after surgery.
• Edema of the stoma is present for 2 to 3 weeks after placement.

A wash and a pat-dry

• When changing the stoma appliance (as needed), record the amount, character, color, and odor of the drainage; wash the stoma with soap and water, rinse, pat dry, apply adhesive material (skin sealant and stoma paste), and reapply the drainage bag.
• Instruct the child and his parents in care of the ostomy.
• If the skin is irritated, apply a protective ointment before applying the appliance.

- An infant's stoma may be left unpouched with a protective wafer around the stoma.

Pouch protector

- In young children, protect the pouch from being pulled off by using one-piece shirt-and-pant outfits.
- To control odor in the appliance, use deodorant drops, aspirin, or mouthwash solutions.
- A low-residue diet may be required; avoid gas-producing foods or foods with strong odors.

Pass the salt

- With an ileostomy, provide a diet high in sodium and potassium; avoid highly seasoned foods.
- Protect the skin around the stoma from enzymes in liquid stool by using a skin protectant or by making sure that the opening to the wafer is cut close to the sides of the stoma.

GI disorders

GI disorders that may affect children include appendicitis, celiac disease, cleft lip and palate, Crohn's disease, hepatitis, Hirschsprung's disease, intussusception, pyloric stenosis, tracheo-esophageal fistula and esophageal atresia, ulcerative colitis, and volvulus.

Appendicitis

Appendicitis is an inflammation and obstruction of the blind sac (vermiform appendix) at the end of the cecum. It's the most common major surgical disease in school-age children and its peak incidence occurs in children between ages 10 and 12 years. Although the appendix has no known function, it does regularly fill and empty itself with food.

What causes it

The appendiceal lumen becomes obstructed with fecal matter, calculi, tumors, or strictures from trauma or infection due to bacteria, viruses, or parasites.

How it happens

The obstruction of the appendiceal lumen sets off an inflammatory process that can lead to infection, thrombosis, necrosis, and perforation. If the appendix ruptures or perforates, the infected contents spill into the abdominal cavity, causing peritonitis.

Advice from the experts

Abdomen assessment tips

Keep these tips in mind when assessing a child's abdomen:
• Warm your hands before beginning the assessment.
• Note guarding of the abdomen and the child's ability to move around on the examination table.
• Flex the child's knees to decrease muscle tightening in the abdomen.
• Have child use deep breathing or distraction during the examination; a parent can help divert the child's attention.

• Have the child "help" with the examination. Place your hand over the child's hand on the abdomen and extend your fingers beyond the child's fingers to decrease ticklishness of palpating the abdomen.
• Before palpation, auscultate the abdomen as palpation can produce erratic bowel sounds; lightly palpate tender areas last.

What to look for

At first, midabdominal cramps and tenderness are diffuse; eventually, they localize in the right lower quadrant (RLQ) at McBurney's point. The child will guard against anyone trying to examine the abdomen. (See *Abdomen assessment tips*.)

He may experience nausea and vomiting and have a low-grade fever. Later complaints include lethargy, irritability, constipation, and, rarely, diarrhea.

Much ado about the RLQ

Auscultation reveals normal bowel sounds. As the inflammation increases, constant pain is noted in the RLQ with rebound tenderness; the pain is exacerbated by coughing and deep breathing.

Calm before the storm

If peritonitis occurs, abdominal distention and rigidity progress. Sudden cessation of abdominal pain signals perforation or infarction.

What tests tell you

Diagnosis of appendicitis is based on physical findings and characteristic clinical symptoms. A moderately elevated white blood cell (WBC) count with increased numbers of immature cells supports the diagnosis.

Complications

The most common complication of appendicitis is peritonitis from appendix rupture, which is a clinical emergency. Signs and symptoms of peritonitis include fever, abdominal

When the pain from appendicitis stops suddenly, it's the calm before the storm—of perforation or infarction, that is.

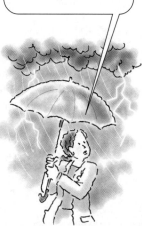

distention and rigidity, sudden relief of pain, decreased bowel sounds, nausea, and vomiting. Other possible complications include ischemic bowel and postoperative wound infection.

How it's treated

Appendectomy is the only effective treatment for appendicitis. Laparoscopic appendectomies decrease recovery time and hospital stay. If peritonitis develops, treatment involves GI intubation, parenteral replacement of fluids and electrolytes, and administration of antibiotics.

What to do

Because appendectomies are usually performed on an emergency basis, there may not be time to formally prepare the child for surgery.

Seize the day

Seize the opportunities that nursing care provides (bedside care, transporting the child, administering medications) to provide brief explanations and answer the child's questions. At the very least, tell the child that he'll be given a special medicine and won't feel anything during surgery.

Tell him where he'll be when he wakes up and when he'll see his parents. Tell the child what to expect when he awakens (I.V. line, NG tube, level of discomfort and what will be done to make him feel better). In addition, follow these steps:
• Position the child preoperatively in a semi-Fowler's or right-side-lying position with knees bent to decrease pain.
• Administer I.V. fluids to prevent dehydration, and keep the patient on NPO status until surgery is performed.
• Never apply heat to the right lower abdomen; this may cause the appendix to rupture.

Postoperative care
• Be aware that the child with a ruptured appendix may have a drain and an NG tube attached to low intermittent suction.
• Keep the incision site clean and dry; change dressings when soiled.

A malodorous sign

• Document the return of bowel sounds, the passing of flatus, and bowel movements—all signs of peristalsis.
• Administer antibiotics and pain medication as ordered.

Infection detection

• Instruct the parents in care of incision and the signs and symptoms of infection.

Celiac disease

Celiac disease is an immune reaction to eating gluten, a protein found in wheat, barley, and rye. The disease usually becomes apparent between ages 6 and 18 months, after gluten-containing foods are introduced into the diet. Family history increases the risk of developing celiac disease. A study done by Mayo Clinic and the National Institutes of Health estimates that about 1 in 141 people in the United States have celiac disease, although the disease often goes undiagnosed. Although celiac disease is most common in Whites, it can affect anyone. It is more common in people who have type 1 diabetes, a family member with celiac disease or dermatitis herpetiformis, Down syndrome or Turner's syndrome, autoimmune thyroid disease, Sjögren syndrome, or microscopic colitis.

> To the child with celiac disease, gluten is the enemy. The child is born with an intolerance of the protein.

What causes it

This disorder probably results from environmental factors and a genetic predisposition, but the exact mechanism is unknown. Some genetic mutations appear to increase the risk of developing the disease.

How it happens

When the body's immune system overreacts to gluten in food, the immune reaction damages the villi that line the small intestine. Villi absorb vitamins, minerals, and other nutrients from food. The damage resulting from celiac disease makes the inner surface of the small intestine unable to absorb nutrients necessary for health and growth. As a result, children with celiac disease may become malnourished if the condition remains undiagnosed.

> Inspection of a child with celiac disease may reveal malnutrition.

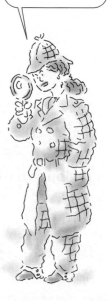

What to look for

Symptoms vary but typically include recurrent attacks of diarrhea and/or constipation, steatorrhea (fatty, foul-smelling stools), abdominal pain and distention, vomiting, anorexia, irritability, and coagulation difficulties from the malabsorption of fat-soluble vitamins. Inspection reveals signs of generalized malnutrition and failure to thrive, such as a potbelly or muscle wasting.

What tests tell you

- Histologic changes seen on small-bowel biopsy specimens confirm the diagnosis.
- A glucose tolerance test shows poor glucose absorption.

- Serum laboratory tests indicate decreases in levels of albumin, calcium, sodium, potassium, cholesterol, and phospholipids.
- Hemoglobin level, hematocrit, WBC counts, and platelet counts may also be decreased.
- Immunologic assay screen (immunoglobulin [Ig] A and IgG antibodies) is positive for celiac disease.
- Stool specimens reveal a high fat content.
- Endoscopy is done to view the small intestine and to take a small tissue biopsy to analyze for damage to the villi.

Complications

If not detected and properly treated, celiac disease can cause malnutrition, loss of calcium and bone density, lactose intolerance, and cancer. People with celiac disease who don't maintain a gluten-free diet have a greater risk of developing several forms of cancer, including intestinal lymphoma and small bowel cancer.

How it's treated

Lifelong elimination of gluten from the child's diet is essential and is the only treatment for managing celiac disease. In addition to wheat, foods that contain gluten include barley, bulgur, durum, farina, graham flour, malt, rye, semolina, spelt (a form of wheat), and triticale.

A high-protein, low-fat, high-calorie diet that includes corn and rice products, soy and potato flour, breast milk or soy-based formula, and all fresh fruits is required. Supportive treatment includes gluten-free vitamins to supplement folic acid, calcium, phosphorus, magnesium, vitamin B_{12}, and iron. Children may also receive administration of vitamins A, E, K, and D in water-soluble forms.

What to do

Because of the need for lifelong adherence to the diet, the child and his parents should be referred to a nutritionist who can help them make informed choices and plan a nutritious diet. (See *Teaching points for celiac disease*, page 480.)

Cleft lip and palate

A cleft lip and palate occur when the bone and tissue of the upper jaw and palate fail to fuse completely at the midline in the first trimester of pregnancy. They may occur separately or together. Cleft deformities usually occur unilaterally or bilaterally but rarely midline. Only the lip may be involved or the defect may extend into the upper jaw and nasal cavity. (See *A look at cleft lip and cleft palate*, page 481.)

It's all relative

Teaching points for celiac disease

Nursing interventions for a child with celiac disease focus primarily on educating the parents about caring for the child at home, with an emphasis on dietary needs:
• Eliminate gluten from the diet.
• Provide a diet that includes corn and rice products, soy and potato flour, and fresh fruits and vegetables; for the infant, give breast milk or soy-based formula.
• Replace vitamins and calories; give small, frequent meals.
• Monitor for steatorrhea; its disappearance is a good indicator that the child's ability to absorb nutrients is improving.
• Read nutrition labels for sources of gluten. Packaged foods should be avoided unless they're labeled as gluten-free or have no gluten-containing ingredients. In addition to cereals, pastas, and baked goods—such as breads, cakes, pies, and cookies—other packaged foods that may contain gluten include beer; candies; gravies; imitation meats or seafood; processed luncheon meats; salad dressings and sauces, including soy sauce; self-basting poultry; and soups. Some hair products and skin products contain also gluten.

What causes it

Cleft lip or palate most commonly occurs as an isolated birth defect. It may also occur as part of a chromosomal abnormality or after prenatal exposure to teratogens, such as anticonvulsant medications and alcohol.

How it happens

Defects originate in the second month of pregnancy, when the front and sides of the face and the palate shelves fuse imperfectly.

What to look for

Inspection reveals abdominal distention from swallowed air and difficulty swallowing or latching on to a bottle or breast. Cleft lip can range from a simple notch on the upper lip to a complete cleft from the lip edge to the floor of the nostril. A cleft palate that occurs alone (without cleft lip) may be partial or complete, involving only the soft palate or extending from the soft palate completely through the hard palate.

What tests tell you

Prenatal ultrasonography may indicate severe defects. A typical clinical picture confirms the diagnosis. Cleft lip with or without cleft palate is obvious at birth. Cleft palate without cleft lip may

A look at cleft lip and cleft palate

These illustrations show the four variations of cleft lip and cleft palate.

Notch with vermilion border	Unilateral cleft lip and cleft palate	Bilateral cleft lip and cleft palate	Cleft palate

not be detected until a mouth examination is done or until feeding difficulties develop.

Complications

Speech difficulties and failure to thrive (due to inadequate oral intake) are possible complications of unrepaired clefts. In addition, dentition problems, nasal defects, increased episodes of otitis media, hearing defects, and appearance are concerns. The infant is also at increased risk for aspiration and upper respiratory infections. Parents' feelings of shock, guilt, and grief may interfere with parent-child bonding.

How it's treated

Cheiloplasty (cleft lip surgery) is performed between birth and age 3 months; it unites the lip and gum edges. It's performed in anticipation of tooth eruption, providing a route for adequate nutrition and sucking. (See *Preoperative cleft lip and cleft palate care*, page 482.)

Advice from the experts

Preoperative cleft lip and cleft palate care

Nursing interventions before cleft lip or cleft palate repair will help to ensure an optimal outcome.

Cleft lip
• Feed the infant slowly and in an upright position to decrease the risk of aspiration.
• Burp the infant frequently during feeding to eliminate swallowed air and decrease the risk of emesis.
• Use gavage feedings if oral feedings are unsuccessful.
• Give a small amount of water after feedings to prevent formula from accumulating and becoming a medium for bacterial growth.

• Give small, frequent feedings to promote adequate nutrition and prevent tiring.
• Hold the infant while feeding, and promote sucking between meals; sucking is important for speech development.

Cleft palate
• Be aware that the infant may be weaned from the bottle or breast before cleft palate surgery; he may be fed by syringe or he may be able to drink from a cup.
• Feed the infant with a cleft palate nipple or a Teflon implant to enhance nutritional intake.
• Teach the parents that the infant is susceptible to pathogens and otitis media from the altered position of the eustachian tubes.

An early start

If cleft lip is detected on sonogram while the infant is in utero, fetal repair may be possible. *Palatoplasty* or staphylorrhaphy (cleft palate repair surgery) is performed between ages 12 and 18 months, before speech patterns develop. The infant must be free from ear and respiratory infections before surgery.

A group effort

Long-term, team-oriented care aims to address speech defects, dental and orthopedic problems, nasal defects, and possible alterations in hearing.

What to do

Parents may experience grief over the "perfect" child they had hoped for and expected. Those feelings may, in turn, cause feelings of guilt. Referral to a counselor or a cleft lip and palate support group may be helpful in working through these feelings so appropriate parent-child bonding can take place.

In addition, follow these steps:
• To help determine an effective feeding method, assess the quality of the infant's sucking by determining if he can form an airtight seal around a finger or nipple that's placed in his mouth; special nipples are available for infants with cleft lip or palate.

A special feeding nipple may be needed for the infant with cleft lip or palate.

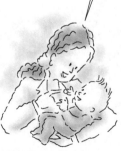

- Assess the child's ability to swallow, assess for abdominal distention from swallowed air, and monitor the child's respiratory status to detect signs of aspiration.
- Monitor vital signs and intake and output to determine fluid volume status.
- Prepare the child and his parents for surgical repair of the defect.
- Monitor for complications and prepare the family to take over the follow-up care postoperatively. (See *Postoperative cleft lip and cleft palate care.*)

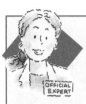

Advice from the experts

Postoperative cleft lip and cleft palate care

Many nursing interventions are needed after surgical repair of a cleft lip or cleft palate.

Cleft lip
- Maintain a patent airway; edema or narrowing of a previously large airway may make the infant appear to be in distress.
- Observe for cyanosis to detect signs of respiratory compromise as the infant begins to breathe through his nose.
- Maintain an intact suture line; keep the infant's hands away from his mouth by using restraints or pinning his sleeves to his shirt.
- Clean the suture line after feedings and apply antibiotic ointment if ordered.
- Anticipate the infant's needs; this will help prevent crying.
- Give extra care and support because the infant's emotional needs can't be met by sucking.
- When feeding resumes, use a syringe with tubing to administer foods at the side of the mouth to prevent trauma to the suture line; never use a straw for feedings.
- Place the infant on his right side after feedings to prevent aspiration. (Don't put the infant in a prone position.)
- Monitor for pain and administer pain medication as prescribed.

Cleft palate
- Position the infant on his abdomen or side to maintain a patent airway.

- Assess for signs of altered oxygenation to promote good respiration.
- Use a syringe or a cup for feeding to prevent injury to the suture line. Breast- or bottle-feeding or use of pacifier are based on surgeon's preference.
- Keep hard or pointed objects (oral thermometers, utensils, straws, frozen dessert sticks) away from the infant's mouth to prevent trauma on the suture line.
- Use elbow restraints to keep the child's hands out of his mouth; remove one restraint at a time.
- Provide soft toys to prevent injury.
- Distract or hold the infant to try to keep his tongue away from the roof of his mouth.
- Start the infant on clear liquids and progress to a soft diet.
- Rinse the suture line by giving the infant a sip of water after each feeding to prevent infection.
- Don't brush the child's teeth for 1 to 2 weeks after surgery.
- Do not run, climb, or play with the mouth for 1 or 2 weeks after surgery.
- Postoperative complications: croup, laryngeal spasm, aspiration, foreign body, hemorrhage, and palate dehiscence.
- Administer decongestants or corticosteroids for congestion. Administer antibiotics to decrease possibility of infection.

Crohn's disease

Crohn's disease is a chronic inflammation and ulceration of the GI tract anywhere from the mouth to the anus, usually involving the terminal ileum, colon, and rectum. The disease extends through all layers of the intestinal wall and may involve regional lymph nodes and the mesentery.

What causes it

Although the exact cause is unknown, possible causes include allergies and other immune disorders and infection (although no infecting organism has been identified). Genetic factors may also play a role.

How it happens

An inflammatory response causes mucosal ulcers to grow in size and depth in the mucosal wall of the GI tract. Fibrosis and stiffening of the mucosal wall can occur. Fistulas can develop between bowel loops or adjoining organs. Healing lesions develop scar tissue, leading to strictures.

What to look for

The child may report a gradual onset of symptoms, marked by periods of remission and exacerbation:
• Acute symptoms include steady, colicky pain in the RLQ (cramping); diarrhea and flatulence; fever; and bloody stool.
• Chronic symptoms, which are more typical of the disease, are more persistent and less severe. These symptoms include diarrhea (four to six stools per day), pain in the RLQ, excess fat in stool, weight loss, weakness and fatigue, cramping, and abdominal distention. Retardation in growth and physical development can also occur.

What tests tell you

Laboratory test findings indicate an increased WBC count and erythrocyte sedimentation rate (ESR). Other findings include hypokalemia, hypocalcemia, hypomagnesemia, hypoalbuminemia, and decreased hemoglobin level.

A string thing

Barium enema shows segments of stricture separated by normal bowel ("string sign"). Sigmoidoscopy and colonoscopy show patchy areas of inflammation. A biopsy is required for definitive diagnosis. Laboratory analysis to detect occult blood in stool is usually positive.

Complications

Complications of Crohn's disease include intestinal obstruction, fistula formation between the small bowel and bladder, perianal and perirectal abscesses and fistulas, intra-abdominal abscesses, bowel perforation, growth retardation, and toxic megacolon.

A toxic outcome

Toxic megacolon is an acute dilation of the colon secondary to severe inflammation of bowel mucosa. Signs and symptoms are spiking fever, acute abdominal pain, and abdominal distention. The bowel mucosa shreds, leading to hemorrhage and peritonitis, and may cause death.

How it's treated

The inflammatory response is controlled by the administration of corticosteroids, aminosalicylates, anti-infectives, antidiarrheal medications, anti–tumor necrosis factor agents, and immunosuppressive agents.

Give the bowel a rest

Effective treatment requires nutritional support with high-protein, high-calorie, low-fiber foods and supplements with iron, zinc, folic acid, and vitamins. Enteral formulas may be used as supplements. TPN may be administered to give the bowel a rest for healing.

A temporary fix

Surgical treatment may involve a bowel resection for obstructions or fistulas or a total colectomy with ileostomy if the bowel perforates or toxic megacolon occurs. Surgery doesn't cure Crohn's disease but relieves symptoms temporarily until the next exacerbation.

What to do

The child with Crohn's disease may need multiple hospitalizations.

Child interrupted

Do everything possible to "normalize" the child's life during hospital stays. Maintain routines to the extent possible. Encourage the child to keep up with schoolwork, provide age-appropriate activities and diversions to maintain development and alleviate boredom, and encourage his family and friends to spend as much time as possible with the child.

In addition, follow these steps:
• Administer analgesics and antispasmodics to decrease abdominal pain and corticosteroids to decrease bowel inflammation.
• Withhold food and fluids, using parenteral nutrition in place of feeding to rest the bowel.

Nutrition 101

- Teach proper nutritional support to the child and his parents, including the need for small, frequent meals that are high-protein, high-calorie, and low-fiber; the use of multivitamin and iron supplements; and the need for bland foods when the child has mouth ulcers.
- Encourage medication compliance even while the child is in remission.
- Promote stress reduction through relaxation and distraction, and promote enhanced self-image and self-esteem; encourage participation in support groups.

Hepatitis

Hepatitis is a communicable, inflammatory condition of the liver; it can be acute or chronic. Hepatitis can be caused by several viruses, and the incubation period differs depending on the type of virus that causes it. Such disease processes as cancer and liver abscesses may also cause hepatitis. Neonatal hepatitis can occur in an infant born to a hepatitis B virus (HBV)–positive mother.

What causes it

There are several different viruses that cause hepatitis.

ABCs (and Ds) of hepatitis

Hepatitis A virus (HAV) is the most common type in children and is transmitted by person-to-person contact (fecal-oral route) or through the ingestion of contaminated food, milk, or water. A child is at an increased risk in day care centers and when traveling to areas with contaminated food or water.

HBV is transmitted by direct contact with contaminated blood, secretions, and feces, most commonly through perinatal exposure from an HBV-positive mother.

Hepatitis C virus (HCV) is transmitted by exposure to blood or blood products, I.V. or intranasal drug use, and sexual contact, and may also be transmitted perinatally. HCV is most commonly transmitted through transfused blood from asymptomatic donors.

Hepatitis D virus (HDV) occurs only in people who also have HBV and is transmitted by intimate contact with a person who also has HBV.

The E and the G

Hepatitis E virus (HEV), not reported in children in the United States, is transmitted by inadequate hand washing or contaminated food and water. HEV is seen in countries with poor sanitation as the virus is shed in stool. Hepatitis G virus (HGV) is a newly recognized virus also not reported in children. HGV is transmitted by blood transfusion, organ transplantation, I.V. drug abuse, and sexual contact.

How it happens

Exposure to the virus or causative agent causes an inflammatory reaction in the liver. Lesions develop and cause necrosis of hepatic cells and scarring. Blood flow becomes obstructed, causing engorgement and hepatomegaly. Bile ducts become obstructed and bile accumulates in the blood, causing jaundice.

In mild forms of hepatitis, the liver cells regenerate and the patient recovers. In severe forms of hepatitis, the liver becomes necrotic and death occurs.

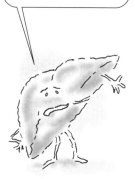

Hepatitis does a real number on me—inflammation, lesions, necrosis, scarring, hepatomegaly, and jaundice. Need I say more?

What to look for

Assessment findings are similar for the different types of hepatitis. Typically, signs and symptoms progress in several stages.

Tired and irritable

In the prodromal stage, the child complains of fatigue, anorexia, mild weight loss, malaise, irritability, headache, weakness, photophobia, and nausea with vomiting. Assessment reveals fever, the onset of clinical jaundice, dark-colored urine, and clay-colored stools. Children younger than age 2 years are commonly asymptomatic with HAV.

Itchy and uncomfortable

During the clinical jaundice stage, the child has itching, abdominal pain, indigestion, skin rashes, and hives. Palpation reveals RUQ discomfort and an enlarged, tender liver.

What tests tell you

Elevated liver enzymes (aspartate aminotransferase, alanine aminotransferase, alkaline phosphatase) are revealed in the prodromal stage. ESR and bilirubin levels are elevated, and prothrombin time is elongated.

A view from the side

A hepatitis profile, which identifies antibodies specific to the causative virus, establishes the type of viral hepatitis. A liver biopsy is performed if chronic hepatitis is suspected.

Complications

Complications of hepatitis include cirrhosis, liver cancer, chronic hepatitis, pancreatitis, myocarditis, pneumonia, aplastic anemia, and life-threatening fulminant hepatitis.

No turning back

Fulminant hepatitis causes unremitting liver failure with encephalopathy, which progresses to coma and usually leads to death within 2 weeks. Signs and symptoms of fulminant hepatitis include:

- vomiting
- anorexia
- jaundice
- ascites
- GI bleeding
- abdominal pain
- lethargy
- progressing disorientation
- coma.

> Fulminant hepatitis is too much for me. All that's left is failure without remission.

Notice of necrosis

A decrease in hepatomegaly is an ominous sign of tissue necrosis. Children with HBV have a much greater chance of becoming chronic carriers than adults and of developing cirrhosis and liver cancer.

How it's treated

Treatment of hepatitis is supportive and focuses on rest, comfort, and good nutrition. Such medications as diphenhydramine (Benadryl) are administered to decrease the inflammatory process and relieve itching from the rash.

Interfering with hepatitis

Alpha-interferon is administered for the treatment of HBV and HCV if the patient is older than age 18 years. Ribavirin (Virazole), a teratogenic drug, is administered for HCV. A liver transplant may be needed for end-stage HBV disease. Prevention of HBV is the treatment for HDV.

Hepatitis prevention

Immunoglobulin is administered within 2 weeks of exposure to HAV or HBV to prevent the disease. The neonate born to an HBV-positive mother should receive the HBV vaccine and hepatitis B immunoglobulin within 12 hours of birth. Additional doses of the hepatitis B vaccine should be administered at ages 1 and 6 months.

A boost of prevention

The HAV vaccine is recommended as part of routine well-child care in areas where the disease is prevalent. The first dose is given between 12 and 18 months, followed by a booster 6 months later.

Come one, come all

The HBV vaccine is recommended for all neonates before they're discharged from the hospital. A second booster is given between 1 and 2 months, a third booster is given between 6 and 18 months.

What to do

Hepatitis is a frightening diagnosis for parents. Provide reassurance and assist parents in getting their questions answered. Prepare the child for blood draws and I.V. line insertions. In addition, follow these steps:
• Promote comfort to decrease abdominal discomfort.

A little here, a little there

• Provide small, frequent meals and snacks to support nutrition.
• Administer antiemetics to decrease nausea and antihistamines to decrease itching; avoid acetaminophen (Tylenol) and other drugs metabolized by the liver.
• Limit activity to promote rest.

Back to school

• Educate the parents about the disease.
• Teach the parents about preventive measures, such as immunizations, good hand-washing habits, and proper disposal of diapers; explain the need to avoid sharing contaminated items.
• Instruct the parents to contact a health care provider before administering medications or over-the-counter products (because of impaired liver function).
• Instruct parents to watch for signs and symptoms that indicate worsening of hepatitis, leading to fulminant hepatitis.

> A few needle sticks is a small price to pay. HAV vaccine is recommended for all children beginning at age 12 months and HBV vaccination is recommended for all neonates.

> When a child has hepatitis, it's the parents who need an education—on everything from hand washing to recognizing signs of worsening disease.

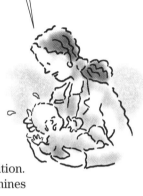

Hirschsprung's disease

Hirschsprung's disease is the absence of parasympathetic ganglionic cells in a segment of the colon, usually at the distal end of the large intestine. The lack of nerve innervation causes an absence of, or alteration in, peristalsis in the affected part of the colon. (See *A look at Hirschsprung's disease*, page 490.)

A look at Hirschsprung's disease

Hirschsprung's disease is a congenital disorder of the large intestine characterized by the absence or marked reduction of parasympathetic ganglion cells in the colorectal wall.

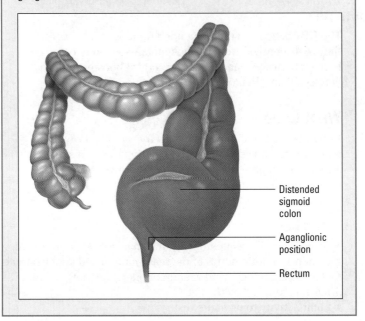

Distended sigmoid colon

Aganglionic position

Rectum

What causes it

Hirschsprung's disease is believed to be the result of a congenital, usually familial, defect. The disease may coexist with other congenital anomalies, particularly Down syndrome and anomalies of the urinary tract.

How it happens

As stool enters the affected part, it remains there until additional stool pushes it through. The affected part of the colon dilates; a mechanical obstruction may result.

What to look for

In a neonate, history commonly reveals a failure to pass meconium and stool within the first 24 to 48 hours after birth. On inspection, the infant may have abdominal distention and easily palpable stool masses. When stool does pass through, it's liquid or ribbonlike.

Suspicious stain

The child may experience bile-stained or fecal vomiting, irritability, lethargy, and weight loss. He may exhibit signs of dehydration, including pallor, dry mucous membranes, and sunken eyes.

What tests tell you
• Rectal biopsy provides definitive diagnosis by showing the absence of ganglion cells.
• Suction aspiration, using a small tube inserted into the rectum, also determines the absence of ganglion cells.
• Full-thickness surgical biopsy under general anesthesia may be performed if findings from suction aspiration are inconclusive.
• Rectal manometry reveals failure of the internal anal sphincter to relax and contract.
• Abdominal X-rays show distention of the colon.

Complications

Disease progression causes the most complications, including severe diarrhea, bowel perforation, sepsis, incontinence, stricture formation, enterocolitis, and hypovolemic shock.

In infants, the main cause of death is enterocolitis (when not treated), caused by fecal stagnation that leads to bacterial overgrowth, production of bacterial toxins, intestinal irritation, profuse diarrhea, hypovolemic shock, and perforation.

How it's treated

Surgery is the treatment of choice in these children and should be performed as soon as the child's fluid and electrolyte imbalances are stabilized.

Out with the bad

Laparoscopic surgery involves pulling the ganglionic segment of bowel through to the anus to remove the affected portion. Surgery is usually delayed until the infant is at least age 10 months. If a total obstruction is present, a temporary colostomy or ileostomy may be necessary to decompress the colon. Next, a second surgery is performed to remove the affected segment of bowel and close the ostomy.

What to do

The infant's parents will need a great deal of emotional support. Prepare them for each procedure, including surgeries, by offering thorough explanations and making sure that their questions are answered. Encourage them to express their feelings and concerns, and encourage their participation in the infant's care to the extent possible.

Preoperative care
• Administer I.V. fluids to maintain fluid and electrolyte balance and prevent dehydration and shock.
• Maintain NPO status and insert an NG tube for gastric decompression.

Forced evacuation

• Administer isotonic enemas (normal saline solution or mineral oil) to evacuate the bowels; don't administer tap water due to the risk of water intoxication.
• Administer antibiotics (and an antibiotic enema) as ordered.

Postoperative care
After colostomy or ileostomy, follow these steps:
• Monitor fluid intake and output; an ileostomy is especially likely to cause excessive electrolyte loss.
• Keep the area around the stoma clean and dry; use colostomy or ileostomy appliances to collect drainage.
• Monitor for return of bowel sounds to begin diet.
    After corrective surgery, follow these steps:
• Keep the wound clean and dry to prevent infection.
• Don't use a rectal thermometer or suppositories.

Bowel sounds = dinner bell

• Begin oral feedings when active bowel sounds begin and NG drainage decreases.
• Educate the parents about suture line care.
• Teach the parents how to recognize the beginning signs of constipation, such as straining during defecation and a distended abdomen, fluid loss and dehydration (decreased urine output, sunken eyes, poor skin turgor), enterocolitis (vomiting, diarrhea, fever, lethargy, sudden marked abdominal distention), and strictures (abdominal distention, constipation, vomiting).

Expert advice

• Before discharge (if possible), arrange for a consultation with an enterostomal therapist who can provide the parents with valuable tips on colostomy or ileostomy care.
• Teach the parents which foods increase the number of stools (raisins, prunes, plums) and tell them to avoid offering these foods. (Reassure them that their child will, in time, probably gain sphincter control and eat a normal diet.)

Patience is a virtue

• Caution the parents that complete continence of stool can take years to develop, and that constipation may occur.

Intussusception

Intussusception is a telescoping or invagination of a bowel segment into itself, the most common site being the ileocecal valve. It usually occurs at about age 6 months but can occur in children up to age 3 years and, rarely, in older children. It's three times more likely to occur in males than in females and is more likely to occur in children with cystic fibrosis.

Intussusception can be fatal, especially if treatment is delayed for more than 24 hours. (See *Understanding intussusception.*)

What causes it

The cause of intussusception is unknown in most cases. It may result from polyps, hyperactive peristalsis, or an abnormal bowel

Understanding intussusception

In intussusception, a bowel section invaginates and is propelled along by peristalsis, pulling in more bowel. In this illustration, a portion of the cecum invaginates and is propelled into the large intestine. Intussusception typically produces edema, hemorrhage from venous engorgement, incarceration, and obstruction.

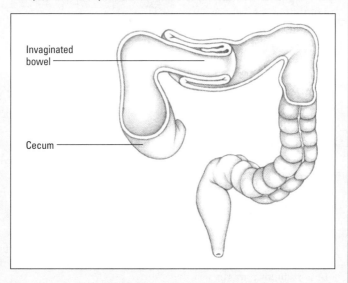

Invaginated bowel

Cecum

lining. It may also be linked to viral infections because seasonal peaks are noted (spring and summer).

How it happens

When a bowel segment invaginates, peristalsis propels it along the bowel, pulling more bowel along with it. Invagination causes inflammation and swelling at the affected site. Edema eventually causes obstruction and necrosis from occlusion of the blood supply to the bowel.

What to look for

The medical history may reveal intermittent attacks of colicky pain characterized by screaming, drawing knees to the chest, sweating, and grunting. Parents report vomitus containing bile or fecal material, which can lead to dehydration, fluid and electrolyte imbalance, and metabolic alkalosis. They also describe the passage of red, "currant jelly–like" stool containing mucus and blood.

Tender to the touch

Inspection and palpation may reveal a distended and tender abdomen with a palpable, sausage-shaped abdominal mass. Other clinical signs include fever, increased pulse, shallow respirations, and decreased blood pressure (shocklike state).

What tests tell you

- Abdominal X-rays and ultrasound or computed tomography show a soft tissue mass and signs of complete or partial obstruction.
- Barium enema confirms colonic intussusception when it shows the characteristic coiled spring sign.
- A WBC count as high as 15,000/µl indicates obstruction.
- A WBC count higher than 15,000/µl indicates strangulation.
- A WBC count higher than 20,000/µl indicates bowel infarction.

Complications

Without proper treatment, strangulation of the intestine may occur, with gangrene, shock, perforation, and peritonitis. These complications can be fatal.

How it's treated

An NG tube is inserted to decompress the intestine and minimize vomiting. Ten percent of children with intussusception may have spontaneous reduction of the bowel. Therapy may include hydrostatic reduction or surgery.

Forceful introduction

During hydrostatic reduction, air pressure or a solution of barium or water-soluble contrast medium is introduced into the rectum. The force from the fluid or air moves invaginated bowel back into its original position.

If at first you don't succeed . . . reduce or resect

Surgery is indicated when hydrostatic reduction fails, intussusception recurs, or signs of shock or peritonitis are present. Manual reduction is attempted first by pulling the intussusception back through the bowel. If manual reduction fails, or if the bowel segment is gangrenous or strangulated, re-section of the affected bowel segment is performed.

What to do

Intussusception is a painful condition; onset of symptoms may be sudden and severe. The child may be inconsolable and the parents are likely to be terrified and distressed from seeing their infant or toddler in so much pain. Provide the parents with as much emotional support and reassurance as possible.

When time is of the essence, use caregiving opportunities to prepare the child for surgery.

Explain on the go

Because intussusception is treated as an emergency, use caregiving opportunities (during bedside care, medication administration, transport to testing areas) to provide as much explanation as possible about tests and procedures, and make sure the parents' questions are answered.

Music to soothe

To the extent possible, allow the parents to remain with the child to comfort him (by holding him, stroking the child's face and hands, singing a soothing song).

Better days ahead

For the child who's old enough to understand, provide simple explanations as procedures are being performed, and reassure him that you're there to help him and he'll feel better soon.
- Prepare for enema insertion (barium or water-soluble contrast medium) to confirm the diagnosis and reduce the invagination by hydrostatic pressure.
- Monitor vital signs; a change in temperature may indicate sepsis.
- Monitor intake and output to prevent dehydration and administer I.V. fluids as ordered.
- Monitor NG tube output and replace volume lost, as ordered.
- Administer pain medication as ordered.

• For the child who has undergone hydrostatic reduction, monitor for the passage of stool (and barium, if used) to determine the need for surgery.

Postoperative care

After surgery, encourage the parents to stay with the child as much as possible. In addition, follow these steps:
• Administer antibiotics as ordered to prevent infection.
• Monitor the incision site for signs of infection, such as inflammation, drainage, and suture separation.
• Monitor for the return of bowel sounds to allow advancement of the diet.
• Continue to offer emotional support and encouragement to the parents.

Pyloric stenosis

Pyloric stenosis is hyperplasia (increased mass) and hypertrophy (increased size) of the circular muscle at the pylorus, the lower opening of the stomach leading to the duodenum. The increased mass and size of the muscle narrows the pyloric canal, preventing the stomach from emptying normally. Pyloric obstruction leads to vomiting and gastritis from prolonged filling of the stomach. It's most commonly seen in boys between ages 1 and 6 months.

What causes it

The exact cause of pyloric stenosis is unknown. It isn't an inherited disorder but may be associated with malrotation, esophageal atresia, and anorectal malformations.

How it happens

Spasms of the pylorus muscle cause the narrowing of the passageway between the stomach and duodenum. Swelling and inflammation further reduce the size of the lumen and could result in complete obstruction. Normal emptying of the stomach is prevented, resulting in vomiting and gastritis.

What to look for

Palpation reveals an olive-shaped bulge below the right costal margin and a distended upper abdomen.

Waving and projecting

The child experiences projectile vomiting during or shortly after feedings. The vomiting is preceded by reverse peristaltic waves (left to right) but not by nausea. Vomitus isn't bile-stained but may be blood-stained due to gastritis.

Déjà lunch

The child will resume eating after vomiting and exhibits poor weight gain. Symptoms of malnutrition and dehydration are present despite the child's apparent adequate intake of food.

What tests tell you

- Vomitus is positive for blood.
- Blood chemistry reveals hypocalcemia, hyponatremia, hypokalemia, and hypochloremia.
- Arterial blood gas analysis may reveal metabolic alkalosis.
- Abdominal ultrasound and endoscopy reveal a hypertrophied sphincter.
- An upper GI series reveals delayed gastric emptying.

Complications

Complications of pyloric stenosis include malnutrition, dehydration, infection, and metabolic alkalosis and failure to thrive.

How it's treated

The child remains on NPO status before surgery. I.V. fluids are administered to correct fluid and electrolyte imbalances and prevent dehydration, and an NG tube is inserted and kept open for gastric decompression. Surgical intervention consists of a pyloromyotomy performed by laparoscopy.

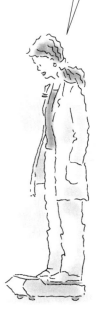

Using the same scale every day ensures that weight measurements for a child with pyloric stenosis will be accurate.

What to do

Provide the child with an age-appropriate explanation of all tests, procedures, and surgery. Make sure the parents' questions are answered. In addition, follow these steps:
- Monitor vital signs and intake and output to assess renal function and check for dehydration.
- Record the amount of vomitus as well as its frequency, characteristics, and relation to feedings.
- Perform daily weight measurements on the same scale to assess growth.
- Assess abdominal and cardiovascular status to detect early signs of compromise.
- Position the child, preferably on his right side, to prevent aspiration of vomitus.

Postoperative care

- Feed the child small amounts of oral electrolyte solution, then increase the amount and concentration of food until normal feeding is achieved.

No need to say "excuse me"

- Burp the child frequently during feedings.
- Provide a pacifier to maintain comfort and satisfy the infant's sucking reflex.
- Monitor intake and output.
- Keep the incision area clean to prevent infection; clean with soap and water and keep the diaper's contents away from the incision.

Going with the flow

- Position the child on his right side, allowing gravity to help the flow of fluid through the pyloric valve; elevate the child's head after feeding.
- Administer analgesics around the clock for pain management.
- Teach the parents proper incision site care and to monitor for signs and symptoms of infection and dehydration.

Tracheoesophageal fistula and esophageal atresia

Tracheoesophageal fistula and esophageal atresia are among the most serious congenital anomalies in neonates. They may develop separately but usually occur together. There's a higher incidence with prematurity and maternal polyhydramnios.

An unhealthy relationship

In tracheoesophageal fistula, an abnormal connection develops between the trachea and the esophagus. In esophageal atresia, the esophagus is closed off at some point, and food can't enter the stomach through the esophagus.

Combo conditions

These conditions may occur in several combinations and may be associated with other anomalies of the heart, anorectal area, or genitourinary system. (See *Types of tracheoesophageal anomalies.*)

What causes it

These conditions are a result of the failure of the embryonic esophagus and trachea to develop and separate correctly.

How it happens

In the fetus, there's a defective separation of the foregut into the trachea and esophagus at about 4 to 5 weeks' gestation. The esophagus fails to meet the stomach and ends in a blind pouch.

What to look for

At delivery, the neonate has frothy saliva in the mouth and choking and coughing due to excessive secretions. With feeding, he experiences sudden coughing and gagging and shows signs of

Types of tracheoesophageal anomalies

Congenital malformations of the esophagus occur in about 1 in 4,000 live births. The American Academy of Pediatrics classifies the anatomic variations of tracheoesophageal anomalies according to type.

Type A
Esophageal atresia without fistula (7.7%)

Type B
Esophageal atresia with tracheoesophageal fistula to the proximal segment (0.8%)

Type C
Esophageal atresia with fistula to the distal segment (86.5%)

Type D
Esophageal atresia with fistula to both segments (0.7%)

Type E (or H-type)
Tracheoesophageal fistula without atresia (4.2%)

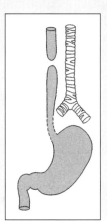 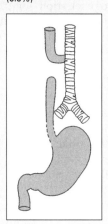 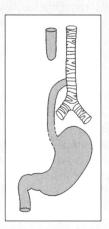 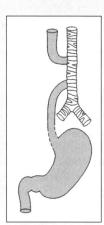 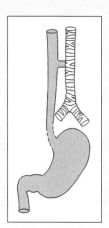

feedings coming out of nose and mouth. He may stop breathing and become cyanotic as the feeding is aspirated into the lungs. Three classic signs are cyanosis, choking, and coughing.

Belly full of air

Stomach distention occurs when air from the trachea enters the esophagus or the stomach directly (through a fistula). Aspiration pneumonia occurs when the esophagus joins the trachea and food regurgitates through the fistula into the lungs.

What tests tell you

A radiopaque catheter is inserted into the esophagus, and an X-ray is taken to see where the catheter goes or what obstruction it hits. Bronchoscopy is performed to visualize the fistula between the trachea and esophagus. Chest X-ray shows pneumonia and a dilated, air-filled upper esophageal pouch.

Complications

Complications include leaking at the anastomosis site, strictures, gastroesophageal reflux, feeding difficulties, and tracheomalacia (weakness of the tracheal wall, allowing the trachea to collapse).

How it's treated

Tracheoesophageal fistula and esophageal atresia require surgical correction and are usually surgical emergencies. (Insertion of an NG tube is impossible in a neonate with esophageal atresia.)

A pump in the pouch

A sump pump may be inserted in the esophageal pouch to remove accumulated secretions, reducing the risk of aspiration. A gastrostomy tube may be placed to decompress the stomach. The child's respiratory status must be closely monitored to maintain a patent airway. I.V. fluids are administered to prevent dehydration, and the patient is placed on NPO status.

Ligate and lengthen

Surgical correction is performed to ligate fistulas and anastomose the esophagus to the stomach. Esophageal lengthening may be needed if the esophagus is too short to join the stomach. A chest tube may be inserted to drain intrapleural fluid and air. Antibiotics are administered to treat aspiration pneumonia.

What to do

Explain all procedures to the parents, make sure their questions are answered, and provide support and reassurance. Allow them to spend as much time as possible with their child. In addition:
• Suction excessive secretions from the mouth and pharynx frequently, and elevate the neonate's head to prevent aspiration.
• Maintain NPO status; begin I.V. fluids.
• Don't allow the infant to suck on a pacifier; this increases saliva secretions.

> The parents of a child who needs emergency surgery will look to the nurse to provide support and answer their questions.

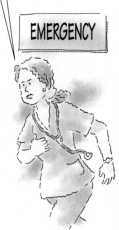

Postoperative care

After surgery, involve the parents in the child's care to help comfort the child, reassure the parents, and prepare them for caring for the child at home. In addition, follow these steps:
• An NG or OG tube is attached to low-suction or gravity drainage; document the amount and character of the drainage at least every 4 hours.
• Gastrostomy feedings may be given until the esophagus heals.

Assess for distress

• Monitor for signs of respiratory distress.
• Monitor chest tube drainage and care of the chest tube site.

• Begin oral feedings with sterile water and advance to normal feedings as tolerated.

Sucking permitted

• Encourage sucking on a pacifier to prevent oral aversion.
• Educate the parents on proper oral or gastrostomy feedings, signs of respiratory distress, and signs of esophageal constriction (such as drooling, difficulty swallowing, or regurgitating undigested food).

Ulcerative colitis

Ulcerative colitis is a chronic, recurrent inflammation of the colon and rectal mucosa with varying degrees of ulceration, bleeding, and edema. It usually begins in the rectum and sigmoid colon and may extend upward into the entire colon.

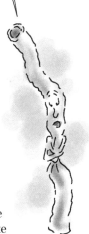

Vasoconstriction starts a painful chain of events—ruptures, ulcers, strictures, and obstructions.

What causes it

Although the etiology of ulcerative colitis is unknown, it may be related to an abnormal immune response in the GI tract, possibly associated with genetic factors. It's more prevalent among people of Jewish heritage and in higher socioeconomic groups.

How it happens

Vasoconstriction initiates an immune response, producing ruptured capillary walls. The swollen bowel then develops ulcers. Healing ulcers can develop scar tissue, which results in strictures and obstructions.

What to look for

The hallmark sign of ulcerative colitis is frequent attacks of watery, bloody diarrhea (in many cases containing pus and mucus) interspersed with asymptomatic remissions. However, one of the earliest signs may be growth failure due to poor nutritional intake resulting from anorexia. Other symptoms include urgency with defecation, abdominal pain, cramping, fever, and chills.

What tests tell you

Sigmoidoscopy confirms rectal involvement in most cases by showing increased mucosal friability, decreased mucosal detail, and thick inflammatory exudate. Colonoscopy may be used to determine the extent of the disease and look for evidence of inflammation. A biopsy performed during the colonoscopy can help confirm the diagnosis.

What's in the stool?

Barium enema is used to evaluate the extent of the disease and detect complications. Stool specimen analysis reveals blood, pus, and mucus but no pathogenic organisms. Other laboratory tests reveal an elevated WBC count, an elevated ESR, decreased hemoglobin level and hematocrit, and elevated C-reactive protein.

Complications

Ulcerative colitis can lead to a variety of complications, depending on the severity and site of inflammation. Nutritional deficiencies are the most common complications, but the disease can also lead to perineal sepsis with anal fissure, anal fistula, perirectal abscess, hemorrhage, iron deficiency anemia, coagulation defects, and toxic megacolon. There's also an increased risk of colorectal cancer.

How it's treated

The goals of treatment are to control inflammation, replace nutritional losses and blood volume, and prevent complications.

Down with inflammation!

Medical treatment begins with the administration of corticosteroids or other anti-inflammatory agent, such as aminosalicylates, to decrease inflammation and probiotics to increase intestinal flora. Supportive treatment includes dietary therapy and bed rest.
• Parenteral nutrition is used for children awaiting surgery or showing signs of dehydration and is intended to give the bowel a chance to rest.
• A low-residue diet may be ordered for the patient with mild signs and symptoms.
• Blood transfusions or iron supplements may be needed to correct anemia.
• Surgery, the treatment of last resort, is performed if the patient has toxic megacolon. (The most common surgical procedure is total proctocolectomy with ileostomy, which may cure the disease.)

What to do

Nursing care focuses on teaching the parents about diet, medications, and stress reduction:
• Encourage small, frequent meals of a diet low in bran and fiber-rich foods. (See *Nutrition by culture.*)
• Stress the importance of compliance with the medication regimen.
• Promote stress reduction through relaxation and distraction.

Cultured pearls

Nutrition by culture

Nutrition varies among cultures and religions because dietary practices differ. Children need a well-balanced diet for growth and development, especially children on specific diets.

   The nurse should do a comprehensive nutrition assessment and teach proper nutrition practices to enhance growth and development in children while respecting the cultural practices and beliefs of the family. Here are some tips on special cultural diet restrictions and characteristics:

• If the child is a vegetarian, the nurse should know proper protein foods to substitute for the lack of meat in the diet.

• Some Jewish children eat kosher meats that are typically high in sodium, which may be a problem in certain disease processes.

• In many cultures, such as Hispanic, Asian, and Black cultures, use of herbal preparations in their diets and as medicinal treatments is common. The nurse should be aware of the types of preparations the child is eating or taking.

• Promote enhanced self-image and self-esteem.
• Instruct in ostomy care, if applicable.

Volvulus

Volvulus is a condition in which the bowel twists around itself at least 180 degrees. This results in vessel compression and ischemia.

What causes it

The twisting in volvulus may result from an anomaly of rotation, an ingested foreign body, or an adhesion. In some cases, the cause is unknown.

How it happens

A prolapsed portion of mesentery causes the bowel to become twisted. The twisted bowel is obstructed, leading to bowel distention and decreased absorption of water and electrolytes. Vomiting also occurs due to the obstruction. A decreased blood supply to the affected bowel leads to necrosis. (See *What happens in volvulus*, page 504.)

What to look for

The child complains of severe abdominal pain and has bilious vomiting, which increases after feedings. Inspection reveals a distended abdomen with absent bowel sounds. The parents may report the passage of bloody stool.

What happens in volvulus

Although volvulus may occur anywhere in a bowel segment long enough to twist, the most common site, as the illustration depicts, is the sigmoid colon, causing edema within the closed loop and obstruction at its proximal and distal ends.

Normal bowel segment

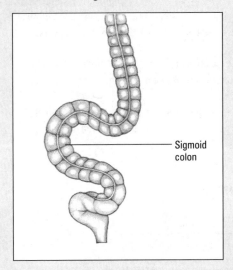

Sigmoid colon

Volvulus

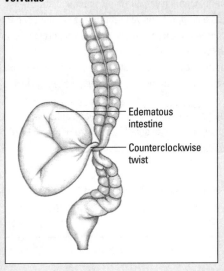

Edematous intestine

Counterclockwise twist

What tests tell you

Abdominal X-rays show multiple distended bowel loops and a large bowel without gas. An upper GI series and barium enema help confirm the diagnosis. Blood chemistry indicates hyperkalemia and hypocalcemia.

Complications

Without immediate treatment, volvulus can lead to strangulation of the twisted bowel loop, ischemia, infarction, perforation, and fatal peritonitis.

Chain of events

Short gut syndrome may develop after surgical correction if an extensive area of bowel is removed. This syndrome results in decreased absorptive surface area which, in turn, leads to decreased absorption of nutrients.

How it's treated

If the bowel is distended but viable, surgery consists of *detorsion* (untwisting). If the bowel is necrotic, surgery includes resection and anastomosis. Prolonged TPN and I.V. administration of antibiotics are usually necessary.

What to do

The child and his parents will need reassurance because the child may be in extreme pain. Because tests may be required on an emergency basis, tell the child what's being done, step-by-step, as each test is being performed.

When the child is relatively comfortable and able to listen, prepare him for surgery with age-appropriate explanations about what will happen. In addition, follow these steps:
• Monitor bowel sounds and bowel movements.
• Give pain medications as ordered.
• Maintain NPO status until surgery is performed; begin administration of I.V. fluids to prevent dehydration.
• Insert an NG tube to decompress the stomach.

Postoperative care
• Maintain the administration of I.V. fluids until the bowel has healed and bowel sounds return.
• Monitor the use of opioid analgesics that decrease GI motility.
• Educate the parents about preventing constipation (for example, increasing the intake of oral fluids, increasing activity, adding high-fiber foods to the diet, and the proper use of stool softeners).

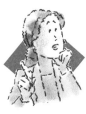

Quick quiz

1. A 2-month-old male infant is admitted with a diagnosis of pyloric stenosis. Due to the projectile vomiting he has had, he's at risk for:
    A.   metabolic acidosis.
    B.   metabolic alkalosis.
    C.   hyperkalemia.
    D.   hypernatremia.

Answer: B. Projectile vomiting causes loss of hydrochloric acid, which results in metabolic alkalosis.

2. A 12-year-old boy is admitted to the pediatric unit with complaints of RLQ abdominal pain and vomiting. When the nurse checks on the child 2 hours later, he states that the pain has stopped. The nurse should suspect that:

    A.   he had indigestion, which has been relieved.

    B.   he's afraid of going to surgery.

    C.   his appendix has ruptured.

    D.   he has irritable bowel syndrome.

Answer: C. Abdominal pain in the RLQ and vomiting are symptoms of appendicitis. When the appendix ruptures, a sudden relief of pain occurs, after which the pain resumes more severely.

3. An 18-month-old child is admitted to the pediatric unit with intussusception. As the nurse is preparing the child for a barium contrast reduction, he passes a soft brown stool. What should the nurse do?

    A.   Notify the doctor in order to cancel the procedure.

    B.   Prepare the child for emergency surgery.

    C.   Take vital signs and monitor for abdominal sounds.

    D.   Administer an enema to clear the rectal area for testing.

Answer: A. Passing a normal-looking brown stool indicates that the child no longer has an invaginated section of bowel.

4. The nurse is completing discharge teaching for a child and her parents regarding her diet to treat celiac disease. Which meal selection would be appropriate for this child?

    A.   A bologna sandwich on whole wheat bread, a chocolate chip cookie, and a glass of milk

    B.   A vegetable pizza, an apple, and a diet cola

    C.   A corn tortilla with hamburger and cooked vegetables and a glass of fruit juice

    D.   A hot dog on a roll, celery and carrot sticks, and a chocolate milk shake

Answer: C. Celiac disease is intolerance to wheat, barley, rye, and oats. Some of these children also have lactose intolerance, especially when they have an acute episode of the disease.

Scoring

☆☆☆   If you answered all four items correctly, congratulations! You've thoroughly digested the material in this chapter.

☆☆   If you answered three items correctly, good job! Your knowledge of GI disorders is unobstructed.

☆   If you answered fewer than three items correctly, don't give yourself an ulcer! Swallow your pride and prepare for the last three quizzes.

13

Endocrine and metabolic problems

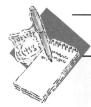

Just the facts

In this chapter, you'll learn:

♦ function of the glands of the endocrine system

♦ tests used to diagnose endocrine and metabolic problems

♦ treatments for children with endocrine and metabolic problems

♦ disorders of the endocrine system and metabolic function.

Anatomy and physiology

The endocrine system is composed of glands that secrete hormones necessary for normal metabolic function. Along with the nervous system, the endocrine system regulates and integrates the body's metabolic activities. (See *Endocrine system components*, page 508.)

Too little, too much

Altered endocrine function involves a hyposecretion or hypersecretion of hormones, which affects the body's metabolic processes and function. Nursing care involves measures to support hormonal secretion, such as hormone replacement, or curtail secretion, such as radiation therapy. Inborn errors of metabolism involve a biochemical alteration that affects metabolism.

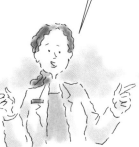

Altered endocrine function involves hyposecretion or hypersecretion of hormones.

Endocrine system components

Endocrine glands secrete hormones directly into the bloodstream to regulate body function. This illustration shows the locations of the major endocrine glands (except the gonads).

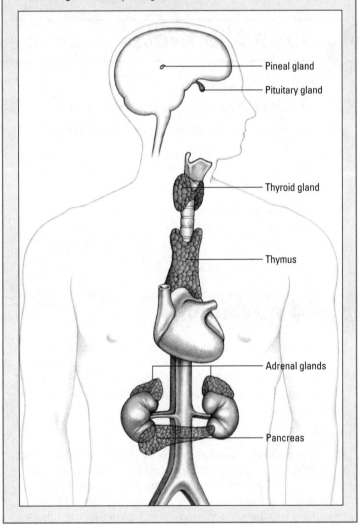

- Pineal gland
- Pituitary gland
- Thyroid gland
- Thymus
- Adrenal glands
- Pancreas

Glands

The major glands of the endocrine system are:
- pituitary gland
- thyroid gland
- parathyroid glands

- adrenal glands
- pancreas
- ovaries and testes.

Pituitary gland

The pituitary gland (also called the *hypophysis* or *master gland*) rests in the sella turcica, a depression in the sphenoid bone at the base of the brain.

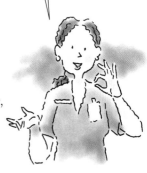

The pituitary may be petite, but it's the master gland of the endocrine system.

Small but mighty

This pea-sized gland connects with the hypothalamus via the infundibulum, from which it receives chemical and nervous stimulation. The pituitary has two main regions:

anterior pituitary

posterior pituitary.

Prolific producer

The anterior pituitary, also called the *adenohypophysis*, makes up 80% of the pituitary gland. It produces seven hormones:

growth hormone (GH), or *somatotropin*

thyroid-stimulating hormone (TSH), or *thyrotropin*

corticotropin

follicle-stimulating hormone (FSH)

luteinizing hormone (LH)

prolactin

melanocyte-stimulating hormone.

Hormones in storage

The posterior pituitary, or *neurohypophysis*, makes up about 20% of the pituitary gland. It serves as a storage area for antidiuretic hormone (ADH), or *vasopressin*, and oxytocin, which are produced by the hypothalamus.

Thyroid gland

The thyroid gland lies directly below the larynx, partially in front of the trachea. Its two lateral lobes—one on either side of the trachea—join with a narrow tissue bridge, called the *isthmus*, to give the gland its butterfly shape.

Thyroid lobe duo

The two lobes of the thyroid gland function as one unit to produce the hormones triiodothyronine (T_3), thyroxine (T_4), and calcitonin. T_3 and T_4 are collectively referred to as thyroid hormones (THs), the body's major metabolic hormones. They regulate metabolism by speeding cellular respiration.

The calcitonin-calcium connection

Calcitonin maintains the blood calcium level by inhibiting the release of calcium from bone. Secretion of calcitonin is controlled by the calcium concentration of the fluid surrounding the thyroid cells.

Parathyroid glands

The parathyroid glands are the body's smallest known endocrine glands. These glands are embedded on the posterior surface of the thyroid, one in each corner.

PTH: A parathyroid production

Working together as a single gland, the parathyroid glands produce parathyroid hormone (PTH). The main function of PTH is to help regulate the blood's calcium balance. This hormone adjusts the rate at which calcium and magnesium ions are removed from urine. PTH also increases the movement of phosphate ions from the blood to urine for excretion.

Adrenal glands

There are two adrenal glands in the body; each gland is situated on top of a kidney. These almond-shaped glands contain two distinct structures—the adrenal cortex and the adrenal medulla—that function as separate endocrine glands.

Adrenal cortex

The adrenal cortex is the large outer layer of the adrenal gland and forms the bulk of the gland. It has three zones, or cell layers:

* *zona glomerulosa*, the outermost zone, which produces mineralocorticoids, primarily aldosterone

* *zona fasciculata*, the middle and largest zone, which produces the glucocorticoids cortisol (hydrocortisone), cortisone, and corticosterone as well as small amounts of the sex hormones androgen and estrogen

* *zona reticularis*, the innermost zone, which produces mainly glucocorticoids and some sex hormones.

Adrenal medulla

The adrenal medulla, or inner layer of the adrenal gland, functions as part of the sympathetic nervous system and produces two catecholamines:

 epinephrine

 norepinephrine.

A leading role

Because catecholamines play an important role in the autonomic nervous system, the adrenal medulla is considered a neuroendocrine structure.

Pancreas

The pancreas, a triangular gland, is nestled in the curve of the duodenum, stretching horizontally behind the stomach and extending to the spleen. The pancreas performs endocrine and exocrine functions. Acinar cells make up most of the gland and regulate pancreatic exocrine function.

Clusters of islets

The endocrine cells of the pancreas are called the *islet cells*, or *islets of Langerhans*. These cells exist in clusters and are found scattered among the acinar cells. The islets contain alpha, beta, and delta cells that produce important hormones:
- Alpha cells produce glucagon.
- Beta cells produce insulin.
- Delta cells produce somatostatin.

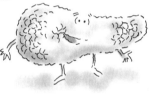

Check out my job description; it includes endocrine functions, exocrine functions, and hormone production. I deserve a raise!

Gonads

The gonads include the ovaries in the female and the testes in the male.

Ovaries

The ovaries are oval-shaped glands in females located on either side of the uterus. They produce ova (eggs) as well as estrogen and progesterone.

It's a girl thing

Estrogen and progesterone are responsible for:
- promoting the development and maintenance of female sex characteristics
- regulating the menstrual cycle
- maintaining the uterus for pregnancy
- preparing the mammary glands for lactation.

Testes

The testes are located in the scrotum. They produce the male hormone testosterone, which stimulates and maintains male sex characteristics. They also produce spermatozoa.

Hormones

Hormones are complex chemical substances that trigger or regulate the activity of an organ or a group of cells. They include pituitary hormones, THs, adrenal hormones, and androgens and estrogens. (See *Effects of altered hormonal function.*)

Pituitary hormones

Pituitary hormones include the anterior pituitary hormones (GH, TSH, FSH, LH, and prolactin) and the posterior pituitary hormones (ADH and oxytocin). Each of these hormones has a particular function:

• GH, secreted by the anterior pituitary gland, affects most body tissues. It triggers growth by increasing protein synthesis and fat mobilization and decreases carbohydrate use.
• TSH is secreted by the anterior pituitary gland and stimulates the thyroid.
• FSH, secreted by the anterior pituitary gland, stimulates the graafian follicles to mature and secrete estrogen in the female. In males, it stimulates development of the seminiferous tubules.
• LH, secreted by the anterior pituitary gland, produces the rupture of the follicle, which results in the discharge of a mature ovum in the female. In the male, it stimulates the production of androgens, particularly testosterone.
• Prolactin is secreted by the anterior pituitary gland and stimulates milk secretion.
• ADH is secreted by the posterior pituitary gland. It controls the concentration of body fluids by altering the permeability of the distal convoluted tubules and collecting ducts of the kidneys to conserve water.
• Oxytocin, secreted by the posterior pituitary gland, stimulates the contraction of the uterus and the letdown reflex in lactating women.

Thyroid hormones

The THs are T_3 and T_4. These hormones are necessary for normal growth and development and act on many tissues to increase metabolic activity and protein synthesis.

Effects of altered hormonal function

This chart shows the effects that may result from excessive or deficient secretion of select hormones.

Hormone	Hypofunction	Hyperfunction
Anterior pituitary hormones		
GH	• Epiphyseal fusion with cessation of growth • Prepubertal dwarfism • Pituitary cachexia (Simmonds' disease) • Generalized growth retardation • Hypoglycemia	• Prepubertal gigantism • Acromegaly (after full growth is attained) • Diabetes mellitus • Postpubertal hypoproteinemia
TSH	• Hypothyroidism • Marked delay of puberty • Juvenile myxedema	• Hyperthyroidism • Thyrotoxicosis • Graves' disease
Corticotropin	• Acute adrenocortical insufficiency (Addison's disease) • Hypoglycemia • Increased skin pigmentation	• Cushing's syndrome
Gonadotropins	• Absent or incomplete spontaneous puberty	• Precocious puberty • Early epiphyseal closure
FSH	• Hypogonadism • Sterility • Absence or loss of secondary sex characteristics • Amenorrhea	• Precocious puberty • Primary gonadal failure • Hirsutism • Polycystic ovary • Early epiphyseal closure
LH	• Hypogonadism • Sterility • Impotence • Absence or loss of secondary sex characteristics • Ovarian failure	• Precocious puberty • Primary gonadal failure • Hirsutism • Polycystic ovary • Early epiphyseal closure
Prolactin	• Inability to lactate • Amenorrhea	• Galactorrhea • Functional hypogonadism
Melanocyte-stimulating hormone	• Diminished or absent skin pigmentation	• Increased skin pigmentation

(continued)

Effects of altered hormonal function *(continued)*

Hormone	Hypofunction	Hyperfunction
Posterior pituitary hormone		
Antidiuretic hormone or vasopressin	• Diabetes insipidus	• Syndrome of inappropriate antidiuretic hormone secretion • Fluid retention • Hyponatremia
Thyroid hormones		
T_4 and T_3	• Hypothyroidism • Myxedema • Hashimoto thyroiditis • Greatly reduced general growth (extent depends on age at which deficiency occurs) • Mental retardation (in infants)	• Exophthalmic goiter (Graves' disease) • Accelerated linear growth • Early epiphyseal closure
Parathyroid gland hormone		
PTH	• Hypocalcemia (tetany)	• Hypercalcemia (bone demineralization) • Hypophosphatemia
Adrenal hormones		
Aldosterone	• Adrenocortical insufficiency	• Electrolyte imbalance • Hyperaldosteronism
Glucocorticoids (cortisol and corticosterone)	• Addison's disease • Acute adrenocortical insufficiency • Impaired growth and sexual function	• Cushing's syndrome • Severe impairment of growth with slowing in skeletal maturation

Adrenal hormones

The adrenal hormones are cortisol, aldosterone, androgens, and estrogen:

• Cortisol is a glucocorticoid that stimulates glucogenesis and increases protein breakdown and free fatty acid mobilization; it also suppresses the immune response and provides for an appropriate response to stress.

• Aldosterone, a mineralocorticoid, regulates the resorption of sodium and the excretion of potassium by the kidneys; it's affected by corticotropin and is regulated by angiotensin II, which, in turn, is regulated by renin. Together, aldosterone, angiotensin II, and renin are involved in the pathogenesis of hypertension.

• Androgens are male sex hormones; they promote male traits, especially secondary sex characteristics, such as facial hair and a low-pitched voice.

• Estrogens are responsible for the development of secondary female sex characteristics.

Pancreatic hormones

The islets of Langerhans are small clusters of endocrine cells in the pancreas. These structures contain cells that produce insulin, glucagon, and somatostatin:
• Insulin: a hormone that raises the blood glucose level by triggering the breakdown of glycogen to glucose
• Glucagon: lowers the blood glucose level by stimulating the conversion of glucose to glycogen
• Somatostatin: inhibits the release of GH, corticotropin, and certain other hormones

Hormone release and transport

Although all hormone release results from endocrine gland stimulation, release patterns of hormones vary greatly.
• Secretion of PTH (by the parathyroid gland) and prolactin (by the anterior pituitary) occurs fairly evenly throughout the day.
• Corticotropin (secreted by the anterior pituitary) and cortisol (secreted by the adrenal cortex) are released in spurts in response to body rhythm cycles; levels of these hormones peak in the morning.
• Secretion of insulin by the pancreas has both steady and sporadic release patterns.

Hormonal action

When a hormone reaches its target site, it binds to a specific receptor on the cell membrane or within the cell. Polypeptides and some amines bind to membrane receptor sites. The smaller, more lipid-soluble steroids and THs diffuse through the cell membrane and bind to intracellular receptors.

Right on target!

After binding occurs, each hormone produces unique physiologic changes, depending on its target site and its specific action at that site. A particular hormone may have different effects at different target sites.

Hormonal regulation

To maintain the body's delicate equilibrium, a feedback mechanism regulates hormone production and secretion. The mechanism involves hormones, blood chemicals and metabolites, and the nervous system. The feedback mechanism may be simple or complex.

For normal function, each gland must contain enough appropriately programmed secretory cells to release active hormone on demand.

Unsupervised cells

Secretory cells need supervision. A secretory cell can't sense on its own when to release the hormone or how much to release. It gets this information from sensing and signaling systems that integrate many messages. Together, stimulatory and inhibitory signals actively control the rate and duration of hormone release.

It's nice to be recognized

When released, the hormone travels to target cells, where a receptor molecule recognizes it and binds to it. The sensitivity of a target cell depends on how many receptors it has for a particular site. The more receptor sites, the more sensitive the target cell.

Diagnostic tests

Diagnostic tests are used to assess endocrine system problems and metabolic function in the pediatric population:

• *Blood glucose tests* are used to diagnose type 1 and type 2 diabetes mellitus. Blood glucose tests commonly used for the pediatric patient include the fasting blood glucose test and the oral glucose tolerance test (OGTT).
• *Growth hormone tests* are used to determine pituitary function. The human growth hormone (hGH) test helps detect hypopituitarism, whereas the growth hormone suppression test is used to diagnose pituitary hyperfunction.
• *Neonatal screening*, which began in the 1960s, is now performed in every state and may consist of tests for a variety of diseases. Typically, neonatal screens are performed for commonly occurring diseases that may cause severe mental retardation or death without early detection and treatment. These tests are all done by dried filter paper blood spots. A very small amount of blood is required and is usually obtained by a heel stick. An example of endocrine and metabolic tests that may be screened for during newborn screening include phenylketonuria (PKU), maple syrup urine disease (MSUD), galactosemia, congenital adrenal hyperplasia, and congenital hypothyroidism.
• *Thyroid function tests* are used to determine thyroid function and include T_4 and T_3 studies.
• Radioimmunoassay is a test used to measure minute quantities of hormones.

Glucose, fasting plasma

The fasting plasma glucose test (also known as the *fasting blood sugar test*) is commonly used to screen for diabetes mellitus. It measures plasma glucose levels after an 8-hour fast.

To fast or not to fast

In the fasting state, plasma glucose levels decrease, stimulating the release of the hormone glucagon. Glucagon then acts to raise plasma glucose by accelerating glycogenolysis, stimulating glyconeogenesis, and inhibiting glycogen synthesis. Normally, secretion of insulin checks this rise in glucose levels. In diabetes, however, absence or deficiency of insulin allows persistently high glucose levels.

And the level is . . .

The normal range for fasting plasma glucose varies according to the laboratory procedure. Normal values after a fast of at least 8 hours differ according to the age of the child:
* premature neonates—40 to 65 mg/dl (SI, 2.2 to 3.6 mmol/L)
* young children (birth to age 2 years)—60 to 110 mg/dl (SI, 3.3 to 6.1 mmol/L)
* children (ages 2 to 18 years)—60 to 100 mg/dl (SI, 3.3 to 5.6 mmol/L).

Glucose tells all

A fasting plasma glucose level of 126 mg/dl or higher obtained on two or more occasions confirms provisional diabetes mellitus. An impaired blood glucose level is 125 mg/dl. A borderline or transiently elevated level requires a 2-hour postprandial plasma glucose test or an OGTT to confirm the diagnosis.

Nursing considerations

* Explain the procedure to the parents and the child, and encourage the parents to stay with the child.
* Determine how long the child must fast.
* Determine if the timing of the patient's medication will interfere with the test results and withhold medication if indicated.

Backup plan

* Apply a topical anesthetic (when possible) to two spots so an alternate puncture site will be available if the first one isn't successful.
* Specify on the laboratory request the time the patient last ate, the sample collection time, and the time he received the last pretest dose of insulin (if applicable).

Glucose tolerance, oral

The OGTT measures carbohydrate metabolism after ingestion of a challenge dose of glucose. A 2-hour OGTT is typically done to diagnose diabetes mellitus in children. (See *Administering oral glucose solutions*, page 518.)

Administering oral glucose solutions

The oral glucose load in a glucose tolerance test usually varies from 50 to 100 g. The American Diabetes Association recommends a glucose dose of 40 g/m^2 of body surface area, as calculated by a nomogram based on height and weight. Other authorities advocate a glucose load of 1.75 g/kg of body weight, which is especially useful in testing pediatric patients.

Glucose in disguise

Many patients become nauseated after drinking the overly sweet glucose solution. One way to make the solution more palatable is to dissolve it in water, flavor it with lemon juice, and chill it. Another way is to substitute Glucola, a carbonated drink, or Gel-a-dex, a cherry-flavored gelatin, for the appropriate amount of glucose.

Up to the challenge?

The body absorbs the challenge dose rapidly, causing plasma glucose levels to rise and peak within 30 minutes to 1 hour. The pancreas responds by secreting more insulin, causing glucose levels to return to normal after 2 to 3 hours.

During this period, plasma and urine glucose levels are monitored to assess insulin secretion and the body's ability to metabolize glucose. Occasionally, glucose levels are monitored for an additional 2 to 3 hours to aid in the diagnosis of hypoglycemia and malabsorption syndrome.

A little intolerant

Some patients with diabetes may have fasting plasma glucose levels in the normal range; however, insufficient secretion of insulin after ingestion of carbohydrates causes plasma glucose levels to rise sharply and return to normal slowly. This decreased tolerance for glucose helps confirm diabetes.

Nursing considerations

Explain to the child and his parents that the test usually requires five blood samples and five urine specimens. Provide the child with coping mechanisms and help him deal with the multiple blood draws by giving him a small reward, such as a sticker, after each blood draw.

In addition, follow these steps:
• Instruct the parents that the child must fast for 8 to 12 hours before the test because the first blood test is a fasting glucose level.
• Send blood and urine samples to the laboratory immediately, or refrigerate them.

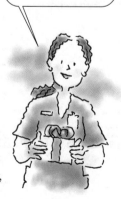

Small rewards, such as stickers, can help make the five needle sticks needed for blood glucose testing a little sweeter.

• Specify blood and urine collection times and the time the child last ate.
• As appropriate, record the time that the child received his last pretest dose of insulin or oral antidiabetic drug.

Blood totals

• If the patient is an infant or young child, keep an ongoing record of repeated specimen collection and a total of the amount of blood collected.
• As ordered, resume administration of medications withheld before the test.

Growth hormone, human

The hGH test is used to detect hypopituitarism. Also known as *growth hormone* and *somatotropin*, hGH is a protein secreted by the anterior pituitary and is the primary regulator of human growth. Children generally have higher hGH levels than adults; these levels can range from undetectable to 16 ng/ml (SI, 16 mcg/L).

The hGH test, a quantitative analysis of plasma hGH levels, is usually performed as part of an anterior pituitary stimulation or suppression test.

The lowdown on levels

Increased hGH levels may indicate a pituitary or hypothalamic tumor (commonly an adenoma), which causes gigantism in children and acromegaly in adults and adolescents.

The highs . . .

Patients with diabetes mellitus sometimes have elevated hGH levels without acromegaly. Suppression testing is necessary to confirm the diagnosis.

. . . and the lows

Pituitary infarction, metastatic disease, and tumors may reduce hGH levels. Dwarfism may be caused by low hGH levels, but confirmation of the diagnosis requires stimulation testing with arginine or insulin.

Nursing considerations

Prepare the child for the test with a simple, developmentally appropriate explanation. Tell the child and his parents that another sample may have to be drawn the following day for comparison. Explain to the parents that the laboratory requires at least 2 days of samples for analysis.

In addition, follow these steps:
• Withhold all medications that affect hGH levels, such as pituitary-based steroids, as ordered. If these medications must be continued, note this on the laboratory request.
• Make sure the patient is relaxed and recumbent for 30 minutes before the test because stress and physical activity elevate hGH levels. Explain that the child must fast and limit physical activity for 10 to 12 hours before the test.
• Between 6 a.m. and 8 a.m. on 2 consecutive days, or as ordered, draw venous blood and send it to the laboratory.

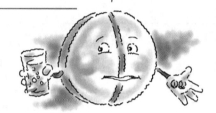

As a pituitary-based steroid, I'm off-limits before a growth hormone test. I do my job so well that I could alter the results.

Growth hormone suppression

The growth hormone suppression test, also known as the *glucose loading test*, is used to diagnose pituitary hyperfunction. It evaluates excessive baseline levels of hGH from the anterior pituitary by measuring the secretory response to a loading dose of glucose.

Failure to suppress

Normally, hGH raises plasma glucose and fatty acid concentrations; in response, insulin secretion increases to counteract these effects. A glucose load should suppress hGH secretion. In a patient with excessive hGH levels, the failure to suppress hGH indicates anterior pituitary dysfunction and confirms a diagnosis of acromegaly or gigantism.

Glucose normally suppresses hGH to levels ranging from undetectable to 3 ng/ml (SI, 3 mcg/L) in 30 minutes to 2 hours. In a patient with active acromegaly, basal hGH levels are elevated to 75 ng/ml (SI, 75 mcg/L) and aren't suppressed to less than 5 ng/ml (SI, 5 mcg/L) during the test. In children, rebound stimulation may occur after 2 to 5 hours.

Rest and repeat

When the hGH levels are unchanged or increased in response to glucose loading, hGH hypersecretion is indicated and may confirm suspected acromegaly or gigantism. This response may be verified by repeating the test after a 1-day rest.

Nursing considerations

Explain the test to the child and his parents. Tell the child that he may experience nausea after drinking the glucose solution, and prepare him for the needle sticks. In addition:
• Withhold all steroids; if these or other medications must be continued, note this on the laboratory request.

• Administer 100 g of glucose solution by mouth; to prevent nausea, tell the child to drink the glucose slowly.

Guthrie screening

The Guthrie screening test, also known as the *phenylalanine test,* is a screening method used to detect elevated levels of serum phenylalanine, a naturally occurring amino acid essential for growth and nitrogen balance.

Metabolic upset

Elevated levels of phenylalanine may indicate PKU, a metabolic disorder inherited as an autosomal-recessive trait. An infant with PKU usually has normal phenylalanine levels at birth, but after he begins feeding with breast milk or formula (both of which contain phenylalanine), levels gradually rise because of a deficiency of the liver enzyme that converts phenylalanine to tyrosine. The resulting accumulation of phenylalanine, phenylpyruvic acid, and other metabolites hinders normal development of central nervous system cells, causing mental retardation.

Three's a charm

The serum phenylalanine screening test detects abnormal phenylalanine levels through the growth rate of *Bacillus subtilis,* an organism that needs phenylalanine to thrive. To ensure accurate results, the test must be performed after 3 full days (preferably 4 days) of breast milk or formula feeding. (In some states, a preliminary test is required 25 hours after birth.)

Danger ahead

Growth of *B. subtilis* on the filter paper indicates that serum phenylalanine levels are high enough to overcome the antagonist. Such a positive result suggests the *possibility* of PKU; diagnosis requires exact serum phenylalanine measurement and urine testing. A positive screening test may also result from hepatic disease, galactosemia (an inherited, autosomal-recessive disorder of galactose metabolism), or delayed development of certain enzyme systems. (See *Confirming PKU.*)

Nursing considerations

Explain the test to the parents. In addition, follow these steps:
• Perform a heel stick and allow the blood to drip onto the filter paper, filling each circle.
• Reassure the parents of a child who may have PKU that early detection and continuous treatment with a low-phenylalanine diet can prevent permanent mental retardation.

Confirming PKU

After the Guthrie screening test detects the possible presence of PKU, serum phenylalanine and tyrosine levels are measured to confirm the diagnosis. Phenylalanine hydroxylase is the enzyme that converts phenylalanine to tyrosine. If this enzyme is absent, increasing phenylalanine levels with concomitant decreasing tyrosine levels indicate PKU.

Samples are obtained by venipuncture. Serum phenylalanine levels greater than 4 mg/dl and tyrosine levels less than 0.6 mg/dl—with urinary excretion of phenylpyruvic acid—confirm PKU.

• Note the infant's name and birth date and the date of the first breast milk or formula feeding on the laboratory request; send the sample to the laboratory immediately.

Neonatal galactosemia

Galactosemia is a genetic disorder. A patient with galactosemia lacks the liver enzyme *galactose-1-phosphate uridyltransferase* (GALT), which converts galactose into glucose. The patient's galactose levels remain abnormally high. Ultimately, galactosemia may cause hepatomegaly, kidney failure, cataracts, or brain damage. If the disorder goes untreated, death may result in 75% of infants with the disorder.

From sea to shining sea

The galactosemia test is mandatory in all 50 states. To detect galactosemia, two tests may be run on the dried filter paper blood spot sample:

☝ First, the level of galactose in the blood is determined.

✌ If this test is abnormally high (usually considered total galactose levels greater than 10 mg/dl), a Beutler assay is performed on the sample to measure GALT enzyme activity.

Where's the GALT?

Galactosemia is diagnosed if there's no detectable GALT enzyme activity. After the positive diagnosis of galactosemia is made, treatment must begin immediately.

Nursing considerations

• Screening will provide the best results if it's done after the infant has received a milk-based feeding.
• Be sure to indicate the infant's feeding and blood transfusion status on the filter paper blood sample.
• Protect the filter paper blood sample from heat, which may damage the GALT enzyme. (See *Galactosemia interference*.)

Neonatal T_4 and TSH blood-spot test

Mandatory in all 50 states, a T_4 test is performed as part of the neonatal screening with the sample placed as a blood spot on filter paper. A low T_4 level (less than 6 mg/dl) must be followed by a TSH level, which may be performed on the same blood sample or from a separate sample. (See *Collecting a filter paper sample*.)

Galactosemia interference

Factors that may alter galactosemia test results include:
• use of aspirin, sulfonamides, nitrofurantoin, vitamin K derivatives, primaquine, and fava beans, which decrease GALT enzyme activity and precipitate hemolytic episodes
• performing the test after a hemolytic episode or a blood transfusion, which can cause false-negative results
• failure to use a collection tube containing the proper anticoagulant or to adequately mix the sample and anticoagulant
• hemolysis caused by rough handling of the sample.

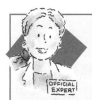

Advice from the experts

OFFICIAL EXPERT

Collecting a filter paper sample

To collect a specimen for neonatal TSH testing using the filter paper method, gather the following equipment and follow the easy steps below.

Equipment
- Alcohol swabs
- Sterile lancet
- Specially marked filter paper
- Sterile 2" × 2" gauze pads
- Adhesive bandage
- Labels
- Gloves

Steps
- Assemble the necessary equipment, wash your hands thoroughly, and put on gloves.
- Wipe the infant's heel with an alcohol swab and then dry it thoroughly with a gauze pad.
- Perform a heel stick and squeeze the infant's heel gently, filling the circles on the filter paper with blood, while making sure the blood saturates the paper.
- Gently apply pressure with a gauze pad to ensure hemostasis at the puncture site.
- Allow the filter paper to dry, label it appropriately, and send it to the laboratory.

The birth surge

Also known as the *neonatal thyrotropin test*, the neonatal TSH test confirms congenital hypothyroidism. TSH levels normally surge after birth and trigger a rise in TH, which is essential for neurologic development. At age 1 to 2 days, TSH levels are normally 25 to 30 µIU/ml (SI, 25 to 30 mU/L). Thereafter, levels are normally less than 25 µIU/ml (SI, 25 mU/L).

Failure to respond

In primary congenital hypothyroidism, the thyroid gland doesn't respond to TSH stimulation, which results in lower TH levels and higher TSH levels. Early detection and treatment of congenital hypothyroidism are critical to prevent mental retardation and cretinism.

Neonatal TSH levels must be interpreted in light of T_4 concentrations. Elevated TSH that's accompanied by decreased T_4 indicates primary congenital hypothyroidism. Depressed TSH and depressed T_4 may be present in secondary congenital hypothyroidism. When TSH is normal and is accompanied by depressed T_4, hypothyroidism due to a congenital defect or transient congenital hypothyroidism due to prematurity or prenatal hypoxia may be the cause. A complete thyroid workup must be done to confirm the cause of hypothyroidism before treatment can begin. (See *Neonatal TSH interference.*)

Neonatal TSH interference

Several factors may alter TSH levels, or the results of tests used to measure TSH levels in the neonate:
- Corticosteroids, T_3, and T_4 lower TSH levels.
- Lithium carbonate, potassium iodide, excessive topical resorcinol, and TSH injection raise TSH levels.
- Failure to let a filter paper sample dry completely may alter results.
- Rough handling of a serum sample may cause hemolysis, which may alter results.

Nursing considerations

Explain the test to the parents. A sample is sent for T_4 and TSH levels. Perform a venipuncture or heel stick, collect and label the sample, and send it to the laboratory immediately.

Thyroxine test

T_4 is an amine secreted by the thyroid gland in response to TSH from the pituitary and, indirectly, to thyrotropin-releasing hormone (TRH) from the hypothalamus.

Cons, pros, and suspects

The rate of secretion is normally regulated by a complex system of negative and positive feedback involving the thyroid, the anterior pituitary, and the hypothalamus. T_4 is the suspected precursor (or prohormone) of T_3 and is converted to T_3 mainly in the liver and kidneys.

The T_4 that binds

Only a fraction of T_4 (about 0.3%) circulates freely in the blood; the rest binds strongly to plasma proteins, primarily to T_4-binding globulin (TBG). This minute fraction of free-circulating T_4 is responsible for the clinical effects of thyroid hormone. TBG binds so tenaciously that T_4 survives in the plasma for a relatively long time, with a half-life of about 6 days. This test measures the total circulating T_4 level when TBG is normal.

More testing ahead

Serum T_4 testing is performed to evaluate thyroid function and to monitor thyroid replacement therapy.

Abnormally elevated levels of T_4 are consistent with primary and secondary hyperthyroidism, including excessive T_4 (levothyroxine [Synthroid]) replacement therapy. Overt signs of hyperthyroidism require further testing, and in doubtful cases of hypothyroidism, the TSH or TRH test may be indicated. (See *Thyroxine levels in children*.)

Nursing considerations

Explain the test to the child and his parents. In addition, follow these steps:
• As ordered, withhold medications that may interfere with test results. If these medications must be continued, note this on the laboratory request. (If the test is being performed to monitor thyroid therapy, the patient should continue to receive daily thyroid supplements.)
• Perform a venipuncture, collect a sample, and send the sample to the laboratory immediately.

Thyroxine levels in children

T_4 levels change as the child grows:
• cord blood—7.4 to 13 mcg/dl (SI, 95 to 168 nmol/L)
• younger than age 1 month—7 to 22.6 mcg/dl (SI, 90 to 292 nmol/L)
• ages 1 month to 1 year—7.2 to 16.5 mcg/dl (SI, 93 to 213 nmol/L)
• ages 1 to 5 years—7.3 to 15 mcg/dl (SI, 94 to 194 nmol/L)
• ages 5 to 10 years—6.4 to 13.3 mcg/dl (SI, 83 to 192 nmol/L)
• ages 10 to 15 years—5.6 to 11.7 mcg/dl (SI, 72 to 151 nmol/L).

Triiodothyronine test (serum)

The T_3 test is a highly specific immunoassay that measures total serum content of T_3 to investigate clinical indications of thyroid dysfunction. It helps diagnose T_3 toxicosis, hypothyroidism, or hyperthyroidism and helps monitor the course of thyroid replacement therapy.

T_3 is the more potent thyroid hormone. At least 50% and as much as 90% of T_3 is thought to be derived from T_4. The remaining 10% or more is secreted directly by the thyroid gland. Like T_4 secretion, T_3 secretion occurs in response to TSH released by the pituitary and, secondarily, to TRH from the hypothalamus.

A little T_3 goes a long way

Although T_3 is present in the bloodstream in minute quantities and is metabolically active for only a short time, its impact on body metabolism dominates that of T_4. T_3 binds less firmly to TBG, so it persists in the bloodstream for a short time; half of it disappears in about 1 day, whereas half of T_4 remains for 6 days.

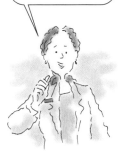

When it comes to potency, T_3 has T_4 beat. Its effect on body metabolism dominates the effect of T_4.

It's all on the level

Normally, serum T_3 levels in children are:
• neonate—70 to 260 ng/dl (SI, 1.16 to 4 nmol/L)
• children ages 1 to 5 years—100 to 260 ng/dl (SI, 1.54 to 4 nmol/L)
• children ages 5 to 10 years—90 to 240 ng/dl (SI, 1.39 to 3.7 nmol/L)
• children ages 10 to 15 years—80 to 210 ng/dl (SI, 1.23 to 3.23 nmol/L).

A tandem rise

Serum T_3 and T_4 levels usually rise and fall in tandem. However, in T_3 toxicosis, only T_3 levels rise, whereas total and free T_4 levels remain normal. T_3 toxicosis occurs in patients with Graves' disease, toxic adenoma, or toxic nodular goiter. T_3 levels also surpass T_4 levels in patients receiving thyroid replacement containing more T_3 than T_4. In iodine-deficient areas, the thyroid may produce larger amounts of the more cellularly active T_3 than T_4 in an effort to maintain the euthyroid state.

Nursing considerations

Explain the test to the child and his parents, and allow a parent to be present during the venipuncture. In addition, follow these steps:
• As ordered, withhold medications that may influence thyroid function, such as steroids and propranolol (Inderal). If such

medications must be continued, record this information on the laboratory request.
• Perform a venipuncture, collect the sample, and send it to the laboratory immediately.
• If a patient must receive thyroid preparations, such as T_3 (liothyronine [Triostat]), note the time of drug administration on the laboratory request.

Treatments and procedures

Common treatments and procedures used in the care of a child with an endocrine and metabolic system disorder include radioactive iodine (^{131}I) therapy and thyroidectomy.

^{131}I therapy

A form of radiation therapy, ^{131}I therapy is used to treat hyperthyroidism in children, particularly Graves' disease. It shrinks functioning thyroid tissue, decreasing circulating TH levels.

After oral ingestion, ^{131}I is rapidly absorbed and concentrated in the thyroid as if it were normal iodine, resulting in acute radiation thyroiditis and gradual thyroid atrophy. ^{131}I causes symptoms to subside after about 3 weeks and exerts its full effect only after 3 to 6 months.

Nursing considerations

Explain the procedure and check the patient's history for allergies to iodine.

Expecting a glow

The idea of ingesting a radioactive material may be frightening to the child and his parents, especially when they hear about the precautions that must be taken. Reassure the child and his parents that this treatment will affect only the thyroid and that all the radioactive material will be excreted from the body.

In addition, follow these steps:
• Unless contraindicated, instruct the patient to stop TH antagonists 4 to 7 days before ^{131}I administration because these drugs reduce the sensitivity of thyroid cells to radiation.
• Tell the child to fast overnight because food may delay ^{131}I absorption.

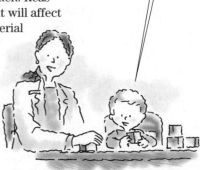

Until my nurse explained my ^{131}I treatment, I thought I was going to be Radioactive Man!

- If the patient received an unusually large dose of ^{131}I or if treatment was for cancer, he may stay in the hospital for monitoring. In such cases, observe radiation precautions for 3 days.
- Don't allow pregnant nurses to care for the child.
- Encourage the patient to drink plenty of fluids for 48 hours to speed excretion of ^{131}I.

At home with radioactive iodine

If the child will be discharged after treatment, instruct the parents about observing radiation precautions at home:
- Tell the parents that the child must urinate into a lead-lined container for 48 hours.
- Tell the parents that the child must use disposable eating utensils, and avoid close contact with young children and pregnant women for 7 days after therapy.
- Advise the parents to dispose of urine, saliva, and vomitus properly; urine and saliva will be slightly radioactive for 24 hours, and vomitus will be highly radioactive for 6 to 8 hours after therapy.

Thyroidectomy

Thyroidectomy (removal of all or part of the thyroid gland) is performed to treat hyperthyroidism and respiratory obstruction from goiter. *Subtotal thyroidectomy*, which reduces secretion of TH, is used to correct hyperthyroidism when drug therapy fails or radiation therapy is contraindicated. After surgery, the remaining thyroid tissue usually supplies enough TH for normal function, although hypothyroidism may occur later.

Nursing considerations

Prepare the child for surgery with an age-appropriate explanation, including the postoperative appearance of the site of surgery. Tell the child that his throat may be sore for a few days after surgery and that medication will be given to make him feel better. Keep in mind that the child may be fearful of having his "throat cut"; provide clarification and answer all questions.

In addition, follow these steps:
- Iodine preparations are typically administered before surgery; to improve the taste of the preparation, mix it with fruit juice.
- Check for laryngeal nerve damage by asking the child to speak as soon as he awakens from anesthesia.
- Watch for signs of respiratory distress. Tracheal collapse, mucus accumulation in the trachea, laryngeal edema, and vocal cord paralysis can all cause respiratory obstruction with sudden stridor and restlessness.

528

Just in case

- Keep a tracheostomy tray at the bedside for the first 24 hours after surgery and be prepared to assist with emergency tracheotomy if necessary.
- Assess for signs of hemorrhage, which may cause shock, tracheal compression, and respiratory distress.
- Check the patient's dressing and palpate the back of his neck (where drainage tends to flow).

Dribbling drainage patrol

- Expect only scant drainage after 24 hours.
- As ordered, administer a mild analgesic to relieve a sore neck or throat; reassure the child that his discomfort should resolve within a few days.
- Test for positive Chvostek's and Trousseau's signs, indicators of neuromuscular irritability from hypocalcemia; keep calcium gluconate available for emergency intravenous (I.V.) administration.

Storm's a'brewin'

- Be alert for signs of thyroid storm, a rare but serious complication in children, characterized by sudden and dangerous signs and symptoms, including severe tachycardia (increased heart rate), severe irritability, vomiting, diarrhea, hyperthermia, and hypertension.

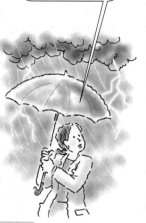

A sudden increase in thyrotoxicosis symptoms is a sign of thyroid storm.

Endocrine and metabolic disorders

Endocrine and metabolic disorders that may affect children include congenital hypothyroidism, Cushing's syndrome, diabetes mellitus, galactosemia, Graves' disease, MSUD, and PKU.

Congenital hypothyroidism

Congenital hypothyroidism is a deficiency of TH secretion during fetal development or early infancy. If left untreated, it will seriously affect mental development. Congenital hypothyroidism is three times more common in girls than in boys.

The early bird catches the best prognosis

Early diagnosis and treatment produces the best prognosis. Infants treated before age 3 months usually grow and develop normally. Athyroid children (born without a thyroid gland) who remain untreated beyond age 3 months and children with acquired hypothyroidism who remain untreated beyond age 2 years suffer irreversible mental retardation. Skeletal abnormalities are reversible with treatment.

What causes it

Congenital hypothyroidism is caused by defective embryonic development (most common cause), causing congenital absence or underdevelopment of the thyroid gland. It can also occur as an inherited autosomal-recessive defect in the synthesis of T_4 (next most common cause).

Mom's meds

Congenital hypothyroidism in infants can result if the mother took antithyroid drugs during pregnancy. Other causes include chronic autoimmune thyroiditis and iodine deficiency during pregnancy.

How it happens

Hypothyroidism in infants and children is related to decreased TH production or secretion, which may result from one of several causes:
• Loss of functional thyroid tissue can be caused by an autoimmune process.
• Defective thyroid synthesis may be related to congenital defects; thyroid dysgenesis (defective development) is the most common defect.
• Hypothyroidism may also be related to decreased TSH secretion or resistance to TSH.
• If left untreated, lack of adequate TH levels seriously affects the nervous system and bone growth.

What to look for

The signs of untreated hypothyroidism usually appear at age 6 weeks:
• The infant with hypothyroidism may sleep more than usual; older children may show signs of lethargy.
• He may have noisy respirations due to tongue enlargement. (The tongue may also be dry.)

Cold to the touch

• The extremities may be cold, and the overall body temperature may be lower due to decreased metabolism.
• The child's neck will be short and thick.
• The extremities appear short and fat; the legs appear shorter in relation to trunk size.

Constipation consternation

- The abdomen becomes enlarged because of intestinal obstruction from constipation (which results from hypotonia of the intestinal tract).
- Other signs include delayed dentition; dry, scaly skin; easy weight gain; and slow pulse.

Whoa, horsey

Infants may have a hoarse cry, persistent jaundice, and respiratory difficulties. Older children may exhibit bone and muscle dystrophy, cognitive impairment (which develops as the disorder progresses), and stunted growth or dwarfism (short stature with the persistence of infant proportions).

What tests tell you

Elevated TSH level associated with low T_3 and T_4 levels points to congenital hypothyroidism. Because early detection and treatment can minimize the effects of congenital hypothyroidism, all states require measurement of infant TH levels at birth through neonate screening tests:

- Thyroid scan and ^{131}I uptake tests show decreased uptake levels and confirm the absence of thyroid tissue in athyroid children.
- Increased gonadotropin levels accompany sexual precocity in older children and may coexist with hypothyroidism.
- An electrocardiogram shows bradycardia and flat or inverted T waves in untreated infants.
- Hip, knee, and thigh X-rays reveal the absence of the femoral or tibial epiphyseal line and delayed skeletal development that's markedly inappropriate for the child's chronological age.

Complications

If hypothyroidism isn't treated by age 3 months, skeletal malformations and irreversible mental retardation can occur; treatment helps to prevent retardation. Learning disabilities and accelerated or delayed sexual maturation may also occur.

How it's treated

The treatment for congenital hypothyroidism is lifelong therapy with synthetic thyroid hormone (levothyroxine, liothyronine). Supplemental vitamin D may also be prescribed to prevent rickets resulting from rapid bone growth. Surgery may be performed for the underlying cause such as a pituitary tumor. The child should have routine monitoring of T_4 and TSH levels as well as periodic evaluation of growth to ensure that thyroid replacement is adequate.

What to do

The child and his parents will need ongoing support and encouragement. They should be encouraged to express their concerns and feelings and may need help to develop effective coping mechanisms. Referral to a support group may be extremely helpful. In addition, follow these steps:
• When caring for a neonate, make sure neonatal screening has been done to allow for early detection of the disorder.
• Stress to the parents the importance of lifelong treatment, including TH replacement therapy as well as routine blood work to adjust the medication as the child grows.
• Administer medications as ordered.
• Offer support and encouragement to the parents.

Too high, too low

• After initiation of treatment for infantile hypothyroidism, monitor blood pressure and pulse rate, and report hypertension and tachycardia immediately. (Normal infant heart rate is approximately 120 beats/minute.) These signs as well as fever, irritability, and sweating indicate that the dose of TH replacement medication is too high.
• Teach the parents to look for signs and symptoms of inadequate treatment (a dose that's too low), including fatigue, lethargy, decreased appetite, and constipation.

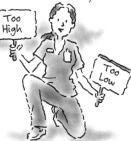

Heed the signs! Parents—and nurses—need to know when the TH replacement dosage is too high or too low.

Plan ahead

• Adolescent girls require future-oriented counseling that stresses the importance of adequate TH replacement during pregnancy.
• If the infant's tongue is unusually large, position him on his side and observe him frequently to prevent airway obstruction.

Don't delay

If treatment is delayed and signs and symptoms develop:
• Help the child and his parents develop effective coping skills.
• Provide meticulous skin and mucous membrane care.
• Check rectal temperature every 2 to 4 hours; keep the patient warm, as needed.

Cushing's syndrome

Cushing's syndrome is a disorder of adrenal hyperfunction. It results from excessive levels of adrenocortical hormones (particularly cortisol) or related corticosteroids and, to a lesser extent, androgens and aldosterone. Cushing's syndrome is most common in females.

Prognosis depends on the underlying cause. The prognosis is poor without treatment and in children with untreatable, ectopic corticotropin-secreting carcinoma or metastatic adrenal carcinoma.

What causes it

Adrenal hyperfunction can be caused by:
- pituitary hypersecretion of corticotropin (Cushing's disease)
- corticotropin-secreting tumor in another organ
- administration of excessive or prolonged synthetic glucocorticoids (most common cause in children)
- adrenal tumor.

How it happens

A loss of normal feedback inhibition by cortisol occurs in Cushing's syndrome. Elevated levels of cortisol don't suppress hypothalamic and anterior pituitary secretion of corticotropin-releasing hormone and corticotropin. The result is excessive levels of circulating cortisol.

What to look for

The unmistakable signs of Cushing's syndrome include adiposity of the face (moon face), neck, and trunk and reddish purple striae on the skin (especially the abdomen). In addition, a child with some or all of the following signs may have Cushing's syndrome:
- weight gain
- muscle weakness
- fatigue
- irritability and emotional instability
- sleep disturbances
- water retention
- amenorrhea
- thin hair and thin, fragile skin (ruddy complexion)
- thinning extremities with muscle wasting and fat mobilization
- bruising, petechiae, and ecchymoses
- delayed wound healing
- buffalo hump
- hirsutism
- truncal obesity.

What tests tell you

A low-dose (overnight) dexamethasone suppression test, elevated 24-hour urine free cortisol levels, and high nighttime cortisol levels (indicating the absence of circadian rhythm) confirm the diagnosis of Cushing's syndrome. The cause can be determined with a plasma corticotropin test and a high-dose dexamethasone suppression test.

Stealth corticotropin

With an adrenal tumor, corticotropin levels aren't detectable and steroid levels aren't suppressed. Ectopic corticotropin syndrome shows elevated corticotropin or unsuppressed steroid levels. Normal to elevated corticotropin with steroid suppressed to less than 50% of baseline indicates Cushing's disease.

Ultrasonography, computed tomography (CT) scanning, or angiography localizes adrenal tumors. CT scanning or magnetic resonance imaging of the head helps localize pituitary tumors.

Complications

Complications of Cushing's syndrome include:
- osteoporosis and pathologic fractures
- peptic ulcer
- impaired glucose tolerance
- frequent infections
- dyslipidemia
- diabetes mellitus
- slow wound healing
- psychiatric problems ranging from mood swings to frank psychosis
- suppressed inflammatory response
- hypertension
- ischemic heart disease, heart failure
- menstrual disturbances.

How it's treated

Radiation, drug therapy, or surgery may be necessary to restore hormone balance and reverse the effects of Cushing's syndrome.

Cushing's combo

These management approaches may be used in combination:
- Drug therapy may include antifungal agents, antihypertensives, diuretics, glucocorticoids, potassium supplements, antineoplastic, or antihormone agents.
- An adrenal tumor is treated with bilateral adrenalectomy.
- Nonendocrine corticotropin-secreting tumors require excision.
- Hypophysectomy may be needed.

Preop prep

Before surgery, the child with cushingoid signs and symptoms needs special management to control hypertension, edema, diabetes, and cardiovascular manifestations and prevent infection.

Glucocorticoid administration on the morning of surgery can help prevent acute adrenal insufficiency during surgery.

What to do

Children with Cushing's syndrome require painstaking assessment and supportive care:
- Frequently monitor vital signs, especially blood pressure; carefully observe the hypertensive child who also has cardiac disease.
- Check laboratory reports for hypernatremia, hypokalemia, hyperglycemia, and glycosuria.

What goes in might not come out!

- Check for edema and carefully monitor daily weight and intake and output; the cushingoid child is likely to retain sodium and water.
- To minimize weight gain, edema, and hypertension, ask the dietitian to provide a diet high in protein and potassium but low in calories, carbohydrates, and sodium.

Infection prevention

- Use protective measures to prevent infection (a significant problem in Cushing's syndrome).
- Carefully perform passive range-of-motion exercises for children who have osteoporosis and are bedridden.

Postoperative care

After hypophysectomy using the transsphenoidal approach:
- Keep the head of the bed elevated at least 30 degrees.
- Maintain nasal packing.
- Provide frequent mouth care.
- Avoid activities that increase intracranial pressure (ICP).
- Monitor for cerebral fluid leaks.
   After bilateral adrenalectomy or hypophysectomy, assess the child for:
- changes in neurologic and behavioral status
- severe nausea, vomiting, and diarrhea
- bowel sounds
- adrenal hypofunction
- increased ICP
- transient diabetes insipidus
- hemorrhage
- shock.

Diabetes mellitus

Diabetes mellitus is a chronic disease of absolute or relative insulin deficiency or resistance.

Absolutely insufficient

Type 1 diabetes mellitus (characterized by absolute insulin insufficiency) is the most common childhood endocrine disorder. No longer rare, the incidence of type 2 diabetes mellitus in childhood is rising dramatically because of the increase in childhood obesity and sedentary lifestyles. Obesity induces resistance to insulin-mediated peripheral glucose uptake. It's characterized by insulin resistance with varying degrees of insulin secretory defects.

Diabetes mellitus (types 1 and 2) can occur at any age, but type 1 has a peak incidence at ages 10 to 15 years.

What causes it

Diabetes mellitus is caused by genetic factors and autoimmune factors (type 1) and may also develop as a result of a viral infection.

Genetic factors

Type 1 isn't inherited, but predisposition plays a part in its development. Type 2 diabetes has strong polygenic (caused by several genes) familial susceptibility.

Blame it on dad

Children born to fathers who have type 1 are about three times more likely to develop diabetes mellitus than children born to mothers with type 1.

Autoimmune factors

About 70% to 85% of newly diagnosed type 1 diabetes mellitus patients are found to have pancreatic islet cell antibodies.

Straggler antibodies

These antibodies disappear in most people after diagnosis. It's thought that the presence of these antibodies makes the immune system vulnerable to a trigger event, such as a virus, bacteria, or chemical irritant.

Viral infection

Several viruses, including coxsackie B, mumps, and congenital rubella, have been associated with the development of type 1 diabetes mellitus.

Vulnerable to viruses

The pancreatic islet cells are susceptible to injury by these viruses and can suffer damage or be changed. This alteration triggers an autoimmune response. The virus becomes a trigger to the development of type 1 diabetes mellitus.

Don't hate me because I'm a virus. Injuring islet cells and triggering type 1 diabetes is my job—it's what I do.

How it happens

Diabetes mellitus is characterized by disturbances in carbohydrate, protein, and fat metabolism. Insulin allows glucose transport into the cells for use as energy or storage as glycogen.

Free the fatty acids!

Insulin stimulates protein synthesis and free fatty acid storage in adipose tissues. Deficiency of insulin or insulin resistance and secretory defects compromise the body tissues' access to essential nutrients for fuel and storage.

What to look for

The three cardinal signs of diabetes mellitus are polyuria, polydipsia, and polyphagia. Other general signs and symptoms may include:
• weakness and fatigue
• nocturia in a child who has already attained nighttime control
• dehydration (dry mucous membranes and poor skin turgor)
• weight loss and hunger
• vision changes (retinopathy or cataract formation)
• frequent skin and urinary tract infections
• skin changes (cool temperature and dry, itchy skin, especially on the hands and feet).

Type 1 in a hurry

A child with type 1 diabetes mellitus will have rapidly developing symptoms, muscle wasting, and loss of subcutaneous fat. A child with type 2 diabetes will have more subtle symptoms of polyuria, polydipsia, polyphagia, weight loss, weakness, fatigue, and frequent infections developing over time.

The pancreas' last stand

A onetime remission of symptoms may occur shortly after insulin treatment is started. It's a last-ditch effort by the pancreas to produce insulin. The child may not need insulin for up to 1 year but may need oral antidiabetic drugs. Symptoms of hyperglycemia will reappear, and the child with type 1 diabetes will be insulin-dependent for life.

Vaguely type 2

In children with type 2 diabetes mellitus, vague, long-standing symptoms develop gradually. These include:
• severe viral infection
• other endocrine diseases
• recent stress or trauma
• use of drugs that increase blood glucose levels
• obesity, particularly in the abdominal area.

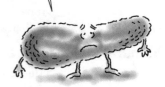

Even in the face of diabetes mellitus, I respond to therapy by making insulin one last time. It's my insulin swan song.

What tests tell you

Two fasting plasma glucose tests above 126 mg/dl or, with normal fasting glucose, two blood glucose levels above 200 mg/dl during a 2-hour glucose tolerance test confirm the diagnosis. Other findings include:
- two-hour postprandial blood glucose level greater than 200 mg/dl
- increased glycosylated hemoglobin level
- urinalysis that may show acetone or glucose
- diabetic retinopathy, which may be revealed by an ophthalmic examination.

Complications

Diabetic ketoacidosis (DKA) and hypoglycemia may occur as well as hyperosmolar hyperglycemic nonketotic syndrome (HHNS). Long-term complications of diabetes mellitus are nephropathy, retinopathy, and neuropathy.

If the diabetes isn't well controlled, complications can occur as early as 2 to 3 years after diagnosis. Therefore, good control and regimen compliance are necessary to postpone or prevent complications.

How it's treated

Treating the child with diabetes mellitus takes a multidisciplinary approach.

Team diabetes

The child, parents, and health care professionals (including an endocrinologist, nutritionist, and a diabetes nurse educator) should all be involved in the treatment plan. It may also be necessary for a mental health professional to be included because the treatment plan can have an impact on the child's emotional and psychological health.

Meal planning, exercise, and, sometimes, insulin or oral antidiabetic agents are prescribed to normalize carbohydrate, fat, and protein metabolism and avert long-term complications while preventing hypoglycemia.

Type 1 diabetes

Patients with type 1 diabetes must take insulin daily because of their absolute insulin deficiency. The insulin need changes and is affected by emotions, nutritional intake, activity, illness, and events such as puberty. (See *Insulin injection sites in children,* page 538.)

Insulin dosages are based on home blood glucose monitoring. Insulin can be administered as one or two injections per day or by insulin pump (continuous S.C. administration).

It's all relative

Insulin injection sites in children

Use this illustration to instruct the child and his parents about the injections sites for insulin administration that are recommended by the American Diabetes Association.

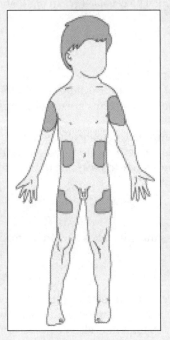 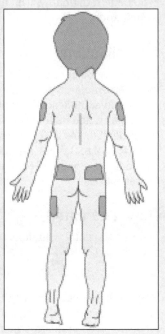

Type 2 diabetes

Patients with type 2 diabetes may require insulin to control blood glucose levels unresponsive to diet and oral antidiabetic agents, or during periods of acute stress. Patients with other types of diabetes commonly require daily insulin therapy to achieve blood glucose control. (See *Insulin therapy*.) The first-line medication used is metformin because of its effects on weight loss and insulin resistance.

What to do

The child with diabetes may be facing lifelong treatment and restrictions for a chronic disease, with the prospect of setbacks (until control is established) and serious complications. The child

Insulin therapy

Insulin is administered as prescribed. There are several routes of administration and devices for injection.

Subcutaneous route

Insulin is usually given by subcutaneous (S.C.) injection with a standard insulin syringe. S.C. insulin can also be given with a penlike injection device that uses a disposable needle and replaceable insulin cartridges, eliminating the need to draw insulin into a syringe.

Jet-propelled

Jet-injection devices are expensive and require special cleaning procedures, but they disperse insulin more rapidly and speed absorption. These devices draw up insulin from standard containers, which enable the patient to mix insulins, if necessary, but require a special procedure for drawing it up. After the insulin is drawn up, it's delivered into the S.C. tissue with a pressure jet.

Pump it up!

Multiple-dose regimens may use an insulin pump to deliver insulin continuously into S.C. tissue. The infusion rate selector automatically releases about half of the total daily insulin requirement evenly over 24 hours. The patient releases the remainder in bolus amounts before meals and snacks.

Ready, set, rotate!

When administering insulin injections S.C., the injection sites should be rotated. Because absorption rates differ at each site, rotating the injection site within a specific area such as the abdomen is recommended.

I.V. and I.M. routes

Regular insulin or insulin lispro may also be administered intramuscularly (I.M.) or I.V. during severe episodes of hyperglycemia. These are the only types of insulin that should ever be administered by these routes.

Investigational routes

Researchers are working on newer, more efficient ways of administering insulin. Two newer methods of insulin administration are the intranasal delivery method and the programmable implantable medication system (PIMS). Both methods are still experimental.

Up your nose with an aerosol

Intranasal administration uses aerosolized insulin combined with a surfactant; it's administered as a nasal spray. Because nasal solutions are less potent than S.C. insulin, dosages are higher.

Batteries included

Now undergoing clinical trials, the PIMS has an implantable infusion pump unit that holds and delivers the insulin, and a delivery catheter that feeds insulin directly into the peritoneal cavity.

The pump, encased in a titanium shell, contains a tiny computer to regulate dosages and runs on a battery with a 5-year life span. The patient uses a handheld external radio transmitter to control insulin release. Because the PIMS has no built-in blood glucose sensor, the patient must monitor his glucose levels several times per day.

and his parents will need a great deal of ongoing support and assistance.

Rebel with restrictions

As the child grows, compliance may become an issue. A child or adolescent may simply become overwhelmed or tired of taking medication and adhering to dietary restrictions. These feelings should be recognized as normal. Referral to a support group will help the child and his parents cope with the diagnosis and its implications.

In addition, follow these steps:
• Emphasize that adherence to the treatment plan is essential; it's crucial to bring the child's blood glucose level within an acceptable range (usually 80 to 120 mg/dl) and alleviate or prevent DKA or hypoglycemia.
• For the child with unstable diabetes who isn't experiencing DKA or HHNS, monitor blood glucose levels several times each day as prescribed until they stabilize.

Like a hawk!

• Monitor the child closely for signs and symptoms of DKA or HHNS. Suspect DKA or HHNS if the child exhibits Kussmaul's respirations, develops a fruity odor to his breath, and shows signs and symptoms of severe dehydration. Notify the doctor immediately if these indications are evident.
• If the child has DKA or HHNS, treatment may include fluid and electrolyte replacement, increased insulin therapy, and therapy to reduce acidosis. Administer doses of I.V. insulin as prescribed. (Monitor blood glucose levels frequently during insulin infusion.)
• Monitor the child closely for signs and symptoms of hyperglycemia and hypoglycemia (caused by an excessively rapid reduction in blood glucose level). Teach these signs and symptoms to the child and his parents and provide specific instructions on how to handle each condition. (See *Hypo or hyper?*)
• Make sure the child and his parents understand that he should base his meal plan on a balanced diet that incorporates the six basic food groups.

Fitting in

• Concentrated sweets are discouraged, so teach the child and his parents about alternate snack ideas to help him feel more like his peers. (See *Diabetes mellitus teaching tips.*)

Show and tell

• Demonstrate to the child how to check his blood glucose; it's especially necessary for the child on a tightly controlled regimen.

Galactosemia

Galactosemia is an inborn error of carbohydrate metabolism and is a rare disorder. Neonate screening for the disorder is required in most states.

What causes it

Galactosemia is inherited as an autosomal-recessive trait. It appears in approximately 1 of every 50,000 births.

Hypo or hyper?

It's generally difficult to distinguish between hypoglycemia and hyperglycemia.

Too little . . .
Hypoglycemia symptoms include:
• lethargy
• hunger
• sweating
• pallor
• seizures
• coma.

. . . too much
Hyperglycemia symptoms include:
• sweet, fruity breath (acetone)
• dehydration
• decreased sodium, potassium, bicarbonate, chloride, and phosphate levels
• vomiting
• abdominal pain
• coma.

Diabetes mellitus teaching tips

Long-term management of diabetes mellitus requires extensive patient—and parent—education:
• Review the prescribed meal plan and teach the child (and his family) how to adjust his diet when engaged in extra activity.
• Advise the child and his parents about aerobic exercise programs; explain how exercise affects blood glucose levels, and provide safety guidelines.
• Instruct the child on insulin administration, if prescribed, including type, peak times, dosage, drawing up the insulin, mixing (if applicable), administration technique, site rotation, sharps disposal, and storage.
• Teach the child (and his parents) how to perform blood glucose monitoring.
• Instruct the child on oral antidiabetic therapy, if prescribed, including dosage, frequency and time of administration, and potential adverse reactions.
• Tell the child and his parents about the Internet as a source of information and about the American Diabetes Association Web site (www.diabetes.org). This site offers accurate information for the child with diabetes, his family, and health care professionals, along with general information about diabetes (advice on exercise, nutrition, and daily meal planning).

How it happens

In galactosemia, the hepatic enzyme GALT is absent. This enzyme is one of three needed to metabolize galactose to glucose. Without GALT, galactose accumulates in the blood, which leads to hepatic dysfunction, cirrhosis, and subsequent jaundice. The jaundice is noticeable during the first few weeks of life. Portal hypertension occurs as the spleen becomes involved.

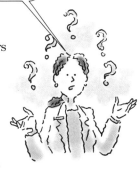

In children with galactosemia, GALT is MIA.

What to look for

Infants with the disorder appear normal at birth. Soon after ingesting milk, which is high in lactose, they begin to vomit and lose weight. Galactosemia is not related to and should not be confused with lactose intolerance. Findings include:
• lethargy
• hypotonia
• diarrhea
• vomiting
• jaundice
• development of bilateral cataracts.

What tests tell you

Genetic screening is positive for the disorder. Galactose levels are increased in the blood and urine (galactosuria), and levels of GALT activity in erythrocytes are decreased or absent.

Complications

Complications of galactosemia include ovarian dysfunction, cataracts, abnormal speech, cognitive impairment, motor delay, and growth retardation.

How it's treated

The disorder is treated by eliminating dietary galactose (generally available as lactose), including breast milk. Lactose-free or soy protein formulas are recommended and, as the child grows, a balanced, galactose-free diet must be maintained. (See *Diet for galactosemia*.)

What to do

Nursing care focuses on education:
• Teach the child and parents about the disorder and provide emotional support and counseling; psychological and emotional problems may result from the difficult dietary restrictions.
• Teach the child and parents about the critical importance of adhering to the diet.
• Teach the parents about normal physical and mental growth and development to help them recognize developmental delay.
• Help the mother deal with feelings of loss, and even guilt, which may result from the inability to breast-feed.

Graves' disease

Graves' disease, also called *hyperthyroidism* in childhood, is associated with exophthalmos and an enlarged thyroid gland. Most cases occur in children between ages 6 and 15 years. The disease may be present in infants whose mothers were thyrotoxic during pregnancy.

What causes it

Graves' disease is caused by an autoimmune response to TSH receptors. However, no specific etiology has been identified. There also seems to be a familial predisposition for the disease.

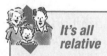

It's all relative

Diet for galactosemia

A patient with galactosemia must follow a lactose-free diet.

Diet do's
• Fish and animal products (except brains and mussels)
• Fresh fruits and vegetables (except peas and lima beans)
• Breads and rolls made from cracked wheat

Diet don'ts
• Dairy products
• Puddings, cookies, cakes, pies
• Food coloring
• Instant potatoes
• Canned and frozen foods (if lactose is listed as an ingredient)

How it happens

In Graves' disease, T_4 production is increased and the thyroid gland is enlarged (called a *goiter*). It's characterized by autoantibodies that attach to and then stimulate TSH receptors on the thyroid gland.

Stimulation overload

A goiter may be the result of increased stimulation of the thyroid gland or a response to increased metabolic demand. The latter occurs in iodine-deficient areas of the world, where the incidence of goiter increases during puberty (a time of increased metabolic demand). These goiters commonly regress to normal size after puberty in males but not in females.

What to look for

Symptoms of Graves' disease begin gradually and develop on and off during a period of 6 to 12 months. Irritability and excessive motion are the most prominent symptoms. The child may also exhibit:
- hyperactivity
- short attention span
- insomnia
- tremors
- weight loss despite a tremendous appetite
- rapid, pounding pulse (even during sleep)
- skin warm and flushed
- widened pulse pressure
- cardiomegaly
- exophthalmos.

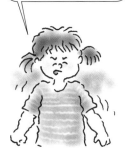

Just because I'm irritable and can't sit still, my parents think I have a behavioral problem! They don't realize these behaviors can be symptoms of Graves' disease.

What tests tell you
- A thyroid scan reveals increased ^{131}I uptake.
- Immunometric assay shows suppressed sensitivity of TSH levels.
- Orbital sonography and CT scans show subclinical ophthalmopathy.
- Radioimmunoassay testing shows elevated T_4 levels.

Complications

Complications of Graves' disease include muscle wasting, atrophy, and paralysis; vision loss or diplopia; and heart failure or cardiac arrhythmias.

How it's treated

Graves' disease is treated with antithyroid medications, such as propylthiouracil (PTU) and methimazole (Tapazole), to suppress the formation of T_4. Hypermetabolic symptoms will subside 4 to 8 weeks after therapy begins, but remission of Grave's disease requires continued therapy for 6 months to 2 years. The child must be monitored closely for signs of leukopenia and thrombocytopenia. If these conditions occur, the medication is discontinued until the counts return to normal levels.

Ablation to the rescue

If the child is unable or unwilling to comply with the medication regimen or if he has a toxic reaction to the medication, ablation therapy with ^{131}I is used to reduce the size of the thyroid gland.

When in doubt, take it out

Surgical removal of all or most of the thyroid may be necessary in the young adult. After ablation or surgical removal of the thyroid, the child must remain on lifelong thyroid replacement therapy.

What to do

Explain the disorder to the child and his parents and prepare the child for all treatments and procedures:
• Teach the parents of a child being treated with antithyroid drugs or radioisotope therapy to identify and report symptoms of hypothyroidism.

Keep it cool

• Encourage a cool, quiet environment that's conducive to rest until there's a response to drug therapy; restrict physical activity.
• Advise the child with exophthalmos or other ophthalmopathy to wear sunglasses or eye patches to protect the eyes from light; moisten the conjunctiva frequently with isotonic eyedrops.
• To meet the child's increased metabolic demand, provide a balanced diet with six meals per day.

Cough with caution

• Tell the child who has had ^{131}I therapy not to expectorate or cough freely because his saliva is radioactive for 24 hours; stress the need for repeated measurement of serum T_4 levels and reassure the child and his parents (who may be frightened by the term "radioactive").
• Instruct the child taking PTU or methimazole (and his parents) to take these drugs with meals to minimize gastrointestinal (GI) distress and to avoid over-the-counter cough preparations because many contain iodine.
• Stress the importance of regular medical follow-up visits after discharge because hypothyroidism may develop 2 to 4 weeks postoperatively and after ^{131}I therapy.

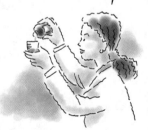

Some over-the-counter products contain iodine. Teach parents to be label-readers and, when in doubt, to ask the pharmacist.

Long-term commitment

- Explain that the child will need lifelong TH replacement. (Encourage him to wear medical identification and to carry his medication with him at all times.)

Maple syrup urine disease

An inborn error of metabolism, MSUD is a rare disorder in which there's a defect in the amino acid metabolism of leucine, isoleucine, and valine. This defect leads to cerebral degeneration.

How sweet it isn't

MSUD derives its name from the sweet, burnt sugar, or maple syrup smell of the urine.

What causes it

MSUD is inherited as an autosomal-recessive trait.

How it happens

In MSUD, the enzymes necessary to break down the branched-chain amino acids (BCAAs) leucine, isoleucine, and valine are either absent, inactive, or only partially active.

Origin of the odor

Because of the enzyme deficiency in MSUD, levels of BCAAs and their by-products, called *ketoacids*, become elevated. These elevations, particularly the elevation in leucine, cause neurologic symptoms. The elevation of plasma isoleucine and ketoacidosis is associated with the maple syrup odor.

> Elevated plasma isoleucine and ketoacidosis cause the maple syrup odor in MSUD.

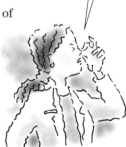

What to look for

Assessment findings of MSUD may be evident within 2 weeks of birth. Findings may include:
- urine with the odor of maple syrup
- feeding difficulties
- absence of Moro's reflex
- irregular respirations
- seizures.

What tests tell you

Genetic screening is positive for the disorder. Amino acid levels in urine and blood will be elevated, and blood gases will show acidosis.

Complications

If not treated, MSUD can lead to mental retardation and death. Early treatment can prevent retardation.

How it's treated

BCAAs, such as leucine, isoleucine, and valine, are restricted. The child is given a diet that's high in thiamine. If necessary, peritoneal dialysis, hemodialysis, or both may be performed.

What to do

The family should be referred to a nutritionist who can teach them about the foods to restrict and encourage. In addition, follow these steps:

• Test urine and blood after the first 24 hours of feeding.
• Check diapers for color, amount, and odor of urine.
• For neonates discharged within 24 hours of birth, ensure home visits by a nurse to obtain blood samples for testing; facilitate rapid test results and refer the parents to the pediatrician if test results are abnormal.
• Stress to the parents the importance of the restricted diet and provide support as necessary.
• Encourage the parents to bring the child for needed follow-up care; frequent appointments are necessary for blood work and to maintain balanced amino acid levels.

Phenylketonuria

PKU is an inborn error in amino acid (specifically phenylalanine) metabolism. It results in high serum levels of phenylalanine, increased urine concentrations of phenylalanine and its by-products, cerebral damage, and mental retardation.

An error by any other name

PKU is also called *phenylalaninemia* and *phenylpyruvic oligophrenia*. The disorder occurs in 1 of approximately 14,000 births in the United States. About 1 person in 60 is an asymptomatic carrier.

The case for early detection

Although blood phenylalanine levels approach normal at birth, they begin to increase within a few days. By the time they reach significant levels (about 30 mg/dl), cerebral damage has begun. Such irreversible damage is probably complete by age 2 or 3 years. Early detection and treatment can minimize cerebral damage.

What causes it

PKU is transmitted through an autosomal-recessive gene.

How it happens

In PKU, an almost totally deficient activity of phenylalanine hydroxylase, an enzyme that acts as a catalyst in the conversion of phenylalanine to tyrosine, results in phenylalanine accumulation in the blood and urine. This accumulation leads to brain damage and mental retardation.

What to look for

The patient may have a family history of PKU. Typically, the history reveals no apparent abnormalities at birth.

Brain on hold

By age 4 months, the untreated child begins to show signs of arrested brain development, including mental retardation and, later, personality disturbances (schizoid and antisocial personality patterns and uncontrollable temper). About one-third of patients have a history of seizures, which usually begin between ages 6 and 12 months. Many patients also show a precipitous decrease in IQ in their first year.

Got the blues?

On inspection, the patient typically has a lighter complexion than unaffected siblings and may have blue eyes. He may also exhibit macrocephaly, eczematous skin lesions, or dry, rough skin.

Hyper, irritable, and repetitive

The child is usually hyperactive and irritable. He exhibits purposeless, repetitive motions, and has an awkward gait. A musty odor from the skin and urinary excretion of phenylacetic acid may also be noted.

In most states, the Guthrie screening test for PKU detection is mandatory in neonates. No studying is required!

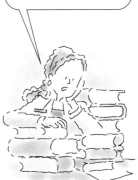

What tests tell you

Most states require screening for PKU at birth; the Guthrie screening test on a capillary blood sample (bacterial inhibition assay) is a reliable indicator of the disorder. Because phenylalanine levels may be normal at birth, the infant should be evaluated after he starts protein feedings; in the infant with PKU, levels are usually abnormally high by day 4. More quantitative fluorometric or chromatographic assays provide additional diagnostic information.

Complications

Phenylalanine accumulation causes mental retardation.

How it's treated

To prevent or minimize brain damage, phenylalanine blood levels are kept between 3 mg/dl and 9 mg/dl by restricting dietary intake of the amino acid phenylalanine.

The lowdown on phenylalanine

During the first month of life, a special, low-phenylalanine amino acid mixture is substituted for most of the protein in the diet, supplemented with a small amount of natural foods. An enzymatic hydrolysate of casein, such as Lofenalac powder or Pregestimil powder, is substituted for milk in the diets of affected infants. Dietary restrictions are required throughout life.

Don't overdo it!

Such a diet calls for close monitoring. The body doesn't make phenylalanine, so overzealous dietary restriction can induce phenylalanine deficiency, causing lethargy, anorexia, anemia, skin rashes, and diarrhea.

What to do

Teach the parents about PKU, and provide emotional support and counseling. Psychological and emotional problems may result from the difficult dietary restrictions. In addition, follow these steps:

• If the child is experiencing seizures or has some mental dysfunction, implement safety measures to prevent injury; refer the parents and child to appropriate community resources.

Just say "no" to chicken and cheese

• Teach the child and his parents about the critical importance of adhering to his diet; the child must avoid breads, cheese, eggs, flour, meat, poultry, fish, nuts, milk, legumes, and aspartame (NutraSweet). Also, the child will need frequent tests for urine phenylpyruvic acid and blood phenylalanine levels to evaluate the effectiveness of the diet.

• Refer the family to a nutritionist.

• Teach the parents about normal physical and mental growth and development to help them recognize developmental delay from excessive phenylalanine intake.

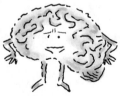

Dietary phenylalanine restriction is the best way to protect me in a child with PKU.

Rebel with a cause

As the child grows older and is supervised less closely, his parents have less control over what he eats. As a result, deviation from the restricted diet becomes more likely, which increases the risk of further brain damage. Encourage the parents to allow the child some choices in the kinds of low-protein foods he eats to help make him feel trusted and more responsible, which will encourage compliance.

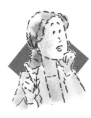

Quick quiz

1. The purpose of the endocrine system is to:
   A. deliver nutrients to the body's cells.
   B. regulate and integrate the body's metabolic activities.
   C. eliminate waste products from the body.
   D. stimulate secondary sex characteristics.

   Answer: B. Along with the nervous system, the endocrine system regulates and integrates the body's metabolic activities.

2. The nurse draws blood from the heel of an infant for a Guthrie screening test. This test is used to diagnose which inborn error of metabolism?
   A. Absence of GALT
   B. PKU
   C. Galactosemia
   D. Hypothyroidism

   Answer: B. The Guthrie screening test is a bacterial inhibition assay used to diagnose PKU. *B. subtilis*, present in the culture medium, grows if the blood contains an excessive amount of phenylalanine.

3. The gland that produces glucagon is the:
   A. pancreas.
   B. thymus.
   C. adrenal.
   D. pituitary.

   Answer: A. The alpha cells of the pancreas produce glucagon, a hormone that raises the blood glucose level by triggering the breakdown of glycogen to glucose.

4. An infant with congenital hypothyroidism shows which sign or symptom?
  A. Shrill cry
  B. Diaphoresis
  C. Hypothermia
  D. Diarrhea

Answer: C. Hypothermia is one common finding in congenital hypothyroidism. Other common findings include lethargy, poor feeding, prolonged jaundice, vomiting, constipation, mottling, coarse facial features, hoarse cry, large fontanels, and hypotonia.

5. Which food shouldn't be eaten by a child with galactosemia?
  A. Instant potatoes
  B. Chicken
  C. Whole wheat bread
  D. Apples

Answer: A. The child with galactosemia must follow a lactose-free diet. Appropriate foods for his diet include fish and chicken, fresh fruits and vegetables (except for lima beans), and bread made from whole wheat. The child should avoid dairy products and other lactose-containing foods such as instant potatoes.

Scoring

☆☆☆ If you answered all five items correctly, astonishing! Your brain cells must be on steroids!

☆☆ If you answered three or four items correctly, wow! You've just won a trip to the islets of Langerhans! Bon voyage!

☆ If you answered fewer than three items correctly, don't moan over these hormones! Two more quick quizzes are ahead.

14

Hematologic and immunologic problems

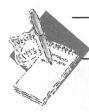

Just the facts

In this chapter, you'll learn:

♦ anatomy and physiology of the hematologic and immune systems

♦ normal function of blood cells and the role of genetics in the hematologic and immune systems

♦ tests used to diagnose hematologic and immunologic problems

♦ treatments and procedures for children with hematologic and immunologic problems

♦ hematologic and immunologic disorders that affect children.

Anatomy and physiology

The hematologic and immune systems are separate but interrelated. They help the body fight infection or invaders through different mechanisms but usually work together for the same goal. Both systems essentially arise from an organ known as *bone marrow* which, although housed within the bones, has little relationship to the skeletal system.

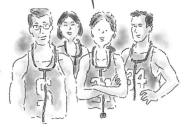

The hematologic and immune systems work as a team to reach the same goal!

Hematologic system

Bone marrow contains the essential element in the hematologic system: the stem cell. The stem cell is sometimes referred to as the *pluripotential stem cell*, meaning it has the ability to transform into more than one type of blood cell. Every blood cell in the body arises from a stem cell.

Did you say organ system?

Although it's a fluid, blood is one of the body's major organ systems. It continually circulates through the heart and blood vessels, carrying vital elements to every part of the body.

Blood formation

> A mother's work is never done! It's from me that new cells are created for all three main blood cell types.

Early in utero, the process of blood formation, called *hematopoiesis*, occurs in the liver and spleen. These organs retain some hematopoietic ability throughout life. After birth, the red bone marrow becomes the main site of hematopoiesis.

Yellow with age

In infants and young children, all bones contain red bone marrow (red from the production of red blood cells [RBCs]) and are, therefore, capable of hematopoiesis. However, as the child approaches adolescence and bone growth ceases, the bone marrow in many bones can't form blood cells because the marrow has transformed to yellow bone marrow (yellow from fat deposits), although it can usually revert to red bone marrow during times of increased blood cell demand. Only the ribs, sternum, vertebrae, and pelvis continue to contain red bone marrow and produce blood cells.

Have a blast

The stem cells contained in the red bone marrow create primitive blood cells called *blast cells*. Blast cells are the least mature form of blood cell and are the precursors to RBCs, white blood cells (WBCs), and platelets. These cells are normal and shouldn't be confused with the blast cells seen in leukemia and other cancers.

Like a fine wine

These blast cells then stay in the bone marrow to mature. The maturation of blood cells, called *differentiation*, occurs in stages; thus, in normal bone marrow, you can see different forms of all the blood cell lines. (See *Human blood cell development*.) Mature blood cells travel by blood throughout the body to perform specific functions.

Blood components

Blood is composed of plasma and cells. Plasma is the fluid portion of the blood. It's 90% water and 10% solutes, such as proteins, electrolytes, albumin, clotting factors, anticoagulants, antibodies,

Human blood cell development

All blood cell types originate from the same stem cell. The chart below shows how this stem cell becomes differentiated, developing into each blood cell type.

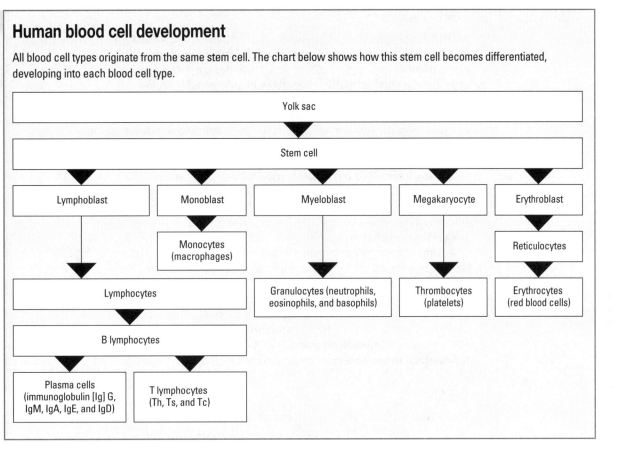

and dissolved nutrients. The three main cell types in the blood originate from blast cells and include:

 RBCs, or *erythrocytes*

 WBCs, or *leukocytes*

 platelets, or *thrombocytes*.

RBCs

In addition to the bone marrow, some RBCs are stored in the liver or spleen. RBCs carry oxygen to the tissues and carry carbon dioxide away from tissues. When tissue is low on oxygen (hypoxia), a hormone from the kidneys called *erythropoietin* stimulates the bone marrow to produce more RBCs. Synthetic forms of erythropoietin are now used to stimulate RBC production in premature neonates and patients receiving chemotherapy to help them maintain higher blood cell levels.

The cycle of life—RBC style

An RBC's life span is approximately 120 days, and an important waste product of RBC death is bilirubin. Bilirubin binds with albumin for transport to the liver cells to conjugate with glucuronide, forming direct bilirubin. Because unconjugated bilirubin is fat-soluble and can't be excreted in urine or bile, it may escape to extravascular tissue, especially fatty tissue and the brain, resulting in hyperbilirubinemia and skin that appears icteric (or jaundiced). Too much bilirubin may result in brain damage—a condition known as kernicterus. In newborns, the normal range of bilirubin levels are determined by the baby's age in hours. For instance, an infant who is 48 hours old will have a different range of acceptable levels than does an infant who is 96 hours old. Other things that may place a newborn at risk for hyperbilirubinemia are being born premature, having a sibling who has had hyperbilirubinemia, or having a blood group incompatibility with the mother (such as the mother having an O+ blood type and the baby having an A+ blood type).

Oxygen is carried in the cell in a protein (globin) and iron (heme) structure known as *hemoglobin*. If adequate amounts of iron aren't available, the protein structure can't be formed and RBCs can't carry their normal amount of oxygen. Lead can also replace iron in the molecule, causing toxicity.

WBCs

WBCs fight different types of infection that occur in or on the body; each type of WBC has its own role in fighting infection. The two main categories of WBCs are granular leukocytes (granulocytes) and nongranular leukocytes (agranulocytes). (See *Two types of leukocytes*.)

Great granulocytes, Batman!

Granulocytes include:
• *neutrophils*, which help devour invading microorganisms, such as bacteria, by phagocytosis
• *eosinophils*, which act in allergic reactions and may defend against large parasites and lung and skin infections
• *basophils*, which release heparin and histamine, are involved in inflammatory and infectious reactions, and are known as *mast cells* when they exist in body tissues.

Not a granule to be found

Agranulocytes include:
• *lymphocytes*, which are the main cells that fight infections and include natural killer (NK) cells, B cells, and T cells

Two types of leukocytes

Leukocytes vary in size, shape, and number and are characterized as granular and nongranular.

Granular

Granular leukocytes (granulocytes) are the most numerous. They include:
- *basophils*, which contain cytoplasmic granules that stain readily with alkaline dyes
- *neutrophils*, which are finely granular and recognizable by their multinucleated appearance
- *eosinophils*, which stain with acidic dyes.

Nongranular

Nongranular leukocytes have few, if any, granulated particles in the cytoplasm. They include:
- lymphocytes
- monocytes.

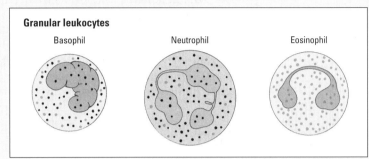

Granular leukocytes

Basophil   Neutrophil   Eosinophil

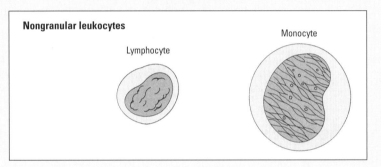

Nongranular leukocytes

Lymphocyte   Monocyte

- *monocytes*, which, along with neutrophils, help devour invading microorganisms by phagocytosis and also form macrophages in the body tissues.

Platelets

Platelets adhere to one another and plug holes in vessels or tissues where there's bleeding. This action is part of a larger coagulation (clotting) process. Platelets also release serotonin at injury sites. Serotonin, a vasoconstrictor, decreases blood flow to the injured area. Nonsteroidal anti-inflammatory drugs (NSAIDs) such as aspirin, ibuprofen, and naproxen may affect platelet aggregation.

Hemostasis

Hemostasis is a complex process by which the body controls bleeding. When a blood vessel ruptures, local vasoconstriction and platelet clumping (aggregation) at the injury site initially help prevent hemorrhaging.

Like a waterfall

Activation of the coagulation system, called the *extrinsic cascade*, involves the release of thromboplastin from the damaged tissue cells. However, formation of a more stable clot requires initiation of the complex clotting mechanism known as the *intrinsic cascade system*.

When endothelial vessel injury or a foreign body in the bloodstream activates the intrinsic cascade, activating factor XII triggers clotting. Finally, prothrombin is converted to thrombin and fibrinogen to fibrin, which is necessary for creation of a fibrin clot.

Immune system

The body protects itself from foreign invaders, such as bacteria, viruses, parasites, and fungi, through the organs and cells of the immune system. The components of the immune system work together to recognize "self" from "non-self" and to rid the body of those substances recognized as "non-self."

> Never fear—the immune system is here! It protects the body from invaders with its army of lymphocytes.

Immune system organs

Immune system organs and tissues are described as *lymphoid* because they're all involved with the growth, development, and dissemination of lymphocytes. These organs and tissues include:
- lymph nodes
- thymus
- spleen
- tonsils
- Peyer patches in the intestine.

Lymph nodes

Lymph nodes are small, oval-shaped structures located along a network of lymph channels. Most abundant in the head, neck, axillae, abdomen, pelvis, and groin, they help remove and destroy antigens (substances capable of triggering an immune response) that circulate in the blood and lymph. Lymph nodes filter lymphatic fluid and return it to the bloodstream.

Lymphocytes in waiting

Lymph nodes filter foreign invaders, such as viruses and bacteria, and can serve as waiting stations for lymphocytes that might be needed in that area to fight infection.

Nodes of concern

In children, the lymphatic system grows rapidly between ages 3 and 6 years. At this age, slightly swollen (less than 0.5 cm) lymph nodes in the neck and groin areas are common. Lymph nodes that should cause concern are:
• enlarged (greater than 1 cm in diameter), firm, painless, and fixed to the skin (malignancy)
• painful, soft, and producing heat (local inflammation or infection)
• nodes in the supraclavicular, infraclavicular, or axillary regions.

Thymus

The thymus is located in the mediastinal area of the chest and may look quite large on the chest X-ray of a neonate. The thymus is largest in the preadolescent period. After adolescence, it begins to shrink in size.

The thymus uses hormones to enable maturation of lymphocytes, produced by the bone marrow, into T lymphocytes (T cells). The mature T cells can then function normally.

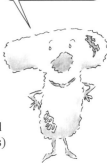

Once I mature in the thymus, I'm ready and willing to function normally.

Spleen

The spleen functions as a reservoir for blood and blood cells. It also acts like a screen to filter out unwanted invaders and help break up old RBCs that lose their elasticity with age and can't squeeze through the fine mesh of the spleen. The spleen is particularly good at filtering out one specific bacterium called *Streptococcus pneumoniae*. Children without a spleen or with a nonfunctioning spleen (such as those with sickle cell disease) are more at risk for invasive streptococcal infections and should be put on prophylactic penicillin (until the age of at least 5 years) and will need immediate antibiotics if they have a fever.

Tonsils

The tonsils consist of lymphoid tissue that serves as a storage site for lymphocytes and can also produce some lymphocytes. In children, the tonsils may normally be slightly enlarged between ages 3 and 6 years (while the immune system is at its peak of development).

Sounds of silence?

Parents of a 3- to 6-year-old child will commonly report that he snores. Snoring at this age is usually due to the enlarged tonsils partially obstructing the airway during sleep.

Immune system cells

All immune system cells are produced in bone marrow. The main cells of the immune system are B cells (B lymphocytes), phagocytes, and T cells (T lymphocytes).

B cells

B cells, which are involved in humoral immunity, produce antibodies. Each B cell is programmed to make a specific antibody. In humoral immunity, a B cell will divide and differentiate into plasma cells when it encounters its triggering antigen. The plasma cells will secrete antibodies to the antigen.

To find and bind

These antibodies then travel in the blood and lymph, which circulate throughout the body. When the antibodies find the antigen, they bind to it to tag it so other immune system cells can destroy it.

Gobs of globulins

Some antibodies are proteins that perform special functions and are called *immunoglobulins*. There are five types of immunoglobulins (Igs) produced by B cells:

IgA defends external body surfaces and is present in colostrum, saliva, tears, and nasal fluids as well as respiratory, gastrointestinal (GI), and genitourinary secretions (neonates have small amounts of this Ig and are more susceptible to an overgrowth of organisms in mucous membranes such as oral *Candida*).

IgD is found on the surface of B cells and functions in controlling lymphocyte activation or suppression.

IgE is the antibody responsible for hypersensitivity reactions; it has an immediate response to an antigen and stimulates the release of heparin and histamine from mast cells.

IgG makes up the majority of plasma antibodies and is the main antibacterial and antiviral antibody; transfusions of IgG specific for viral diseases, such as varicella (chickenpox), are useful in treating children who are exposed but have decreased immune function (such as those on chemotherapy).

IgM is the first Ig produced during an immune response; because it's very large, IgM is usually seen only in the blood and can't pass into tissues to fight infections.

Memory jogger

If humoral immunity is all Greek to you, you're right! To remember what humoral immunity is, think Greek. B-cell antibodies travel in the blood and lymph, which the ancient Greeks called the humors of the body.

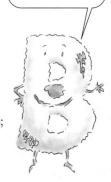

I'm the great antigen hunter. I release the hounds (antibodies) on invading forces!

Phagocytes

Phagocytes are immune cells that engulf, kill, and digest particulate matter and foreign invaders. Phagocytes include neutrophils, monocytes, and macrophages. Macrophages are a type of monocyte; they're versatile scavenger cells found in tissues throughout the body. In addition to their phagocytic action, macrophages:

 activate T cells

secrete various blood products, including clotting factors, enzymes, and regulatory molecules.

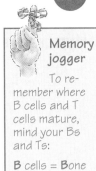

> Memory jogger
>
> To remember where B cells and T cells mature, mind your Bs and Ts:
>
> B cells = Bone marrow
>
> T cells = Thymus

T cells

T cells are responsible for cell-mediated immunity. Lymphocytes derived from bone marrow migrate to the thymus, where they mature into T cells. In cell-mediated immunity, T cells directly attack antigens, including bacteria, viruses, and other pathogens. They have the ability to identify an antigen (target cell) and produce lymphokines that attack the target directly. Cell-mediated immunity is also responsible for tissue and transplant incompatibility rejections and delayed hypersensitivity reactions (such as a positive tuberculin test response).

There's definitely a T in team

Different types of T cells work together to create the best immune response possible. Helper T cells (CD4$^+$ cells) stimulate B cells to mature into plasma cells that produce Igs to fight antigens and to also remember them if they occur again in the future.

Search and destroy

The helper T cells also help the killer T cells (CD8$^+$ cells) to more readily recognize the antigen and attack directly. Killer T cells bind to the surface of the invading antigen and disrupt the cell membrane, causing the antigen's destruction.

> Immunoglobulins are like me—they never forget! Once they fight an antigen, they remember it as the enemy if it ever has the nerve to show up again.

Complement system

The *complement system* is composed of several proteins that are important in the inflammatory process. It's activated by the antigen-antibody complexes (classic pathway) or toxins released by antigens (alternate pathway). The complement system is one of the body's primary defenses; it immediately assists in mast cell degradation, which enhances vascular permeability and assists in attracting neutrophils to the site.

Hypersensitivity

Hypersensitivity reactions are one of the body's immune responses to an antigen and may be immediate (occurring within minutes) or delayed (may take several hours). There are four types of hypersensitivity reactions, each serving a specific function.

Type I: Atopy or anaphylaxis

In some people, certain antigens (allergens) induce B-cell production of IgE, which binds to receptors on mast cell surfaces. The mast cells degranulate and release various mediators, including heparin, histamine, and prostaglandins. These mediators cause vasodilation, bronchospasm, edema, and mucus secretion, leading to such symptoms as wheezing, hives, and rhinorrhea.

Second time around

IgE is produced in sufficient quantities only with repeated exposure and, therefore, may have little effect with occasional allergic reactions. Because severe reactions may not occur with the first exposure to a drug or allergen, the body may only produce antibodies, which will react with the second exposure. In severe reactions, anaphylaxis may occur, resulting in respiratory and cardiac arrest. Someone may not react to an antibiotic the first time—even if they are allergic—but react the second or third time.

Type II: Cytotoxic response

IgG and IgM are involved in tissue-specific hypersensitivity reactions (type II). The type II hypersensitivity response generally involves the destruction of a target cell by an antibody directed against cell-surface antigens.

Deadly complement

Binding of an antigen and an antibody activates the complement system, which ultimately disrupts the cellular membranes, causing cell death. Cytotoxic T cells and NK cells also contribute to tissue death in type II hypersensitivity. Examples of type II hypersensitivity include transfusion reactions and hemolytic disease in the neonate.

Type III: Immune complex

Immune complex–mediated (type III) reactions are similar to type II in that the complex recognizes the same type of antigen. However, in type II, the antigen is found on the cell or organ surface, whereas in type III, the antigen is free-floating and is attacked regardless of where it's located. If the antigens are left in the circulatory system, they may cause inflammatory reactions that can result in vessel wall damage and changes in permeability.

Attack first, ask questions later

Autoimmune disorders are caused by type III reactions in which the immune complexes have difficulty distinguishing between normal and abnormal tissue and may attack both. These disorders include systemic lupus erythematosus (SLE), juvenile rheumatoid arthritis, and glomerulonephritis.

Type IV: Cell-mediated hypersensitivity

In type IV hypersensitivity, antigen is processed by macrophages and presented to T cells.

Release the lymphokines!

T cells function by releasing *lymphokines*, which recruit and activate other lymphocytes, monocytes, macrophages, and polymorphonuclear leukocytes. The coagulation (kinin) and complement pathways also contribute to tissue damage in this type of reaction. The most serious reactions occur with transplantation when the transplanted tissue is perceived as foreign and attacked. Type IV reactions also occur with exposure to plants or substances that trigger a response resulting in contact dermatitis.

Diagnostic tests

Tests used to diagnose hematologic and immunologic problems in children include allergy skin testing, bone marrow aspiration and biopsy, and CBC with differential.

Allergy skin testing

Children commonly have short-term allergic problems that may disappear as the child grows older. A child older than age 2 years with a history of chronic allergic symptoms, such as coughing, runny nose, watery eyes, and upper respiratory congestion, may need to be evaluated for allergies. Symptom management with medications (such as antihistamines) is recommended until the child reaches age 4 years or older. If symptoms persist beyond this age, allergy testing may be warranted.

RAST to the rescue

Allergy skin testing examines specific allergic antigens. The radio-allergosorbent test (RAST) identifies antigens in the blood that are causing an immunologic reaction mediated by IgE. The quantity of circulating IgE correlates well with the clinical severity of the allergic symptoms.

The family tree of allergy

When testing is started, a pediatric allergist obtains a detailed history from the family and the child in an attempt to identify the specific antigen. Allergy skin testing entails injecting small amounts of common allergic antigens under the skin (intradermal) to assess for localized reaction. RAST is recommended when there's a strong suspicion that a specific substance is responsible for the allergy problem.

Nursing considerations

Allergy shots run the risk of causing an anaphylactic reaction, and the nurse should be prepared to provide emergency care. The child should remain in the facility for at least 15 minutes after the shot to be monitored for an injection site reaction and signs of an impending anaphylactic reaction.

A song and a wiggle

The child should be prepared for injections (for testing and treatment) and given a "job" to do such as holding very still. Distraction techniques (such as telling the child to wiggle his toes or sing a song) may help reduce the child's anxiety and enhance cooperation.

Bone marrow aspiration and biopsy

Bone marrow aspiration and bone marrow biopsy are slightly different tests that are usually done for the same reason. Both tests are done to view the integrity of function of the bone marrow as an organ.

Bone bank withdrawal

In bone marrow aspiration, a specially designed needle with a stylet is inserted into the center of the bone to withdraw bone marrow. The front and back crests of the iliac bone are most commonly sampled in children. In a bone marrow biopsy, a section of bone is taken, revealing all levels of bone and bone marrow.

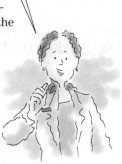

Bone marrow aspiration is used to withdraw a small amount of bone marrow. In bone marrow biopsy, a small section of bone is removed.

To aspirate or biopsy—that is the question

Ideally, the marrow should show a wide variety of cell types in various stages of maturation. Primary, malignant, blast leukemic cells with few normal cells are seen in leukemia. When a solid tumor, such as neuroblastoma or rhabdomyosarcoma, has metastasized to the bone marrow, a biopsy may be more helpful in showing the clumps of tumor cells among some normal cells. Both tests show whether the bone marrow is functioning normally.

Nursing considerations

Bone marrow aspiration or biopsy can be performed under light general anesthesia or with a local injection to numb the area. An oral or intravenous (I.V.) sedative may be given before the procedure. Prepare the child for the test with an age-appropriate explanation, and monitor for sedation or adverse effects of anesthesia. Tell the child that a parent may stay with him during the test.

In addition, follow these steps:
• Apply a pressure dressing after the procedure, which should be sufficient to stop blood loss.
• Be aware of the proper handling and labeling of the specimens to prevent the need to repeat the aspiration; multiple tests may be performed on the specimens obtained.
• Provide a mild analgesic as ordered; postprocedure pain is short-term after aspiration and consists of a dull ache for about 24 hours after biopsy.

CBC with differential

One of the most important tests for general screening for hematologic and immune problems is the complete blood count (CBC). An additional test that may be ordered is the *differential*, which is used to determine the percentage of WBCs that are present.

Decrease = disorder

In general, the CBC reveals the numbers of the three main blood cells (WBCs, RBCs, and platelets). Decreased values in any cell line may be an indication of a disorder related to the bone marrow or the immune system or may be the result of infection.

What's up with the whites?

WBC counts vary with age.
• A healthy neonate typically has higher counts of 15,000 to 20,000/µl, with 60% to 70% being lymphocytes.
• The typical adult WBC count of 5,000 to 10,000/µl is generally present in children after age 2 years.

Don't be alarmed! A WBC count of 15,000 to 20,000/µl is normal in a healthy neonate like me.

15,000 TO 20,000

• Counts over 15,000/µl in children older than age 6 months should be considered high and abnormal (although this doesn't necessarily indicate serious illness).

Seeing red

Although the RBC count is included in the CBC, the hemoglobin level and hematocrit are usually used as a gauge of the number of RBCs present:

• *Hemoglobin* is a molecule responsible for carrying oxygen to the tissue and is somewhat affected by age. Higher levels of 15 to 20 g/dl are present in the neonate but, within 2 months, the normal range will be 12 to 15 g/dl.

• *Hematocrit* is approximately three times the level of hemoglobin, and normal ranges are 35% to 45%. This level is affected by hydration level and may be elevated with dehydration and decreased if the child has fluid overload.

Pediatric and parental platelets

Platelet counts should be between 150,000 and 500,000/mm^3, regardless of age.

Nursing considerations

Prepare the child for venipuncture and allow the parent to be present to comfort the child. After the venipuncture, monitor the site for signs of continued bleeding.

Treatments and procedures

Treatments and procedures used for children with hematologic and immunologic problems include blood transfusion and bone marrow transplantation.

Blood transfusion

Blood transfusion is necessary if levels of blood cells become too low or if the child is experiencing symptoms caused by a decrease in the number of available cells.

Pump up the vascular volume

Generally, transfusions are aimed at increasing volume within the vascular system, increasing RBCs to improve oxygenation, or increasing the number of platelets to reduce or correct bleeding problems:

• Whole blood is transfused if trauma with bleeding occurs and the risk of shock is present because of decreased intravascular volume. Blood loss from surgery may also require whole blood to replace cells and plasma.

• In children who have decreased levels of RBCs only, transfusion with packed RBCs is indicated. Because plasma is removed from these concentrated RBCs, transfusion increases intravascular volume only minimally (only small amounts of WBCs and platelets are contained in the transfused RBCs).

• Platelets are transfused when counts are below 60,000/mm^3 with symptoms of active bleeding. If the count is below 20,000/mm^3, transfusion with platelets is recommended due to the risk of spontaneous intracranial bleeding, which can lead to death.

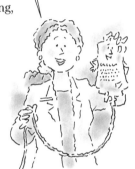

Blood product screening has come a long way, baby! Reassure the child and his parents that the blood used for transfusion is safe.

Nursing considerations

Prepare the child and his parents for the procedure. Reassure the parents (and the child, if old enough) about the measures that are taken to ensure the safety of transfused blood products.

In addition, follow these steps:

• Double-check the child's name, identification number, name bracelet, ABO group, and Rh status with another nurse to help prevent hemolytic transfusion reactions. If there's a discrepancy, don't administer the blood product and notify the blood bank immediately.

• Start the blood transfusion within 30 minutes after it arrives from the blood bank. If you can't start the transfusion in this time-frame, return the blood product to the blood bank.

• Take baseline vital signs just before the start of the transfusion and every 15 minutes during the transfusion.

Bone marrow transplantation

Bone marrow transplantation is used to treat such diseases as acute leukemia, aplastic anemia, and severe combined immunodeficiency disease. The hematopoietic stem cells may be malignant themselves or may have been destroyed by aggressive therapy for malignant disease. Sometimes the stem cells are absent or just don't work like aplastic anemia.

We're compatible in every way . . .

. . . right down to our HLA!

Share and share alike

With transplantation, marrow or stem cells are transplanted from a twin or another human leukocyte antigen (HLA)–identical donor (usually a sibling) in the hope that the new stem cells will produce normal, healthy cells. Autologous bone marrow transplantation is another option for some patients. In this procedure, the patient's own marrow or stem cells are harvested from healthy tissues or harvested and then treated to remove malignant cells. The cells are then returned to the patient.

A harvest of plenty

During bone marrow harvest, marrow is extracted from a matched donor with multiple bone marrow aspirations; 200 to 500 ml of marrow are collected, processed, and purified.

Getting ready to receive

The recipient is given high-dose chemotherapy to destroy the malignant marrow and WBCs that might cause a reaction. On the day of the transplant, the recipient is given total-body radiation to further destroy components of the malignant bone marrow and to destroy WBCs throughout the body that may identify the transfused cells as foreign and destroy them.

From harvest to seed

The collected donor marrow, which looks like a blood product, is then transfused through an I.V. line. If the transfusion is successful, the transplanted stem cells will reseed the bone marrow and start producing normal blood cells.

Graft battles host

A great risk after bone marrow transplantation is that the new bone marrow may produce B cells that interpret the normal body tissue as being foreign and attack it. This is commonly seen in the skin, eyes, liver, and other organs and is known as *graft-versus-host disease* (GVHD). The donated cells must be HLA-matched to prevent GVHD. Typically, this complication will start after the stem cells have engrafted (about 2 weeks after the transplant).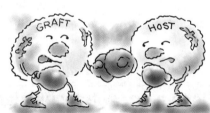

Although some GVHD may not be harmful, if the stem cells continue to produce cells that attack tissue, the effect can be dramatic, with sloughing of skin, organ malfunction or failure, and eventual death.

Nursing considerations

The donor and the recipient should be prepared for the procedure with age-appropriate explanations. In addition, follow these steps:
• Administer immunosuppressants, such as steroids and cyclosporine (Sandimmune), as ordered to control GVHD.

- Monitor the child for signs of GVHD, such as changes in skin color or appearance, hematuria, diarrhea, jaundice, and a change in mental status (even after they leave the facility).
- Because the child is at high risk for infection immediately after the transplantation, monitor closely for signs of infection.
- Prevent skin breakdown by using pressure-relieving or pressure-reducing beds or mattresses; turn the child frequently.
- Support the child and his family throughout this stressful time because the child will be critically ill with the potential for life-threatening complications.

Hematologic and immunologic disorders

Hematologic and immunologic disorders that may affect children include acquired immunodeficiency syndrome (AIDS), allergic rhinitis, aplastic anemia, atopic dermatitis, hemophilia, Hodgkin's disease, iron deficiency anemia, leukemia, sickle cell anemia, SLE, and thalassemia.

HIV/AIDS

The identification of the human immunodeficiency virus (HIV) in the 1980s foreshadowed a worldwide epidemic that crosses all ethnic, cultural, and age barriers. Although the initial cases were primarily among gay men, the virus then expanded into all groups, including infants and children.

What causes it

HIV, a retrovirus, has the ability to enter a cell and incorporate itself into the cell's ribonucleic acid, essentially changing the genetic structure and causing the cell to slowly die.

A stranger in friend's clothing

Because HIV becomes part of the cell, the body's normal defense mechanisms (from the immune system) don't recognize it as foreign, and the virus goes unchallenged.

Out of control

From the first single cell, the virus replicates and then enters other cells, eventually infecting several cells and rendering them nonfunctional. When a large number of cells become infected, the normal ability to control common organisms is compromised, and the person develops AIDS.

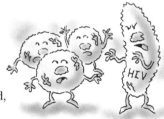

After I enter a single cell, I replicate—and the rest fall like dominoes!

How it happens

Transmission of HIV occurs by contact with infected blood or body fluids and is associated with identifiable, high-risk behaviors, including sexual intercourse with multiple partners, I.V. drug use, and pregnancies in HIV-infected women.

It's different for kids

The mode of transmission in children has always been different from that in adults. Although transmission in adolescents may occur from sexual contact or I.V. drug use, these issues aren't common factors in transmission to the younger child. Potential sources of infection in children include:
• being born to an untreated, infected mother
• breast-feeding from an infected mother
• blood transfusions with HIV-tainted blood products (hemophiliacs with contaminated factor VIII or other factor products that were pooled from multiple donors before blood donations were routinely screened).

Destructive domino effect

HIV has a particular affinity for the $CD4^+$ helper T cell as well as monocytes and macrophages. The virus invades these cells and renders them nonfunctional, resulting in suppressed cell-mediated and humoral immunity. The degree of immunosuppression will progress and, eventually, result in opportunistic infection and even death.

Diagnosing HIV/AIDS

HIV was historically suspected when a person developed an indicator disease listed in the following chart and a $CD4^+$ count was monitored and the antibody was detected. The current method for diagnosing a person as being HIV positive is to detect the virus itself and look at the "viral load" to determine the extent of the infection. This allows for quicker diagnosis because the body takes time to develop an antibody. A person now is considered to have AIDS if the $CD4^+$ lymphocyte count is below 200.

What to look for

In adults, the diagnosis of AIDS was historically based on $CD4^+$ counts and the presence of *indicator diseases*, which are opportunistic infections associated with HIV disease. (See *Indicator diseases and HIV.*)

In children, these diseases are less common until the infection is more severe. However, infants and children are particularly susceptible to fungal diseases. Children who are HIV-positive tend to have repeated bacterial infections, such as otitis media, that don't respond to antibiotics.

Indicator diseases and HIV

This chart describes some common infections associated with HIV disease in children, along with their characteristic signs and symptoms, and their treatments. They are no longer required to diagnose AIDS.

Infection	Signs and symptoms	Treatment
Bacterial *Mycobacterium avium* complex A primary infection acquired by oral ingestion or inhalation; can infect the bone marrow, liver, spleen, GI tract, lymph nodes, lungs, skin, brain, adrenal glands, and kidneys; is chronic and may be localized and disseminated in its course of infection	Multiple, nonspecific symptoms consistent with systemic illness (fever, fatigue, weight loss, anorexia, night sweats, abdominal pain, and chronic diarrhea); *physical examination findings:* emaciation, generalized lymphadenopathy, diffuse tenderness, jaundice, and hepatosplenomegaly; *laboratory findings:* anemia, leukopenia, and thrombocytopenia	Treatment regimens vary and can include two to six drugs. The Centers for Disease Control and Prevention currently recommend that every patient take either azithromycin (Zithromax) or clarithromycin (Biaxin). Many experts prefer ethambutol (Myambutol) as a second drug. Additional drugs include rifabutin (Mycobutin), rifampin (Rifadin), ciprofloxacin (Cipro), and, sometimes, amikacin (Amikin).
Fungal Candidiasis A disease caused by the fungus *Candida albicans* that exists on teeth, gingivae, and skin and in the oropharynx, vagina, and large intestine; majority of infections are endogenous and related to interruption of normal defense mechanisms; possible human-to-human transmission, including congenital transmission in neonates (who develop thrush after vaginal delivery)	*Thrush* (the most prevalent form in HIV-infected individuals): creamy, curdlike, white patches surrounded by an erythematous base, found on any oral mucosal surface; *nail infection:* inflammation and tenderness of tissue surrounding the nails or the nail itself; *vaginitis:* intense pruritus of the vulva and curdlike vaginal discharge	Nystatin suspension (Mycostatin) and clotrimazole troches (Lotrimin) are administered for thrush; nystatin suspension or pastilles, clotrimazole troches, fluconazole (Diflucan), or itraconazole (Sporanox) for esophagitis; topical clotrimazole, miconazole (Micatin), or ketoconazole (Nizoral) for cutaneous candidiasis; oral fluconazole or ketoconazole for candidiasis of nails; and topical clotrimazole, miconazole, or oral fluconazole for vaginitis.
Protozoan *Pneumocystis jirovecii* pneumonia Pneumonia caused by *P. jirovecii*; also has properties of fungal infection; exists in human lungs and is transmitted by airborne exposure; the most common life-threatening opportunistic infection in individuals with AIDS	Fever, fatigue, and weight loss for several weeks to months before respiratory symptoms develop; *respiratory symptoms:* dyspnea (usually noted initially on exertion and later at rest) and cough (usually starting out dry and nonproductive and later becoming productive)	Co-trimoxazole (Bactrim) may be given orally or I.V., although about 20% of patients with AIDS are hypersensitive to sulfa drugs. I.V. pentamidine may be given but can cause many adverse effects, including permanent diabetes mellitus. Dapsone (DDS) with trimethoprim (Primsol), clindamycin (Cleocin), primaquine, atovaquone (Malarone), or corticosteroids are also used. Prophylaxis for disease prevention and following treatment includes co-trimoxazole, atovaquone, or dapsone.

(continued)

Indicator diseases and HIV *(continued)*

Infection	Signs and symptoms	Treatment
Protozoan *(continued)* Cryptosporidiosis An intestinal infection caused by the protozoan *Cryptosporidium;* transmitted by person-to-person contact, water, food contaminants, and airborne exposure; small intestine is the most common site	Abdominal cramping; flatulence; weight loss; anorexia; malaise; fever; nausea; vomiting; myalgia; and profuse, watery diarrhea	No treatment currently exists that can eradicate the infecting organism. Treatment consists mainly of supportive measures to control symptoms. These measures may include fluid replacement; total parenteral nutrition (occasionally); correction of electrolyte imbalances; and administration of analgesic, antidiarrheal, and antiperistaltic agents. Paromomycin (Humatin) and octreotide (Sandostatin) are used.
Viral Herpes simplex virus Chronic infection caused by a herpes virus; usually a reactivation of an earlier herpes infection	Red, blisterlike lesions occurring in oral, anal, and genital areas; also found on the esophageal and tracheobronchial mucosa; pain, bleeding, and discharge	Acyclovir (Zovirax), famciclovir (Famvir), or valacyclovir (Valtrex) are given I.V. or orally. Low maintenance dosages may be given to prevent recurrence of symptoms.
Cytomegalovirus (CMV) A viral infection of the herpes virus that may result in serious, widespread infection; most common sites are the lungs, adrenal glands, eyes, central nervous system, GI tract, male genitourinary tract, and blood	Unexplained fever; malaise; GI ulcers; diarrhea; weight loss; swollen lymph glands; hepatomegaly; splenomegaly; blurred vision; floaters; dyspnea (especially on exertion); dry, nonproductive cough; and vision changes leading to blindness in patients with ocular infection	Ganciclovir (Cytovene) or foscarnet (Foscavir) is used to treat CMV. Ganciclovir has shown some anti-HIV properties. Foscarnet or intraocular ganciclovir implants may be used to treat CMV retinitis.

The incubation period for children averages only 17 months, and the signs and symptoms of HIV resemble those in adults. Initially, the child may have flulike symptoms and then may remain asymptomatic for years. As the disease progresses, neurologic signs from HIV encephalopathy and symptoms of an opportunistic infection may manifest. (See *HIV classification in children.*)

What tests tell you

Virologic assays that directly detect HIV (such as HIV DNA polymerase chain reaction and HIV RNA assays) must be used to diagnose HIV infection in infants younger than 18 months. Virologic diagnostic testing in infants with known perinatal HIV exposure is recommended at ages 14 to 21 days, 1 to 2 months, and 4 to

HIV classification in children

The Centers for Disease Control and Prevention's revised classification system for HIV-infected children is based on four categories.

Category	Symptoms and criteria
Category A	A child is *mildly symptomatic* when he has two or more symptoms, such as enlarged lymph nodes, liver, or spleen or recurrent or persistent upper respiratory infections, sinusitis, or otitis media.
Category B	A child is *moderately symptomatic* if he has developed more serious illnesses, such as oropharyngeal candidiasis, bacterial meningitis, pneumonia, sepsis, cardiomyopathy, cytomegalovirus infection, hepatitis, herpes simplex virus infection, bronchitis, pneumonitis or esophagitis, herpes zoster (shingles), lymphoid interstitial pneumonia, pulmonary lymphoid hyperplasia complex, or toxoplasmosis.
Category C	A child is *severely symptomatic* if he has developed serious bacterial infections, such as septicemia, pneumonia, meningitis, bone or joint infections, or abscess of an internal organ or body cavity or infections, such as candidiasis (esophageal or pulmonary), encephalopathy, herpes simplex lasting longer than 1 month, histoplasmosis, lymphoma, mycobacterium tuberculosis, or *Pneumocystis jirovecii* pneumonia. Unlike adults, children rarely develop Kaposi's sarcoma.
Category N	A child is *not symptomatic* if he or she has no signs or symptoms considered to be the result of HIV infection or if he or she has only one of the conditions listed in Category A.

6 months. Virologic diagnostic testing at birth should be considered for infants at high risk of HIV infection. A positive virologic test should be confirmed as soon as possible by a repeat virologic test on a second specimen. HIV antibody assays alone can be used for diagnosis of HIV infection in children with perinatal exposure who are 18 months of age or older and in children with nonperinatal exposure.

Screen with ELIZA, confirm with the blot

In children and adolescents with nonperinatal exposure to HIV, the recommended protocol is initial screening with an enzyme-linked immunosorbent assay (ELISA). After checking and rechecking the results, findings are confirmed by the Western blot test or an immunofluorescence assay.

Back-up blood tests

Other blood tests support the diagnosis and are used to evaluate the severity of immunosuppression:
• The $CD4^+$ and $CD8^+$ cell subset counts determine the risk of HIV being converted to AIDS. As the $CD4^+$ level lowers, the risk of AIDS conversion increases, with levels below 200 cells/µl considered diagnostic of AIDS (with or without the presence of another disease or condition).

- CD8$^+$ killer T cell counts are monitored, as is the ratio of CD4$^+$ to CD8$^+$, which may give an indication of decreased percentage of CD4$^+$ cells, and AIDS conversion.
- A CBC may provide an overall view of the health of the child but a special test is required to distinguish between types of lymphocytes.

Complications

Complications of HIV infection may include opportunistic infections, failure to thrive and nutritional deficits, malignancies, and HIV encephalopathy. In addition to treatment for HIV itself, the patient may be on various drugs to treat or control opportunistic infections, including antibiotics for bacterial infection, steroids for control of symptoms, and chemotherapy if malignancies are present. These drugs can cause an array of severe adverse reactions, including peripheral neuropathy, seizures, nausea, vomiting, neutropenia, and thrombocytopenia.

How it's treated

There's no cure for HIV infection; however, several types of drugs are used to treat the disease and prolong life. Many treatment protocols combine three or more drugs to produce the maximum benefit with the fewest adverse reactions. Combination therapy also helps to inhibit the production of mutant HIV strains resistant to particular drugs.

The 076 study (named after research number)

In the late 1980s, the National Institutes of Health conducted a study involving several medical centers across the country designed to reduce the incidence of HIV-positive babies born to HIV-positive mothers. Historically, about 33% of babies born to HIV-positive mothers would be infected with the virus. By treating the mother in the last month of pregnancy and the baby upon birth, the risk was reduced to about 8%. This dramatic decrease established the need to identify and treat all HIV pregnant women.

Do-good drugs

Several drugs are known to be effective against HIV and can be used in different combinations. Current treatment may depend on several factors including renal status and resistance patterns. Detailed preferred and alternative regimens are outlined in the Centers for Disease Control and Prevention (CDC) Web site (http://www.aidsinfo.nih.gov/guidelines).

Preferred regimens include:
- efavirenz (EFV)/tenofovir disoproxil fumarate (TDF)/ emtricitabine (FTC)
- atazanavir/ritonavir (ATVr) + TDF/FTC

- darunavir/ritonavir + TDF/FTC
- raltegravir (RAL) + TDF/FTC

What to do

Many parents and children equate this diagnosis with a death sentence. Despite the increasing numbers of people who are living with AIDS (because of new treatments), the diagnosis is likely to be terrifying and devastating to the entire family. People who are HIV positive may live long lives and HIV may be considered a chronic disease in some persons.

A listening ear

The diagnosis is also profoundly distressing because of the disease's social impact and the discouraging prognosis. Listen to the child and his parents because they may feel alone and isolated and may need a safe person with whom they can talk.

In addition, follow these steps:
- Use standard precautions to reduce the risk of HIV transmission.
- Monitor the child for changes in vital signs, especially low-grade fevers of above 100.4° F (38° C).

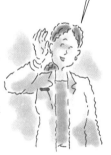

Sometimes, having someone just listen is the best medicine for a family dealing with HIV/AIDS.

Infection detection

- Observe for evidence of infection or lesions, including signs of skin breakdown, cough, sore throat, and diarrhea.
- Maintain strict confidentiality as a stigma remains with this disease and the family may not want the diagnosis to be common knowledge.
- Refer the family to counselors and agencies that can help them cope with the diagnosis as well as provide concrete forms of assistance (such as help with finances and transportation and educating day care or school personnel).
- Educate family members on symptoms of infections that may be of concern and make everyone aware of standard precautions (use of gloves) when dealing with the child's bodily fluids.

Allergic rhinitis

Inhaled airborne antigens, such as dust and pollen, may cause an immune response that results in watery eyes (allergic conjunctivitis) or an inflammation of the nasal mucosa (rhinitis). Depending on the allergen, allergic rhinitis may occur seasonally (hay fever) or year-round (perennial allergic rhinitis).

What causes it

Allergic rhinitis is a type I hypersensitivity reaction mediated by IgE. Hay fever occurs in the spring, summer, and fall and is usually induced by airborne pollens from trees, grass, and weeds. In the summer and fall, mold spores may also cause it.

It may be difficult to identify the exact source of allergic rhinitis. Major perennial allergens and irritants include:

- house dust and dust mites
- feathers
- molds and fungi
- animal dander
- processed materials or industrial chemicals
- tobacco smoke, directly or from clothes worn while smoking (a major offender in children).

Hope for the future

Children who have allergic symptoms beginning before age 2 years may outgrow them or may have reduced symptoms with time.

How it happens

Once the antigen is recognized by the immune system, a type I hypersensitivity reaction occurs. IgE is created by the conversion of B cells to plasma cells. Histamine release results in the swelling of the mucous membranes. Secondary sinus infections and middle ear infections may be triggered, and nasal polyps caused by edema and infection may increase nasal obstruction.

What to look for

Allergic rhinitis may produce symptoms that vary by age and may be difficult to distinguish from viral upper respiratory infections:

- The patient complains of sneezing attacks, rhinorrhea (profuse, watery nasal discharge), nasal obstruction or congestion, itching nose and eyes, and headache or sinus pain.
- Allergic rhinitis doesn't normally cause fever unless a secondary infection is present; fever with viral illnesses, such as an upper respiratory infection, isn't uncommon.
- A family history of allergies, asthma, and atopic dermatitis (eczema) may indicate that symptoms are IgE mediated.
- Symptoms lasting longer than 2 weeks may indicate a more allergic than infective cause, especially if the child hasn't had a fever. (See *Allergic shiners*.)

What tests tell you

Most laboratory tests aren't helpful in determining if a short-term illness is an allergy. A large number of eosinophils are seen in specimens of sputum and nasal secretions. The activity of the eosinophils isn't completely understood, but they're known to destroy parasitic organisms and play a role in allergic reactions.

Allergic shiners

In allergic shiners, blood circulation around the eye backs up around the orbit, resulting in dark circles under the eyes or *Dennie's sign* (a peculiar horizontal line).

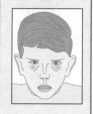

Sneezing in your sleep

CBC will be normal with either short- or long-term allergic problems but may be helpful in ruling out a more serious illness if fever is present. Skin testing for allergies, or *RAST*, is helpful after the symptoms are present for several weeks and begin to affect the quality of life, especially by causing sleep disturbances. Short-term or less severe allergic rhinitis remains primarily a clinical diagnosis in children.

Complications

Complications of allergic rhinitis are rarely serious but affect the quality of life of the child and his family. The child may have sleep disturbances from a runny nose, frequent sneezing, or coughing caused by postnasal drip.

The nose knows

Nosebleeds (epistaxis) may occur as a result of the allergic rhinitis itself or from overuse of medications, which dries mucous membranes. Children with allergic rhinitis are more susceptible to otitis media, sinusitis, bacterial conjunctivitis, and other infections of the upper respiratory tract.

How it's treated

Treatment of allergic rhinitis is aimed at controlling the symptoms and preventing infection. Treatment may include removing the environmental allergen and administering drug therapy. Antihistamines block histamine release and decrease the overall reaction and swelling of the tissue. This action reduces the inflammation of the mucous membranes and decreases nasal drainage. Overuse of antihistamines may dry out the mucous membranes, causing sneezing and nosebleeds.

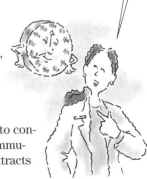

Antihistamines at bedtime help a child be bright-eyed, bushy-tailed, and ready (if not willing) for school in the morning.

Timing is everything

One adverse effect of antihistamines (diphenhydramine [Benadryl]) in children is sedation. Use of antihistamines should be avoided before going to school and are usually more appropriate at bedtime or naptime. Newer antihistamines, such as loratadine (Claritin) and cetirizine (Zyrtec), have been approved for use in older children and are nonsedating.

Up your nose with a nasal spray!

Other therapies may include topical nasal corticosteroids to control exacerbations. Long-term management may include immunotherapy or desensitization with injections of allergen extracts administered preseasonally, seasonally, or annually.

What to do

Stress the importance of taking daily antihistamines, and teach the parents and child about their potential adverse effects and ways to reduce the child's exposure to the identified environmental allergen:
• Monitor a child who has received an allergy injection for at least 30 minutes to detect adverse reactions.
• Determine if family history is consistent with allergic problems and be aware that asthma is more common with familial history of allergies.
• Because many of the allergy medications are over-the-counter, make sure the parent is giving the correct dose.

Atopic dermatitis

Atopic dermatitis, also called *eczema*, is a chronic condition of the skin characterized by superficial skin inflammation and intense itching. The skin doesn't hold moisture or oil and becomes dry, scaly, and itchy. Although this disorder may appear at any age, it typically begins during infancy or early childhood.

What causes it

The exact cause is unknown but an allergic component is strongly suspected. A family history commonly reveals adults with childhood histories of atopic dermatitis, other forms of allergies, or asthma.

To make matters worse . . .

Exacerbating factors include irritants, skin infections (commonly caused by *Staphylococcus aureus*), and some allergens. Exposure to food allergens (such as milk proteins, soybeans, fish, or nuts) may coincide with flare-ups of atopic dermatitis.

> Atopic dermatitis sets up a vicious cycle. Itching leads to scratching, which causes vasoconstriction and makes itching even worse!

How it happens

Scratching the skin causes vasoconstriction and intensifies itching, resulting in reddened, weeping lesions. Eventually, the lesions become scaly and lichenified. Usually, they're located in areas of flexion and extension, such as the neck, antecubital fossa, popliteal folds, and behind the ears. In infants, the lesions are also common on the cheeks and may look like a windburn.

What to look for

Atopic dermatitis begins with skin drying and then cracking, eventually leading to open sores with bleeding. These open sores are susceptible to secondary infections. Children commonly scratch in their sleep and can do most of the skin damage at that time if the itching isn't controlled. Heat, sweating, dry skin, and clothing with wool or coarse materials tend to worsen the itching sensation. (See *Infant with atopic dermatitis*.)

What tests tell you

Elevated levels of IgE and eosinophils are seen in this disorder, but routine laboratory values, such as CBC, aren't affected. Allergy testing may be warranted in the older child, but avoiding the allergen may not affect the course of atopic dermatitis.

Complications

Atopic dermatitis may disrupt the family in general because it's a chronic condition that requires daily care. The child may have sleep difficulties from constant pruritus (itching).

From scratching to scarring

Skin damage from scratching leaves the child susceptible to secondary infection that may require either topical treatment with antibiotic ointment or systemic antibiotics. Scarring may occur due to excoriations from scratching.

How it's treated

Measures to ease this chronic disorder include meticulous skin care with moisturizers such as petroleum jelly, environmental control of offending allergens, and drug therapy (often topical steroids). The overall treatment plan is aimed at controlling the symptoms—particularly the pruritus—and restoring moisture to the skin to prevent further drying.

Too clean, too dry

Excessive bathing leads to further reduction of skin oils and worsens the dryness. Once-daily bathing in warm water with cream-based soaps, such as Tone, Dove, Caress, or Ivory cream, can relieve symptoms. Frequent application of nonirritating topical lubricants is important, especially after bathing or showering. Vaseline and Crisco shortening have been used in the past with some positive results and may be alternatives for families with limited budgets.

Wash, then wear—hold the bleach

Minimizing exposure to irritants, such as wool and harsh detergents, also helps control symptoms. New clothes should be washed before wearing to avoid exposure to irritating dyes or chemicals. Clothes washed with bleach should be double-rinsed to ensure that all bleach is removed (because it dries

Infant with atopic dermatitis

Children with atopic dermatitis have papular and vesicular skin eruptions with surrounding erythema. The vesicles rupture and exude yellow, sticky exudate. The secretions form crusts on the skin as they dry.

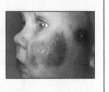

To manage atopic dermatitis, there's a "laundry" list of do's and don'ts.

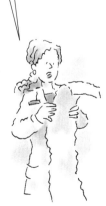

and irritates the skin). Hypoallergenic soaps should be used for all laundry, and starch should be avoided.

Down with itch and inflammation!

Drug therapy involves the use of topical corticosteroids and antipruritics. A mild steroid cream, such as hydrocortisone 1%, can relieve the inflammation and associated itching and may be massaged into the affected area two to three times per day for 1 week.

Diphenhydramine or hydroxyzine (Atarax) are effective antipruritics but may cause sedation. These medications are especially useful at bedtime to reduce nighttime scratching and resulting skin damage.

What to do

The nurse plays an important role in the management of atopic dermatitis and is commonly the key source of critical daily care plans for minimizing the impact of this condition on the child and his family:

• Instruct all caretakers about the management of the skin lesions.
• Make the family aware that atopic dermatitis is a chronic condition that isn't usually related to an identifiable allergen.
• Make sure the parents are aware of such serious complications as infection and emphasize the need for evaluation of any open, draining areas.

Hemophilia

A hereditary bleeding disorder, hemophilia results from a deficiency of specific clotting factors. Hemophilia A (classic hemophilia) results from deficiency of factor VIII; hemophilia B (Christmas disease) results from deficiency of factor IX. There are two less common types of hemophilia. Hemophilia C is a deficiency of factor XI. Von Willebrand's disease includes a deficiency in von Willebrand's factor, an important protein necessary for platelet adhesion.

What causes it

The inheritance pattern is X-linked recessive in about 80% of all hemophilia cases. Hemophilia C is transmitted by an autosomal recessive trait in both sexes. Von Willebrand's disease is transmitted as an autosomal dominant disorder.

> Ho, ho, hemophilia B is known as Christmas disease. (Don't expect any factor IX under the tree.)

How it happens

Hemophilia produces mild to severe abnormal bleeding. After a platelet plug develops at a bleeding site, the lack of clotting factor prevents a stable fibrin clot from forming. Although hemorrhaging usually doesn't occur immediately, delayed bleeding is common.

A matter of degrees

Hemophilia may be severe, moderate, or mild, depending on the degree of normal clotting (factor VIII) activity:
- In severe disease, there's less than 1% normal clotting activity.
- In moderate disease, there's 1% to 5% normal clotting activity.
- In mild disease, there's 5% to 50% normal clotting activity.

Most children with hemophilia (60% to 70%) demonstrate the severe form.

What to look for

There's usually a family history of hemophilia or bleeding problems in men.

The circumcision clue

Bleeding can occur spontaneously, and the neonate may have prolonged bleeding times with routine blood collection for neonate tests. It's also common to diagnose hemophilia when the child has excessive and prolonged bleeding after circumcision.

Mountain out of a molehill

Later, spontaneous or disproportionately severe bleeding after minor trauma may produce large subcutaneous and deep intramuscular hematomas. Signs and symptoms of decreased tissue perfusion include restlessness, anxiety, confusion, pallor, cool and clammy skin, chest pain, decreased urine output, hypotension, and tachycardia.

What tests tell you

- A coagulation screen shows a normal prothrombin time (PT) with a prolonged partial thromboplastin time (PTT).
- Factor VIII coagulant activity is decreased in hemophilia A and is normal in hemophilia B.
- Factor IX is decreased in hemophilia B and normal in hemophilia A.
- Platelet aggregation and platelet count is normal in both hemophilia A and B.

Complications

Any type of hemophilia puts the child at risk for bleeding—even with normal activities—making it extremely important to take safety precautions during activities that could place the child at risk.

> Parents of a child with hemophilia must become safety experts!

Head's up!

The greatest risk is with a head injury with intracranial bleeding or bleeding into joints. Joint mobility may be affected with repeated joint injury and may cause decreased range of motion. Any injury may cause bleeding into tissue that may require clotting factor transfusion and hospitalization for monitoring.

The incredible expanding spleen

Injury of the spleen with resulting bleeding may be life-threatening as the spleen expands with blood, causing hypovolemic shock. Historically, hemophiliacs were infected in large numbers with HIV and hepatitis C before screening for these viruses in blood products was started.

How it's treated

Hemophilia isn't curable, but treatment can prevent crippling deformities and prolong life. Increasing plasma levels of deficient clotting factors helps prevent disabling deformities caused by repeated bleeding into muscles, joints, and organs.

Everyone in the pool!

Hemophilia A or B can be treated with pooled factor obtained from blood products. Historically, these products ran a risk of transmitting viral illness, but current recombinant factor VIII and IX are safe and free from viral infection. Desmopressin acetate (DDAVP) is a synthetic vasopressin analog. It has a minimal antidiuretic effect but does increase the factor VIII level up to fourfold. It has no effect on factor IX. Hemophilia C and von Willebrand's disease are treated with DDAVP, and factor VIII replenishment may also help in von Willebrand's disease.

What to do

The nurse's role involves educating the parents about safety issues while monitoring the child for acute problems. The child must become accustomed to restrictions in activities and precautions that may make him feel different from his peers. Counseling may be needed to help the child deal with these issues and to help ensure compliance. In addition, follow these steps:
• Observe for evidence of bruising, bleeding, or change in mental status.

- If transfusions are ordered, monitor for blood product reactions, such as fever, chills, or irritability.

Do try this at home

- Because home infusions are commonly done (minimizing the need for hospitalization), educate the parents about the process and refer them to a home care infusion agency.
- Teach the family about age-appropriate safety measures, including padding hard surfaces and, later, wearing a bicycle helmet and other protective gear during sports activities.
- Teach the parents to recognize signs of bleeding by monitoring for nosebleeds and color of stool. Fresh blood in stool or black, tarry stools are signs of gastric bleeding; excessive swallowing during sleep may be a sign of bleeding and swallowing the blood.

Quash the rebellion

- As the child grows older, assess his participation in new activities and reinforce the need for safety measures. Including the child in these discussions and allowing him as much choice as possible will help keep the growing child's normal tendency to rebel against restrictions in check.
- Make families aware of such support groups as the National Hemophilia Foundation, and inform them about any local support sources.

Hodgkin's lymphoma

Hodgkin's lymphoma, formerly known as Hodgkin's disease, is a malignancy of the lymphatic system. In the pediatric age-group, it affects primarily adolescents, although children as young as age 3 years have been diagnosed with the disease. This type of cancer causes painless, progressive enlargement of the lymph nodes, spleen, and other lymphoid tissue.

And the good news is . . .

Although the disease is fatal if untreated, recent advances have made Hodgkin's lymphoma potentially curable, even in advanced stages. With appropriate treatment, more than 90% of patients live at least 5 years.

What causes it

Like most malignancies, the exact cause is unknown. It's found worldwide and can occur at any age but is most common after the second decade of life. It is known that most Hodgkin's lymphoma occurs when B cells develop a mutation in the DNA. The mutation causes a large number of oversized, abnormal B cells to accumulate in the lymphatic system, where they crowd out healthy cells and cause the signs and symptoms of Hodgkin's lymphoma.

How it happens

Lymph nodes, most typically in the chest and neck area, take a malignant turn and don't grow into normal lymphatic tissue. The malignant nodes become hard and enlarged, leading to firm-to-hard masses in the neck and chest.

Bigger isn't better

Enlargement of the lymph nodes, spleen, and other lymphoid tissues results from proliferation of lymphocytes, histiocytes and, rarely, eosinophils. Patients also have distinct chromosome abnormalities in their lymph node cells.

What to look for

Hard, swollen lymph nodes of the supraclavicular, axillary, or groin areas that aren't erythematous or tender are classic characteristics of Hodgkin's lymphoma. Imaging tests used to diagnose Hodgkin's lymphoma include X-rays, computed tomography (CT) scan, magnetic resonance imaging (MRI), and positron emission tomography (PET).

Spreading swelling

The painless swelling of the lymph nodes progresses to the axillary, inguinal, mediastinal, and mesenteric regions. (See *Staging Hodgkin's lymphoma.*)

In addition to the symptoms of the primary disease, secondary symptoms associated with Hodgkin's lymphoma (any of which warrants bone marrow biopsy to assess for more extensive disease) may include:
- unexplained fever above 100.4° F (38° C)
- night sweats without fever
- unexplained weight loss of more than 10% of total body weight in the previous 6 months
- severe pruritus causing skin excoriation.

What tests tell you

CBC is usually normal unless the child has anemia from malnutrition or bone marrow involvement. The erythrocyte sedimentation rate (ESR) may be elevated, but this test is nonspecific and ESR may be elevated with any infection. Bone marrow biopsy may rule out or confirm metastatic disease.

Staging Hodgkin's lymphoma

Treatment of Hodgkin's lymphoma depends on its stage (the number, location, and degree of involved lymph nodes). The Ann Arbor classification system, adopted in 1971, divides Hodgkin's lymphoma into four stages, which are then subdivided into categories. Category A includes patients without defined signs and symptoms, and category B includes patients who experience such defined signs as recent, unexplained weight loss, fever, and night sweats.

Stage I
Hodgkin's lymphoma appears in a single lymph node region or a single extralymphatic organ.

Stage II
Hodgkin's lymphoma appears in two or more nodes on the same side of the diaphragm and in an extralymphatic organ.

Stage III
Hodgkin's lymphoma spreads to both sides of the diaphragm and, perhaps, to an extralymphatic organ, the spleen, or both.

Stage IV
Hodgkin's lymphoma disseminates, involving one or more extralymphatic organ or tissues, with or without associated lymph node involvement.

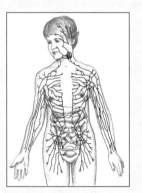
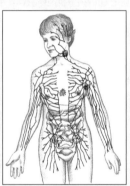
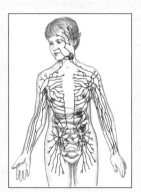
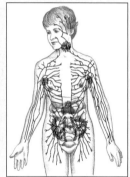

Verify, then confirm

Chest radiography that verifies the presence of a mediastinal mass remains the easiest way to confirm the diagnosis, but further evaluation with enhanced CT scanning or MRI will confirm the presence of other enlarged nodes throughout the body. Bone, liver, and spleen scans may help determine whether metastatic disease is present.

It's a hoot!

A lymphangiogram has historically been used to identify enlarged nodes but is less valuable now that improved radiologic studies are available. The diagnosis must be confirmed by lymph node biopsy showing the presence of *Reed-Sternberg cell* (a double nucleus cell that looks like an owl) or malignant lymphatic tissue consistent with a histologic type of Hodgkin's lymphoma.

> Chest X-ray makes diagnosis of a mediastinal mass a snap. CT scanning and MRI can confirm enlarged nodes in other areas.

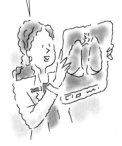

Complications

Hodgkin's lymphoma will cause enlarging nodes that may restrict lung movement and create respiratory distress. The nodes may also press against the heart, causing cardiac arrhythmias if the mass is large and untreated. Metastatic disease may cause anemia and decreased blood counts if bone marrow disease is extensive. It may invade and compromise bone, the liver, or the spleen.

When treatment gets complicated

Today, most complications are related more to therapy, with short- and long-term consequences:
• Short-term radiation may cause severe, localized skin reactions, although usually less severe than those seen in adult malignancies as doses are lower in children.
• Immunosuppression with decreased ability to fight all types of infection is common with decreased blood counts from chemotherapy.
• Anemia is common, although transfusion may not be required.
• Lowered platelet counts are seen but usually aren't severe and rarely cause major bleeding problems. If the platelet count is below 60,000/mm^3 or hemoglobin is below 8 g/dl, transfusion with a specific blood product may be considered.

Long-term legacy

One of the most severe, long-term problems of Hodgkin's lymphoma is secondary malignancies, which develop in up to 5% of long-term survivors. Acute myelocytic leukemia is the most common. Sterility is another severe long-term complication and is caused by chemotherapeutic agents. Radiation may cause decreased bone and tissue growth, which can be a major cause of scoliosis and kyphosis in childhood survivors.

> Combination therapy with the COPP/MOPP protocol is the mainstay of chemotherapy for Hodgkin's lymphoma. COPP = cyclophosphamide [or mechlorethamine (MOPP)], Oncovin, procarbazine, and prednisone.

How it's treated

Hodgkin's disease was one of the first malignancies to demonstrate the superiority of treatment with multiple chemotherapeutic agents (versus a single agent).

Mopping the floor with Hodgkin's

The mechlorethamine, Oncovin (vincristine), procarbazine, and prednisone (MOPP) research protocol of the mid-1960s immediately changed the prognosis for Hodgkin's disease to a survival rate of more than 50% in adults and children. The drugs from the MOPP protocol remain staples of therapy, although the less toxic cyclophosphamide (Cytoxan) may be used in place of mechlorethamine in children. Several other drugs may be effective, including doxorubicin (Adriamycin), bleomycin (Blenoxane), and vinblastine (Velban).

What to do

Care of children with malignancies is usually coordinated through one of several pediatric oncology centers. Nursing care is based on the treatment protocol and understanding the adverse effects of the drugs and therapies used:
• Watch for and promptly report adverse effects of radiation and chemotherapy (particularly anorexia, nausea, vomiting, diarrhea, fever, and bleeding).
• Minimize adverse effects of radiation therapy by maintaining good nutrition, encouraging fluid intake, pacing activities to counteract therapy-induced fatigue, and keeping the skin dry in irradiated areas.
• Prepare the child (and his parents) for all tests and treatments, including adverse effects of therapy. Encourage the child to express his feelings, which may include fear and anger.
• Provide emotional support and offer appropriate reassurance. Make sure the family knows that the local chapter of the American Cancer Society is available for information, financial assistance, and supportive counseling.

Iron deficiency anemia

Iron deficiency anemia is a disorder of oxygen transport in which the amount of hemoglobin circulating in the blood is inadequate. Without sufficient iron, the body can't produce the hemoglobin molecule because the heme component is primarily iron.

Some heavy competition

Excesses of other heavy metals (such as lead) may compete for iron-binding sites and cause a lack of hemoglobin that may lead to iron deficiency. Iron deficiency anemia is most common in the youngest and oldest children in the pediatric age range (infants and toddlers, and adolescents).

Heavy metals compete for iron-binding sites and lack of hemoglobin can lead to iron deficiency. I think I'll stick with folk music!

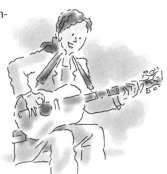

What causes it

Iron deficiency anemia can be caused by inadequate intake of iron in the diet, malabsorption of iron through the GI tract, or chronic blood loss.

A gift from mom

In the last trimester of pregnancy, the fetus draws what iron it needs from the mother. In the last month, it draws enough iron stores for approximately 6 to 12 months. If the mother is deficient in iron or the neonate is more than 4 weeks premature, the infant may not have sufficient iron stores and, eventually, becomes anemic. This condition is usually evident by 9 to 12 months of life but can occur earlier if the child is more premature, especially less than 32 weeks' gestation.

How it happens

Anytime there is blood loss, there is loss of iron. Adolescents with heavy menses are at risk for iron deficiency anemia because they lose blood during menstruation. GI bleeding can result from regular use of some over-the-counter pain relievers, especially aspirin. If too little iron is consumed, over time, children can become iron deficient. Iron from food is absorbed into the bloodstream in the small intestine. An intestinal disorder, such as celiac disease, which affects the intestine's ability to absorb nutrients from digested food, can lead to iron deficiency anemia. If part of the small intestine has been bypassed or removed surgically, that may affect the body's ability to absorb iron and other nutrients. In developing countries, a leading cause of iron deficiency is infestation from parasitic worms (hookworms, whipworms, roundworms).

> Who knew? Most of the iron used to build hemoglobin comes from the GI tract, where it's resorbed from dead RBCs.

Got milk?

Cow's milk allergy (common in Blacks and Asians), due to heat-labile protein in cow's milk, causes inflammation of the GI tract with chronic blood loss and decreased absorption. This allergy is a common source of iron deficiency anemia. In adolescents, iron deficiency anemia is commonly related to fad dieting and overconsumption of snack foods containing little or no iron.

You are what you eat

Adolescent girls are at risk for iron deficiency anemia during their growth spurt and at the beginning of menses, especially if periods are irregular. Adolescent boys are at a lower risk, although boys and girls may have poor dietary habits or eat fad diet foods. Vegetarians and vegans aren't at increased risk if they plan their diets with adequate sources of iron.

What to look for

Clinical symptoms may be mild until anemia is severe, causing a pale appearance and decreased activity. Toddlers may have a history of prematurity and poor weight gain. Other symptoms include:

- fatigue
- inability to concentrate
- palpitations
- dyspnea on exertion
- craving for nonnutritive substances such as ice, dirt, or starch
- tachycardia
- dry, brittle nails
- concave, or "spoon-shaped," fingernails.

What tests tell you

Hemoglobin, hematocrit, red cell distribution width (RDW), and ferritin tests may be used in diagnosing iron deficiency anemia. Lower than normal hemoglobin levels indicate anemia. The normal ranges for children vary depending on the child's age and sex. Hematocrit is the percentage of the blood volume made up by RBCs. Like hemoglobin, the hematocrit values differ according to the child's age. The RDW will show RBCs that are smaller and paler in color than normal cells in children with iron deficiency anemia. Ferritin is a protein that helps the body store iron. A low level of ferritin usually indicates a low level of stored iron.

Bleached out bull's eye

Iron deficiency anemia is a microcytic, hypochromic anemia, meaning the RBCs are small and pale. RBCs with decreased iron appear bleached out, resembling a bull's eye target. Because the cells are small, the mean corpuscular volume, the mean corpuscular hemoglobin, and the mean corpuscular hemoglobin concentration are low. Serum iron levels are decreased.

Complications

Untreated iron deficiency anemia can cause stress on all body tissue, with decreased oxygenation. Severe anemia poses the greatest risk to the respiratory and cardiovascular systems. Increasing evidence suggests that children with even mild iron deficiency have less ability to concentrate and greater difficulty in school. Overtreatment with replacement iron can occur when toxic levels of iron build up, which may cause excessive iron deposits, affecting the liver, heart, pituitary glands, and joints. Pica may lead to eating lead-based paint and can result in lead poisoning.

How it's treated

The main treatment is correction of the underlying problem. If chronic blood loss or GI bleeding is suspected, appropriate intervention is needed.

In with the iron

If the problem is nutritional, the child's diet should be adjusted to increase iron intake. Good sources of dietary iron include red meat, organ meat, legumes (such as kidney and pinto beans), green leafy vegetables, raisins, and dried apricots as well as iron-fortified cereals and formula. Milk has little iron and may actually cause the anemia by preventing the intake of other iron-rich foods (if the child fills up on milk).

It's supplementary, my dear Watson!

In addition to dietary changes, the child may be placed on oral iron supplementation, although iron supplements aren't absorbed as well as iron from dietary sources. The American Academy of Pediatrics recommends that children with hematocrit below 34% (hemoglobin level less than 11.3 g/dl) be placed on supplemental iron.

Ascorbic acid (vitamin C) may be added to the supplement because it helps with iron absorption. Breast milk has low levels of iron, but the iron that is present is extremely well absorbed and is adequate for most infants. If an infant is drinking formula, it should be iron-fortified.

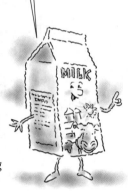

Contrary to popular belief, I'm not a good source of iron. Check back with me when you need some calcium.

What to do

Nursing care focuses on educating the parents about diet and treatment regimens:
- Monitor the child's compliance with the prescribed iron supplement therapy.
- Teach the parents of infants the importance of using iron-fortified infant cereals or iron-fortified formula.
- Teach the parent or adolescent about good iron sources in the normal diet; if the child is a vegetarian, explain the importance of incorporating iron-rich vegetable sources into the diet.
- Caution the child and parents that taking iron supplements may result in dark green or black stool; supplements can also cause constipation and this may need to be treated with prunes or a laxative.
- Make sure the parents understand the dosage and administration of oral iron supplements; stress the importance of storing the supplements safely because they're a major source of poisoning in children.
- Taking iron supplements with vitamin C sources (like orange juice) may help absorption.

Leukemia

Leukemia is cancer of the body's blood-forming tissues, including the bone marrow and the lymphatic system. Leukemia usually starts in the WBCs with an abnormal, uncontrolled overproduction of WBCs by the stem cells in bone marrow. The nonfunctional, leukemic cells infiltrate the tissues of the body and replace normal cells. Children are most commonly diagnosed with acute lymphocytic leukemia (ALL), which involves the lymphocytic WBC cell line, or acute myelogenous leukemia (AML), which involves the granulocytic-myelocytic WBC cell line.

What causes it

The exact cause of leukemia is unknown. It seems to develop from a combination of genetic and environmental factors. There's an increased incidence of ALL in children with Down syndrome (trisomy 21). Other risk factors include exposure to large doses of ionizing radiation or drugs that suppress bone marrow. Certain viruses, such as human T-cell lymphotrophic virus type I, are also associated with an increased risk for leukemia.

How it happens

Leukemia is thought to occur when some blood cells acquire mutations in their DNA. This causes a rapid production of WBCs which results in the accumulation of immature, nonfunctional cells called *blast cells*. The blast cells multiply continuously, regardless of the body's needs. However, the proliferating blast cells don't attack and destroy normal cells. Rather, they crowd out other healthy, functional cells, robbing them of nutrition essential for metabolism, leading to *pancytopenia* (reduction in the number of blood cells being produced by all cell lines).

Needed: Crowd control

Eventually, the bone marrow becomes packed with the malignant cells, and they spill out into the peripheral blood where they can be seen on microscopic slides.

In leukemia, the malignant cells crowd out my buddies—the WBCs and platelets—and me until we become the minority.

What to look for

Signs and symptoms of ALL and AML are similar and are related to suppression of elements of the bone marrow:
• RBC and platelet levels are reduced as the stem cells are no longer producing them, which leads to anemia with decreased hemoglobin.
• A low platelet count leads to bruising, bleeding, and multiple nosebleeds; minor trauma, such as bumping into furniture, may cause large bruises.
• Because the WBCs are immature and nonfunctioning, the ability to fight infection is diminished, and the child may experience high fevers and show signs of sepsis.

What tests tell you

• Blood counts show thrombocytopenia and neutropenia. The WBC count in a CBC will be very high (usually over 25,000/µl) and the differential determines cell type.
• Lumbar puncture is performed to detect meningeal involvement; cerebrospinal fluid analysis reveals abnormal WBC invasion of the central nervous system (CNS).
• Bone marrow aspiration and biopsy confirm the disease, showing mostly malignant blast cells present in large numbers. (These tests are also used to determine whether the leukemia is lymphocytic or myelogenous, which will help determine treatment and prognosis.)

Complications

Because leukemia and its treatment affect all blood cell lines and the immune system, complications vary and can be severe. Infections are of particular concern.

Fungus alert

Children on long-term immunosuppressive therapy may have overgrowth of fungal infections, such as candidiasis, or little resistance to severe fungal infections such as aspergillosis. Disruptions in the child's and the family's routine may cause major problems with school or socialization as well as stress and anxiety.

How it's treated

Both forms of acute leukemia are treated with combinations of I.V. chemotherapy drugs aimed at killing the malignant stem cells plus leukemia cells that may have migrated to other areas of the body. AML is more resistant; therefore, the treatment regimens are more severe, usually requiring more hospitalizations. Because I.V. chemotherapy can't penetrate the CNS and spinal fluid, treatment of the CNS involves intrathecal chemotherapy and low-dose radiation of the spine and head.
    Treatment may also include:
• antibiotic, antifungal, and antiviral drugs
• colony-stimulating factors, such as filgrastim (Neupogen), to spur the growth of granulocytes, RBCs, and platelets
• transfusions of platelets to prevent bleeding and RBCs to prevent anemia.

> Bone marrow transplantation improves long-term survival. Its use during remission is the standard of care for children with AML.

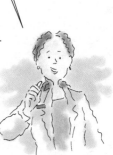

Transplant to the rescue

Bone marrow transplantation has become a standard treatment for AML when the child is in remission because a transplant improves long-term survival. In ALL, bone marrow transplantation is used after relapse if a second remission can be achieved because a relapse signifies more resistant disease.

What to do

Leukemia is a devastating diagnosis for the child and his family. The child must deal not only with the disease but also with the adverse effects of treatment. The child should be prepared for all tests and treatments, and emotional support should be offered to his family. Referral to additional support services may be needed.

In addition, follow these steps:
• Educate the child and his family about the disease and treatments (including treatment-related problems).
• Assess for bleeding, bruising, fatigue, or signs and symptoms of an impending infection.
• To control infection, place the patient in a private room and institute reverse isolation. Coordinate care so the child doesn't come in contact with staff members who also care for patients with infections or infectious diseases.
• Provide guidelines for reducing such adverse effects of chemotherapy as nausea, vomiting, and diarrhea. Make sure the parents understand how to administer medications to treat these adverse effects.
• Make the parents aware that any fever is serious and may be life-threatening; a health care provider should immediately evaluate the child with a fever.

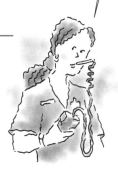

Any fever is cause for concern in a child with leukemia.

Sickle cell anemia

Sickle cell anemia is an inherited, autosomal-recessive genetic disease that affects the RBCs, which become acutely sickle-shaped. They occlude small vessels, causing pain and decreased function. The two common variants of sickle cell anemia are hemoglobin SS (Hgb SS) and hemoglobin SC (Hgb SC) disease. Symptoms are usually severe with Hgb SS and moderate or undetectable in Hgb SC.

What causes it

The child must receive the autosomal-recessive gene from both parents to have the condition. The defective hemoglobin (hemoglobin S) takes on the classic sickle shape with decreased oxygen-carrying capacity and inability to flow through capillaries. Carriers of sickle cell trait have few symptoms and only on rare occasions.

How it happens

Sickle cell anemia occurs as a result of a mutation in the gene that encodes the beta chain of hemoglobin. This mutation causes a structural change in hemoglobin. A single amino acid change from glutamic acid to valine occurs in the sixth position of the betahemoglobin chain.

Hemoglobin S is for sickle

When hypoxia (oxygen deficiency) occurs, the hemoglobin S in the RBCs becomes insoluble. As a result, the blood cells become rigid and rough, forming an elongated crescent, or sickle, shape. Sickling can cause hemolysis (cell destruction).

Capillary traffic jam

Sickle cells accumulate in capillaries and smaller blood vessels, causing occlusions and increasing blood viscosity. This increased viscosity impairs normal circulation, causing pain, tissue infarctions (tissue death), swelling, and anoxic changes that lead to further sickling and obstruction.

Low on O$_2$

Sickle cell crisis occurs when a patient with sickle cell anemia experiences cellular oxygen deprivation from, for example, an infection, exposure to cold or high altitude, or overexertion. A chain of events then ensues. (See *Understanding sickle cell crisis.*)

What to look for

All infants are screened for sickle cell on the newborn screening test so children with sickle cell disease and sickle cell trait should be identified early. Signs and symptoms of sickle cell anemia usually don't develop until after age 6 months because large amounts of fetal hemoglobin protect infants until then. Fetal hemoglobin has a higher oxygen concentration and inhibits sickling. Swollen hands and feet (hand-foot syndrome) may be the first signs of sickle cell anemia in babies. The swelling is caused by sickle-shaped RBCs blocking blood flow out of their hands and feet. Periodic episodes of pain, called sickle cell crises, are a major symptom of sickle cell anemia. Pain develops when sickle-shaped RBCs block blood flow through tiny blood vessels to the chest, abdomen, and joints. Sickle cells can damage the spleen, an important organ in fighting infection—making children more vulnerable to infections. Children with sickle cell anemia usually receive prophylactic antibiotics until the age of 5 years to prevent potentially life-threatening bacterial infections. Children with sickle cell disease may have delayed growth and anemia because the sickle cells have a shortened life span compared to normal RBCs (20 days for sickle cells versus 120 days for normal RBCs).

A telling history

The patient's history includes chronic fatigue (due to chronic anemia), unexplained dyspnea or dyspnea on exertion, joint swelling, aching bones, severe localized and generalized pain, leg ulcers (rare in children), and frequent infections. Inspection of the skin

Understanding sickle cell crisis

Sickle cell crisis is triggered by infection, cold exposure, high altitudes, overexertion, dehydration, and other conditions that cause cellular oxygen deprivation. Here's what happens:
• Deoxygenated, sickle-shaped erythrocytes adhere to the capillary wall and to one another, blocking blood flow and causing cellular hypoxia.

• The crisis worsens as tissue hypoxia and acidic waste products cause more sickling and cell damage.
• With each new crisis, organs and tissues are destroyed and areas of tissue die slowly (especially in the spleen and kidneys).

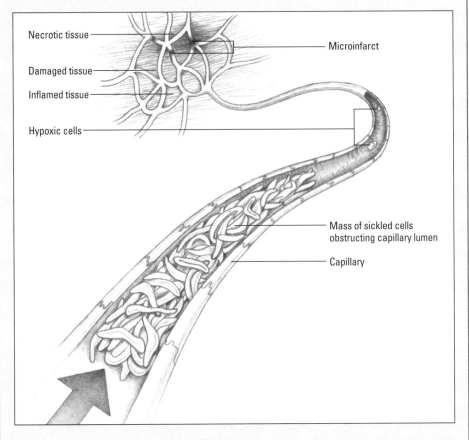

Necrotic tissue

Damaged tissue

Inflamed tissue

Hypoxic cells

Microinfarct

Mass of sickled cells obstructing capillary lumen

Capillary

may reveal jaundice or pallor. A young child may appear small for his age. The spleen will usually be enlarged and palpable.

Sickle cell crisis

In sickle cell crisis, symptoms include severe pain, hematuria, lethargy, irritability, and pale lips, tongue, palms, and nail beds.

Isn't one enough?

Four different types of crisis can occur:

In *painful crisis*, patients report severe abdominal, thoracic, muscle, or bone pain and, possibly, increased jaundice, dark urine, or a low-grade fever.

Aplastic crisis results from bone marrow depression and is characterized by pallor, lethargy, sleepiness, dyspnea, markedly decreased bone marrow activity, RBC hemolysis, and possible coma.

Acute sequestration crisis, occurring in infants, may cause sudden, massive entrapment of RBCs in the spleen and liver; if untreated, lethargy and pallor progress to hypovolemic shock and death.

Hemolytic crisis results from complications of the disease rather than the disease itself; degenerative changes cause liver congestion and enlargement, and chronic jaundice develops and worsens. The spleen is often nonfunctioning from being infarcted by sickle cells.

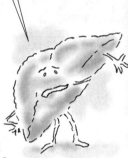

Being trapped inside me definitely qualifies as a crisis—an acute sequestration crisis, to be specific.

What tests tell you

• Hemoglobin levels will be low, and sickle cells will be seen on microscopic slide.
• Additional blood tests show low RBC counts, elevated WBC and platelet counts, a decreased ESR, increased serum iron levels, decreased RBC survival, and reticulocytosis.
• Genetic tests will help identify the status of the parents and can be used to assess sibling status. Because of the importance of early diagnosis, it has become standard for all neonates to be tested at birth for both carrier and disease state.

Complications

Clinical manifestations of sickle cell anemia vary, resulting in a wide range of complications related to occlusion of the blood vessels. Complications include stroke, acute chest syndrome, organ damage, retinal damage/blindness, and priapism. A stroke can occur if the sickle cells block blood flow to the brain. Acute chest syndrome is a life-threatening complication of sickle cell anemia that causes chest pain, fever, and difficulty breathing. Acute chest syndrome can be caused by a lung infection or by sickle cells blocking blood vessels in the lungs. It may require emergency medical treatment with antibiotics and other treatments.

Sickle cells can block blood flow through blood vessels, immediately depriving an organ of blood and oxygen. Chronic deprivation of oxygen-rich blood can damage nerves and organs, including the kidneys, liver, and spleen. Organ damage can be fatal.

The blood vessels that supply the eyes can get blocked by sickle cells and, over time, can damage the retina and lead to blindness. Sickle cells can block the blood vessels in the penis. As a result, boys with sickle cell anemia may experience painful, long-lasting erections—a condition called priapism. This can damage the penis and eventually lead to impotence.

How it's treated

Bone marrow transplant offers the only potential cure for sickle cell anemia. Transplants are recommended only for people who have significant symptoms and problems from sickle cell anemia. As a result, treatment for sickle cell anemia is usually aimed at avoiding crises, relieving symptoms, and preventing complications. Treatments may include medications to reduce pain and prevent complications and blood transfusions and supplemental oxygen. To prevent life-threatening bacterial infections, children with sickle cell anemia may begin taking the antibiotic penicillin when they're about 2 months of age and continue taking it until they're 5 years old. To relieve pain during a sickle crisis, over-the-counter or prescription pain relievers may be recommended.

When taken daily, hydroxyurea reduces the frequency of painful crises and may reduce the need for blood transfusions. Hydroxyurea seems to work by stimulating production of fetal hemoglobin—a type of hemoglobin found in newborns that helps prevent the formation of sickle cells. Long-term use of hydroxyurea may increase the risk of infection. In children with sickle cell anemia at high risk of stroke, regular blood transfusions can decrease their risk of stroke but may cause an excess amount of iron to build up in the body. Excess iron can damage the heart, liver, and other organs. Therefore, people who undergo regular transfusions may need iron-chelating treatment with deferasirox (Exjade) to reduce iron levels. Because infections can be very serious in children with sickle cell anemia, children should be up-to-date on all of their immunizations.

What to do

A child who experiences the pain of a crisis will likely be fearful of future crises, as will his parents. This may have a significant impact on the child's life. He may be afraid to participate in normal activities for fear of bringing on a crisis, and his parents may become overprotective. Pain is often severe. Always believe the patient about their level of pain.

In pursuit of normal

Prevention and education are the keys to leading a normal life, and participation in a support group may be extremely helpful in this regard. To prevent sickle crisis, the goal is to maintain as high a state of oxygenation as possible:

• Be aware that excessive exercise or activity may precipitate crisis.

• Avoid tight or restricting clothes such as elastic at the end of sleeves.

• Promote relaxation and stress-reducing activities because mental stress may play a role in crisis.

• Encourage the child to attend school and social functions while being aware that he may be more susceptible to infection.

• Explain the need to avoid flying in unpressurized aircrafts.

• Stress the importance of immediate evaluation of fever; children with sickle cell anemia are functionally asplenic and are at risk for pneumococcal sepsis.

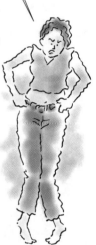

No one has to convince me that tight clothing has an adverse effect on oxygenation. Yeeouch!

Systemic lupus erythematosus

SLE is an autoimmune disease. For unknown reasons, the body turns on itself and attacks healthy cells and tissues leading to inflammation and damage.

It generally affects adolescent girls and women between ages 15 and 45, but it can be seen at other ages. Neonatal lupus is seen in infants of women with SLE. Lupus is more common in African Americans, Hispanics, and Asians.

What causes it

The exact cause of SLE is unknown, although there are likely genetic, environmental, and, possibly, hormonal influences. Exposure to ultraviolet light, infections, stress, and pregnancy are known precipitating factors.

How it happens

The formation of autoantibodies in lupus occurs for unknown reasons. These autoantibodies join together with antigens to form soluble immune complexes and are deposited in multiple body tissues, including the skin, joints, lungs, heart, kidneys, brain, and blood vessels.

A complex reaction

Symptoms appear due to inflammatory reactions and tissue damage that occur after the deposition of these immune complexes. Defects in the body's production of complement and cellular and humoral responses cause increased B-lymphocyte production and autoantibody reactions against T-lymphocytes, rendering them ineffective.

What to look for

SLE is a multisystem inflammatory disease of the joints, serous linings, kidneys, skin, and CNS; therefore, symptoms may be widespread. Symptoms vary depending on the severity of the organ involvement. Common findings include:
• painful and swollen joints
• muscle pain
• unexplained fever
• extreme fatigue
• weight loss
• alopecia
• skin rashes, including the characteristic "butterfly" (malar) rash over both cheeks and the nasal bridge, which are extremely sensitive to sun
• peripheral vasospasm (Raynaud's phenomenon).

Getting involved

As the disease progresses, systemic involvement increases. Hepatosplenomegaly and lymphadenopathy may occur. Inflammation of the lung and heart linings may cause chest pain and dyspnea. CNS involvement can produce seizures, coma, hemiplegia, and behavioral disturbances, including psychosis. Renal SLE can progress rapidly and is the leading cause of death in people affected with this disease.

What tests tell you

Antinuclear antibody test (ANA) is positive in patients who have active untreated disease; however, a negative test doesn't completely exclude SLE. A CBC may be ordered. People with lupus are prone to developing anemia. Low WBC counts and low platelets may also occur. Kidney and liver function tests may be ordered to assess the function of these organs because they can be adversely affected by lupus.
• ESR is usually elevated; anemia, leukopenia, and thrombocytopenia are commonly seen.
• Proteinuria may be noted on urinalysis and is one of the initial signs of renal involvement.
• Imaging tests such as a chest X-ray and echocardiogram may be ordered. A chest X-ray may reveal inflammation in the lungs and an echocardiogram may reveal problem with heart valves that may be associated with lupus. CT scan or MRI may identify pathologic conditions of the brain due to SLE.

Complications

Complications from SLE are commonly related to inflammation and treatment. The inflammation can affect many parts of the body including the kidneys, brain, blood vessels, heart, and lungs. Lupus can cause serious kidney damage, and kidney failure is one of the leading causes of death among people with lupus. Many people with lupus experience memory problems and may have difficulty expressing their thoughts.

Lupus may lead to blood problems, including anemia and increased risk of bleeding or blood clotting. It can also cause vasculitis (inflammation of the blood vessels). Having lupus increases the chances of developing an inflammation of the chest cavity lining (pleurisy). Lupus can also cause pericarditis (inflammation of the heart muscle, arteries, or heart membrane). The risk of cardiovascular disease and heart attacks is increased in patients with lupus.

People with lupus are more vulnerable to infection because both the disease and its treatments weaken the immune system. Infections that most commonly affect people with lupus include urinary tract infections, respiratory infections, yeast infections, salmonella, herpes, and shingles. Toxicity from the medications can cause growth failure, adrenal suppression, Cushing's syndrome, osteoporosis, and aseptic necrosis. Liver damage and bone marrow suppression can occur with immunosuppressant use. Retinal damage may occur with the use of hydroxychloroquine (Plaquenil). Amenorrhea may result either from the disease itself or from the medications used to treat it.

How it's treated

Although SLE can't be cured, people with the disease can achieve remission and lead a high-quality life. Treatment may include drugs and other approaches:
- Corticosteroids are a mainstay of SLE treatment; they've been shown to significantly reduce mortality and should be used in all patients with renal, cardiac, and CNS involvement. Side effects include weight gain, easy bruising, thinning bones (osteoporosis), high blood pressure, diabetes, and increased risk of infection.
- Immunosuppressants may be added if disease control is inadequate with steroids. Potential side effects may include an increased risk of infection, liver damage, decreased fertility, and an increased risk of cancer.
- Anti-inflammatory medications, such as NSAIDs and cyclooxygenase-2 (COX-2) inhibitors, may be used to help decrease pain and inflammation associated with SLE.

As a corticosteroid, I'm the go-to guy for treatment of SLE.

• Hydroxychloroquine is an antimalarial drug used to treat the inflammation associated with this disease. Side effects can include GI upset and, very rarely, damage to the retina.
• Holistic treatment approaches include fostering healthy behaviors, such as diet, rest, and exercise.

What to do

Nursing care aims to promote the best possible outcome for the child with a chronic illness. Interventions are directed toward preventing flare-ups, maintaining growth and development, preventing infection, and preserving skin integrity. In children with lupus, the nurse should:
• Teach the child to avoid such precipitating factors as sun exposure and stress.
• Promote self-esteem, especially in adolescents. The use of hypoallergenic make-up, wigs, and other aids will help cover up the disfiguring effects of this disease.
• Instruct the child to layer clothing and use mittens and sock liners to help decrease the discomfort associated with Raynaud's phenomenon.
• If needed, refer the child and her family to support groups or for mental health treatment to help them cope with the diagnosis.

Thalassemia

Thalassemia is an inherited blood disorder characterized by less hemoglobin and fewer RBCs in the body than normal. Several types of thalassemia exist, including alpha-thalassemia, beta-thalassemia, Cooley's anemia, and Mediterranean anemia.

Phi beta defective synthesis

Beta-thalassemia is the most common form of this disorder, resulting from defective beta-polypeptide chain synthesis. It occurs in three clinical forms: major, intermedia, and minor, and the prognosis depends on which form of beta-thalassemia the child has.
• Children with *thalassemia major* may survive into adulthood but generally have reduced life spans.
• Children with *thalassemia intermedia* develop normally into adulthood, although puberty is usually delayed.
• People with *thalassemia minor* can expect a normal life span. (See *Ethnicity and thalassemia*.)

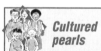

Cultured pearls

Ethnicity and thalassemia

Thalassemia is most common in people of Mediterranean ancestry (especially Italians and Greeks) but also occurs in people from southern China, India, and Southeast Asia.

What causes it

Thalassemia major and thalassemia intermedia result from homozygous inheritance of the partially dominant autosomal gene responsible for this trait. Thalassemia minor results from heterozygous inheritance of the same gene.

How it happens

In each disorder, total or partial deficiency of beta-polypeptide chain production impairs hemoglobin synthesis and results in continual production of fetal hemoglobin, lasting even past the neonatal period.

What to look for

In thalassemia major, the infant is well at birth but develops severe anemia, bone abnormalities, failure to thrive, and life-threatening complications. In many cases, the first signs are pallor and yellow skin and sclera in infants ages 3 to 6 months.

Large but not in charge

Later clinical features include splenomegaly or hepatomegaly with abdominal enlargement, frequent infections, bleeding tendencies, and anorexia. These signs and symptoms are also found:
• Children usually have small bodies and large heads.
• If untreated, older children may have an enlarged maxilla, depressed bridge of the nose, and protruding lips.
• Children become susceptible to pathologic bone fractures as well as cardiac arrhythmias, heart failure, and other complications that result from iron deposits in the heart and other tissues due to repeated blood transfusions.
• Patients with thalassemia intermedia show some degree of anemia, jaundice, and splenomegaly; thalassemia minor may cause mild anemia but usually produces no symptoms and is commonly overlooked.

What tests tell you

Hemoglobin levels and RBC counts are low, and reticulocyte and bilirubin levels are elevated. X-rays of the skull and long bones show thinning and widening of the marrow space because of overactive bone marrow. (See *Skull changes in thalassemia major.*) Quantitative hemoglobin studies show a significant rise in hemoglobin F. With prolonged disease, there may be increased levels of serum ferritin from RBC lysis and chronic transfusion.

Complications

Possible complications of thalassemia include iron overload and infection. People with thalassemia can get too much iron

---

Skull changes in thalassemia major

This illustration of an X-ray shows a characteristic skull abnormality in thalassemia major: diploetic fibers extending from internal lamina, resembling hair standing on end.

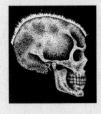

in their bodies, either from the disease itself or from frequent blood transfusions. Too much iron can result in damage to the heart, liver, and endocrine system. They also have an increased risk of infection—especially if they have had a splenectomy. In cases of severe thalassemia, children can develop bone deformities, splenomegaly, slowed growth, and heart problems. Thalassemia can cause the bone marrow to expand, which causes bones to widen. This can result in abnormal bone structure, especially in the face and skull. Bone marrow expansion also makes bones thin and brittle, increasing the chance of fractures. Splenomegaly can worsen anemia by reducing the life of RBCs. Some patients may require a splenectomy. Anemia can contribute to a decreased rate of growth. Puberty also may be delayed in children with thalassemia. Heart problems such as congestive heart failure and arrhythmias may be associated with severe thalassemia.

How it's treated

Thalassemia intermedia and thalassemia minor generally don't require treatment. Treatment for thalassemia major generally involves repeated packed RBC transfusions to maintain higher hemoglobin levels. Transfusions may be needed as frequently as every 3 weeks. A stem cell transplant may be used to treat severe thalassemia in select cases.

Don't overdo it!

These transfusions must be administered judiciously to minimize iron overload. Deferoxamine (Desferal) is a chelating agent commonly given to eliminate excess iron from the body. Increased demand for folic acid requires supplements to help maintain normal levels.

What to do

Provide emotional support to the parents; encourage them to express their feelings and concerns and make sure that their questions are answered. Explain all tests and procedures. In addition, follow these steps:
• Monitor for adverse reactions during packed RBC transfusions, such as fever, chills, and irritability.
• Make the parents aware of the inherited nature of the disorder so they can seek genetic counseling.
• Educate the parents on the nature of the disease and the symptoms of low hemoglobin, such as fatigue and paleness, and the risk of failure to thrive.
• Encourage a normal lifestyle to the extent possible.
• Provide education about adequate diets, which can reduce the risk of further complications, including anemia and growth problems.

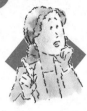

Quick quiz

1. The main function of platelets is to:
   A. provide oxygen to tissue.
   B. fight viral infections and provide immunity.
   C. fight bacterial infections.
   D. form a blood clot.

Answer: D. Platelets adhere to one another and plug holes in vessels or tissues where there's bleeding.

2. Which type of cell induces cell-mediated immunity?
   A. T lymphocytes
   B. Monocytes
   C. Reticulocytes
   D. B lymphocytes

Answer: A. T lymphocytes and macrophages are the chief participants in cell-mediated immunity.

3. What causes ALL?
   A. RBCs are defective and can't fight infection.
   B. Bone marrow stem cells are defective and produce ineffective blast cells.
   C. WBCs mature into only one cell line and fight only one type of infection.
   D. Platelets can't form clots, leading to severe hemorrhaging.

Answer: B. Stem cells start to produce nonfunctional blast cells for no apparent reason. The blast cells compete with and deprive normal cells of their essential nutrients and gradually replace them.

4. An example of a type I hypersensitivity reaction is:
   A. anaphylaxis.
   B. transfusion reaction.
   C. autoimmune disorder.
   D. GVHD.

Answer: A. Examples of type I hypersensitivity reactions are anaphylaxis, hay fever (allergic rhinitis) and, in some cases, asthma.

Scoring

✩✩✩ If you answered all four items correctly, bravo! You're obviously immune to incorrect answers.

✩✩ If you answered three items correctly, great work! Your knowledge of hematologic and immunologic systems is

✩ coursing through your blood.

If you answered fewer than three items correctly, don't have an adverse reaction. There's only one more quiz to go!

Dermatologic problems

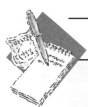

Just the facts

In this chapter, you'll learn:

♦ anatomy and physiology of the integumentary system

♦ tests used to diagnose dermatologic problems in children

♦ treatments and procedures for children with skin problems

♦ dermatologic disorders that may affect infants, children, and adolescents.

Anatomy and physiology

The integumentary system, which consists of the skin and its components, is the largest organ system in the body. At birth, the skin is only 1 mm thick; the dermal layer of the skin doubles in thickness at maturity.

The great protector

The skin protects most of the other organ systems by acting as a mechanical barrier. Other functions include sensory perception, temperature regulation, vitamin synthesis, and excretion of wastes through sweating.

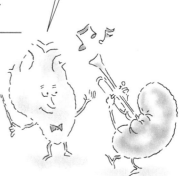

This one's for you, Mr. Skin—our protector and barrier to the outside world. Without you, we'd be out there for the whole world to see!

Structures of the skin

The skin is composed of layers of tissue. Appendages of the skin include the hair and glands.

Skin layers

The skin consists of two layers and a sublayer, the hypodermis or subcutaneous tissue:
• The *epidermis*, or outermost covering, provides a protective barrier to external trauma and limits the loss

of body contents to the environment; dermatologic problems are characteristically evident on the epidermis.
• The *dermis* consists of connective tissue that gives the skin strength and elasticity; it contains blood vessels, lymphatics, and nerves.
• The *hypodermis* lies below the dermis and is composed of loose connective tissue, or *adipose tissue.* It contains larger blood vessels, lymph channels, and nerve trunks. This layer attaches the skin to the underlying bones, acts as a cushion and temperature insulator, and determines the skin's contours. (See *Structure of the skin.*)

Thin-skinned

Skin layers act to prevent water loss, which varies with environmental temperature and humidity as well as the proportion of body surface exposed. Thus, fluid loss in the preterm neonate is greater than in an adult because the neonate's skin is thinner.

Hair

Hair changes markedly during the stages of development.

Fetal comb-over

Fine body hair, or *lanugo*, is found in utero over most of the fetus but decreases as the fetus approaches full-term. The neonate's scalp hair varies greatly in amount and is usually lost before growth of permanent hair, which gradually thickens.

Growth spurt

Puberty causes additional growth of hair in the axilla and pubic regions of both genders; boys experience facial hair growth.

Glands

The main glands of the skin are:
• *sebaceous glands*, or sebum-producing glands, which contain the hair follicles and keep the skin supple by minimizing water loss. They're more prevalent on the scalp, forehead, nose, chin, and genitalia.
• *sweat glands*, which may be *eccrine* (function as the body's heat-regulating mechanism by producing sweat) or *apocrine* (mature at puberty and cause the unpleasant body odor associated with sweating).

Structure of the skin

Major components of the skin include the epidermis, dermis, and epidermal appendages (hair and glands).

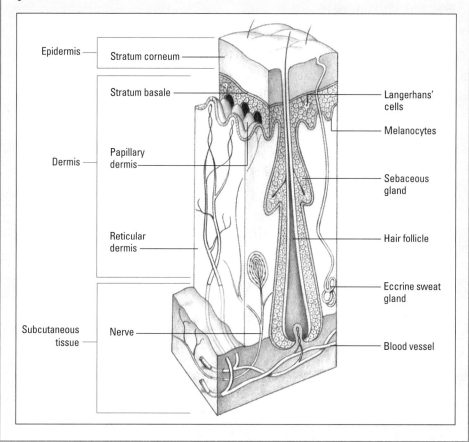

Epidermis

Stratum corneum

Stratum basale

Langerhans' cells

Melanocytes

Papillary dermis

Dermis

Sebaceous gland

Reticular dermis

Hair follicle

Eccrine sweat gland

Subcutaneous tissue

Nerve

Blood vessel

Diagnostic tests

Various tests are used to help diagnose skin problems and related systemic diseases and to identify the causes of the disorder.

Potassium hydroxide preparation

Potassium hydroxide (KOH) preparation is an alkalinizing agent that's used to prepare clinical specimens for microscopic examination needed to help diagnose fungal disorders.

Fungus finder

A drop of 20% KOH is added to skin scrapings to dissolve debris before the scrapings are placed on a slide. When the slide is heated, the skin cells dissolve, leaving fungal elements visible on microscopic examination.

Nursing considerations

Explain the procedure to the parents and the child. Tell the child what to expect, including discomfort he may experience, and suggest coping strategies such as distraction techniques.

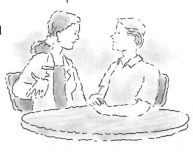

There's no closer shave than a shave biopsy! The part of the growth that protrudes is shaved off at skin level.

Skin biopsy

Skin biopsy is the removal of a section or an entire lesion for microscopic analysis to determine its cell structure and make a diagnosis. (See *Recognizing skin lesions*.) A skin biopsy specimen can be obtained by:
• shave biopsy
• punch biopsy
• excisional biopsy.

The closest shave

In a shave biopsy, the protruding portion of the growth is excised at skin level and the specimen is sent for microscopic examination.

Pulled and punched

In a punch biopsy, the skin surrounding the lesion is pulled taut, and the punch is introduced firmly into the lesion. The punch is then rotated to obtain a tissue specimen, or *plug*. The plug is lifted with forceps or a needle and the surgeon severs as deeply as possible into the fat layer. The wound is then sutured closed.

Out, out, darn lesion

In an excisional biopsy, a scalpel is used to excise the lesion completely.

Nursing considerations

Explain the procedure to the parents and child. Tell the child what to expect, including discomfort he may experience, and suggest coping strategies such as distraction techniques.

Post punch, shave, and excise

After the procedure:
• Apply a pressure dressing to the site.
• Observe the site for bleeding.
• Administer analgesics for pain as ordered.

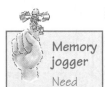

Memory jogger

Need help remembering what to assess when evaluating a skin lesion? Just think about your ABCDs.

Asymmetry

Border

Color and configuration

Diameter and drainage.

Recognizing skin lesions

These illustrations depict the most common primary and secondary skin lesions.

Macule
Flat, pigmented, circumscribed area less than 1 cm in diameter (freckle, rubella, petechiae)

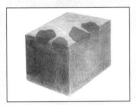

Patch
Flat, pigmented, circumscribed area more than 1 cm in diameter (herald patch [pityriasis rosea], Mongolian spots, vitiligo)

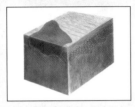

Wheal
Raised, firm lesion with intense localized skin edema, varying in size and shape; color ranging from pale pink to red, disappears in hours (hive [urticaria], insect bite)

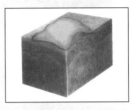

Vesicle
Raised, circumscribed, fluid-filled lesion less than 0.5 cm in diameter (chickenpox, herpes simplex)

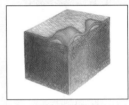

Papule
Firm, inflammatory, raised lesion up to 0.5 cm in diameter, may be same color as skin or pigmented (acne papule, lichen planus, wart, basal cell carcinoma)

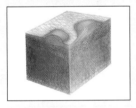

Nodule
Firm, raised lesion; deeper than a papule, extending into the dermal layer; 0.5 to 2 cm in diameter (intradermal nevus, keloid, lipoma)

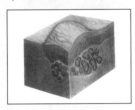

Comedo
Plugged pilosebaceous duct, exfoliative, formed from sebum and keratin (blackhead [open comedo], whitehead [closed comedo])

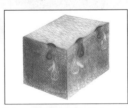

Pustule
Raised, circumscribed lesion usually less than 1 cm in diameter; containing purulent material that makes it a yellow-white color (acne pustule, impetigo, furuncle)

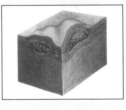

Plaque
Circumscribed, solid, elevated lesion more than 1 cm in diameter; elevation above skin surface occupies larger surface area compared with height (psoriasis, mycosis fungoides)

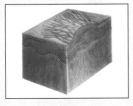

Tumor
Elevated, solid lesion more than 2 cm in diameter, extending into dermal and subcutaneous layers (dermatofibroma, hemangioma)

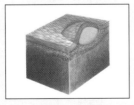

Cyst
Semisolid or fluid-filled encapsulated mass extending deep into the dermis (sebaceous cyst, cystic acne)

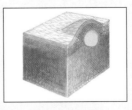

Bulla
Fluid-filled lesion more than 2 cm in diameter; also called a *blister* (severe poison oak or ivy dermatitis, bullous pemphigoid, second-degree burn)

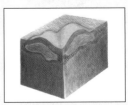

(continued)

Recognizing skin lesions (continued)

Atrophy
Thinning of skin surface at site of disorder (striae, aging skin)

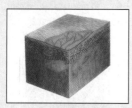

Scale
Thin, dry flakes of shedding skin (psoriasis, dry skin, newborn desquamation)

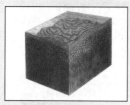

Excoriation
Linear scratched or abraded area, usually self-induced (abraded acne, eczema)

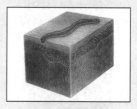

Lichenification
Thickened, prominent skin markings from constant rubbing (chronic atopic dermatitis)

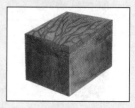

Erosion
Circumscribed lesion involving loss of superficial epidermis (rug burn, abrasion)

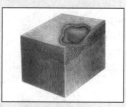

Crust
Dried sebum, serous, sanguineous, or purulent exudate overlying an erosion or weeping vesicle, bulla, or pustule (impetigo, secondarily infected dermatitis)

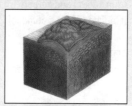

Fissure
Linear cracking of the skin extending into the dermal layer (hand dermatitis [chapped skin], interdigital tinea pedis)

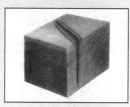

Scar
Fibrous tissue caused by trauma, deep inflammation, or surgical incision; red and raised (recent), pink and flat (6 weeks), and depressed (old) (on a healed surgical incision)

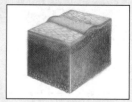

Ulcer
Epidermal and dermal destruction may extend into subcutaneous tissue; usually heals with scarring (pressure ulcer)

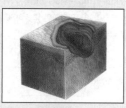

Tzanck test

Tzanck test is a microscopic examination of cells taken from skin lesions to aid in the diagnosis of vesicular diseases. Cells are scraped from the base of a vesicle to obtain moist, cloudy debris, or *exudate*. The cells are then placed on a slide, air-dried, and stained with Wright's or Giemsa stain. Multinucleated giant cells are indicative of either herpesvirus or varicella.

Nursing considerations

Explain the procedure to the parents and the child. Tell the child what to expect, including discomfort he may experience, and suggest coping strategies such as distraction techniques.

Treatments and procedures

Management of skin disorders may include a variety of therapeutic procedures, including laser surgery and skin grafting.

Laser surgery

Laser is the common term for light amplification by simulated emission of radiation. Lasers are used in surgery to divide adhesions or to treat lesions of the skin. The most common types of lasers used are the pulsed dye laser, the argon laser, and the carbon dioxide laser, each of which emits light at a different wavelength.

Complications

Complications associated with laser surgery include secondary infections, keloid or pyrogenic granuloma formation, localized dermatitis, and hyperpigmentation or hypopigmentation.

Nursing considerations

Explain the procedure to the parents and the child and prepare the child for discomfort he may experience. Make sure to prepare the child (and the parents) for the appearance of the treated area after laser surgery because it will probably look much worse than it does before treatment (some laser treatments leave skin raw and oozing). Reassure the child that this is normal and the area will heal quickly.

After the laser

After laser surgery:
• Apply dressings as ordered.
• Instruct the parents in care of the treated area.

• Stress to the child and parents the importance of avoiding trauma to the lesion or picking at the scab.

Skin grafting

During skin grafting, a section of skin is separated from its blood supply and implanted over an area where skin has been lost due to burns, injury, or surgical debridement of diseased tissue.

'Tis better to give than receive

The area from which the skin is removed is referred to as the *donor site*. For donor areas in which appearance or joint movement is important, the graft is transplanted intact. In flat areas where appearance is less critical, the graft may be meshed (fenestrated) to cover up to three times its original size. It's then placed on what's known as the *recipient site*.

A healthy loan

Skin from the patient's own healthy skin (autograft) may be used. If an autograft isn't available, a *homograft* (cadaver skin) or *xenograft* (pigskin) may be surgically attached.

Keys to success

The skin graft may be a *split-thickness graft* (involving the epidermis and superficial dermis) or a *full-thickness graft* (involving the epidermis and all layers of dermis). To be successful, grafts must have a sufficient blood supply, have contact with the recipient area, be free from infection and mechanical trauma, and have minimal bleeding or fluid accumulation.

Nursing considerations

Explain the procedure to the parents and the child. Prepare the child for the postgrafting appearance of the donor site and the recipient site. Reassure the child that the sites will heal, but tell him that this may take some time.

After graft

After grafting, follow these steps:
• Observe the donor and graft sites dressings for fluid drainage and odor; if these occur, notify the doctor.
• Observe the child for pain at the graft sites because this may indicate infection.
• Monitor the child's temperature every 4 hours because a rise in temperature may also indicate the present of infection.
• Instruct the parents on the care of the donor and recipient sites and include them in the child's care as much as possible (including dressing changes).

• Teach parents to recognize the signs of infection (such as pain, a rise in temperature, fluid drainage and odor) and instruct them to report these signs immediately.
• Stress to the parents (and the child) the importance of protecting the donor and recipient sites from trauma.
• Encourage the parent to hold and comfort the child despite the presence of the bulky dressings; reassure them that the dressings allow them to hold their child without hurting him.

> After skin grafting, the parents may need to be reassured that holding and cuddling their child won't hurt him.

Dermatologic disorders

Dermatologic disorders that may affect children and adolescents include acne, burns, contact dermatitis, and scabies.

Acne

Acne is a chronic skin disorder of the *pilosebaceous unit*, which consists of sebaceous glands that produce sebum (an oily substance) and open onto the skin surface. Comedones, pustules, nodules, and nodular lesions characterize this inflammatory disease.

Facing up to acne

Acne is the most prevalent pediatric skin condition especially among adolescents and is typically observed on the face, chest, upper arms and back, and neck, where a large number of sebaceous glands are located. It appears predominantly during middle to late adolescence often paralleling puberty and with a peak incidence at ages 16 to 17 in girls and ages 17 to 18 in boys. It's a common skin problem in all ethnic populations and affects males more severely than females. Neonatal acne takes approximately 1 month to resolve spontaneously.

Lasting legacy

Even though acne is self-limiting, the psychosocial impact and significance of acne on the quality of life of adolescents can have a negative effect on their self-esteem.

What causes it

Although the exact etiologic mechanism remains unknown, many factors affect the pathogenesis of the inflammatory response that's evident in acne:
• Androgenous hormones play a role in the development of acne; circulating androgens stimulate the production of sebum.
• Many adolescent girls have an increased incidence of acne before their menstrual periods, also suggesting a hormonal link.

- Genetic factors seem to play a role because acne appears to run in families.
- Certain medications are known to aggravate acne, including corticosteroids, phenytoin, lithium, androgens, and hormonal contraceptives containing norethindrone and norgestrel.
- Adolescents commonly cite stress as a precipitating factor, but there's no evidence of a clear association.
- Ingestion of specific foods, such as chocolate, hasn't been found to be associated with the tendency to develop acne.

> Go ahead— indulge! Contrary to popular belief, there's no evidence linking chocolate, nuts, fried foods, or carbonated beverages to the tendency to develop or increase the severity of acne.

How it happens

Acne results from a combination of factors causing a keratin plug to develop within the follicular canal that opens onto the skin's surface.

During adolescence, androgens stimulate sebaceous gland growth and production of sebum, which is secreted into dilated hair follicles that contain bacteria. The resulting environment permits the overgrowth of gram-positive bacteria known as *Propionibacterium acnes* and *Staphylococcus epidermidis*.

Volcanic eruption

Continued accumulation of follicular contents results in perforation of the follicular wall; the contents leak into surrounding tissue and cause an inflammatory reaction and the characteristic skin lesions of acne.

What to look for

Patients with acne usually exhibit two types of lesions:

Noninflammatory lesions consist of *closed comedones* (whiteheads) or *open comedones* (blackheads).

Inflammatory lesions consist of papules, pustules, and nodules or cysts that may result in permanent scarring of the skin.

> It figures! A pimple's favorite place to be is where everyone can see.

In full view

Inspection reveals acne lesions, most commonly on the face, neck, shoulders, chest, and upper back. The area around the infected follicle may appear red and swollen. The rupture or leakage of an enlarged plug into the dermis produces inflammation and characteristic acne pustules, papules, or, in severe forms, acne cysts or abscesses. If the patient has previously picked or squeezed the lesions, scars may be visible.

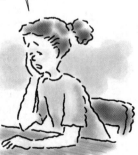

Acne classification

Classification of acne is based on the type of lesions observed. *Mild acne* involves primarily noninflammatory lesions with or without a limited number of inflammatory papules or pustules. *Moderate acne* involves noninflammatory lesions with more inflammatory papules and pustules present. Scarring is usually nonexistent or mild. *Severe acne* involves noninflammatory lesions along with numerous extensive inflammatory papules, pustules, and nodules. Scarring is more prevalent and usually dictates oral therapy.

What tests tell you

The diagnosis of acne is typically based solely on clinical appearance of the lesions.

Complications

Adolescents typically perceive acne as distressing and may need additional emotional support from the nurse as well as the family. In severe cases, the child may become withdrawn or depressed. Additional complications may occur:

• Permanent scarring can result from compulsive picking of acne lesions.

• Isotretinoin (Accutane) causes teratogenicity and can't be taken if the adolescent is pregnant or lactating; two negative pregnancy test results must occur before initiating treatment and effective contraception must be used by the sexually active adolescent girl starting at least 1 month before starting Accutane. Informed consent is necessary, and registration with the federally mandated iPLEDGE program requires monthly laboratory studies and office visits.

• Systemic antibiotics can interfere with the effectiveness of hormonal contraceptives; sexually active adolescent girls using hormonal contraceptives should use a backup method of contraception for the first 2 weeks of systemic antibiotic therapy to prevent unwanted pregnancies.

• Sun exposure may cause excessive burning in a child taking certain medications (such as tetracycline [Sumycin] and Accutane) and should be avoided.

How it's treated

Various treatments are used and may be topical or systemic, depending on such factors as history, severity, types of lesions, psychological impact, cost-effectiveness, and benefit-risk assessment. Usually, several treatments are used simultaneously.

On the skin or in the mouth

Mild acne usually requires only topical therapy such as benzoyl peroxide, which is available over the counter. Adolescents with persistent acne may need follow-up with a primary care provider or dermatologist for further treatment. Moderate acne generally requires topical and oral medications. Severe acne is treated initially with topical and oral medications, and isotretinoin (Accutane) is added if the acne fails to resolve. Acne lesions may be slow to resolve, with improvements typically taking up to 6 weeks. The patient should be taught to observe for adverse effects specific to these preparations, such as lethargy, insomnia, nausea, vomiting, and abdominal pain.

Skin care 101

The child can help ensure successful acne treatment by:
• developing health-promoting behaviors, such as getting adequate rest, participating in moderate exercise, eating a well-balanced diet, and reducing stress
• using good hygiene practices, including washing with mild soap and water twice per day, and avoiding abrasive and drying cleansers or aggressive measures (such as scrubbing)
• resisting the temptation to pick or squeeze blemishes
• avoiding the use of aggravating agents, such as oil-based cosmetics, face creams, and hair sprays and gels.

A referral to a dermatologist is necessary for further treatment. (See *Teaching about acne*.)

Topical therapy

Lotions and creams tend to be less drying than topical medications in gels or solutions. There are three main categories of topical acne therapy:

Keratolytics include benzoyl peroxide (Benoxyl), azelaic acid (Azelex), salicylic acid (Propa pH), and sulfur (Novacet).

Retinoids include adapalene (Differin), tretinoin (Vesanoid), and tazarotene (Tazorac).

Topical antibiotics include erythromycin (Erygel), clindamycin (Cleocin), sodium sulfacetamide (Klaron), and dapsone (Aczone).

Systemic therapy

Adolescents who have moderate to severe inflammatory acne that isn't successfully controlled with topical medications or those with widespread acne will generally require additional therapy with systemic oral medications. Antibiotic resistance

It's all relative

Teaching about acne

Be sure to include these points in your teaching plan for the child with acne:
• myths about the causes of acne
• predisposing factors
• how acne develops
• stages of severity
• medications (such as benzoyl peroxide, tretinoin, antibiotics, and isotretinoin)
• other care measures, including hygiene and cosmetic use.

may be minimized when used for short-term therapy or combined with topical agents rather than used as a monotherapy. All of these medications, except isotretinoin, may be used along with the topical acne preparations.

The dope on drugs

Acne is treated systemically with antibiotics, such as tetracycline, erythromycin, co-trimoxazole (Bactrim), clindamycin, cephalexin (Keftab), doxycycline (Periostat), and minocycline (Dynacin). Instruct the adolescent that tetracycline and minocycline should be taken on an empty stomach but is using doxycycline, it should be taken with food. (Tetracycline is contraindicated during pregnancy and in children younger than age 8 because it discolors developing teeth; erythromycin is an alternative for these patients.) Antibiotics should be discontinued once the acne is under good control.

Other systemic acne treatments include isotretinoin, hormonal contraceptives, and oral spironolactone. Oral contraceptives and spironolactone are used solely to treat female adolescents.

Intralesional therapy

Acne may also be treated with intralesional injections of corticosteroids. This procedure involves injection of a corticosteroid (usually triamcinolone [Kenalog]) into the acne cysts with a fine needle. This therapy reduces skin inflammation and may help prevent scarring.

What to do

Be prepared to discuss psychosocial concerns and self-esteem issues while reinforcing that acne is self-limiting and slow to resolve. Severe acne can lead to serious emotional problems. The child may endure teasing by her peers, leading to feelings of embarrassment or humiliation. He may become withdrawn and, in severe cases, clinically depressed. In these cases, referral to a psychologist, social worker, or other professional is indicated.

In addition, follow these steps:
- Encourage compliance with specific treatment regimens.
- Monitor the child for potential adverse effects associated with the prescribed drug therapy.

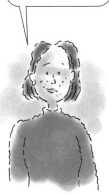

Acne is more than skin deep. It causes me to be depressed sometimes.

A gentle touch

- Encourage the child to avoid vigorous scrubbing and picking at lesions and to eliminate mechanical irritation to lesions such as bicycle helmet straps.
- Help the child select safe, noncomedogenic, water-based skin care products.

• Reinforce teaching about the adverse effects of isotretinoin, including increased cardiovascular risk, hepatotoxicity, and teratogenicity.

Myth busters

• Focus teaching on key aspects of good hygiene, information about specific medications and their adverse effects, and dispel myths about the causes of acne.
• Instruct the child not to take vitamin A supplements due to the risk of hepatotoxicity.
• Caution the child about a potential decrease in tolerance to wearing contact lenses.

Burns

Burns are caused by excessive heat but are also related to exposure to cold, chemicals, electricity, or radiation. When the skin is burned, it loses its ability to perform its normal physiologic functions.

Educational efforts aimed at burn prevention have significantly decreased the number of burn injuries and deaths among children. However, fire and burn injuries remain a leading cause of unintentional, injury-related death in children younger than age 14 years.

What causes it

Burn injuries result from various causes and represent a severe trauma to the body. Exposure to thermal, chemical, and electrical and radioactive sources can cause burn injuries.

Thermal burns

Thermal burns, the most common type, are usually the result of residential fires, automobile accidents, children playing with matches, improperly stored gasoline, space heater or electrical malfunctions, or arson. Other causes include improper handling of firecrackers, scalding accidents, kitchen accidents (such as a child climbing on top of a stove), and access to dangerous items (such as a hot iron).

Chemical burns

Chemical burns result from contact, ingestion, inhalation, or injection of acids, alkalis, vesicants, or noxious agents commonly used in cleaning products.

Electrical burns

Electrical burns usually occur after contact with faulty electrical wiring or from inserting conductive objects into electrical outlets.

Many infants and toddlers sustain electrical burns by chewing on electric cords.

Other burns
Burns also may occur from:
• skin being rubbed harshly against a coarse surface (called *friction* or *abrasion burns*)
• sun exposure (minor burns)
• child abuse (intentionally inflicted injuries from such actions as immersion in hot water and contact with hot objects such as cigarettes).

How it happens

Children, especially those younger than age 5 years, are at greater risk for burn injuries. Developmentally, children have a limited ability to act promptly and properly in a dangerous situation, such as a fire and an explosion, or when they're exposed to dangerous items (such as a pot on the stove and a hot iron).

Thermal and chemical burns disrupt the normal protective function of the skin, leading to various sequelae. In an electrical injury, the heat generated by the electricity passes through the body, causing injury to the tissues.

Two levels of response to the burn injury occur:

 local

 systemic.

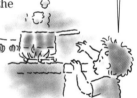

Hey, I'm just a kid! I can't be trusted to make adult decisions about dangerous situations.

Local response
Local response represents local tissue damage to the skin:
• Edema results from increased capillary permeability and increased hydrostatic pressure forcing water, protein, and electrolytes into the interstitial spaces.
• Fluid loss from the burn-injured skin is a result of the inflammatory response.
• Significant circulatory alterations cause capillary stasis in the burned area.
• Thrombi develop, leading to tissue ischemia and necrosis, causing pain and edema.

Systemic response
Systemic response to burns may involve various body systems:
• Cardiovascular changes occur, such as burn shock caused by dramatic alterations in circulation; tachycardia and tachypnea occur to compensate for decreasing vascular volume and increased oxygen needs.

A tight squeeze

• Compartment syndrome, requiring surgical correction, may occur when severe edema causes a tourniquet-like effect that compromises circulation and entraps nerves.
• The respiratory system may be compromised by smoke inhalation; injuries can range from tissue edema of upper respiratory airways to impaired gas exchange in the alveoli.

Constricted and depressed

• Renal changes occur, such as renal vasoconstriction, reduced renal plasma flow, and depressed glomerular filtration.
• Gastrointestinal (GI) ischemia may occur as perfusion to the GI tract and liver is decreased.
• Gastric ileus may occur, with digestion almost ceasing.
• Metabolism is greatly increased, which can lead to prolonged starvation and extensive energy needs.

Changing spaces

• Fluid shifts from the vasculature to the extravascular spaces and altered concentrations of potassium, sodium, chloride, and bicarbonate occur.
• Elevated body temperature occurs as a result of increased metabolism, even in the absence of infection.
• The neuroendocrine system attempts to restore equilibrium by secreting trophic hormones to stimulate various organs.

> Burns can make you hot all over! When burns occur, metabolism increases and body temperature rises.

Fragile: Handle with care

• Increased cell fragility and loss of circulatory red blood cells leads to anemia and the production of lactic acid.
• Growth and development are retarded with severe burn injuries due to growth hormone suppression.
• The patient is prone to infections, such as nosocomial infections, due to loss of skin and tissue integrity and an immature immune system.

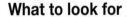

What to look for

Assessment of the child with a burn injury should begin with a thorough history. A description of events surrounding the burn injury should include the cause and the duration the agent was in contact with the skin. The history also consists of how and when the injury occurred, treatment of the burn, and history of previous burns.

A matter of degree

Burns are assessed according to degree (depth of damage), extent (percentage of body surface area), and specific body part involved.

Gauging burn depth

One method of assessing burns is determining their depth. As shown in this illustration, a partial-thickness burn damages the epidermis and part of the dermis, whereas a full-thickness burn damages the epidermis, dermis, subcutaneous tissue, and muscle.

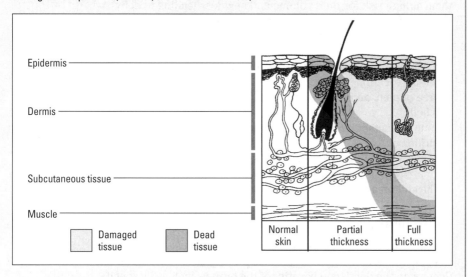

Epidermis

Dermis

Subcutaneous tissue

Muscle

| Damaged tissue | Dead tissue | | Normal skin | Partial thickness | Full thickness |

One goal of assessment is to determine the depth of skin and tissue damage:

In *first-degree burns*, damage is limited to the epidermis, causing erythema and pain.

In *second-degree burns* (partial thickness), the epidermis and part of the dermis are damaged, producing blisters and mild to moderate edema and pain.

In *third-degree burns* (full thickness), the epidermis and the dermis are damaged; no blisters appear, but white, brown, or black leathery tissue and thrombosed vessels are visible.

Fourth-degree burns are rare, and damage extends through deeply charred subcutaneous tissue to muscle and bone. (See *Gauging burn depth*.)

TBSA or not TBSA

Another assessment goal is to estimate the size of a burn, which is usually expressed as a percentage of the total body surface area (TBSA). The TBSA, together with the body part affected, determines morbidity, mortality, and management strategies.

10% of TBSA = a hospital stay

For children, burns that make up 10% or more of TBSA are considered critical and require hospitalization. In addition, significant burns of the hands, feet, face, ears, and genitalia also require immediate hospitalization. Children's larger body surface areas put them at high risk for fluid volume and heat loss leading to dehydration. (See *Estimating the extent of a burn.*)

Inspect to detect

Inspection reveals other characteristics of the burn as well, including location, pattern, and extent. Assess for sensation and degree of pain, and check for blanching and capillary refill of the nail beds.

• Lung auscultation may reveal respiratory compromise, tachypnea, or stridor.

• Assessment of the cardiovascular system may reveal tachycardia, narrow pulse pressure, and hypotension.

• The child may have decreased urine output.

Complications

Nursing care of a burn patient is challenging because many organ systems are affected by the burn injury. Potential complications depend on the depth and severity of the burn as well as its specific cause. The most common complications and leading causes of death are respiratory complications and sepsis. Other possible complications include:

• burn shock
• fluid and electrolyte deficits
• hypothermia
• hypermetabolism
• hypovolemic shock
• infections
• scarring and disfigurement
• contractures
• multisystem organ failure.

How it's treated

Superficial first-degree burn injuries and partial-thickness burns heal spontaneously with reasonable care.

Minor burns

Management of minor burns includes removing burned clothing, cleaning with mild soap and tepid water, and leaving blisters intact. In addition:

• Nothing should be applied to the burn except a clean cloth that is (usually) treated with antimicrobial ointment or cream.

Advice from the experts

Estimating the extent of a burn

To estimate the extent of a burn in a pediatric patient, use the Lund and Browder chart. To use the chart:
- Mentally transfer your patient's burns to the body chart shown here.
- Then add up the corresponding percentages for each burned body section.

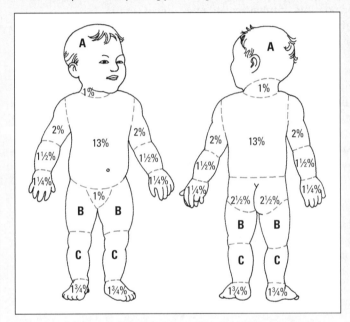

Relative percentages of areas affected by growth

	At birth	0 to 1 yr	2 to 4 yrs	5 to 9 yrs	10 to 15 yrs
A: Half of head	9½%	8½%	6½%	5½%	4½%
B: Half of thigh	2¾%	3¼%	4%	4¼%	4½%
C: Half of leg	2½%	2½%	2¾%	3%	3¼%

- Tetanus prophylaxis is necessary if no history of immunization is available, if more than 5 years has passed since the last immunization, or if the child has not completed the full vaccine series.
- A mild analgesic or moist soaks may be administered to relieve pain.

Moderate or severe burns

If the burn involves a large area of the body surface or critical body parts, it represents severe trauma and usually requires treatment at a specialized burn center. Emergency management of major burns begins with stopping the burning process and placing the child in a horizontal position. In addition:
- Establish and maintain a patent airway, initiating cardiopulmonary resuscitation if necessary.
- Remove burned clothing and jewelry while keeping the child warm.

• Cover the burn to prevent contamination.
• Until transported to a medical facility or burn center, don't allow the patient to eat or drink anything; intravenous (I.V.) fluids with lactated Ringer's or normal saline solution should be started and oxygen therapy provided at 100%.

In the unit

Initial management of the major burn in the burn unit includes maintenance of an adequate airway. I.V. fluid replacement should be started as soon as possible. Intubation and mechanical ventilation may be necessary. In addition:
• A urinary catheter is inserted to adequately measure urine output.
• A nasogastric tube may be necessary to decompress the stomach; later, it may be used to administer a high-protein, high-calorie diet or total parenteral nutrition (which may be necessary if the GI tract is dysfunctional).
• Baseline laboratory studies are performed.
• I.V. pain medication is administered.
• Topical wound cleaning is begun to prevent infections.
• Tetanus prophylaxis is administered if required.

In general

General wound management includes wound debridement, hydrotherapy for dressing removal and debridement, topical antimicrobial therapy, nutritional therapy, physiotherapy focusing on range of motion and contracture prevention, and skin grafting.

What to do

Burns are one of the most painful injuries a child can sustain. Severe burns are life-threatening. The child and his parents will need a great deal of emotional support and reassurance.

Every effort should be made to make the child as comfortable as possible during such painful procedures as debridement. Depending on the child's age, it may be difficult for him to understand why doctors and nurses are inflicting pain during such procedures. The reasons for these treatments should be explained repeatedly, and the child should be encouraged to express his feelings, which may include fear and anger.

Referral to a therapist and a support group may be needed to help the child and parents deal with the traumatic injury and any altered body image because such traumas can have long-lasting psychological effects. Similar referrals are needed if severe scarring or disfigurement is anticipated.

In the heat of the moment

During the acute phase—the first 24 to 48 hours after the burn occurs—nursing care includes:
- treating burn shock
- monitoring respiratory status
- maintaining a patent airway
- monitoring vital signs and fluid status every hour
- maintaining adequate fluid and electrolyte balance
- caring for the burn wound
- managing pain
- providing emotional support.

When the fire dies down

Ongoing management and rehabilitation should include preventing wound infections and complications (such as heat loss and contractures), promoting wound healing, managing the child's pain and promoting comfort, promoting adequate nutrition, and providing psychosocial support for the child and his family. The child and his family should be educated about long-term needs and follow-up care. Education about safety issues, including prevention of future burns, should be conducted in a nonjudgmental manner with genuine interest and concern, making appropriate referrals as needed.

Contact dermatitis

Contact dermatitis occurs as an acute or chronic inflammatory response due to a hypersensitivity reaction to a natural or synthetic chemical substance resulting in a localized flare. The irritating substance can be a primary irritant or a sensitizing agent or allergen.

What causes it

Irritant dermatitis is caused by the toxic effect of the substance directly on the skin. The extent of the rash and itching depends on the length of exposure and the concentration of the irritant. Common irritants include:
- detergents, harsh soaps, fabric softeners, bubble bath, and baby wipes
- bathing too frequently
- saliva, urine, and feces. (*Diaper dermatitis*, the most common form of irritant dermatitis, is a reaction to urine and by-products of feces.)

Diaper dermatitis is one reaction to irritation caused by urine and by-products of feces.

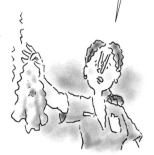

Allergic annoyances

Allergic dermatitis occurs with exposure to substances that cause an immunologic response triggered by an allergen to which the child has become sensitized. Sensitizing reactions occur with repeated or prolonged exposure to such substances as:
• plant oils (poison ivy, oak, and sumac)
• nickel-containing jewelry
• clothing with woolen or rough textures
• topical medications, such as neomycin (Mycifradin) and lanolin
• perfumed soaps or cosmetics
• latex.

How it happens

In primary irritant dermatitis, the toxic substance causes damage to the stratum corneum and the skin's lipid film, impairing the protective barrier mechanism of the skin. The toxic substance is then absorbed into the skin, resulting in vasodilatation, edema of the upper dermis, inflammatory infiltrates, and breakdown of epidermal cells. Vesicles or bullae that rupture ooze and crust may develop as a result of the fluid accumulating between the epidermal cells that act as a sponge.

Not immune to an immune response

Allergic dermatitis is due to an immune response caused by the sensitizing chemical entering the dermis and combining with epidermal proteins to form a new molecule that acts as an antigen. This antigen enters the local cutaneous lymphoid tissue, causing an inflammatory reaction.

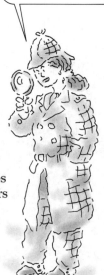

Following the clues from a thorough history will lead you to the prime suspect— the offending substance in contact dermatitis.

What to look for

A thorough history should elicit information about:
• exposure to new or unusual substances
• repeated exposure to a substance
• history of diarrhea or infrequent diaper changes
• location and distribution of the rash related to specific areas of the body
• treatments or forms of at-home management.

Oozing, scaling, and itching—Oh, my!

Mild irritants and allergens produce erythema and small vesicles that ooze, scale, and itch. Strong irritants may also cause blisters and ulcerations.

It's a classic

A classic allergic response produces clearly defined lesions with straight lines following the points of contact. A severe allergic reaction also produces marked edema of the affected area.

What tests tell you

Tests should be reserved for a time when the child isn't experiencing acute, active dermatitis. There are two methods used to determine allergy:
• The *patch test* identifies specific allergens. The suspected substance is applied to a patch left in place on the child's skin for a specified period. If the area under the patch is red and swollen when the patch is removed, the test is positive and the child is considered allergic to the offending substance.
• In *skin testing*, the suspected allergen is introduced intradermally on the child's back or upper arm.

Complications

Complications of contact dermatitis include secondary infections and trauma from scratching. The child may have serious concerns about his appearance and body image.

How it's treated

The keys to successful treatment are identification and removal or elimination of the causative agent and appropriate skin care and management. Resolution of contact dermatitis typically takes 2 to 3 weeks.

How offensive!

When the offending substance has been identified and eliminated from the child's environment, management consists primarily of treating and preventing worsening of symptoms:
• For diaper dermatitis, change diapers frequently, use air-drying if possible, and avoid rubber pants.
• Hydrocortisone cream 1% (Dermacort) should be used sparingly for no more than 5 days.
• Antifungal agents may be necessary if secondary infection develops.

A soak in the tub

• Burrow solution soaks, Aveeno or oatmeal baths, and cool compresses may soothe itching and vesicular rashes.
• Petroleum-based or lanolin and petroleum-based emollients may be applied to dry and chaffed skin but must be avoided if the skin is inflamed.

Ditch the itch!

• Topical corticosteroids may be administered two to three times per day; oral antihistamines are commonly prescribed for itching.
• Referral to a dermatologist for patch testing may be necessary.

What to do

Management requires problem solving to determine the cause of the skin reaction and to find a mutually agreeable solution:
• Educate the child and his family about hygiene practices to prevent infections.
• Teach the parents about antipruritic agents and their proper use to relieve discomfort and itching.

Replace; don't recycle

• Discuss proper use and regular replacement of skin care and make-up products.
• Educate the parents and the child about ways to prevent future exposures, such as wearing protective clothing and using such blocking agents as Ivy Block for prevention of plant oil contact dermatitis.

Leave the judging to Judy

• Establish a professional rapport with the child and his parents and provide education in a nonjudgmental manner; parents may become defensive and are less likely to listen when they feel they're being judged or their parenting skills are being questioned.
• Encourage the child to express concerns about his appearance and body image.

> It's human nature. Parents are more likely to listen (and learn) when they aren't put on the defensive.

Scabies

Scabies, a highly transmissible parasitic skin infestation, is characterized by burrows, pruritus, and excoriations with secondary infections. It characteristically spreads by skin-to-skin contact to family members, intimate contacts, and among school children. Prolonged contact is needed to become infected.

What causes it

Scabies is a contagious disease caused by the scabies mite, *Sarcoptes scabiei*, which burrows into the stratum corneum of the epidermis and deposits eggs and feces. (See *Scabies: Cause and effect.*)

How it happens

The female scabies mite burrows under the skin and forms a small tunnel that's evident as a fine, wavy, dark line with a black dot at the end. The mite extends the burrow, laying up to three eggs per day as she travels. The eggs hatch in about 2 weeks, thus continuing the process.

What to look for

- The lesions initially produce no symptoms, but sensitization to the mites occurs in about 3 weeks. At that time, intense itching occurs, becoming more severe at night.

Loads of lesions

- Infants have dozens of lesions, whereas older children commonly have fewer than 10. Children younger than age 2 years usually have lesions on the feet and ankles; in older children, most lesions are found on the hands and wrists.
- Inspection reveals characteristic gray-brown burrows, which may appear as erythematous nodules when excoriated; secondary excoriation and bacterial infections commonly obscure the burrows and papules.
- Papules of various sizes may exist simultaneously and are typically distributed in such areas as the finger webs, flexor surfaces of the wrist, elbows and axillary folds, along the belt line, and on the lower buttocks.

What tests tell you

- Microscopic examination reveals the characteristic eight-legged scabies mite, eggs, or feces. (Scrapings from an unscratched burrow should be placed in saline or mineral oil. The scrapings shouldn't be placed in KOH because it can dissolve the mites, eggs, or feces.)
- The burrow ink test reveals the presence of burrows. This test involves applying a drop of ink or a blue or black felt–tipped pen to a suspected burrow, wiping off the excess ink with an alcohol pad, and examining the area with a magnifying glass for an ink-stained burrow.

Complications

A secondary bacterial infection from scratching is one possible complication of scabies. Postscabetic syndrome may occur, characterized by lesions and itching that commonly persist for days to weeks following treatment.

How it's treated

Pharmacologic treatment with a thin layer of scabicide (applied after a soap and water bath) to the entire body (except the eyes) is usually recommended:

- Be especially careful to gently massage the cream into the fingernails, scalp, behind the ears, all folds and creases, and the feet and hands; in 7 days, reapply the cream to the child and all symptomatic contacts.

Scabies: Cause and effect

Infestation with *S. scabiei*—the itch mite—causes scabies. The top illustration shows the mite (enlarged); it has a hard shell and measures a microscopic 0.1 mm. The bottom illustration depicts the erythematous nodules with excoriation that appear in patients with scabies.

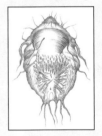

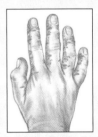

- Permethrin 5% cream (Elimite) is safer and more effective than lindane and is safe for infants as young as age 2 months; the cream should be left on for 8 to 14 hours and then removed with bathing and shampooing. The use of mitts for the hands and socks to cover the feet may reduce the chance of the young child sucking and ingesting the scabicide during the time that the cream is on the skin.

Fighting the mighty mite

- Lindane 1% cream (Kwell) is contraindicated for children younger than age 6 months and for those with seizure disorders because it has potential central nervous system effects. If used, the cream is applied from the neck down and is left on for 8 to 12 hours before bathing. Treatment is then repeated in 1 week.

What to do

All family members, friends, and school and day care contacts should undergo treatment simultaneously with the infected individual, even if they're asymptomatic. Parents should be educated about the course of the disease and told that the rash and itching commonly persist for up to 3 weeks. Oral antihistamines (such as Benadryl or Atarax) may be necessary if itching is pronounced. Children are no longer infectious 24 hours after treatment has started and may return to school or day care.

Instruct the parents to:

- Wash all bed linens and clothing with hot water and then dry for 40 minutes in a hot dryer.

Hoover Whole House

- Vacuum the entire house.
- Store nonwashable items in sealed plastic bags for 2 weeks.
- Use meticulous hand washing and good hygiene to avoid secondary infections.
- Trim the child's fingernails short to avoid excoriation from scratching.
- Use soothing lotions and bathe with Aveeno or a similar product to control itching.

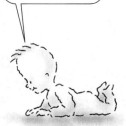

Hmmm . . . looks like Mom vacuumed just like the nurse told her to!

Tinea capitis (ringworm of the scalp)

Tinea capitis is a superficial cutaneous fungal infection of the scalp and hair. It characteristically spreads through direct and indirect contact with infected humans and animals such as dogs and cats and sharing of personal items, such as hats, combs, and brushes, in addition to close contact with infected fomites such as bedding, couches, and soft stuffed toys. It occurs more frequently in hot, humid climates and among individuals living in overcrowded conditions and in disadvantaged areas. It is important to allay the child's misperception that tinea capitis is caused by worms. Fungi are commonly found in the environment.

What causes it

Tinea capitis is the most common contagious fungal infection in children younger than 12 years old. It is caused predominately by the dermatophyte *Trichophyton tonsurans* and involves both the scalp and hair shaft.

How it happens

Dermatophytes attach to the epidermis skin layer of the scalp and may invade the hair shaft, often resulting in hair breakage and temporary alopecia. An exaggerated cell-mediated response occurs and results in severe inflammation, leading to varying degrees of itching, scaling, pustules, and papules.

What to look for

- Erythema and scaling of the scalp
- Pustules, papules, and often yellow honeycomb crusts
- Varying degrees of pruritus
- Broken hairs at the scalp level resembling a dotted black stubbled appearance or patchy hair loss
- Adenopathy may occur.

What tests tell you

Microscopic examination of hair and scalp scrapings using KOH wet mount can detect and immediately confirm the dermatophytes. The use of a fungal culture is more sensitive but does take additional time to obtain the results.

Complications

In severe cases of tinea capitis, permanent alopecia may result. If symptoms do not improve, refer to a dermatologist.

How it's treated

- Oral antifungal medication such as griseofulvin for a minimum of 8 weeks but may be extended to 12 to 16 weeks and should continue for 1 to 2 weeks after resolution of symptoms; medication absorption is enhanced if given with whole milk or other foods high in fat.
- Selenium sulfide (Selsun Blue) shampoo two to three times weekly, leaving it on the scalp for 10 minutes before rinsing to eradicate the scalp spores

What to do

• Use shampoo with selenium sulfide for all family members for several weeks to prevent infection.
• Clean all potentially contaminated objects that came into contact with the infected child's head.
• Avoid sharing personal items, such as hats, combs, brushes, towels, bedding, etc., or anything that may have had close physical contact with the infected child's head.
• Discourage scratching or touching of scalp and hair.

Tinea corporis (ringworm of the body)

Tinea corporis is a superficial dermatophyte fungal skin infection commonly known as *ringworm* because of the characteristic pattern of annular (ring-shaped), scaling, erythematous plaques with sharply defined borders. It is found on the trunk and limbs, excluding hands, feet, head, and groin.

What causes it

Tinea corporis is most prevalent during the preadolescent years. It is caused by *Trichophyton rubrum*, *Trichophyton mentagrophytes*, *Microsporum canis*, and *Epidermophyton floccosum*. Contact with these dermatophytes occurs typically with infected humans, infected animals, fomites (such as wrestling mats and towels), and, less frequently, from the soil or from infection on other anatomic locations on the same individual such as tinea pedis (athlete's foot).

How it happens

Dermatophytes that are transmitted from an infected person, animal, or fomite attach to the superficial epidermis skin layer and release keratinases that invade and multiply within the stratum corneum. About 1 to 3 weeks later, the dermatophytes invade the epidermis peripherally and increase the proliferation of the basal cell layer. This results in epidermal thickening, and the lesion begins to appear as a ring-shaped lesion with an erythematous, scaly border with a healthy center.

What to look for

• Slightly raised ring-shaped lesions with pink boarders ranging in size from 5 mm to 3 cm
• Lesions may be singular or multiple but usually not very numerous.
• Lesions are more commonly found on exposed areas of the body.
• Mild pruritus or burning sensation may be present.

What tests tell you

KOH scraping of the lesion's border can confirm the dermatophyte's hyphae and spores but cannot identify the specific species of dermatophyte involved. Dermatophyte test medium (DTM) is used for selective recognition of the dermatophytic fungus, which is the causative agent in ringworm. A fungal culture is more sensitive but takes more time to obtain results.

How it's treated

• Treat with topical antifungal medications (creams) such as clotrimazole, miconazole, econazole, terbinafine, tolnaftate, naftifine, ciclopirox, or ketoconazole for up to 8 weeks before resolution. Apply cream once or twice daily as prescribed.
• Do not use topical corticosteroids or combination antifungal/corticosteroid preparations, which can cause infections to persist or recur.
• Use oral antifungal agents if unresponsive to topical therapy or the ringworm recurs or is extensive. Griseofulvin is often the drug of choice.

What to do

• Avoid sharing of personal items to prevent the spread of the lesions.
• Wash hands before and after applying the cream to the lesions.
• Avoid touching or scratching the lesions.
• Wash clothing that comes in contact with affected areas once removed.
• Clean wrestling mats after use.
• Discourage athletes from practice until at least 72 hours after treatment begins and lesions should be covered before resumption of any contact sport.

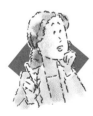

Quick quiz

1. Which statement about the integumentary system and its components is true?
    A.   It's the largest organ in the body and serves primarily as an insulator.
    B.   It can only protect the body from trauma that's mechanical in nature.
    C.   It consists of just the dermis and epidermis.
    D.   Its main function is to act as an organ of excretion.

Answer: A. The integumentary system, which consists of the skin and its components, is the largest organ system in the body. It functions to shelter most of the other organ systems, protecting them while acting as a mechanical barrier.

2. The glands that are primarily responsible for the odor associated with sweating are known as the:
- A. endocrine sweat glands.
- B. eccrine sweat glands.
- C. cutaneous sweat glands.
- D. apocrine sweat glands.

Answer: D. The sweat glands consist of the eccrine sweat glands, which function as the body's heat-regulating mechanism by producing sweat, and the apocrine sweat glands, which mature at puberty and cause the unpleasant body odor associated with sweating.

3. The proportion of a child's body that's burned is typically estimated according to:
- A. Rule of Nines.
- B. TBSA.
- C. depth of injury.
- D. three-dimensional analysis.

Answer: B. One goal in assessing burns is to estimate its size, which is usually expressed as a percentage of TBSA. The TBSA and body part affected determines morbidity, mortality, and management strategies.

4. When assessing a child with a rash consistent with irritant dermatitis, which question should the nurse ask?
- A. "Has your child been playing with children who may have chickenpox?"
- B. "Has your child been ill lately?"
- C. "Has your child been exposed to new or unusual substance?"
- D. "Has your child visited mountainous regions?"

Answer: C. Irritant dermatitis is caused by the toxic effect of the substance directly on the skin. Common irritants include detergents, harsh soaps, bubble bath, baby wipes, saliva, urine or feces, or overbathing.

5. Pruritus caused by contact dermatitis can usually be treated at home with:
- A. oatmeal or Aveeno baths.
- B. soothing scented bath oils.
- C. ice and heat alternately.
- D. patch skin applications.

Answer: A. Burrow solution soaks, Aveeno or oatmeal baths, and cool compresses may soothe itching and vesicular rashes.

6. Which of the following is true about scabies?
   A. Tzanck testing is done immediately to confirm the scabies mite.
   B. Infants usually have very few lesions on their bodies.
   C. Characteristic lesions are raised grayish brown linear burrows.
   D. Itching is worse during the daytime hours when the child is awake.

Answer: C. Inspection of scabies reveals characteristic grayish brown burrows, which may appear as erythematous nodules when excoriated.

7. What are the functions of the integumentary system? Select all that apply.
   A. Temperature regulation
   B. Vitamin synthesis
   C. Protective barrier
   D. Gas exchange

Answer: A, B, and C. The integumentary system's functions include sensory perception, temperature regulation, vitamin synthesis, mechanical protection, and excretion of wastes through sweating.

8. What type of skin lesion is commonly observed in a child with second-degree burns?
   A. Vesicle
   B. Bulla
   C. Macule
   D. Wheal

Answer: B. Bullae are fluid-filled lesions more than 2 cm in diameter and are often referred to as blisters, which occur in second-degree burns.

9. Classification of acne is based on:
   A. the amount of scarring involved.
   B. the type of hormone involvement.
   C. the type of lesions observed.
   D. the presence of scarring.

Answer: C. Classification of acne is based on the type of lesions observed.

10. Patient teaching for the adolescent who has acne should include which of the following? Select all that apply.

    A. Getting adequate rest and hydration
    B. Scrubbing using an alcohol-based cleanser
    C. Resist squeezing blemishes
    D. Using oil-based cosmetics often

Answer: A and C. The adolescent should develop health-promoting behaviors and resist squeezing blemishes. Scrubbing with drying or abrasive cleansers is not recommended. Using oil-based cosmetics and face creams are to be avoided.

11. For the adolescent who has been diagnosed with acne, which of the following is true?

    A. Poor hygiene often leads to developing acne.
    B. Acne causes clinical depression.
    C. Acne affects males more severely than females.
    D. Acne can be aggravated by ingesting chocolate.

Answer: C. Acne affects males more severely than females.

12. Which of the following is caused by a parasitic skin infestation?

    A. Impetigo
    B. Cellulitis
    C. Dermatitis
    D. Scabies

Answer: D. Scabies is caused by a highly transmissible parasitic skin infestation.

13. Steve is a wrester at his high school. He has a few abdominal lesions that are scaly, irregular-shaped plaques with skin-colored centers and erythematous borders that are slightly itchy. What type of skin infection would you suspect?

    A. Impetigo
    B. Acne
    C. Tinea corporis
    D. Contact dermatitis

Answer: C. Tinea corporis or ringworm is a fungal infection of the trunk and limbs often contacted during sports such as wrestling.

14. Patient teaching for the child who has tinea caputis should include:

    A. shampooing with selenium sulfide twice a week.
    B. using mineral oil to loosen crusts on scalp.
    C. avoiding exposure to the sun.
    D. limiting touching of the scalp and hair.

Answer: D. Avoid touching the scalp and hair to prevent spread of the infection.

15. When trying to assess and describe a skin lesion, which of the following applies? Select all that apply.
  A.   Asymmetry
  B.   Border
  C.   Configuration
  D.   Duration

Answer: A, B, and C. Asymmetry, border, color, configuration, diameter, and drainage are key to describing lesions of the skin.

16. Important information that leads to a diagnosis of irritant dermatitis includes which of the following? Select all that apply.
  A.   The length of exposure to the irritant
  B.   Failure to bath
  C.   Type of detergents used
  D.   Use of bubble bath

Answer: A, C, and D. The length of exposure and the concentration of the irritant such as detergents, bubble baths, and baby wipes lead to irritant dermatitis.

Scoring

☆☆☆   If you answered all six items correctly, hooray! Your knowledge of dermatologic problems is more than skin deep.

☆☆   If you answered four or five items correctly, congratulations! The material in this chapter has gotten under your skin.

☆   If you answered fewer than four items correctly, take an oatmeal bath, relax, and then re-read the chapter! This is the last quick quiz to irritate you.

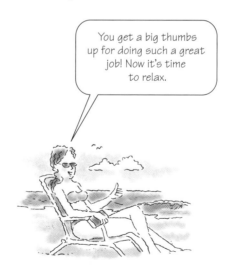

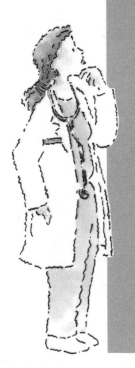

Glossary

accessory muscles: thoracic and abdominal muscles used during respiratory distress to help expand and contract the chest so the patient can inhale and exhale

allergic shiners: dark circles under the eyes from edema and congestion related to histamine

allergy: hypersensitivity to normal environmental antigens

alveoli: small, saclike structures in the lungs where the exchange of oxygen for carbon dioxide takes place

anemia: decrease in the number or quality of circulating red blood cells from hemorrhage, hemolysis, or lack of production

anorexia: lack or loss of appetite for food

anorexia nervosa: voluntary control of hunger characterized by a refusal to eat and a loss of 25% of body weight without an organic cause

antigen: a substance that stimulates the body to produce antibodies

anuria: absence of urine formation, manifested by no urine output

arteries: large, thick-walled blood vessels that distribute oxygenated blood to the capillaries

astrocytoma: slow-growing tumor in the cerebellum

atelectasis: failure of a portion of the lung to expand, preventing respiratory exchange in that area

atresia: termination or absence of a normal anatomic passageway

azotemia: excess nitrogenous waste products, such as urea, in the blood

bulimia: multiple episodes of compulsive overeating followed by forced emesis; also called *the binge-purge cycle*

cancer: multiple and varying alterations in cell function resulting from overproduction of immature and nonfunctional cells or tissue enlargement for no physiologic reason

cardiac output: amount of blood ejected by the heart in 1 minute

cephalocaudal: head-to-toe direction

chemotherapy: medical treatment with highly toxic doses of medications aimed at interfering with the mitotic division of cancerous cells

chordae tendineae: thin, fibrous bands that attach the leaflets of the tricuspid and mitral valves of the heart to the papillary muscles in the ventricles

chorea: purposeless, rapid, involuntary movements seen as a consequence of rheumatic fever and lasting for months

colic: daily period of crying for 3 hours or more during which the infant is virtually inconsolable; occurs in 10% to 20% of infants

debridement: removal of eschar (dead skin) to allow granulation

dehydration: deficiency in body fluid from decreased intake, output greater than intake, or loss of fluids by vomiting, diarrhea, or diaphoresis

development: acquisition of skills and abilities occurring throughout life

developmental assessment: measurement of physical (motor), cognitive, psychosocial, and psychosexual

parameters compared to norms for one's chronologic age

diaphoresis: excessive sweating

diffusion: passage of molecules from an area of higher concentration to an area of lower concentration

ductus arteriosus: fetal cardiac structure that connects the pulmonary artery to the aorta, allowing blood to bypass the fetal lungs; when this structure remains patent after birth, it creates an abnormal heart condition known as *patent ductus arteriosus*

ductus venosus: fetal structure that carries oxygenated blood from the umbilical vein to the inferior vena cava, bypassing the liver

echolalia: verbal pattern of one who repeats whatever is said

electrocardiography: graphic representation of the heart's electrical activity

enuresis: involuntary urination after the age at which control should have been attained

ependymoma: ventricular tumor that results in a noncommunicating hydrocephalus; usually benign, but pressure can damage vital organs

epiglottis: a flaplike structure that overhangs the entrance to the trachea

erythropoiesis: red blood cell formation

ethnicity: belonging to or believing in a group with customs, languages, and characteristics different from the general population

failure to thrive: failure of an infant to maintain weight, and sometimes length, above the 5th percentile on age- and gender-appropriate growth charts

family: structure or relationship of individuals to one another to provide financial and emotional support and for social functioning

family-centered care: incorporating parental and family input and involvement into a child's care

fine motor skills: skills requiring the use of small muscles (primarily those in the hand), such as using the hands and fingers to grasp or manipulate an object

fontanel: space covered by membranous tissue at the juncture of cranial sutures

foramen ovale: septal opening between the atria of the fetal heart

glioma: slow-growing tumor that's usually inoperable because of its location in the brain stem

glomerular filtration: process of filtering blood as it flows through the kidneys

gross motor skills: skills requiring the use of large muscle groups, such as head control, sitting, standing, and walking

growth: increase in size, such as in height or weight

head circumference: measurement of the largest diameter of the head; taken by placing a measuring tape around the head at the level of the frontal bone of the forehead to the occipital prominence at the back of the head

Healthy People 2020: national health initiative aimed at continuing to increase healthy life expectancy and eliminate differences in health care availability to all individuals

hemarthrosis: bleeding into a joint

hematuria: blood in the urine

human leukocyte antigen: genetically transferred antigenic marker on the cell surface of all nucleated cells that allows the body to recognize self and non-self

hypertrophy: increase in the size of a body organ or structure, sometimes because of an increase in cell size

hypoxia: deficiency of oxygen to the tissue

immunotherapy: using specially treated white blood cell immunopotentiators to replace immunocompetent lymphoid tissue, such as bone marrow and thymus

incubation period: time between the reception of an antigen and initiation of clinical symptoms

infant mortality: number of infant deaths during the first year of life per 1,000 live births in any given year

infratentorial: below the plate that's under the cerebellum

interstitial compartments: spaces between tissues

intravascular compartments: spaces within blood vessels

left-to-right shunt: pressure from the left side of the heart pushing blood through a septal defect to the right side, thereby increasing blood flow to the lungs

medulloblastoma: highly malignant, fast-growing tumor in the cerebellum

metastasize: growing and spreading of malignant cells from the primary site to other tissues

morbidity: number of people in a population who are faced with a specific health problem at a particular point in time

mortality: number of deaths from a specific cause in a given year

nephron: functional unit of the kidney responsible for the formation of urine

neurogenic bladder: dribbling of urine from the lack of spontaneous bladder emptying

nystagmus: involuntary, rapid, jerky movement of the eye

object permanence: awareness that objects exist while not in view

oligohydramnios: abnormally decreased amount of amniotic fluid in utero

oliguria: decreased urine formation manifested by low urine output

opisthotonos: spasmodic body posturing in which the back arches and the head and heels bend back

peer: individual who's the same as another in age, class, or rank

polycythemia: overproduction of red blood cells, resulting in increased blood viscosity and hematocrit

poverty: lack of money or resources necessary for survival

priapism: painful, prolonged, and abnormal erection of the penis, usually unrelated to sexual desire

pruritus: itching

puberty: physical changes resulting in reproductive maturity

rumination: voluntary regurgitation and reswallowing

scoliosis: lateral curvature of the spine

separation anxiety: manifested by crying and withdrawal; occurs when an infant or child recognizes that his attachment figure isn't present

sinoatrial node: pacemaker of the heart; located within the right atrial wall near the opening of the superior vena cava

status asthmaticus: acute asthma exacerbation in which there's unrelenting, severe respiratory distress and bronchospasm

steatorrhea: more than normal amounts of fat in the feces resulting in foamy, light-colored, bulky, foul-smelling, greasy stools

strabismus: condition in which the eyes are misaligned when fixating on the same object from a muscle imbalance

stroke volume: amount of blood ejected by the heart with each heartbeat (or contraction)

subluxation: partial dislocation of any joint

sudden infant death syndrome: sudden death of a previously healthy infant in which a postmortem examination fails to confirm the cause of death

supratentorial: within the cerebrum and above the tentorial plate

surfactant: phospholipid that lines the alveoli, preventing them from collapsing during exhalation

talipes: clubfoot; inability of the foot or ankle to attain correct alignment from twisting in any of multiple directions

toxoid: toxin that's rendered nontoxic

tracheostomy: surgically created opening in the anterior neck leading directly to the trachea; this opening is cannulated with a tracheostomy tube to serve as an airway

transitional object: object or comfort measure that represents parental security

umbilical arteries: two of the three blood vessels in the umbilical cord that carry deoxygenated blood from the fetus to the placenta; the other blood vessel is the umbilical vein

umbilical vein: one of the three blood vessels in the umbilical cord that carries oxygenated blood from the placenta to the fetus; the other two blood vessels are the umbilical arteries

veins: small, thin-walled blood vessels that carry deoxygenated blood from the capillaries to the heart

Selected references

Alencar, A., Sanudo, A., Sampaio, V., Góis, R., Benevides, F., & Guinsburg, R. (2012). Efficacy of tramadol versus fentanyl for postoperative analgesia in neonates. *Archives of Disease in Childhood: Fetal and Neonatal Edition, 97,* F24–F29.

American Academy of Pediatric Dentistry, Clinical Affairs Committee—Infant Oral Health Subcommittee. (2012). *Guideline on infant oral health care.* Chicago, IL: American Academy of Pediatric Dentistry.

American Academy of Pediatrics. (2010). Clinical report—Diagnosis and prevention of iron deficiency and iron-deficiency anemia in infants and young children (0–3 years of age). *Pediatrics, 126,* 1–11.

American Academy of Pediatrics. (2011). Policy statement—Child passenger safety. *Pediatrics, 127,* 788–793.

American Academy of Pediatrics, Task Force on Sudden Infant Death Syndrome. (2011). SIDS and other sleep-related infant deaths: Expansion of recommendations for a safe infant sleeping environment. *Pediatrics, 138,* 1030–1039.

American Academy of Pediatrics. (2012). Policy statement: Breastfeeding and use of human milk section on breastfeeding. *Pediatrics, 129,* e827–e841.

Balk, S. J., Fisher, D. E., & Geller, A. C. (2013). Teens and indoor tanning: A cancer prevention opportunity for pediatricians. *Pediatrics, 131,* 772–785.

Bor, N., Herzenberg, J., & Frick, S. (2006). Ponseti management of clubfoot in older infants. *Clinical Orthopaedics and Related Research, 444,* 224–228.

Brailsford, J., Smith, D. D., Lizarraga, A. K., & Bermudez, L. E. (2010). Surgical management of patients with cleft palate. *OR Nurse, 4*(3), 16–25.

Centers for Disease Control and Prevention. (2013). *2013 Recommended immunizations for children from birth through 6 years old.* Retrieved from http://www.cdc.gov/vaccines/parents/downloads/parent-ver-sch-0-6yrs.pdf

Cole, S. Z., & Lanham, J. S. (2011). Failure to thrive: An update. *American Family Physician, 83,* 829–834.

Franck, L., Ridout, D., Howard, R., Peters, J., & Honour, J. (2011). A comparison of pain measures in newborn infants after cardiac surgery. *Pain, 152,* 1758–1765.

George, H., Unnikrishnan, P., Garg, N., Sampath, J., & Bruce, C. (2011). Unilateral foot abduction orthosis: Is it a substitute for Denis Browne boots following Ponseti technique? *Journal of Pediatric Orthopaedics, 20,* 22–25.

Hasler, C., & Krieg, A. (2012). Current concepts of leg lengthening. *Journal of Children's Orthopaedics, 6,* 89–104.

Heard, L. (2008). Taking care of the little things: Preparation of the pediatric endoscopy patient. *Gastroenterology Nursing, 31*(2), 108–112.

Jarrett, D., Matheney, T., & Kleinman, P. (2013). Imaging SCFE: Diagnosis, treatment and complications. *Pediatric Radiology, 43,* S71–S82.

Karpoff, S., Levine, J., & Thompson, G. (Eds.). (2008). *Straight A's in pediatric nursing* (2nd ed.). Philadelphia, PA: Wolters Kluwer Health/Lippincott Williams & Wilkins.

Larson, N. (2011). Early onset scoliosis: What the primary care provider needs to know and implications for practice. *Journal of the American Academy of Nurse Practitioners, 23,* 392–403.

London, M. L., Laedwig, P. W., Ball, J. W., Bindler, R. C., & Cowen, K. J. (2011). *Maternal & child nursing care* (3rd ed.). Upper Saddle River, NJ: Pearson Education, Inc.

Maffulli, N., Longo, U., Spiezia, F., & Denaro, V. (2010). Sports injuries in young athletes: Long-term outcome and prevention strategies. *The Physician and Sports Medicine, 38,* 29–34.

Mak, W., Yuen, V., Irwin, M., & Hui, T. (2011). Pharmacotherapy for acute pain in children: Current practice and recent advances. *Expert Opinion on Pharmacotherapy, 12,* 865–881.

Ogden, C., Carroll, M., Kit, B., & Flegal, K. (2012). Prevalence of obesity and trends in body mass index among US children and adolescents, 1999-2010. *Journal of the American Medical Association, 307,* 483–490.

O'Malley Olsen, E., Shults, R. A., & Eaton, D. K. (2013). Texting while driving and other risky mother vehicle behaviors among US High School Students. *Pediatrics, 131,* e1708–e1715.

Porth, C. M. (2011). *Essentials of pathophysiology* (3rd ed.). Philadelphia, PA: Wolters Kluwer Health/Lippincott Williams & Wilkins.

Sullivan, J., & Farrar, H. (2011). Fever and antipyretic use in children. *Pediatrics, 127*(3), 580–587.

Tully, M. (2008). Pediatric celiac disease. *Gastroenterology Nursing, 31,* 132–140.

U.S. Department of Health and Human Services. (2012). *Preventing tobacco use among youth and young adults.* Rockville, MD: U.S. Department of Health and Human Services, National Center for Chronic Disease Prevention and Health Promotion, Office of the Surgeon General.

Walker, W. A., & Heintz, K. (2012). Protective nutrients: Are they here to stay? *Nutrition Today, 47*(3), 110–122.

Wiener, L., McConnell, D., Latella, L., & Ludi, E. (2013). Cultural and religious considerations in pediatric palliative care. *Palliative and Supportive Care, 11,* 47–67.

Web resources

Alateen
www.al-ateen.org

American Academy of Allergy, Asthma & Immunology
www.aaaai.org

American Academy of Dermatology
www.aad.org

American Academy of Neurology
www.aan.com

American Academy of Ophthalmology
www.aao.org

American Academy of Pediatrics
www.aap.org

American Association of Kidney Patients
www.aakp.org

American Burn Association
www.ameriburn.org

American Cancer Society
www.cancer.org

American Heart Association
www.heart.org

American Lung Association
www.lung.org

American Nurses Association
www.nursingworld.org

Asthma and Allergy Foundation of America
www.aafa.org

Autism Society
www.autism-society.org

Centers for Disease Control and Prevention
www.cdc.gov

Cystic Fibrosis Foundation
www.cff.org

Dermatology Foundation
www.dermfnd.org

Emedicine
www.emedicine.medscape.com

Heart Center Online
www.heartcenteronline.com

Hydrocephalus Association
www.hydroassoc.org

InteliHealth
www.intelihealth.com

Mayo Clinic
www.mayoclinic.org

Narcotics Anonymous
www.na.org

National Association for Children of Alcoholics
www.nacoa.net

National Association of Anorexia Nervosa and Associated Disorders
www.anad.org

National Association of Pediatric Nurse Practitioners
www.napnap.org

National Asthma Education and Prevention Program
*www.nhlbi.nih.gov/about/*naepp

National Cancer Institute
www.cancer.gov

National Center for Learning Disabilities
www.ncld.org

National Council on Alcoholism and Drug Dependence
www.ncadd.org

National Down Syndrome Society
www.ndss.org

National PKU News
www.pkunews.org

Sickle Cell Disease Association of America
www.sicklecelldisease.org

Society of Pediatric Nurses
www.pedsnurses.org

Index

Note: i refers to an illustration; t refers to a table; **bold** refers to color pages.

Note: i refers to an illustration; t refers to a table; **bold** refers to color pages.

Note: i refers to an illustration; t refers to a table; **bold** refers to color pages.

Note: i refers to an illustration; t refers to a table; **bold** refers to color pages.

Note: i refers to an illustration; t refers to a table; **bold** refers to color pages.

Note: i refers to an illustration; t refers to a table; **bold** refers to color pages.

Muscles affected by Duchenne's muscular dystrophy

Duchenne's muscular dystrophy, also known as *pseudohypertrophic dystrophy*, is a congenital disorder characterized by progressive wasting of skeletal muscles (without neural or sensory deficits) that strikes during childhood and is typically fatal during the second decade of life. It has an insidious onset and initially affects the legs, pelvis, and shoulders. Children with Duchenne's muscular dystrophy have difficulty climbing stairs, fall frequently, and exhibit Gower's sign when standing from a sitting position. They also toe-walk and have a waddling gait and lumbar lordosis.

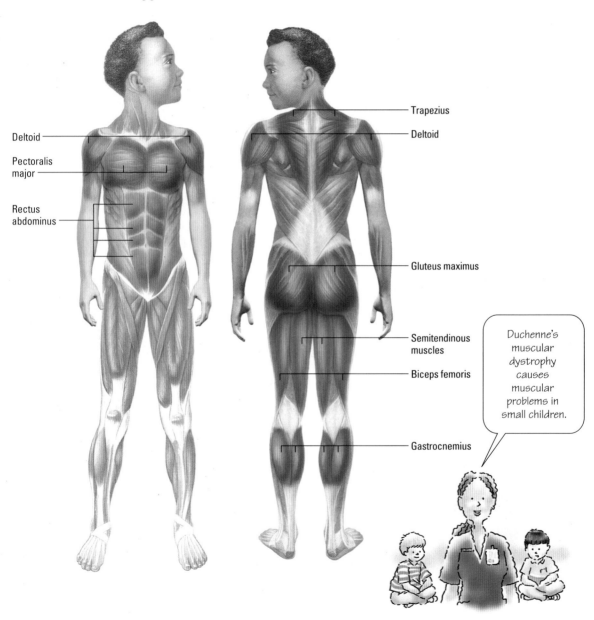

Deltoid

Pectoralis major

Rectus abdominus

Trapezius

Deltoid

Gluteus maximus

Semitendinous muscles

Biceps femoris

Gastrocnemius

Duchenne's muscular dystrophy causes muscular problems in small children.

Classifications and complications of otitis media

Otitis media is one of the most common disorders of childhood. It occurs most commonly in children ages 6 months to 2 years, and primarily results from eustachian tube dysfunction. Otitis media can be classified as acute otitis media or otitis media with effusion. Complications may include atelectasis, perforation, or cholesteatoma.

Classifications

Otoscopic view

Acute otitis media
In acute otitis media, there's infected fluid in the middle ear, and rapid onset of symptoms such as pain; symptoms, however, have a short duration.

Otitis media with effusion
In otitis media with effusion, there's usually asymptomatic fluid in the middle ear. It may be acute, subacute, or chronic in nature.

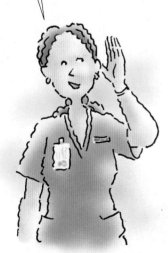

Listen up! Complications of otitis media can cause permanent ear damage.

Complications

Atelectasis

Atelectasis occurs as the tympanic membrane becomes thin and can potentially collapse.

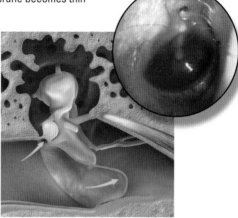

Perforation

A hole in the tympanic membrane signals perforation. It's caused by chronic negative pressure in the middle ear, inflammation, or trauma.

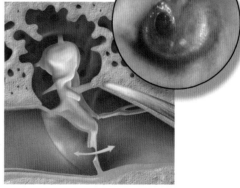

Cholesteatoma

Cholesteatoma is a mass of entrapped skin in the middle ear or temporal lobe.

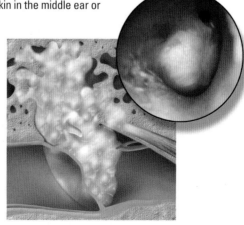

Hydrocephalus

Hydrocephalus is an excessive accumulation of cerebrospinal fluid within the ventricle spaces of the brain. In infants, hydrocephalus causes the head to grow at an abnormal rate. In infants and children, it may cause signs of increased intracranial pressure, such as a tense and bulging anterior fontanel, irritability, and lethargy.

Normal brain—Lateral view

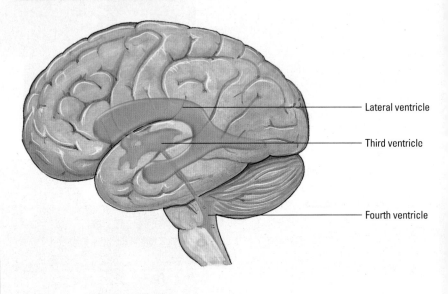

Lateral ventricle

Third ventricle

Fourth ventricle

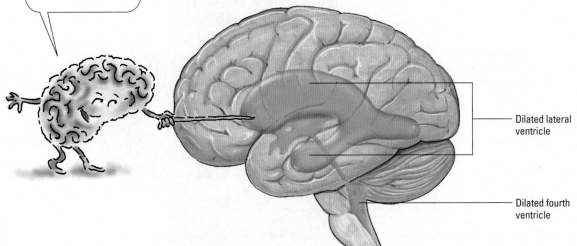

So, in other words . . . if I had extra fluid, it would most definitely NOT be a good thing!!

Ventricular enlargement in hydrocephalus

Dilated lateral ventricle

Dilated fourth ventricle

Hirschsprung's disease

Also called *congenital megacolon* or *congenital aganglionic megacolon,* this congenital disorder of the large intestine is characterized by absence or marked reduction of parasympathetic ganglionic cells in the colorectal wall.

The resulting impaired intestinal mobility causes severe intractable constipation. Colonic obstruction then occurs, dilating the bowel and occluding the surrounding blood and lymphatic vessels.

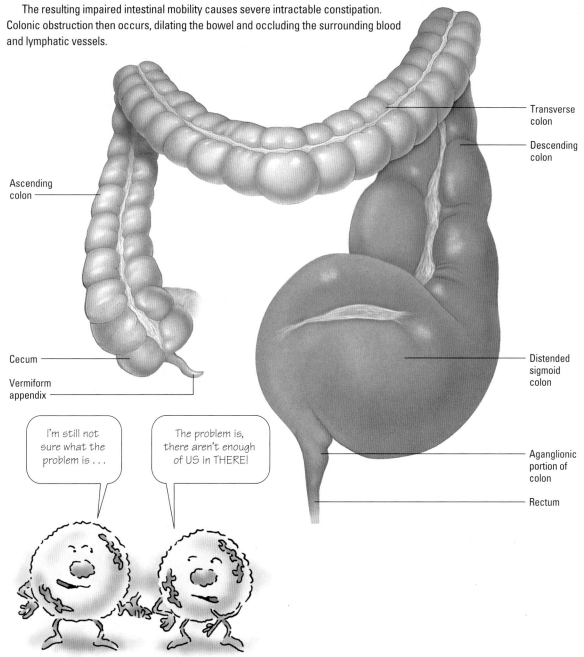

Acne

Acne is a chronic inflammatory disease of the sebaceous glands, associated with a high rate of sebum production. When sebum blocks a hair follicle, one of two types of acne occurs.

In *inflammatory acne*, bacteria grow in the blocked follicle and lead to inflammation and eventual rupture of the follicle. In *noninflammatory acne*, the follicle remains dilated by accumulating secretions but doesn't rupture.

Acne develops in 80% to 90% of adolescents or young adults, primarily between ages 15 and 18; however, the lesions can appear as early as age 8.

How acne develops

Excessive sebum production

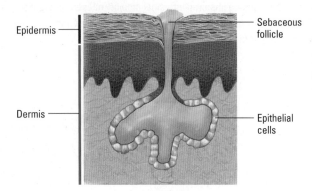

Epidermis

Dermis

Sebaceous follicle

Epithelial cells

Increased shedding of epithelial cells

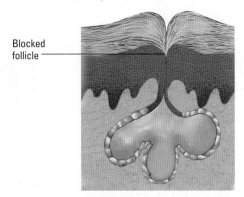

Blocked follicle

Inflammatory response in follicle

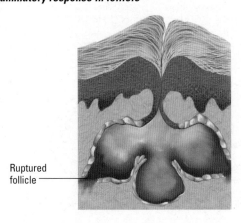

Ruptured follicle

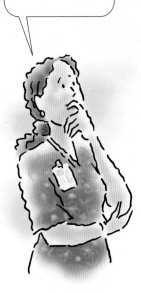

Boy, when those sebaceous glands get inflamed, it's not a pretty sight!

Comedones of acne

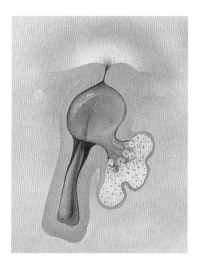

Closed comedo (whitehead)
A closed comedo doesn't protrude from the follicle and is covered by the epidermis.

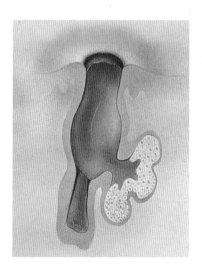

Open comedo (blackhead)
An open comedo protrudes from the follicle and isn't covered by the epidermis.

Melanin or pigment of the follicle causes the black color.

> The combination of bacteria and blocked follicles is like a green light for inflammatory acne.

Rheumatic heart disease

Rheumatic fever is an inflammatory disease of childhood; it develops after an infection of the upper respiratory tract with group A beta-hemolytic streptococci. It mainly involves the heart, joints, central nervous system, skin, and subcutaneous tissues.

The antigens of group A streptococci bind to receptors in the heart, muscle, brain, and synovial joints, causing an autoimmune response. Because of a similarity between the antigens of the streptococcus bacteria and the antigens of the body's own cells, antibodies may attack healthy body cells by mistake.

Rheumatic heart disease refers to the cardiac manifestations of rheumatic fever and includes pancarditis (myocarditis, pericarditis, and endocarditis) during the early acute phase and chronic valvular disease later.

Just hearing rheumatic heart disease makes me shudder!

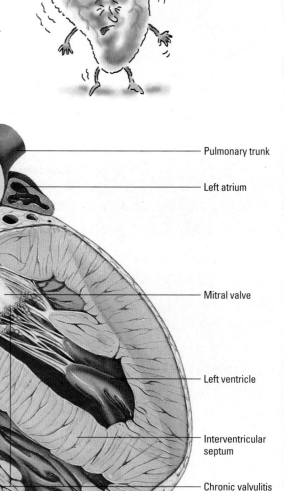

Aorta

Superior vena cava

Aortic valve

Right atrium

Tricuspid valve

Right ventricle

Pulmonary trunk

Left atrium

Mitral valve

Left ventricle

Interventricular septum

Chronic valvulitis or insufficiency due to vegetations